Holistic Approaches to Health Recovery

Adérito Seixas
Escola Superior de Saúde Fernando Pessoa, Portugal

Rita Alegria
Escola Superior de Saúde Fernando Pessoa, Portugal

Daniela Vieira
Escola Superior de Saúde Fernando Pessoa, Portugal

IGI Global
Scientific Publishing
Publishing Tomorrow's Research Today

Vice President of Editorial	Melissa Wagner
Director of Acquisitions	Mikaela Felty
Director of Book Development	Jocelynn Hessler
Production Manager	Mike Brehm
Cover Design	Jose Rosado

Published in the United States of America by
IGI Global Scientific Publishing
701 East Chocolate Avenue
Hershey, PA, 17033, USA
Tel: 717-533-8845
Fax: 717-533-7115
Website: https://www.igi-global.com E-mail: cust@igi-global.com

Library of Congress Cataloging-in-Publication Data

Names: Seixas, Adérito, 1979- editor
http://id.loc.gov/rwo/agents/n2025015538 | Alegria, Rita, 1975- editor
http://id.loc.gov/rwo/agents/n2025015539 | Vieira, Daniela, 1983- editor
http://id.loc.gov/rwo/agents/n2025015540
Title: Holistic approaches to health recovery / edited by Adérito Seixas, Rita Alegria, Daniela Vieira.
Description: Hershey, PA : IGI Global Scientific Publishing, [2026] | Includes bibliographical references and index. | Summary: "This publication serves as a catalyst for advancing research in the rehabilitation domain by fostering a holistic and integrated framework. By showcasing the interconnectedness of diverse rehabilitation disciplines, it encourages researchers to explore new paradigms, identify innovative intervention strategies, and contribute to a more comprehensive understanding of holistic health recovery"-- Provided by publisher.
Identifiers: LCCN 2024058278 (print) | LCCN 2024058279 (ebook) | ISBN 9798369364321 hardcover | ISBN 9798369364338 paperback | ISBN 9798369364345 ebook
Subjects: LCSH: Medical rehabilitation
http://id.loc.gov/authorities/names/n99043710 | Holistic medicine
http://id.loc.gov/authorities/subjects/sh85061482
Classification: LCC RM930 .H65 2025 (print) | LCC RM930 (ebook) | DDC 615.5--dc23/eng/20250407
LC record available at https://lccn.loc.gov/2024058278
LC ebook record available at https://lccn.loc.gov/2024058279
British Cataloguing in Publication Data
A Cataloguing in Publication record for this book is available from the British Library.

Table of Contents

Detailed Table of Contents

Population ageing presents a profound challenge to global health systems, necessitating innovative, integrative, and multidimensional responses to support recovery and optimise well-being in older adults. This chapter explores a holistic framework for health recovery tailored to the ageing population, incorporating physical, emotional, cognitive, social, environmental, and spiritual dimensions. The chapter emphasises evidence-based approaches in falls prevention, emotional intelligence, integrative medicine, and person-centred care strategies. It presents a synthesis of Western and traditional health paradigms—including Traditional Chinese Medicine and naturopathy—while addressing rehabilitation, functional restoration, and dignity in ageing. A particular focus is given to practices that foster resilience, autonomy, and long-term recovery in both clinical and community contexts. Through theory, policy, and practice, the chapter advocates for a paradigm shift from disease management to holistic recovery and flourishing in later life.

Communication and language development are key to a child's cognitive, social, and overall well-being. While many children develop language skills despite risk factors, language development is vulnerable to various challenges, impacting academic performance, employment, and mental health. Early identification and intervention are crucial for achieving positive outcomes for children at risk of atypical language development. Such approaches must be collaborative, involving families, healthcare

in the US affected. This has led to increased research into effective interventions. Today, many individuals with ASD have better outcomes than in the past, with more becoming verbal, reading, and living in the community. This progress is due in part to improved knowledge and evidence-based treatments. Alongside traditional therapies, complementary therapies—used alongside conventional treatments—have gained attention. This chapter provides an overview of ASD's defining traits and explores innovative interventions, including water-based speech therapy, music therapy, and animal-assisted therapy. These approaches not only enhance speech, sensory integration, and social skills but also support relaxation and inclusion, empowering individuals with ASD to achieve their full potential and contributing to a more inclusive future.

Food allergies are a major global health concern that affect millions of people. The intricacy of the food supply chain and the range of allergens cannot be fully accommodated by traditional methods, such as labeling laws and manufacturing procedures. In response, new approaches and cutting-edge technologies are being developed to improve the management of food allergies. By enhancing the identification, management, and dissemination of allergen risks, these strategies hope to boost consumer confidence and safety. This review examines recent developments in food allergen management, such as innovative food processing techniques, state-of-the-art detection methods, and regulatory advancements. In order to address the changing issues surrounding food allergies and safeguard the public's health, the review highlights how crucial it is for stakeholders to keep coming up with new ideas and working together.

This chapter investigates the role of Emotional Intelligence (EI) as a proactive strategy to enhance caregiver well-being and mitigate burnout in geriatric settings. As the ageing population grows globally, professional and informal caregivers face

The perception of patients, ENT doctors and speech therapists about the experience of living with dysphagia and dysphonia after chemoradiotherapy (CRT) for oropharyngeal cancer is little studied. This perception is essential for improving care and influencing health policies. A descriptive qualitative study was carried out using semi-structured interviews. The interviews were recorded, transcribed and analysed thematically using NVivo®. The themes 'swallowing and dysphagia' and 'voice and dysphonia' emerged, with sub-themes related to quality of life, eating, socialising and communication. The most frequently reported difficulties were hoarseness, choking, thick saliva and coughing when drinking liquids. The need for a holistic approach and continuous monitoring from the start of treatment, involving patients and families, is emphasised.

The concept of vulnerability is commonly used to refer to people's susceptibility to environmental problems, health damage and the degree of risk to which a population tends to suffer damage from natural disasters. Urban areas are vulnerable to climate change. The propensity of a given population/location can be adversely affected by climate change, based on three fundamental elements: sensitivity, adaptive capacity and exposure. The degree of vulnerability of a area, depends on indicators of exposure, sensitivity and adaptive capacity in a stepwise manner. Vulnerability is thus presented as the degree of susceptibility or risk to which a population is exposed to suffering damage from natural disasters. This vulnerability concept is explained through the application of a case study carried out in the city of Rio de Janeiro, Brazil, to produce maps that have made it possible to identify the most vulnerable areas in the

Preface

Health and healing are deeply personal, context-dependent, and complex experiences. While modern medicine has advanced rapidly, its conventional focus on pathology often overlooks the integrated nature of human well-being, leaving gaps in patient care and recovery processes. In contemporary healthcare, the recognition of this complexity has given rise to a renewed interest in holistic approaches—those that consider the individual as a whole, integrating physical, emotional, social, cognitive, environmental, and spiritual dimensions of well-being. *Holistic Approaches to Health Recovery* brings together diverse perspectives and evidence-based strategies that aim to reframe health not merely as the absence of illness, but as a dynamic process of recovery, adaptation, and flourishing across the lifespan.

This volume aims to inspire students, educators, professionals, and decision-makers to adopt more integrative, human-centered approaches to promoting global health and well-being by bridging research, practice, and policy. Reflecting the collaborative efforts of clinicians, researchers, and educators from various disciplines and international contexts, this edited volume highlights the value of integrative care models and innovative methodologies, interdisciplinary partnerships, and person-centered practices that respond to some of today's most pressing health challenges, from ageing and neurodevelopmental disorders to communication impairments and public health policy. It emphasizes the importance of integrated care models and showcases innovative methodologies, interdisciplinary partnerships, and person-centered practices that address some of today's most urgent health issues, ranging from ageing and neurodevelopmental disorders to communication impairments and public health policy. The volume is organized into thirteen chapters, each addressing a key dimension of integrative health.

CHAPTER OVERVIEW

Chapter 1 introduces a comprehensive, multidimensional model of health recovery for older adults, emphasizing a shift from disease management to holistic well-being. It integrates perspectives from conventional and traditional medical systems and promotes dignity and autonomy in ageing.

Chapter 2 explores the early identification of communication disorders in children, offering a nuanced understanding of the risk and protective factors that influence language development. This chapter advocates proactive, collaborative interventions that involve families and professionals alike.

Chapter 3 examines the intersection of clinical assessments and patient perception in the treatment of mechanical dysphagia post-head and neck cancer. It presents evidence that supports aligning therapeutic strategies with patient-reported outcomes to improve quality of care.

Chapter 4 presents a bibliometric and visual analysis of global trends in Complementary and Alternative Medicine (CAM) for the mental health of older adults. It identifies research gaps and suggests opportunities for integrating CAM into mainstream public health strategies.

Chapter 5 focuses on communication-enabling materials in healthcare settings. It provides a narrative review of tools that reduce barriers between professionals and patients, reinforcing communication as a cornerstone of effective and humane care.

Chapter 6 reviews complementary approaches to autism spectrum disorder intervention. Highlighting therapies such as music, water-based, and animal-assisted therapy, it affirms the potential of holistic strategies to enhance quality of life and inclusiveness for individuals with ASD.

Chapter 7 explores emerging innovations in managing food allergens, highlighting technological advancements, improved detection methods, and collaborative approaches aimed at enhancing consumer safety and confidence.

Chapter 8 delves into the role of emotional intelligence in preventing caregiver burnout in geriatric care. By promoting emotional awareness and empathy, it offers practical frameworks for supporting those who care for an ageing population.

Chapter 9 discusses the empowerment of patients through education in rehabilitation settings. It demonstrates how tailored educational strategies can enhance motivation, engagement, and long-term health outcomes.

Chapter 10 presents a qualitative study on the lived experiences of patients and healthcare professionals managing dysphagia and dysphonia post-treatment. The findings call for holistic, continuous care that addresses both clinical and psychosocial dimensions.

Chapter 11 introduces the concept of vulnerability in public health and the use of sensitivity indices to guide decision-making. Using a case study from Rio de Janeiro, it illustrates how data-driven tools can inform targeted interventions and policy.

Chapter 12 highlights the role of Speech-Language Pathologists in empowering parents and caregivers as communicative partners during early childhood. It supports a family-centered model that nurtures developmental outcomes and emotional resilience.

Chapter 13 concludes the volume by presenting the integrative role of physiotherapy in women's health across the lifespan. It reinforces the importance of holistic, multidisciplinary care in addressing diverse health conditions, including those that are often underrepresented.

Together, these chapters present a compelling case for holistic recovery as a guiding principle in 21st-century healthcare. It is our hope that this collection not only serves as a current resource but also stimulates further inquiry and innovation in these critical areas.

Adérito Seixas
Escola Superior de Saúde Fernando Pessoa, Portugal

Rita Alegria
Escola Superior de Saúde Fernando Pessoa, Portugal

Daniela Vieira
Escola Superior de Saúde Fernando Pessoa, Portugal

Chapter 1
Holistic Health Recovery for the Ageing Population: A Multidimensional Approach

Tiago Manuel Horta Reis da Silva
https://orcid.org/0000-0001-5220-1718
King's College, London, UK

ABSTRACT

Population ageing presents a profound challenge to global health systems, necessitating innovative, integrative, and multidimensional responses to support recovery and optimise well-being in older adults. This chapter explores a holistic framework for health recovery tailored to the ageing population, incorporating physical, emotional, cognitive, social, environmental, and spiritual dimensions. The chapter emphasises evidence-based approaches in falls prevention, emotional intelligence, integrative medicine, and person-centred care strategies. It presents a synthesis of Western and traditional health paradigms—including Traditional Chinese Medicine and naturopathy—while addressing rehabilitation, functional restoration, and dignity in ageing. A particular focus is given to practices that foster resilience, autonomy, and long-term recovery in both clinical and community contexts. Through theory, policy, and practice, the chapter advocates for a paradigm shift from disease management to holistic recovery and flourishing in later life.

DOI: 10.4018/979-8-3693-6432-1.ch001

1. INTRODUCTION

Population ageing is increasingly recognised as a global phenomenon, influencing various facets of society, economy, and healthcare systems (Reis da Silva, 2025a). As life expectancy rises and birth rates decline, countries around the world are experiencing a demographic shift towards an older population. This transition is particularly significant in high-income nations, where the proportion of individuals aged 65 and older is set to increase dramatically in the coming decades (Yue, 2023; Maestas et al., 2016). The implications of this shift are profound, necessitating a comprehensive approach to understanding and managing the challenges associated with an ageing populace. This context sets the stage for exploring the concept of "holistic recovery," particularly as it pertains to older adults.

Defining "holistic recovery" in the context of ageing involves addressing physical, emotional, social, and psychological well-being, which are integral to the recovery processes of the older adults. Holistic recovery recognises that health is not merely the absence of illness but a state of complete physical, mental, and social well-being (Adetunji et al., 2023). Effective models of recovery-oriented care emphasise the importance of empathy, compassion, and support from healthcare providers, who must be attuned to the multifaceted needs of older individuals (Reis da Silva, 2024a). Moreover, the necessity for transdisciplinary approaches in geriatric care illustrates the imperative for collaboration across various healthcare fields to enhance recovery outcomes for older patients (Chia et al., 2016; Reis da Silva, 2025b).

The significance of holistic recovery is underscored by the increasing complexity of health issues faced by the older population, such as multimorbidity and frailty (Reis da Silva, 2024b; Reis da Silva, 2024c). These conditions require not only medical interventions but also comprehensive care strategies that integrate social support systems (Wang et al., 2022). For instance, recognising the psychosocial needs of older adults is critical, as unmet emotional and social needs can greatly impede recovery and contribute to poorer health outcomes (Adetunji et al., 2023; Reis da Silva, 2024d). Therefore, adopting a holistic framework is essential in developing effective interventions that not only focus on biological or medical outcomes but also encompass the broader determinants of health.

The objectives of this chapter are threefold: First, to articulate the pressing challenges of population ageing on healthcare systems and society; second, to define and elaborate on the concept of holistic recovery, illustrating its relevance to the geriatric population; and third, to highlight the significance of integrating holistic approaches within healthcare practices to improve quality of life and recovery outcomes for older individuals. Understanding these dimensions will help inform policymakers, healthcare providers, and researchers about effective strategies to address the multidimensional aspects of ageing and recovery.

2. THEORETICAL AND CONCEPTUAL FOUNDATIONS

In elucidating the implications of an ageing population, it is vital to examine how countries are responding to the healthcare needs of their older citizens through policies and programs (Reis da Silva, 2025a; Reis da Silva, 2023a). Emerging evidence indicates that countries such as the UK and China are implementing strategies aimed at enhancing the health outcomes and quality of life for older individuals through tailored healthcare services and community support initiatives (Yue, 2023; Reis da Silva, 2205a). This includes innovations in healthcare delivery systems that promote continuity of care and integrate various services to cater to the unique needs of older adults (Zhang et al., 2024). The drive towards patient-centred care further highlights the importance of recognising older individuals as active participants in their healthcare decisions, fostering a sense of agency and empowerment crucial for holistic recovery (Adetunji et al., 2023).

2.1 Holistic Health Paradigms: From Biomedical to Integrative Models

In recent decades, the discourse surrounding health and healthcare paradigms has transitioned from a predominantly biomedical model focused on disease treatment to one that embraces holistic and integrative approaches (Reis da Silva, 2024e). This shift acknowledges the multifaceted nature of health, emphasising the interplay of physical, emotional, social, and environmental factors. The biomedical model, traditionally characterised by its focus on pathology and symptom management, often neglects the individual's overall well-being and contextual circumstances (Agarwal, 2018). Conversely, integrative health models promote the understanding of health as a dynamic equilibrium influenced by various determinants, reflecting a comprehensive view that aligns well with the complexities of aging populations (Rahmani et al., 2020; Dallinger et al., 2022).

Central to the integrative approach is the concept of holistic health, which calls for addressing health on multiple levels—biological, psychological, social, and environmental (Reis da Silva, 2024e). Unlike the biomedical model's reductionist view, holistic health paradigms encourage practitioners to consider patient narratives, lifestyle choices, and psychosocial factors that contribute to overall well-being (Choo et al., 2019). As healthcare services continue adopting this integrative paradigm, the promotion of mental health and functionality alongside physical health has become increasingly vital (Dallinger et al., 2022), demonstrating a recognition that effective recovery goes beyond mere disease management (Chester et al., 2016).

The eclectic nature of holistic health also extends into therapeutic practices where complementary and alternative medicine (CAM) signifies an integral part of contemporary health conversations (Reis da Silva, 2024e). CAM integrates traditional, cultural, and non-conventional health practices that resonate with patients' beliefs and values, providing a more personalised and culturally sensitive approach to care (Agarwal, 2018). This is particularly significant in the context of an ageing population, where chronic conditions and multimorbidity necessitate broader perspectives on health recovery (Gouvernet & Brisson, 2024; Reis da Silva, 2024d).

2.2 Definitions of Health Recovery vs. Disease Management

Health recovery and disease management often coexist in healthcare settings but serve distinctly different objectives. Disease management primarily focuses on controlling symptoms and reducing the burden of diseases through treatment protocols (Reis da Silva, 2024c). It relies heavily on clinical guidelines and often views health as a linear process wherein specific interventions target identifiable pathologies (Chester et al., 2016). In contrast, health recovery encompasses a wider lens, concentrating on the individual's journey to regain control over their health, enhancing resilience, and promoting overall wellness (Dallinger et al., 2022; Reis da Silva, 2025c). The recovery paradigm promotes a shift in focus from merely treating symptoms to supporting individuals in attaining optimal health outcomes. This model emphasises patient empowerment and a collaborative partnership between providers and patients, allowing healthcare to respect individual choices and experiences (Rahmani et al., 2020). In contexts such as mental health, for instance, recovery has been articulated as a personal, subjective process that involves developing meaning from one's experiences, which can enable more profound healing and reintegration into everyday life (Chester et al., 2016; Reis da Silva, 2025d).

This differentiation becomes even more critical in geriatric care, where older adults often face challenges that extend beyond physical health. A holistic recovery approach integrates various aspects of life—social engagement, mental acuity, and emotional stability—into the recovery process, thus enabling older individuals to restore their functionality and improve their quality of life (Choo et al., 2019; Dallinger et al., 2022). In this light, relationship-building and fostering hope become imperative components of holistic recovery.

2.3 Salutogenesis and Resilience Theory

Salutogenesis, a term coined by Aaron Antonovsky, shifts the focus of health studies from pathology to the factors that promote human health and well-being (Gouvernet & Brisson, 2024). The concept of salutogenesis explores how individuals manage stress and maintain well-being despite various stressors encountered throughout life. This perspective supports the view that health is not merely the absence of disease; rather, it is a dynamic state that can be cultivated through effective coping strategies and supportive environments (Gouvernet & Brisson, 2024).

Linked closely with salutogenesis is resilience theory, which posits that individuals have the capacity to adapt to adversity and recover after stress (Reis da Silva, 2025c). In the context of ageing, resilience becomes vital as older adults often confront various life transitions, including loss, chronic illness, and changing social roles (Reis da Silva, 2025e; Reis da Silva, 2024f). The focus on building resilience through community support, social networks, and personal agency aligns well with holistic recovery strategies aimed at promoting well-being (Gouvernet & Brisson, 2024). As healthcare systems increasingly recognise the significance of resilience, interventions designed to bolster coping mechanisms can enhance recovery outcomes, particularly in older populations navigating the complexities of ageing (Hernandez et al., 2021).

2.4 Ageing Through the Lens of Complex Systems Thinking

Complex systems thinking offers a profound framework for understanding health and ageing, recognising that health outcomes are the result of intricate interactions between various components of health, society, and environment. This approach emphasises the interdependence of these elements, which influences individual health trajectories and experiences (Gouvernet & Brisson, 2024). In terms of ageing, complex systems thinking illustrates how older adults do not exist in isolation; their health can be substantially affected by social determinants, cultural contexts, and community resources (Nyatuka & Harpe, 2021).

From a systems perspective, ageing can be viewed as a phenomenon characterised by multiple dimensions—biological functioning, social connectivity, psychological resilience, and environmental factors—all of which contribute to health outcomes (Reis da Silva, 2025a). This model of thought encourages healthcare providers to adopt adaptive strategies that foster collaboration across disciplines and sectors, leading to more effective interventions (Nyatuka & Harpe, 2021). For instance, recognising that mental health, nutrition, and physical activity are interconnected facets of a person's health may encourage healthcare systems to promote integrated care pathways that consider the holistic nature of health recovery (Math et al., 2015; Reis da Silva, 2023b; Reis da Silva, 2024g).

Moreover, the complexity inherent in health systems parallels that found in ageing dynamics, where constant change and adaptation are essential for promoting resilience and well-being among older adults (Reis da Silva, 2024h). Thus, adopting a complexity lens in geriatric care can facilitate a deeper appreciation of the multi-dimensional nature of aging and the nuanced strategies required to enhance recovery and quality of life in older populations.

2.5 Resilience, Recovery and Systems of Thinking

In addressing the multifaceted domain of holistic health recovery for the ageing population, particularly concerning the linking concepts of resilience, recovery, and systems thinking, insights from a diverse spectrum of literature will be used. These concepts not only reinforce each other but also interconnect in practical frameworks that can significantly enhance health outcomes in older adults.

Resilience, fundamentally defined as the ability to recover from adversity, is paramount for the ageing population, who often confront a myriad of health challenges, including chronic diseases and mental health issues (Amin & Pinilih, 2024). As highlighted by Amin and Pinilih (2024), resilience necessitates a holistic approach, which integrates factors that influence an individual's capacity to withstand and recover from health-related adversities. This perspective on resilience emphasises the importance of contextual factors, such as social isolation and economic instability, which can significantly impact older populations (Reis da Silva, 2025e; Reis da Silva, 2024f).

Integrating resilience into recovery models provides a framework that acknowledges the strengths and capacities within individuals and communities (Reis da Silva, 2025c). The recovery-oriented approach emphasises healing not merely as the absence of disease but as a holistic and empowering process (Bilgin, 2023). As underscored by Bilgin (2023), this model fosters autonomy and encourages individuals to actively participate in shaping their recovery journeys. Moreover, the importance of community support systems and peer interventions, as outlined by Lyons et al. (2021), provides evidence that collaborative and supportive environments enhance resilience and, ultimately, recovery processes.

Systems thinking, characterising a holistic view of health recovery, is critical to understanding the complexities of the ageing population (Karthika et al., 2025). This approach necessitates consideration of multiple interactions within health systems, encompassing medical, psychological, and social dimensions occurring simultaneously. For instance, Karthika et al. (2025) emphasise how mental health recovery benefits from a systems approach that integrates various sectors, such as healthcare and community supports, to create a cohesive support structure for individuals with mental health concerns. By employing systems thinking, practitioners can design interventions that systematically address the interdependencies between health, social structure, and personal resilience (Gomes et al., 2023).

The integration of resilience and systems thinking has particular implications for palliative care in ageing individuals (Reis da Silva, 2024c). Research conducted by Gomes et al. (2023) illustrates that a humanised approach in palliative care—rooted in a robust understanding of individuals' needs and preferences—facilitates a supportive environment conducive to resilience, thereby enhancing recovery. This aligns with the broader understanding of recovery-focused interventions, which highlight the necessity of embedding resilience within supportive recovery frameworks (Insalaco & Hobelmann, 2023).

Addressing mental health recovery within the context of holistic approaches invites broader recognition of the environmental and lifestyle factors inherent to the ageing process (Amin & Pinilih, 2024). Amin and Pinilih (2024) further emphasise that recovery from mental health challenges necessitates a holistic perspective, incorporating both individual resilience capacities and systemic supports. This interconnectedness underscores the pivotal role that caregivers, healthcare systems, and community resources play in enabling older adults to cultivate resilience in their recovery efforts.

Furthermore, as highlighted by Pasupuleti (2024), learning from systems-based innovations in disaster management can also inform health recovery strategies by promoting resilience among vulnerable populations, including seniors. Such applications reflect an understanding of health maintenance that transcends traditional medical models, emphasising the need for interdisciplinary collaboration in addressing the health needs of the ageing population.

In addition to improving resilience and recovery, adopting systems thinking encourages practices that enhance overall quality of life. For instance, Elmajee et al. (2021) assert that interventions addressing various dimensions of health—including physical, mental, and social aspects—can significantly aid in the recovery from complex health issues prevalent in older demographics. By creating integrated health models that respect these interconnections, the potential for improved patient outcomes is substantially heightened (Elmajee et al., 2021).

Moreover, evidence from the literature shows that individuals' perceptions of their strengths play a crucial role in recovery endeavours (Pasupuleti, 2024). Recovery should be characterised not just by the reduction of symptomatology but by meaningful engagement in life pursuits and adaptive functioning within community settings—both core to resilience (Heveran & Andrewes, 2020). Thus, recovery narratives are not linear but consist of repetitive cycles of challenge and rebirth, reinforcing the necessity of systems perspectives in crafting continuous care pathways (Bayuo et al., 2020).

Finally, the transitional phases between health states in older adults necessitate flexible systems that adapt to evolving needs. This aspect is echoed in the work of Bayuo et al. (2020), which illuminated the need for comprehensive support mechanisms for individuals following hospital discharge, reinforcing the argument that health recovery cannot be perceived in isolation from systemic factors. As recovery journeys unfold, understanding the familial, communal, and systemic interactions becomes fundamental in nurturing resilience and meaningful recovery outputs.

3. PHYSICAL RECOVERY AND FUNCTIONAL RESTORATION

As the global population continues to age, strategies for physical recovery and functional restoration in older adults have garnered increasing attention (Reis da Silva, 2023b). Among the most pressing health concerns for this demographic are falls, which are a leading cause of injury and declining functional capacity (Reis da Silva, 2024g). This section discusses falls prevention and rehabilitation, active movement and ergonomic considerations, as well as the role of nutrition in recovery. It also presents a case study illustrating the efficacy of community-based falls prevention programs.

3.1 Fall Prevention and Rehabilitation

Falls prevention is critical in maintaining independent living among older adults. With increasing age, the risk of falls escalates due to factors like muscle weakness, balance impairments, and environmental hazards (Vincenzo et al., 2021; Reis da Silva, 2023b). A study found that older adults often do not engage in falls prevention practices due to fears related to reduced physical function and self-management (Wen et al., 2021). In response to these challenges, effective rehabilitation strategies have been developed, emphasising the importance of tailored interventions that consider individual capabilities and preferences (Tsai et al., 2020; Cardozo-Stolberg et al., 2023).

Physical therapy (PT) has been shown to play a pivotal role in fall prevention through strength and balance training programs (Wingood et al., 2024; Reis da Silva, 2024g). A study by Gell and Patel (2018) revealed that a significant proportion of older adults engaged in rehabilitation services displayed improved functional outcomes. Such programs need to communicate the role of physical therapists in educating clients about fall risks and prevention strategies to enhance awareness among older adults (Vincenzo et al., 2021). A fear of falling can lead to self-imposed activity restrictions, which subsequently reduce physical strength and overall mobility (Reis da Silva, 2023b; Shelton et al., 2024).

Thus, the implementation of community-based falls prevention initiatives is essential. These programs often focus on exercise interventions, education about environmental modifications, and the promotion of safety awareness among older adults (Moreland et al., 2018; Olij et al., 2019; Reis da Silva, 2023b).

3.2 Moving and Handling: Ergonomics, Safety, and Autonomy

The principles of ergonomics are essential in promoting safety and autonomy for older adults in various settings, including domestic and healthcare environments (Reis da Silva, 2023c). Proper ergonomic practices can help mitigate the risk of injuries during mobility tasks, facilitating better movement capability and independence. For instance, utilising assistive devices correctly can enhance stability and confidence in older adults, significantly reducing fall risk (Lee et al., 2018; Reis da Silva, 2023c).

Educational seminars focused on moving and handling principles can empower older individuals to understand how their physical capabilities influence their safety (Kiyoshi-Teo et al., 2020). Incorporating ergonomic assessments into physical therapy sessions can provide personalised recommendations that enhance both safety and comfort during daily activities (Cardozo-Stolberg et al., 2023). Autonomy is a core concept in falls prevention, as older adults who feel empowered to manage their care and make informed decisions about their health are more likely to participate in physical activity and rehabilitation (Yang et al., 2024). Ensuring that caregivers and healthcare providers respect this autonomy is vital in encouraging an environment that promotes independence (Fernandes et al., 2021).

3.3 Nutrition, Mobility, and Physical Therapy in Recovery

Nutrition plays a critical role in supporting the physical recovery and mobility of older adults. Reports highlight that adequate nutrient intake is associated with improved muscle strength and mobility, both essential components for falls prevention (Reis da Silva, 2023b). Specifically, diets rich in fruits, vegetables, and macronutrients help combat malnutrition, which is prevalent among this demographic (Khor et al., 2021).

The interaction between nutritional health and physical therapy interventions is crucial; studies indicate that combined strategies of restoring adequate nutrition alongside rehabilitation yield significant improvements in functional outcomes (Kirn et al., 2015). Moreover, structured physical activity programs, when complemented by nutritional education, can significantly enhance mobility and restore functional independence in older adults (Neil-Sztramko et al., 2022).

Involving nutritionists in geriatric rehabilitation programs allows for a comprehensive strategy that addresses both physical and nutritional needs (Khor et al., 2021). Such holistic approaches increase the likelihood of achieving favourable recovery results and minimising the risk of future falls (Neil-Sztramko et al., 2022).

3.4 Case Study: Community-Based Falls Prevention in Older Adults

A community-based program targeting falls prevention provides practical insights into the efficacy of localised interventions. One such program used a multi-faceted approach, combining exercise sessions tailored to older adults, environmental assessments, and educational workshops on fall awareness (Vendramini et al., 2017). Participants engaged in supervised exercises that emphasised balance, coordination, and strength training.

The results demonstrated a significant reduction in fall incidence among participants while concurrently enhancing their functional mobility and self-efficacy regarding fall-related fears (Shelton et al., 2024). Furthermore, older adults reported improvements in their overall quality of life and expressed increased confidence in their ability to engage in daily activities without the fear of falling (Yang et al., 2024). This case study underscores how community involvement and tailored interventions can effectively address the complex issue of falls among older adults.

4. EMOTIONAL AND COGNITIVE DIMENSIONS OF RECOVERY

The emotional and cognitive dimensions of recovery for older adults are of paramount importance, as these factors significantly influence health behaviours and overall recovery processes (Reis da Silva et al., 2025). Emotional intelligence, psychological resilience, and effective coping strategies play a critical role in managing mental health challenges, enhancing life satisfaction, and promoting successful ageing (Reis da Silva, 2024i). This section explores the interplay of these elements, addressing issues such as loneliness, elder abuse, depression, anxiety, and cognitive decline, while also presenting effective interventions like narrative therapy, meditation, mindfulness, and reminiscence therapy.

4.1 The Role of Emotional Intelligence in Health Behaviour and Recovery

Emotional intelligence (EI) refers to the ability to recognise, understand, manage, and utilise emotions effectively in oneself and others (da Silva, 2022; Reis da Silva, 2025f). In older adults, higher emotional intelligence has been linked to improved health behaviours and better recovery outcomes. Individuals with strong EI are more adept at navigating social environments and responding to health-related challenges (Duan et al., 2024; Reis da Silva et al., 2025). For older adults facing the complexities of ageing, such as chronic illnesses or social isolation, utilising emotional intelligence skills can not only enhance their self-regulation but also contribute positively to their interactions with healthcare professionals and peers (Reis da Silva, 2024f).

Research has shown that older adults with higher levels of emotional intelligence tend to engage in healthier lifestyle choices and are more likely to adhere to treatment regimens, thereby improving their recovery trajectories (Shuang-Shuang & Ma, 2023). Through enhanced emotional regulation, these individuals may experience greater resilience against stressors and an increased ability to cope with the emotional repercussions of health decline, thus facilitating a more supportive recovery environment.

4.2 Mental Peace, Grief Processing, and Psychological Resilience

Mental peace and the ability to process grief are critical components of psychological resilience (Reis da Silva, 2025g). For older adults, coping with loss—be it the death of a spouse, friends, or a decline in physical health—can lead to a complex emotional landscape marked by sadness, anxiety, and sometimes depression (Reis da Silva, 2024j). Psychological resilience, which comprises an individual's capacity to adapt and recover from setbacks, offers a protective factor against these emotional challenges (Upasen et al., 2024). The theme of resilience is particularly pertinent in evaluating how older adults experience grief and loss. Studies indicate that higher levels of resilience are associated with more effective grief processing, which in turn correlates with improved mental health outcomes (Herrera et al., 2021). Resilience allows older adults to foster a sense of meaning and purpose, promoting a positive outlook even amid adversity. It enhances emotional well-being, enabling them to engage in social activities and maintain cognitive functions, thereby contributing to overall recovery (Lee, 2023).

4.3 Addressing Loneliness, Elder Abuse, Depression, Anxiety, and Cognitive Decline

The emotional dimensions of recovery are further challenged by social isolation, elder abuse, and prevalent psychological issues like depression and anxiety. Loneliness is particularly common among older adults, leading to detrimental effects on both mental and physical health (Reis da Silva, 2024f; Reis da Silva, 2025e). Research suggests that loneliness is closely linked to cognitive decline and increased morbidity (Cleofas, 2024). Interventions targeting social connectedness can significantly mitigate these issues, fostering an environment where older adults feel supported and valued.

Furthermore, elder abuse remains a crucial concern that not only impacts emotional health but can also result in severe psychological trauma (Reis da Silva, 2024k). Studies indicate that victims of elder abuse frequently experience heightened levels of depression and anxiety, underscoring the necessity for preventative measures and education surrounding this issue (Ávila et al., 2016). Addressing these threats through community awareness and comprehensive support systems is vital for enhancing emotional recovery.

4.4 Interventions

Several therapeutic interventions have been identified as effective in promoting emotional and cognitive recovery among older adults. Narrative therapy encourages individuals to explore and reshape their personal stories, allowing them to reframe negative experiences, including those related to loss and trauma. This process can enhance self-identity and resilience, facilitating a sense of control over one's life narrative (Landi et al., 2020). Meditation and mindfulness practices have also gained traction for their ability to reduce anxiety and improve emotional regulation (Reis da Silva, 2024e). Through practices that promote present-moment awareness, older adults may achieve greater mental clarity and emotional stability, thereby enhancing their overall well-being (Lim et al., 2021). Studies indicate that regular mindfulness practice can significantly alleviate symptoms of anxiety and depression, fostering a more positive outlook on ageing.

Additionally, reminiscence therapy, which involves recalling past experiences, has proven beneficial in facilitating emotional expression and reducing feelings of loneliness. It allows older adults to connect with their memories and share these narratives with others, fostering a sense of community and belonging (Li et al., 2023). Engaging in collective reminiscence activities can also diminish the impacts of loneliness and enhance life satisfaction, demonstrating the interconnectedness of social support and emotional health in recovery (Reis da Silva, 2024f).

5. SOCIAL ENGAGEMENT AND SUPPORTIVE NETWORKS

The importance of social engagement and supportive networks for older adults cannot be overstated, especially as they navigate the complexities of ageing (Reis da Silva, 2025e). Community connectedness and intergenerational engagement significantly influence physical and mental health outcomes for older individuals. Caregivers, peer networks, and informal care systems serve as essential pillars of support in promoting well-being, alongside the built environment, which includes housing, transport, and age-friendly settings (Reis da Silva, 2024f). This section explores these aspects, highlighting how public health strategies can foster social capital and create an enabling environment for older adults.

5.1 Community Connectedness and Intergenerational Engagement

Community connectedness primarily revolves around relationships and interactions that bind individuals within their local constructs. Intergenerational engagement facilitates the sharing of knowledge, resources, and emotional support between different age groups, significantly enhancing the mental health and social well-being of older adults (Zhu et al., 2025). Studies have indicated that when older individuals participate in intergenerational programs, they report lower levels of loneliness and greater overall satisfaction with life (Reis da Silva, 2024f). For instance, an analysis of various intergenerational programs highlighted their effectiveness in reducing isolation among seniors and strengthening community ties (Zhu et al., 2025).

Intergenerational interactions serve as a reciprocal mechanism where younger generations gain valuable insights and wisdom, while older adults benefit from youthful energy and perspectives. This symbiotic relationship can be especially beneficial in cultures where filial piety is highly valued, enhancing support for older adults within their families and communities (Xu et al., 2024). Programs designed to cross age boundaries, such as mentorship initiatives or shared community activities, have proven fruitful, fostering environments that celebrate shared experiences and mutual respect (Mahoney et al., 2019).

5.2 Role of Caregivers, Peer Networks, and Informal Care

Caregivers—whether family members, friends, or professional support workers—play a pivotal role in the health and well-being of older adults. Peer networks also provide significant informal care that complements formal healthcare services, creating a system of support that addresses practical, emotional, and social needs (Yan et al., 2023). Numerous studies have shown that older adults engaged with informal networks experience improved mental health, greater stability, and resilience against stressors (Yan et al., 2023).

Moreover, collaborative caregiving can reduce the burden on individual family caregivers, allowing for a distribution of responsibilities that enhances the quality of care. The significance of recognising and supporting informal networks, such as community groups or volunteering programs, has been underscored in public health frameworks, demonstrating their contributions to overall wellness outcomes for older adults (Dunn et al., 2021).

5.3 Housing, Transport, and Age-Friendly Environments

The built environment significantly influences older adults' social connectivity and mobility. Age-friendly environments—typically characterised by accessible housing, reliable public transport, and inviting communal spaces—empower seniors to remain engaged with their communities, thus mitigating social isolation (Gibson et al., 2022; Reis da Silva, 2025a). Research indicates that communities designed with the needs of older adults in mind not only improve their quality of life but also enhance their sense of security and belonging (Gibson et al., 2022).

Accessible transportation options are critical, enabling older adults to participate in community activities and healthcare visits. Initiatives aimed at creating walkable neighbourhoods or accessible public transit systems have shown positive correlations with improved health outcomes among seniors (Shu et al., 2021). In addition, age-friendly housing that incorporates universal design practices, such as barrier-free entrances and adaptable features, fosters independence and facilitates social interactions within the community (Melo et al., 2023; Reis da Silva, 2023a).

5.4 Promoting Social Capital Through Public Health Strategies

Public health strategies are crucial in promoting social capital—essentially the networks of relationships and norms that enable collective action for mutual benefit (Cowley et al., 2023). Traditional healthcare interventions often overlook the social determinants of health; however, integrating social capital development into public health strategies can substantially impact well-being (Fu & Ji, 2020). For instance, incorporating social engagement and support into health policies encourages community participation and creates opportunities for older individuals to build and maintain relationships. Policy frameworks can promote funding for intergenerational programs and community centres that foster social interactions among various age groups (Betancourt et al., 2020). Moreover, facilitating partnerships between healthcare organisations and community groups can lead to the implementation of local initiatives that enhance connectedness and build resilience within older populations (Ward et al., 2018).

Public health messaging that emphasises the importance of social ties enhances awareness around mental health, combating stigma and promoting pro-social behaviour. Interventions leveraging digital platforms to foster virtual community support during crises—such as the COVID-19 pandemic—illustrate how technology can be harnessed to maintain connections, thereby mitigating potential declines in mental and emotional health (Reis da Silva, 2025h).

6. INTEGRATIVE AND TRADITIONAL APPROACHES TO HEALING

The integration of traditional and complementary approaches to health care is becoming increasingly prominent in addressing the multifaceted needs of older adults. As healthcare systems evolve, the understanding of well-being expands beyond conventional biomedical models, incorporating holistic frameworks involving various traditional practices (Reis da Silva, 2024e). This section will examine key areas, including Naturopathy, Traditional Chinese Medicine (TCM) and herbal pharmacology, acupuncture, Qi Gong, and energy medicine, focusing on their integration with Western models. Furthermore, it will address the associated risks, ethical considerations, and regulatory challenges faced when delivering integrative care to older populations.

6.1 Naturopathy, Traditional Chinese Medicine, and Herbal Pharmacology

Naturopathy is a holistic healthcare approach that emphasises preventive care and the body's inherent ability to heal itself through natural remedies (Reis da Silva, 2024e). Practitioners use various modalities, including nutrition, herbal medicine, and physical therapies (Corso et al., 2022). In the context of elder care, Naturopathy is particularly beneficial for managing chronic conditions, promoting self-care practices, and enhancing overall wellness without relying heavily on pharmaceuticals.

Traditional Chinese Medicine (TCM) encompasses various therapeutic practices based on principles that view health as a harmonious balance of body, mind, and spirit (Reis da Silva, 2024e). Key components of TCM involve Tuina (massage), herbal medicine and nutrition, acupuncture and moxibustion, and Qi Gong. Herbal medicine within TCM utilises a diverse array of natural substances that have been empirically tested over centuries. For example, saponins from plants like *Panax ginseng* have shown potential cardioprotective benefits, highlighting the ability of

TCM herbalists to offer comprehensive management strategies for health issues common in older adults (Wang et al., 2021).

Incorporating herbal pharmacology into gerontological care requires qualified practitioners who understand both the efficacy and potential interactions of herbal treatments with prescribed medications. As such, the integration of TCM's herbal knowledge can offer powerful adjuncts to conventional therapies in managing conditions such as hypertension or diabetes (Zhao et al., 2022).

Acupuncture is a key therapeutic modality within TCM, involving the insertion of fine needles into specific points along meridian pathways to restore balance and improve health (Reis da Silva, 2024e). Research suggests that acupuncture may be particularly effective in alleviating chronic pain, which is often prevalent in the geriatric demographic. Studies have noted significant reductions in pain levels and improvements in functional outcomes for older adults using acupuncture as part of their integrative care plan (Shropshire et al., 2018).

Qi Gong, a mind-body practice combining physical movement, meditation, and controlled breathing, has shown considerable promise in enhancing the quality of life for older individuals. This practice promotes relaxation, mental clarity, and physical strength—all crucial factors for the aging population. Regular engagement in Qi Gong has been linked to improvements in mobility, balance, and mental well-being, potentially lowering risks of falls among seniors (Allen et al., 2020).

Energy medicine encompasses various modalities, including therapeutic touch and Reiki, which focus on the body's energy fields to promote healing. Although empirical validation for energy medicine often lags behind that of more conventional approaches, anecdotal evidence and emerging clinical studies suggest potential benefits for relaxation and stress management, contributing to overall psychological resilience and emotional health among the older population (Corso et al., 2022).

6.2 Evidence-Based Integration with Western Models

The integration of traditional healing practices with evidence-based Western models requires rigorous evaluation processes to establish credibility and safety. Collaborative care models that incorporate traditional therapies such as Naturopathy and TCM not only provide holistic perspectives but also enrich clinical practices within conventional biomedical systems (Doucette et al., 2024).

A successful integration model often involves interdisciplinary collaboration between traditional practitioners and healthcare providers. For instance, training in cultural safety and knowledge-sharing between Indigenous conceptions of health and Western practices can foster understanding and improve health outcomes for Indigenous older populations (Doucette et al., 2024). Additionally, studies have shown that primary healthcare settings that integrate traditional healing practices can enhance patient engagement and satisfaction (Harfield et al., 2018), illustrating a tangible pathway for integrating complementary approaches into routine gerontological care.

Moreover, the growing emphasis on personalised medicine aligns with the principles of traditional approaches, which often emphasise individualised treatment plans (Reis da Silva, 2024e). Implementing evidence-based practices alongside traditional therapies may yield synergistic effects, enhancing recovery trajectories for older adults with multifactorial health challenges (Drost, 2019).

6.3 Risks, Ethics, and Regulation in Integrative Care for Elders

While the integration of traditional healing practices into geriatric care presents numerous benefits, it also poses challenges, including potential risks and ethical considerations. One significant concern is the risk of ineffective or unsafe treatments, particularly if practitioners lack appropriate training or background knowledge. Proper education and certification processes for integrative care practitioners are essential to ensure safe practices and patient well-being (Drost, 2019).

Ethical issues arise when these integrative treatments do not align with evidence-based guidelines or when patients seek alternative therapies after foregoing conventional medical advice (Reis da Silva, 2024e). A transparent dialogue between healthcare providers and patients is crucial to navigate these complexities. Educating patients about the efficacy and safety profiles of various treatments can empower decision-making and minimise risks (Allen et al., 2020).

Regulation of integrative care practices poses another significant challenge. Regulatory frameworks must evolve to encompass traditional and holistic practices without compromising patient safety or care quality. Legal standards should address the qualifications of practitioners, the safety of treatments, and the necessity for informed consent for all interventions. Policymakers must prioritise establishing guidelines that validate and protect both patients and practitioners in the integrative health domain (Corso et al., 2022).

7. SPIRITUAL AND EXISTENTIAL RECOVERY

Spirituality plays a vital role in the holistic healing process for older adults, serving as a source of comfort, strength, and resilience during the challenges of ageing. As individuals enter later life, many seek deeper meaning and purpose, often turning to spirituality as a pathway for understanding and coping with existential issues (Reis da Silva, 2024b). This section explores the significance of spirituality in later life, the processes of life review and meaning-making, cross-cultural perspectives on aging and spirituality, and the role of rituals and spiritual care, including institutional chaplaincy.

7.1 Spirituality in Later Life and Its Role in Holistic Healing

As individuals age, spirituality often becomes more pronounced, acting as a stabilising force that can enhance overall well-being. Spirituality is deeply personal and may encompass a range of beliefs, including religiosity, but also includes secular perspectives on meaning and fulfilment (Chen et al., 2018). The search for spiritual meaning is linked to improved quality of life, particularly among older adults facing terminal illnesses (Chen et al., 2018).

Studies illustrate that spirituality can foster resilience and coping capabilities among the older population. Spiritual practices such as prayer, meditation, and reflection have been linked to reduced levels of anxiety and depression, contributing to a more positive outlook on life (Reis da Silva, 2024d). Naturopathy and other holistic healing systems often emphasise the importance of the spiritual dimension as a critical component of health. When older adults engage with their spirituality, they often report feeling a renewed sense of hope, peace, and connection, which can bolster their ability to manage chronic illness or cope with the loss of loved ones (Reis da Silva, 2024e).

7.2 Life Review, Meaning-Making, and Transcendence

The process of life review is significant during later life, allowing individuals to reflect on their experiences and extract meaning from their past. Engaging in the life review process can facilitate understanding and acceptance of life events, enhancing self-worth and contributing to personal growth (Guo et al., 2023). Research indicates that meaningful life reviews often lead to the recognition of personal strengths, fostering a sense of transcendence and purpose beyond the physical limitations of aging (Guo et al., 2023).

Meaning-making is closely intertwined with life review; it involves interpreting past experiences to construct a coherent narrative of one's life. This cognitive reframing allows older adults to integrate memories—both positive and negative—into a meaningful framework, often catalysing personal transformation and existential fulfilment (Reis da Silva et al., 2025). Such processes can promote emotional healing, reduce feelings of despair, and encourage social engagement, which can be particularly beneficial when coping with grief or loss (Reis da Silva, 2024e; Reis da Silva, 2024f).

Moreover, transcendent experiences—those that go beyond the self and create a connection to something greater—can be pivotal for older adults as they search for purpose (Jones et al., 2024). Many individuals report that during times of crisis or significant life changes, such as retirement or the death of a spouse, spirituality and transcendence provide profound comfort and guidance, thus facilitating emotional healing (Jones et al., 2024).

7.3 Cross-Cultural Perspectives on Ageing and Spirituality

Spirituality and its role in ageing can vary significantly across cultural contexts. For example, in Pacific cultures, such as among Tongan and Samoan elders, spirituality is often seen as integral to overall wellness (Ihara, and Vakalahi, 2011). It encompasses a balance between the physical, mental, and spiritual domains of life (Reis da Silva, 2024e). Indigenous cultures frequently emphasise spirituality as a means of connection to ancestors and the environment, fostering community ties and support systems that empower older individuals (Chen et al., 2018).

In contrast, Western perspectives may focus primarily on individualistic concepts of spirituality, often linked to personal growth and psychological well-being. Understanding spirituality from diverse cultural frameworks can enhance healthcare delivery by tailoring spiritual care initiatives that resonate with the values and beliefs of specific populations (Chen et al., 2018). Cross-cultural perspectives on ageing and spirituality reinforce the necessity for healthcare providers to adopt culturally competent practices that respect and incorporate the spiritual values of older adults.

7.4 Rituals, Spiritual Care, and Institutional Chaplaincy

Rituals play a significant role in the spiritual lives of older adults, often providing structure and meaning in transitioning life stages. Engaging in rituals—whether religious or personal—affords individuals opportunities to express their spirituality, commemorate significant events, and reinforce community bonds (Memaryan et al., 2016).

Spiritual care in clinical settings has gained recognition as an essential aspect of holistic health. Institutional chaplaincy, for example, involves trained professionals who provide spiritual support within healthcare environments, addressing the spiritual and existential concerns of patients. Research indicates that the incorporation of spiritual care within healthcare settings can improve patients' mental health outcomes and enhance overall quality of life (Memaryan et al., 2016).

Furthermore, spiritual care training for healthcare providers underscores the importance of perception and competence in delivering effective spiritual care. This training is essential in enabling staff to recognise and respond to the spiritual needs of older adults, who may be seeking guidance, comfort, or hope in times of crisis (Guo et al., 2023). As healthcare increasingly embraces holistic practices, aligning with the spiritual dimensions of patient care will be paramount in fostering comprehensive well-being.

8. POLICY, PRACTICE, AND EDUCATIONAL IMPLICATIONS

The evolving landscape of gerontological healthcare necessitates a shift toward more holistic approaches that acknowledge the multifactorial needs of older adults. Training health professionals in holistic gerontology, designing recovery-oriented health systems, integrating holistic recovery into nursing curricula, and formulating policy recommendations for health equity are critical components to improving care for this demographic. This section discusses these areas, providing insights into how they can be implemented in practice and education.

8.1 Training Health Professionals in Holistic Gerontology

To provide effective care to older adults, health professionals must be trained in holistic gerontology, which encompasses a comprehensive understanding of physical, psychological, social, and spiritual dimensions of health (Reis da Silva, 2024b). Holistic care prioritises the patient as a whole, moving beyond merely treating specific ailments to understanding the broader contexts of their lives. This approach fosters relational empathy and improves the interactions healthcare providers have with older individuals, ultimately enhancing patient satisfaction and health outcomes (LaVela et al., 2015).

Educational programs should incorporate training that emphasises empathy and include simulation-based learning to increase practitioners' emotional intelligence (Reis da Silva, 2024a). For example, a study demonstrated that physiotherapy interns trained within a holistic framework reported enhanced empathy towards older adults, leading to better care experiences (Lin et al., 2022). Such training programs should also emphasise interdisciplinary collaboration, as holistic care often requires input from various health professionals to meet the diverse needs of older patients (Jasemi et al., 2017).

To effectively cater to the diverse health challenges faced by older adults, educational reforms must encompass a holistic approach to training healthcare professionals in gerontology (Reis da Silva, 2024a). Specifically, the incorporation of recovery-based practices into nursing and other healthcare curricula is crucial. As indicated by Sreeram et al. (2021), providing specific and practical training enables healthcare workers to cultivate more positive attitudes towards recovery-oriented practices, ultimately leading to improved care outcomes for older adults. By embedding recovery-focused educational components, candidates can better understand the multifactorial aspects of health affecting older populations, including physical, social, and psychological factors (Souza et al., 2023).

Moreover, the integration of interprofessional education—as highlighted by Souza et al.—is an essential strategy whereby future healthcare providers engage collaboratively across various disciplines (Reis da Silva, 2024a). This synergy enhances teamwork and drives the implementation of comprehensive health strategies tailored to the needs of geriatric populations, thus effectively supporting recovery-oriented systems (Souza et al., 2023). Such educational reforms can produce healthcare professionals who are knowledgeable about the ageing process and skilled in fostering supportive, multidimensional care environments (Reis da Silva, 2025i). Additionally, initiatives geared toward improving communication skills are essential, as effective interactions can lead to better treatment adherence and patient outcomes (Reis da Silva, 2024a). Training modules should focus on culturally competent communication, ensuring healthcare providers can engage with diverse populations and understand the specific cultural contexts influencing health behaviours and beliefs (Reis da Silva, 2025i).

8.2 Designing Recovery-Oriented Health Systems

Recovery-oriented health systems aim to support individuals in achieving their highest potential for well-being and functioning (Wiklander et al., 2023). This paradigm shifts the focus from illness management to promoting recovery through integrative practices and supportive environments. Designing such systems for older adults involves several key elements, including comprehensive assessments, trained professionals, and a focus on patient-centred care (Reis da Silva, 2024b). Incorporating recovery-oriented practices into health systems involves understanding the various obstacles older adults face, such as cognitive decline, mobility limitations, and social isolation. Interventions should be personalised, addressing the unique goals and preferences of individuals. For instance, community-based programs that integrate social and therapeutic activities have demonstrated significant success in enhancing recovery outcomes among older adults (Wiklander et al., 2023).

There needs to be a strong emphasis on building supportive networks—both formal and informal—that assist older adults in maintaining their independence. This includes healthcare providers and community resources such as elder support groups that can reinforce recovery and personal agency (Hohenberg et al., 2021). Moreover, incorporating feedback loops into these systems ensures that the voices of older adults are heard, allowing for continuous improvement in service delivery (Reis da Silva, 2024j). Regularly assessing the effectiveness of these recovery-oriented approaches can facilitate the refinement of practices based on the lived experiences of older patients.

The successful application of recovery-oriented practices in healthcare settings mandates a system-wide commitment to patient-centred care. According to Lyons et al. (2021), existing frameworks for implementing recovery-based interventions have shown that educating healthcare professionals in innovative recovery-focused strategies leads to significant improvements in service delivery and patient experiences. Recovery-oriented systems must operationalise these insights by ensuring that healthcare settings incorporate principles learned through training initiatives. This symbiosis between educational reform and practice can create an environment conducive to healing and empowerment for older adults (Lyons et al., 2021).

A pivotal component of this ecosystem is the emphasis on training that fosters effective communication skills (Kang & Joung, 2020). Programs designed to enhance cultural competence among health professionals are vital for addressing the diverse backgrounds of older adults, as emphasised by Kang and Joung (2020), who argue that culturally attuned care is associated with stronger recovery outcomes. With curricula that prioritise these essential interpersonal skills, healthcare professionals can better navigate the complexities of gerontological care, enabling them to build stronger patient-provider relationships essential for successful recovery trajectories (Kang & Joung, 2020).

8.3 Integrating Holistic Recovery into Nursing Curricula

To equip future nurses with the knowledge and skills necessary for holistic care, nursing curricula must incorporate educational components that emphasise holistic recovery principles (Reis da Silva, 2024a; Reis da Silva, 2025i). This integration should cover various aspects of health, including emotional, social, and spiritual dimensions. Incorporating modules that focus on gerontological nursing and holistic assessments can enhance the competence of nursing students in addressing the complex needs of older adults (Jasemi et al., 2017).

As older adults compose a significant population of patients in nursing practice, nursing programs should prioritise geriatrics and gerontology as a field of specialisation (Reis da Silva, 2024a). Addressing ageism within nursing education is also critical, as stigma against older adults can deter students from pursuing careers in geriatric nursing. Creative exposure to this field, through placements and community engagement with older populations, can motivate students and promote respect for the ageing process (Dahlke & Hunter, 2021). Educators must engage nursing students in reflective practices that challenge stereotypes about ageing, encouraging a therapeutic approach that values the experiences and identities of older adults. This aligns with findings that suggest a gap in nursing education regarding gerontological content, leading to a lack of confidence in nursing graduates when caring for older patients (Poulos et al., 2020).

8.4 Policy Recommendations for Health Equity and Inclusive Care

Progressing from educational reforms to policy-level considerations necessitates a deliberate focus on health equity and comprehensive care strategies that address systemic barriers faced by older adults. According to Lima et al. (2024), policies must foster access to training programs that emphasise holistic and recovery-oriented care principles. These strategies need to converge with broader health equity initiatives, ensuring that policies are designed to reduce disparities affecting older adult populations across various socio-economic backgrounds (Lima et al., 2024). For example, strategies aimed at increasing accessibility to healthcare resources, including transportation and community services, are crucial in bridging gaps in health equity (Lima et al., 2024).

Effective health policies are needed to promote equity and ensure that all older adults have access to comprehensive and holistic care. First, policymakers should advocate for the funding of programs that enhance the training and development of healthcare professionals in gerontology, emphasizing holistic care principles (Turner, 2018). Ensuring that the workforce is equipped to meet the diverse needs of older adults is crucial for improving health outcomes. Furthermore, addressing social determinants of health plays a vital role in reducing health disparities. Policies should focus on ensuring equitable access to resources such as transportation, housing, and healthcare services for all older adults, regardless of socioeconomic status, race, or geographic location (Pappa et al., 2015). This requires cross-sector collaboration among healthcare providers, social workers, and community organizations to bolster support for older adults facing systemic barriers (Blakey & Aveyard, 2017). Further, integrating feedback mechanisms into recovery-oriented health systems allows for continuous refinement and improvement based on the lived experiences of older adults. Such adaptive approaches champion consumer involvement, as noted by Kang and Joung (2020), which enhances recovery outcomes and service delivery. This reflection not only bolsters individual recovery but also shapes policy and practice at multiple levels, thereby improving systemic responses to the needs of older adults (Kang & Joung, 2020).

Lastly, integrating a framework that emphasises culturally appropriate care can help ensure inclusivity in gerontological care (Jasemi et al., 2017). Policymakers should promote the establishment of community health initiatives that recognise and honour the diverse cultural contexts of older populations, enabling tailored health interventions that are respectful of individual identities and beliefs (Jasemi et al., 2017).

8.5 The Role of Collaborative Frameworks

The efficacy of recovery-oriented systems hinges on the establishment of collaborative frameworks that umbrella various health disciplines. As suggested by Regenhardt et al. (2020), collaborative networks among professionals focused on integrating community resources with healthcare services can significantly enhance recovery outcomes for older populations. Developing organisational structures that support interprofessional collaboration, training, and shared goals is crucial for creating holistic health systems that can respond effectively to the complex needs of older individuals (Regenhardt et al., 2020; Reis da Silva, 2025i).

Collectively, training focused on recovery-oriented practices, combined with holistic educational reforms, emphasises the interdependencies present in the care landscape for older adults (Reis da Silva, 2024a; Reis da Silva, 2025i). As healthcare organisations strive to implement integrated treatment paths, multifaceted strategies that align educational initiatives with systemic reforms can create resilient health frameworks capable of supporting diverse recovery journeys. Ultimately, these steps contribute to a health system that not only addresses the immediate needs of older adults but also promotes sustained wellbeing and resilience within this demographic (Reis da Silva, 2025i).

9. CONCLUSION AND FUTURE DIRECTIONS

As the healthcare landscape evolves to meet the demands of an ageing population, a multidimensional approach to gerontological care emerges as a critical identity for practitioners and policymakers alike. This approach encapsulates a range of physical, emotional, social, and spiritual dimensions of health, reflecting the complexity inherent in the ageing experience. By recognising the interconnectedness of these dimensions, healthcare systems can shift from a primarily biomedical model to an integrative model that prioritises the holistic needs of older adults.

9.1 Summarising the Multidimensional Approach

The multidimensional approach underscores the necessity for healthcare providers to engage with older adults comprehensively, focusing not only on physical ailments but also on fostering emotional well-being and spiritual fulfilment. This involves a paradigm shift toward person-centred care, where health professionals consider factors such as life history, cultural backgrounds, and individual preferences. By adopting this perspective, healthcare becomes more personalised and effective, ultimately enhancing the quality of life for older adults and their families.

Furthermore, this approach highlights the importance of collaboration among healthcare providers from various disciplines, including traditional methods and modern evidence-based practices. For instance, the integration of Traditional Chinese Medicine (TCM) with Western medical practices exemplifies a collaborative framework that respects cultural perspectives while optimizing patient outcomes. Such synergies provide pathways for innovation, leading to holistic care models that can be both flexible and adaptable to the diverse needs of aging populations.

9.2 Calls for Research, Innovation, and Practice Development

There exists a pressing need for further research into innovative practices that promote holistic recovery for older individuals. As healthcare systems increasingly strive to integrate traditional practices with modern science, controlled studies examining the efficacy of various holistic interventions are essential. For example, exploring the impact of combining herbal remedies with conventional pharmaceuticals could yield valuable insights, particularly for managing chronic diseases that disproportionately affect older adults.

In addition to scientific inquiry, practice development should emphasise the importance of interdisciplinary teamwork in designing effective care pathways. Educational initiatives, such as training programs for healthcare providers on the application of holistic practices, can foster a culture of collaboration and empower practitioners to address the complex needs of older adults effectively. The development of fluid and adaptable health systems will be crucial for accommodating the ongoing changes in demographics and advancing care models that prioritise integrative approaches.

REFERENCES

Adetunji, O., Bishai, D., Pham, C., Taylor, J., Thi, N., Khan, Z., & Bachani, A. (2023). Patient-centered care and geriatric knowledge translation among health-care providers in vietnam: Translation and validation of the patient-centered care measure. *BMC Health Services Research*, *23*(1), 379. Advance online publication. DOI: 10.1186/s12913-023-09311-z PMID: 37076905

Agarwal, V. (2018). Complementary and alternative medicine provider knowledge discourse on holistic health. *Frontiers in Communication*, *3*, 15. Advance online publication. DOI: 10.3389/fcomm.2018.00015

Allen, L., Hatala, A., Ijaz, S., Courchene, E., & Bushie, E. (2020). Indigenous-led health care partnerships in Canada. *Canadian Medical Association Journal*, *192*(9), E208–E216. DOI: 10.1503/cmaj.190728 PMID: 32122977

Amin, M. and Pinilih, S. (2024). Exploring recovery-focused health workers for advancing mental health: literature review., 881-890. https://doi.org/DOI: 10.2991/978-2-38476-273-6_90

Ávila, M., Lucchetti, A., & Lucchetti, G. (2016). Association between depression and resilience in older adults: A systematic review and meta-analysis. *International Journal of Geriatric Psychiatry*, *32*(3), 237–246. DOI: 10.1002/gps.4619 PMID: 27805730

Bayuo, J., Wong, F., & Agyei, F. (2020). "on the recovery journey:" an integrative review of the needs of burn patients from immediate pre-discharge to post-discharge period using the Omaha system. *Journal of Nursing Scholarship*, *52*(4), 360–368. DOI: 10.1111/jnu.12563 PMID: 32445507

Betancourt, T., Keegan, K., Farrar, J., & Brennan, R. (2020). The intergenerational impact of war on mental health and psychosocial wellbeing: Lessons from the longitudinal study of war-affected youth in Sierra Leone. *Conflict and Health*, *14*(1), 62. Advance online publication. DOI: 10.1186/s13031-020-00308-7 PMID: 32884581

Bilgin, H. (2023). Mental Health. *Mental Health (Detroit, Mich.)*, •••, 199–211. DOI: 10.69860/nobel.9786053359135.11

Blakey, E., & Aveyard, H. (2017). Student nurses' competence in sexual health care: A literature review. *Journal of Clinical Nursing*, *26*(23-24), 3906–3916. DOI: 10.1111/jocn.13810 PMID: 28328169

Cardozo-Stolberg, S., Szydziak, E., Angus, L., Blake, R., Marsden, D., Venkatesh, S., & Mon, N. (2023). Geospatial mapping to target injury prevention for older adult ground-level falls: A feasibility study. *Journal of Trauma Nursing*, *30*(6), 340–345. DOI: 10.1097/JTN.0000000000000753 PMID: 37937875

Chen, J., Lin, Y., Yan, J., Wu, Y., & Hu, R. (2018). The effects of spiritual care on quality of life and spiritual well-being among patients with terminal illness: A systematic review. *Palliative Medicine*, *32*(7), 1167–1179. DOI: 10.1177/0269216318772267 PMID: 29708010

Chester, P., Ehrlich, C., Warburton, L., Baker, D., Kendall, E., & Crompton, D. (2016). what is the work of recovery oriented practice? a systematic literature review. *International Journal of Mental Health Nursing*, *25*(4), 270–285. DOI: 10.1111/inm.12241 PMID: 27381002

Chia, C., Mantoo, S., & Tan, K. (2016). 'start to finish trans-institutional transdisciplinary care': A novel approach improves colorectal surgical results in frail elderly patients. *Colorectal Disease*, *18*(1). Advance online publication. DOI: 10.1111/codi.13166 PMID: 26500155

Choo, C., Chew, P., Tan, P., Choo, J., Choo, A., Ho, R., & Quah, T. (2019). Health-related quality of life in pediatric patients with leukemia in Singapore: A cross-sectional pilot study. *International Journal of Environmental Research and Public Health*, *16*(12), 2069. DOI: 10.3390/ijerph16122069 PMID: 31212740

Cleofas, J. (2024). National resilience and mental well-being among Filipino emerging adults at risk for depression: the parallel mediating role of peace of mind and life satisfaction. https://doi.org/DOI: 10.21203/rs.3.rs-5450577/v1

Corso, M., DeSouza, A., Brunton, G., Yu, H., Cancelliere, C., Mior, S., Taylor-Vaisey, A., MacLeod-Beaver, K., & Côté, P. (2022). Integrating indigenous healing practices within collaborative care models in primary healthcare in Canada: A rapid scoping review. *BMJ Open*, *12*(6), e059323. DOI: 10.1136/bmjopen-2021-059323 PMID: 35710234

Cowley, S. A., Tzouvara, V., & Horta Reis da Silva, T. (2023). Public Health: healthy ageing and well-being. In *Redfern's Nursing Older People*. Fifth edition. Editors: Ross, Harris, Fitzpatrick and Abley. Elsevier.

da Silva, T. H. R. (2022). Emotional awareness and emotional intelligence. *British Journal of Community Nursing*, *27*(12), 573–574. DOI: 10.12968/bjcn.2022.27.12.573 PMID: 36519463

Dahlke, S., & Hunter, K. (2021). Harnessing nursing to diminish ageism. *International Journal of Older People Nursing*, *17*(2), e12417. Advance online publication. DOI: 10.1111/opn.12417 PMID: 34420260

Dallinger, V., Krishnamoorthy, G., Burton, L., Plessis, C., Pillai-Sasidharan, A., & Ayres, A. (2022). Internet-based interventions to support recovery in youth: A systematic review. *Digital Health*, *8*, 205520762211290. DOI: 10.1177/20552076221129094 PMID: 36211796

Doucette, M., Bove, C., & Hill, S. (2024). Healing through tradition: The role of indigenous elder support in child and youth mental health in Canada. *Alternative an International Journal of Indigenous Peoples*, *20*(4), 670–681. DOI: 10.1177/11771801241289999

Drost, J. (2019). Developing the alliances to expand traditional indigenous healing practices within Alberta health services. *Journal of Alternative and Complementary Medicine (New York, N.Y.)*, *25*(S1), S69–S77. DOI: 10.1089/acm.2018.0387 PMID: 30870024

Duan, A., Zhao, H., & Zhou, C. (2024). The effects of a healthy lifestyle on depressive symptoms in older Chinese adults: The mediating role of psychological resilience. *Cureus*. Advance online publication. DOI: 10.7759/cureus.57258 PMID: 38686246

Dunn, A., Startup, H., & Cartwright-Hatton, S. (2021). Adult mental health service engagement with patients who are parents: Evidence from 15 English mental health trusts. *British Journal of Clinical Psychology*, *61*(2), 335–348. DOI: 10.1111/bjc.12330 PMID: 34609005

Elmajee, M., Munasinghe, C., Aljawadi, A., Elawady, K., Shuweihde, F., & Pillai, A. (2021). Posterior stabilisation without formal debridement for the treatment of non-tuberculous pyogenic spinal infection in frail and debilitated population – a systematic review and meta-analysis. *Journal of Clinical Orthopaedics and Trauma*, *15*, 9–15. DOI: 10.1016/j.jcot.2020.11.009 PMID: 33717910

Fernandes, J., Fernandes, S., Almeida, A., Vareta, D., & Miller, C. (2021). Older adults' perceived barriers to participation in a falls prevention strategy. *Journal of Personalized Medicine*, *11*(6), 450. DOI: 10.3390/jpm11060450 PMID: 34070987

Fu, Y., & Ji, X. (2020). Intergenerational relationships and depressive symptoms among older adults in urban China: The roles of loneliness and insomnia symptoms. *Health & Social Care in the Community*, *28*(4), 1310–1322. DOI: 10.1111/hsc.12964 PMID: 32115795

Gell, N., & Patel, K. (2018). Rehabilitation services use of older adults according to fall-risk screening guidelines. *Journal of the American Geriatrics Society*, *67*(1), 100–107. DOI: 10.1111/jgs.15625 PMID: 30295320

Gibson, G., Quirke, M., & Lovatt, M. (2022). The role of environmental design in enabling intergenerational support for people with dementia – what lessons can we learn from Japan. *Working with Older People (Brighton, England)*, *26*(3), 226–237. DOI: 10.1108/WWOP-12-2021-0064

Gomes, V., Cajaíba, R., Costa, J., Damasceno, P., Souza, A., Goto, L., … & Figueira, S. (2023). Palliative care for the elderly in a long-stay institution in a municipality in west Pará: an experience report based on Arco de Maguerez.. https://doi.org/DOI: 10.56238/interdiinovationscrese-059

Gouvernet, B., & Brisson, J. (2024). Menstrual health under the scientific microscope: Text mining analysis. *Women's Health (London, England)*, *20*, 17455057241290895. Advance online publication. DOI: 10.1177/17455057241290895 PMID: 39449243

Guo, W., Liu, X., Zhang, Y., Chen, R., Qi, W., Deng, J., & Cui, J. (2023). Competence and perceptions of spiritual care among clinical nurses: A multicentre cross-sectional study. *Journal of Clinical Nursing*, *33*(4), 1432–1443. DOI: 10.1111/jocn.16932 PMID: 37994280

Harfield, S., Davy, C., McArthur, A., Munn, Z., Brown, A., & Brown, N. (2018). Characteristics of indigenous primary health care service delivery models: A systematic scoping review. *Globalization and Health*, *14*(1), 12. Advance online publication. DOI: 10.1186/s12992-018-0332-2 PMID: 29368657

Hernandez, R., Pyatak, E., Vigen, C., Jin, H., Schneider, S., Spruijt-Metz, D., & Roll, S. (2021). Understanding worker well-being relative to high-workload and recovery activities across a whole day: Pilot testing an ecological momentary assessment technique. *International Journal of Environmental Research and Public Health*, *18*(19), 10354. DOI: 10.3390/ijerph181910354 PMID: 34639654

Herrera, M., Elgueta, R., Fernández, M., Giacoman, C., Leal, D., Marshall, P., Rubio, M., & Bustamante, F. (2021). A longitudinal study monitoring the quality of life in a national cohort of older adults in Chile before and during the Covid-19 outbreak. *BMC Geriatrics*, *21*(1), 143. Advance online publication. DOI: 10.1186/s12877-021-02110-3 PMID: 33637054

Heveran, L., & Andrewes, T. (2020). Nursing measures to support the needs of haematological cancer survivors post-treatment: A literature review. *British Journal of Nursing (Mark Allen Publishing)*, *29*(3), S18–S24. DOI: 10.12968/bjon.2020.29.3.S18 PMID: 32053451

Hohenberg, M., Metri, N., Firdaus, R., Simmons, D., & Steiner, G. (2021). What we need as we get older: needs assessment for the development of a community geriatrics service in an Australian context. https://doi.org/DOI: 10.21203/rs.3.rs-156168/v1

Ihara, E., & Vakalahi, H. (2011). Spirituality: The essence of wellness among Tongan and Samoan elders. *Journal of Religion & Spirituality in Social Work*, *30*(4), 405–421. DOI: 10.1080/15426432.2011.619916

Insalaco, W. and Hobelmann, J. (2023). Behavioral and self-directed treatments for opioid use disorder., 730-758. https://doi.org/DOI: 10.1093/oxfordhb/9780197618431.013.26

Jasemi, M., Valizadeh, L., Zamanzadeh, V., & Keogh, B. (2017). A concept analysis of holistic care by hybrid model. *Indian Journal of Palliative Care*, *23*(1), 71. DOI: 10.4103/0973-1075.197960 PMID: 28216867

Jones, K., Kearney, M., & Best, M. (2024). Effect of a spiritual care training program to build knowledge, competence, confidence and self-awareness among Australian health and aged care staff: An exploratory study. *Journal of Religion and Health*, *63*(1), 274–288. DOI: 10.1007/s10943-023-01990-6 PMID: 38206559

Kang, K., & Joung, J. (2020). Outcomes of consumer involvement in mental health nursing education: An integrative review. *International Journal of Environmental Research and Public Health*, *17*(18), 6756. DOI: 10.3390/ijerph17186756 PMID: 32948052

Karthika, S., b, a., & Bakker, C. (2025). A qualitative study on psychiatric social workers in mental health profession., 150-156. https://doi.org/DOI: 10.26524/royal.228.31

Khor, P., Vearing, R., & Charlton, K. (2021). The effectiveness of nutrition interventions in improving frailty and its associated constructs related to malnutrition and functional decline among community-dwelling older adults: A systematic review. *Journal of Human Nutrition and Dietetics*, *35*(3), 566–582. DOI: 10.1111/jhn.12943 PMID: 34494314

Kirn, D., Koochek, A., Reid, K., Berens, Å., Travison, T., Folta, S., & Fielding, R. (2015). The vitality, independence, and vigor in the elderly 2 study (vive2): Design and methods. *Contemporary Clinical Trials*, *43*, 164–171. DOI: 10.1016/j.cct.2015.06.001 PMID: 26044464

Kiyoshi-Teo, H., Northrup-Snyder, K., Davis, M., Garcia, E., Leatherwood, A., & Izumi, S. (2020). Qualitative descriptions of patient perceptions about fall risks, prevention strategies and self-identity: Analysis of fall prevention motivational interviewing conversations. *Journal of Clinical Nursing*, *29*(21-22), 4281–4288. DOI: 10.1111/jocn.15465 PMID: 32810908

Landi, G., Pakenham, K., Boccolini, G., Grandi, S., & Tossani, E. (2020). Health anxiety and mental health outcome during Covid-19 lockdown in Italy: The mediating and moderating roles of psychological flexibility. *Frontiers in Psychology*, *11*, 2195. Advance online publication. DOI: 10.3389/fpsyg.2020.02195 PMID: 32982888

LaVela, S., Heinemann, A., Etingen, B., Mišković, A., Locatelli, S., & Chen, D. (2015). Relational empathy and holistic care in persons with spinal cord injuries. *The Journal of Spinal Cord Medicine*, *40*(1), 30–42. DOI: 10.1080/10790268.2015.1114227 PMID: 26833180

Lee, S. (2023). Exploring the role of resilience and optimism during the covid-19 pandemic in older European adults. *Research on Aging*, *45*(9-10), 643–653. DOI: 10.1177/01640275231152570 PMID: 36696282

Lee, S., Oh, E., & Hong, G. (2018). Comparison of factors associated with fear of falling between older adults with and without a fall history. *International Journal of Environmental Research and Public Health*, *15*(5), 982. DOI: 10.3390/ijerph15050982 PMID: 29757960

Li, C., Tang, N., Yang, L., Zeng, Q., Yu, T., Pu, X., Wang, J., & Zhang, H. (2023). Effect of caregiver burden on anticipatory grief among caregivers of elderly cancer patients: Chain mediation role of family functioning and resilience. *Frontiers in Psychology*, *13*, 1020517. Advance online publication. DOI: 10.3389/fpsyg.2022.1020517 PMID: 36704702

Lim, X., Yap, A., Mahendran, R., & Yu, J. (2021). The interplay between anxiety, fear, protective behaviors, compassion, and resilience among older adults during a covid-19 lockdown: A structural equation modeling study. *Translational Behavioral Medicine*, *11*(5), 1172–1178. DOI: 10.1093/tbm/ibaa143 PMID: 33793946

Lima, A., Nóbrega, H., Filho, J., Cordeiro, A., Sobral, R., & Oliveira, K. (2024). Evolution and challenges of telemedicine in children's health: an integrative review.. https://doi.org/DOI: 10.56238/sevened2023.007-086

Lin, I., Wang, C., Lin, Y., Chen, H., & Lin, L. (2022). Simulation-based holistic education in physiotherapy interns to increase empathy toward older adults and individuals with disabilities. *BMC Geriatrics*, *22*(1), 795. Advance online publication. DOI: 10.1186/s12877-022-03500-x PMID: 36224529

Lyons, N., Cooper, C., & Lloyd-Evans, B. (2021). A systematic review and meta-analysis of group peer support interventions for people experiencing mental health conditions. *BMC Psychiatry*, *21*(1), 315. Advance online publication. DOI: 10.1186/s12888-021-03321-z PMID: 34162340

Maestas, N., Mullen, K., & Powell, D. (2016). The effect of population aging on economic growth, the labor force and productivity.. https://doi.org/DOI: 10.3386/w22452

Mahoney, N., Wilson, N., Buchanan, A., Milbourn, B., Hoey, C., & Cordier, R. (2019). Older male mentors: Outcomes and perspectives of an intergenerational mentoring program for young adult males with intellectual disability. *Health Promotion Journal of Australia*, *31*(1), 16–25. DOI: 10.1002/hpja.250 PMID: 30959560

Math, S., Nirmala, M., Moirangthem, S., & Kumar, N. (2015). Disaster management: Mental health perspective. *Indian Journal of Psychological Medicine*, *37*(3), 261–271. DOI: 10.4103/0253-7176.162915 PMID: 26664073

Melo, L., Silva, B., Nitschke, R., & Viegas, S. (2023). Virtual social networks and health technologies in the daily life of clients and households: Care and health promotion. *Ciencia & Saude Coletiva*, *28*(8), 2193–2202. DOI: 10.1590/1413-81232023288.05252023 PMID: 37531528

Memaryan, N., Rassouli, M., & Mehrabi, M. (2016). Spirituality concept by health professionals in Iran: a qualitative study. *Evidence-Based Complementary and Alternative Medicine*, 2016(1). https://doi.org/DOI: 10.1155/2016/8913870

Moreland, B., Durbin, L., Kasper, J., & Mielenz, T. (2018). Rehabilitation utilization for falls among community-dwelling older adults in the United States in the national health and aging trends study. *Archives of Physical Medicine and Rehabilitation*, *99*(8), 1568–1575. DOI: 10.1016/j.apmr.2018.02.009 PMID: 29545001

Neil-Sztramko, S., Teggart, K., Moore, C., Sherifali, D., Fitzpatrick-Lewis, D., Coletta, G., Phillips, S. M., Newbold, K. B., Alvarez, E., Kuspinar, A., Kennedy, C. C., Santaguida, P. L., & Ganann, R. (2022). Community-based group physical activity and/or nutrition interventions to promote mobility in older adults: An umbrella review. *BMC Geriatrics*, *22*(1), 539. Advance online publication. DOI: 10.1186/s12877-022-03170-9 PMID: 35768770

Nyatuka, D., & Harpe, R. (2021). Service design as a catalyst for patient-centered ehealth innovation. *International Journal of Information System Modeling and Design*, *12*(3), 62–85. DOI: 10.4018/IJISMD.20210701.oa1

Olij, B., Barmentloo, L., Smilde, D., Velde, N., Polinder, S., Schoon, Y., & Erasmus, V. (2019). Factors associated with participation of community-dwelling older adults in a home-based falls prevention program. *International Journal of Environmental Research and Public Health, 16*(6), 1087. DOI: 10.3390/ijerph16061087 PMID: 30917618

Pappa, E., Chatzikonstantinidou, S., Chalkiopoulos, G., Papadopoulos, A., & Niakas, D. (2015). Health-related quality of life of the Roma in Greece: The role of socio-economic characteristics and housing conditions. *International Journal of Environmental Research and Public Health, 12*(6), 6669–6681. DOI: 10.3390/ijerph120606669 PMID: 26075724

Pasupuleti, M. (2024). Resilient innovations: leading the way in disaster management and recovery., 1-25. https://doi.org/DOI: 10.62311/nesx/77639

Poulos, R., Boon, M., George, A., Liu, K., Mak, M., Maurice, C., Palesy, D., Pont, L. G., Poulos, C. J., Ramsey, S., Simpson, P., Steiner, G. Z., Villarosa, A. R., Watson, K., & Parker, D. (2020). Preparing for an aging Australia: The development of multidisciplinary core competencies for the Australian health and aged care workforce. *Gerontology & Geriatrics Education, 42*(3), 399–422. DOI: 10.1080/02701960.2020.1843454 PMID: 33252017

Rahmani, A., Lai, J., Jafarlou, S., Yunusova, A., Rivera, A., Labbaf, S., . . . Borelli, J. (2020). Personal mental health navigator: harnessing the power of data, personal models, and health cybernetics to promote psychological well-being. https://doi.org//arxiv.2012.09131DOI: 10.48550

Regenhardt, R., Takase, H., Lo, E., & Lin, D. (2020). Translating concepts of neural repair after stroke: Structural and functional targets for recovery. *Restorative Neurology and Neuroscience, 38*(1), 67–92. DOI: 10.3233/RNN-190978 PMID: 31929129

Reis da Silva, T. H. (2023a). Ageing in place: Ageing at home and in the community. *British Journal of Community Nursing, 28*(5), 213–214. DOI: 10.12968/bjcn.2023.28.5.213 PMID: 37130715

Reis da Silva, T. H. (2023b). Falls assessment and prevention in the nursing home and community. *British Journal of Community Nursing, 28*(2), 68–72. DOI: 10.12968/bjcn.2023.28.2.68 PMID: 36735363

Reis da Silva, T. H. (2023c). Moving and Handling in the Community. *British Journal of Community Nursing, 28*(8), 369. DOI: 10.12968/bjcn.2023.28.8.369 PMID: 37527217

Reis da Silva, T. H. (2024a). Chapter 8 – Emotional Intelligence in Teaching Geriatric Nursing: Humanising Technology for Compassionate Care in Higher Education. In Tikadar, S.; Liu, H.; Bhattacharya, P.; Bhattacharya, S. *Humanizing Technology With Emotional Intelligence*. Pp. 141-160. IGI Global Scientific Publishing. https://doi.org/DOI: 10.4018/979-8-3693-7011-7.ch008

Reis da Silva, T. (2024b). The Evolution of Nursing for Older Adult: A Historical Perspective. *Associative J Health Sci.* 3(3). AJHS. 000561. 2024. DOI: . Link: https://crimsonpublishers.com/ajhs/pdf/AJHS.000561.pdfDOI: 10.31031/AJHS.2024.03.000561

Reis da Silva, T. H (2024c). Oncology and Cancer Medicine: Understanding the complexities in Older Patients. *Biomed J Sci & Tech Res* 55(3)-2024. DOI: https://doi.org/DOI: 10.26717/BJSTR.2024.55.008720

Reis da Silva, T. H. (2024d). Enhancing the mental health of refugees and asylum seekers through music interventions. *Mental Health Practice*. Advance online publication. DOI: 10.7748/mhp.2024.e1717

Reis da Silva, T. H. (2024e). Chapter 12 – Emotional Intelligence in Integrative Medicine: Enhancing Patient-Centred Care Through Humanised Technology. In Tikadar, S.; Liu, H.; Bhattacharya, P.; Bhattacharya, S. *Humanizing Technology With Emotional Intelligence*. Pp. 263-280. IGI Global Scientific Publishing. https://doi.org/DOI: 10.4018/979-8-3693-7011-7.ch012

Reis da Silva, T. H. (2024f). Loneliness in older adults. *British Journal of Community Nursing*, *29*(2), 60–66. DOI: 10.12968/bjcn.2024.29.2.60 PMID: 38300245

Reis da Silva, T. H. (2024g). Falls prevention in older people and the role of nursing. *British Journal of Community Nursing*, *29*(7), 335–339. DOI: 10.12968/bjcn.2024.0005 PMID: 38963269

Reis da Silva, T. H. (2024h). Chapter 11 - Integrating business essentials into Gerontological Nursing: Enhancing Care for Older Adults in Diverse Settings. In Sedky, A. *Resiliency Strategies for Long-Term Business Success*. Pp. 283-316. IGI Global. DOI: https://doi.org/DOI: 10.4018/979-8-3693-9168-6.ch011

Reis da Silva, T. H. (2024i). Chapter 6 – Navigating Healthcare Complexity: Integrating Business Fundamentals into Nursing Leadership. In Sedky, A. *Resiliency Strategies for Long-Term Business Success*. Pp. 145-168. IGI Global. https://doi.org/DOI: 10.4018/979-8-3693-9168-6.ch006

Reis da Silva, T. H. (2024j). Death and Its Significance in Nursing Practice. *Palliat Med Care Int J.* 2024; 4(3): 555640. DOI: https://juniperpublishers.com/pmcij/pdf/PMCIJ.MS.ID.555640.pdf

Reis da Silva, T. H. (2024k). Prevalence of elder abuse: A narrative review. *British Journal of Community Nursing, 29*(9), 442–446. DOI: 10.12968/bjcn.2024.0004 PMID: 39240800

Reis da Silva, T. M. (2025a). Designing for Longevity: Economic Perspectives on Age-Friendly Housing and Urban Development. In Gölçek, A. (Ed.), *Perspectives on the Economics of Aging* (pp. 151–176). IGI Global Scientific Publishing., DOI: 10.4018/979-8-3693-7753-6.ch006

Reis da Silva, T. H. (2025b). Emotional Intelligence and AI in Geriatric Nursing: Bridging Technology and Compassionate Care. In Jermsittiparsert, K., & Marzo, R. R. (Eds.), *Physical Health, Mental Health, and Human Well-Being in the Age of AI.* IGI Global Scientific Publishing., DOI: 10.4018/979-8-3693-6190-0.ch10

Reis da Silva, T. M. (2025c). Fostering Emotional Resilience and Mindful Leadership in Gerontology Nursing: A Model for Change and Innovation. In Baez, M. (Ed.), *Strategic Approaches to Mindful Leadership and Change Management* (pp. 259–280). IGI Global Scientific Publishing., https://doi.org/10.4018/979-8-3693-7066-7.ch009

Reis da Silva, T. H. (2025d). Integrating Artificial Intelligence in Geriatric Care: Enhancing Physical and Mental Health Outcomes. In Jermsittiparsert, K., & Marzo, R. R. (Eds.), *Physical Health, Mental Health, and Human Well-Being in the Age of AI.* IGI Global Scientific Publishing., DOI: 10.4018/979-8-3693-6190-0.ch11

Reis da Silva, T. H. (2025e). Exploring loneliness: Conceptualisation and impact in older adults. *British Journal of Community Nursing, 30*(4), 188–195. DOI: 10.12968/bjcn.2024.0025

Reis da Silva, T. M. (2025f). Fostering Emotional Intelligence for Competency Development in Nursing Education. In Aldosemani, T., Lytras, M., & Ordóñez de Pablos, P. (Eds.), *Innovative Educational Frameworks for Future Skills and Competencies* (pp. 39–62). IGI Global Scientific Publishing., https://doi.org/10.4018/979-8-3693-7555-6.ch002

Reis da Silva, T. M. H. (2025g). The Role of Emotional Intelligence in Promoting Mental Peace, Healthy Work Environments, and Emotional Well-Being Among Entrepreneurs. In Tunio, M. N. (Ed.), *Supporting Psychological and Emotional Well-being Among Entrepreneurs.* IGI Global Scientific Publishing., DOI: 10.4018/979-8-3693-3673-1.ch21

Reis da Silva, T. H. (2025h). AI-Powered Emotional Intelligence in Nursing: Bridging the Gap in Older People Care. In Jermsittiparsert, K., & Marzo, R. R. (Eds.), *Physical Health, Mental Health, and Human Well-Being in the Age of AI*. IGI Global Scientific Publishing., https://doi.org/10.4018/979-8-3693-6190-0.ch9

Reis da Silva, T. M. (2025i). Teaching With Adaptability: Cognitive and Pedagogical Strategies for Geriatric Nursing. In Yalçın, M., Uslukaya, A., & Demirdiş, B. (Eds.), *Holistic Approaches to Teacher Development: Leadership, Pedagogical Practices, and Cognitive Insights* (pp. 205–234). IGI Global Scientific Publishing., DOI: 10.4018/979-8-3373-0472-4.ch009

Reis da Silva, T. M., Hammett, R., & Low, G. (2025). Emotional Intelligence in Business: Enhancing Leadership, Collaboration, and Performance. In Sedky, A. (Ed.), *Building Business Knowledge for Complex Modern Business Environments* (pp. 149–178). IGI Global Scientific Publishing., DOI: 10.4018/979-8-3693-6447-5.ch006

Shelton, A., Allen, J., Mercer, V., Crenshaw, J., & Franz, J. (2024). Questionnaires of self-perception poorly correlate with instability elicited by walking balance perturbations. *PLoS One*, *19*(12), e0315368. DOI: 10.1371/journal.pone.0315368 PMID: 39666738

Shropshire, M., Stapleton, S., Dyck, M., Kim, M., & Mallory, C. (2018). Nonpharmacological interventions for persistent, noncancer pain in elders residing in long-term care facilities: An integrative review of the literature. *Nursing Forum*, *53*(4), 538–548. DOI: 10.1111/nuf.12284 PMID: 30242833

Shu, Z., Xiao, J., Dai, X., Yu, H., & Liu, Y. (2021). Effect of family "upward" intergenerational support on the health of rural elderly in China: Evidence from Chinese longitudinal healthy longevity survey. *PLoS One*, *16*(6), e0253131. DOI: 10.1371/journal.pone.0253131 PMID: 34143838

Shuang-Shuang, X., & Ma, X. (2023). Mechanisms of physical exercise effects on anxiety in older adults during the covid-19 lockdown: An analysis of the mediating role of psychological resilience and the moderating role of media exposure. *International Journal of Environmental Research and Public Health*, *20*(4), 3588. DOI: 10.3390/ijerph20043588 PMID: 36834282

Souza, A., Santos, P., Cachoeira, F., & Beal, S. (2023). Interprofessionality in health care.. https://doi.org/DOI: 10.56238/globalhealthprespesc-037

Sreeram, A., Cross, W., & Townsin, L. (2021). Effect of recovery-based interventions on recovery knowledge and attitudes of mental health professionals, regarding recovery-oriented practice: A quantitative narrative review. *International Journal of Mental Health Nursing*, *30*(5), 1057–1069. DOI: 10.1111/inm.12897 PMID: 34109703

Tsai, Y., Yang, P., Yang, Y., Lin, M., & Wang, Y. (2020). Prevalence and risk factors of falls among community-dwelling older people: Results from three consecutive waves of the national health interview survey in Taiwan. *BMC Geriatrics*, *20*(1), 529. Advance online publication. DOI: 10.1186/s12877-020-01922-z PMID: 33297968

Turner, P. (2018). Facilitators and barriers to holistic practice, an osteopathic perspective. *IJCAM*, *11*(2). Advance online publication. DOI: 10.15406/ijcam.2018.11.00355

Upasen, R., Saengpanya, W., Awae, W., & Prasitvej, P. (2024). The influence of resilience and social support on mental health of older adults living in community: A cross-sectional study. *BMC Psychology*, *12*(1), 397. Advance online publication. DOI: 10.1186/s40359-024-01892-6 PMID: 39020436

Vendramini, A., Azevedo, R., Reiners, A., Mendes, P., & Segri, N. (2017). Factors associated with fall prevention practices in older adults. *Escola Anna Nery*, *21*(2). Advance online publication. DOI: 10.5935/1414-8145.20170044

Vincenzo, J., Patton, S., Lefler, L., Falvey, J., McElfish, P., Curran, G., & Wei, J. (2021). Older adults' perceptions regarding the role of physical therapists in fall prevention: A qualitative investigation. *Journal of Geriatric Physical Therapy*, *45*(3), E127–E136. DOI: 10.1519/JPT.0000000000000304 PMID: 33782360

Wang, M., Sung, H., & Liu, J. (2022). Population aging and its impact on human wellbeing in China. *Frontiers in Public Health*, *10*, 883566. Advance online publication. DOI: 10.3389/fpubh.2022.883566 PMID: 35419339

Wang, R., Wang, M., Zhou, J., Wu, D., Ye, J., Sun, G., & Sun, X. (2021). Saponins in Chinese herbal medicine exerts protection in myocardial ischemia–reperfusion injury: Possible mechanism and target analysis. *Frontiers in Pharmacology*, *11*, 570867. Advance online publication. DOI: 10.3389/fphar.2020.570867 PMID: 33597866

Ward, R., Clark, A., Campbell, S., Graham, B., Kullberg, A., Manji, K., & Keady, J. (2018). The lived neighborhood: Understanding how people with dementia engage with their local environment. *International Psychogeriatrics*, *30*(6), 867–880. DOI: 10.1017/S1041610217000631 PMID: 28462764

Wen, G., Singh, D., Mesbah, N., Hanafi, A., & Azwan, A. (2021). Fall awareness behaviour and its associated factors among Malaysian community dwelling older adults. https://doi.org/DOI: 10.21203/rs.3.rs-54230/v2

Wiklander, P., Fröberg, A., & Lundvall, S. (2023). Searching for the alternative: A scoping review of empirical studies with holistic perspectives on health and implications for teaching physical education. *European Physical Education Review*, *29*(3), 351–368. DOI: 10.1177/1356336X221147813

Wingood, M., Kiyoshi-Teo, H., Scott, A., Caulley, J., Wilson, B., Council, S., & Vincenzo, J. (2024). Demographic comparisons of self-reported fall risk factors among older adults attending outpatient rehabilitation. *Clinical Interventions in Aging*, *19*, 1287–1300. DOI: 10.2147/CIA.S456894 PMID: 39050519

Xu, J., Wang, Y., Cheung, J., & Yin, Y. (2024). Analysis of the chain mediation effect between intergenerational support and mental health of older adults in urban China: A structural equation model. *BMC Geriatrics*, *24*(1), 323. Advance online publication. DOI: 10.1186/s12877-024-04883-9 PMID: 38589808

Yan, X., Wu, W., Chen, X., Xu, G., Yu, S., & Li, S. (2023). Intergenerational caregiving on mental health of middle-aged and older adults in China: Empirical insights. *Frontiers in Public Health*, *11*, 1224062. Advance online publication. DOI: 10.3389/fpubh.2023.1224062 PMID: 37483932

Yang, Y., Yao, M., Yang, Y., & Lin, T. (2024). Self-management experiences in fall prevention among community-dwelling older adults in China: A descriptive qualitative study. *Annals of Medicine*, *56*(1), 2392878. Advance online publication. DOI: 10.1080/07853890.2024.2392878 PMID: 39320983

Yue, X. (2023). Exploring the economic implications and challenges of an ageing population in the UK and China. *Lecture Notes in Education Psychology and Public Media*, *9*(1), 358–367. DOI: 10.54254/2753-7048/9/20230260

Zhang, M., Chen, C., Zhou, X., Wang, X., Wang, B., Huan, F., & Liu, J. (2024). The impact of accelerating population aging on service industry development: Evidence from China. *PLoS One*, *19*(6), e0296623. DOI: 10.1371/journal.pone.0296623 PMID: 38843199

Zhao, M., Yi, L., & Wang, Z. (2022). Mercury and mercury-containing preparations: History of use, clinical applications, pharmacology, toxicology, and pharmacokinetics in traditional Chinese medicine. *Frontiers in Pharmacology*, *13*, 807807. Advance online publication. DOI: 10.3389/fphar.2022.807807 PMID: 35308204

Zhu, X., Du, Q., Li, Y., Zhu, Y., Ge, C., & Chen, J. (2025). Activating the souls of the older adults: Insights into the psychological well-being of older adults through social interactions in the Guangdong - Hong Kong - Macao greater bay area. *Frontiers in Public Health*, *13*, 1461481. Advance online publication. DOI: 10.3389/fpubh.2025.1461481 PMID: 40109420

Chapter 2
A Holistic Perspective on Risk and Protective Factors for Language Development in the Early Years and Early Identification of Communication Disorders

Vânia Peixoto
https://orcid.org/0000-0002-8212-2137
Centro de Investigação em Estudos da Criança, Instituto de Educação, Universidade do Minho, Portugal

Anabela Cruz-Santos
https://orcid.org/0000-0002-9985-8466
Centro de Investigação em Estudos da Criança, Instituto de Educação, Universidade do Minho, Portugal

Paula Martins
https://orcid.org/0000-0002-0160-5066
Centro de Investigação em Estudos da Criança, Universidade do Minho, Portugal

DOI: 10.4018/979-8-3693-6432-1.ch002

ABSTRACT

Communication and language development are key to a child's cognitive, social, and overall well-being. While many children develop language skills despite risk factors, language development is vulnerable to various challenges, impacting academic performance, employment, and mental health. Early identification and intervention are crucial for achieving positive outcomes for children at risk of atypical language development. Such approaches must be collaborative, involving families, healthcare professionals, and educators. A literature review explored the impact of risk and protective factors on language development in children aged 0-3 years, emphasizing the skills that predict early language growth. Understanding these factors is vital for effective prevention, early identification, and targeted interventions, which help prevent long-term issues by addressing language development challenges early. These interventions are essential for mitigating the compounded risks many children face, promoting healthier communication skills and better life outcomes.

INTRODUCTION

Language is of pivotal importance to human development, functioning as the principal means of creating and exchanging meaning (Wells, 2007). It is a primary determinant of social preferences, inclusion and social participation from infancy through to childhood, with a greater influence than other cues such as age, race and gender (Esseily et al., 2016). The development of language is inextricably linked to communication within a socio-cultural context. Linguistic structures emerge from authentic interactions between learners and their environment (Abrar-ul-Hassan, 2011). This emergentist perspective places significant emphasis on the pivotal role of communication in language acquisition. Moreover, language plays a pivotal role in collective learning and cultural achievements, enabling teamwork and the sharing of ideas (Owens, 2014; Turnbull & Justice, 2016). From a sociocultural perspective, understanding is a dialogical phenomenon, and its development is fundamentally a social and collaborative process (Tomasello, 2003; Eilan, Hoerl, McCormack & Roessler, 2005). Given the importance of language in human development, research has moved beyond a narrow focus on linguistic competence to an investigation of communicative competence in diverse social contexts (Owens, 2014).

Existing literature on the importance of communication and language in human development reveals a complex interplay between sociocultural influences, neuropsychological factors, and individual experiences. Tomasello's seminal work (Tomasello, 2003) highlights the critical role of prelinguistic communication as a precursor to language acquisition, suggesting that higher cognitive functions emerge through socially mediated processes. His research shows how early communication abilities in infants provide the foundation for complex linguistic interactions, supporting Vygotsky's assertion that cultural tools, particularly language, mediate cognitive development. These findings indicate that the evolution of human cognition is enhanced by foundational social cognitive skills, which facilitate unique forms of interaction (Tomasello, 2003; Liszkowski, 2011).

Building on this foundation, several authors (Hoff, 2006; Clegg & Ginsborg, 2006; Owens, 2016; Snow, 2021) examine a range of factors that influence language development, including the home environment, bilingualism and early intervention strategies. Attention is drawn to the importance of language in both receptive and expressive skills and connect language skills to wider developmental outcomes. These authors also highlight the detrimental impact of language delays on overall development, underscoring the need for early intervention to support children with speech and language impairments. This convergence of environmental influences and individual developmental pathways reinforces the idea that language is a fundamental aspect of learning and cognitive development.

Jethava et al. (2022) further expands this discourse by examining the role of early attachment in shaping social communication through a neuropsychological lens. The research demonstrates the impact of attachment relationships on the development of socio-cognitive, socio-emotional, and socio-linguistic skills. By characterizing the attachment relationship as a template for future interactions, the authors elucidate how early caregiving can either facilitate or impede neuropsychological development. The study highlights the significance of responsive caregiving in promoting self-regulation and executive functioning, which are intimately associated with language development. The relationship between language and self-regulation is worthy of particular attention, as the authors posit that language serves as a cognitive instrument that facilitates mental organization and behavioral planning.

Taken together, they present a comprehensive view of communication and language as not just tools for expression, but as deeply embedded in the fabric of human development, influencing cognitive processes, social interactions and emotional regulation. The interplay between socio-cultural factors and neuropsychological development highlights the intricate nature of language acquisition and its central role in influencing human experience.

The objective of this review is to synthesize the insights gained from the aforementioned studies in order to provide a comprehensive understanding of the factors influencing language development in children around 36 months of age.

COMMUNICATION AND LANGUAGE DEVELOPMENT

Commonly discussed initial stages of language acquisition refers to approximately 12 months of age, with the emergence of the first words. Nevertheless, the evolution of communication and language commences well before the inaugural words are uttered. This process unfolds through instances of alternating turns (approximately four months of age), moments of joint attention (from around nine months of age), the intentional use gestures, and the comprehension of the initial words and expressions (also from around nine months of age). Subsequently, vocabulary expansion occurs as children begin to combine two words, typically around their second birthday. This is followed by the development of various grammatical elements, including syntax and morphology (Owens, 2016).

The study of language development in children from birth to three years of age represents a crucial area of enquiry, given that this period encompasses a number of significant milestones which serve to establish the foundation for future communication skills. Several milestones have been identified by research as typical of children during this developmental stage, which can be categorized into expressive and receptive language skills.

From birth to six months of age, infants primarily engage in pre-linguistic communication, which is characterised by the production of sounds such as cooing and babbling. By approximately three months of age, infants begin to recognize their caregivers' voices and respond to them, indicating the onset of social engagement through language (Bochane et al., 2020; Owen, 2016). From six to nine months of age, infants typically produce a variety of sounds and begin to understand simple words, such as "no" or their name (Perrin, 2013; Owens, 2016; Turnbull & Justice, 2016; Sheldrick &). This initial stage is of great importance, as it establishes the foundation for more sophisticated language abilities.

Between the ages of six months and one year, infants typically begin to develop their first words, usually around the age of twelve months. At this stage, infants begin to use simple words in a meaningful manner, often referring to familiar people or objects (Bochane et al., 2020; Flensborg-Madsen et al., 2019). This period also marks the emergence of joint attention, whereby infants follow the gaze of adults in order to share experiences, which is essential for language learning (Tomasello, 2003; Walle & Campos, 2014). The capacity to engage in joint attention has been demonstrated to correlate with subsequent language development, as it facilitates the acquisition of vocabulary and enhances comprehension skills (Guédeney et al., 2016; Sheldrick & Perrin, 2013; Wetherby, Warren & Reichle, 1998).

The extant literature on communication and language development in children, particularly those around 18 months of age, underscores the intricate interplay between cultural influences, parental interactions, and educational environments.

Scribner (2013) posits that culture plays a pivotal role in language acquisition, suggesting that effective language learning extends beyond grammatical proficiency to encompass cultural competence. This highlights the necessity of establishing an environment that is conducive to cultural diversity and sensitive to its nuances. It is therefore proposed that exposure to a diverse range of cultural contexts can prove beneficial in promoting children's language skills. However, potential limitations are also recognized, particularly when there is a discrepancy between parents' beliefs and the cultural characteristics introduced into educational contexts. This paves the way for further research into the potential impact of cultural diversity on young children's language development (Visser-Bochane et al, 2019; Owens, 2014; Sheldrick et al, 2013).

From one to two years of age, children typically experience a significant increase in vocabulary acquisition, whereby they may learn new words at an accelerated rate. By the age of two, many children are capable of producing two-word combinations, such as “more juice” or “mummy go”, which demonstrate an understanding of basic grammar (Owens, 2014; He et al., 2015; Turnbull & Justice, 2016; Flensborg-Madsen et al., 2019; Bochane et al., 2020). This stage is typified by an expansion in both expressive and receptive language abilities, as children commence to comprehend and utilize language to articulate their needs and thoughts with greater efficacy (He et al., 2015; Libertus & Violi, 2016; Flensborg-Madsen et al., 2019).

Between the ages of two and three, children continue to expand their vocabulary and begin to form more complex sentences. By the age of three, children are typically able to use three- to four-word sentences and have a vocabulary of approximately 200 to 1,000 words (Owens, 2014; Turnbull & Justice, 2016; McKean et al., 2017; Bochane et al., 2020). During this period, children also begin to demonstrate a growing understanding of language rules, as evidenced by the emergence of more sophisticated grammatical structures, such as plurals and past tense (Owens, 2014; Turnbull & Justice, 2016; McKean et al., 2017; Flensborg-Madsen et al., 2019). Moreover, the capacity to engage in discourse and comprehend the dynamics of turn-taking in conversation becomes more pronounced, reflecting their evolving social communication abilities (Guédeney et al., 2016; Sheldrick & Perrin, 2013; Owens, 2014; McKean et al., 2017).

Building upon this foundation, Thurman (2017) explores the role of parent-child interactions in fostering language and literacy skills. The article highlights the significance of engaging children in open-ended conversations and daily literacy activities, proposing that these interactions are vital for the development of critical thinking and vocabulary.

Thurman (2017) accentuates that the formative years are a crucial period for establishing a robust foundation in academic and social skills. The author cautions that insufficient interaction during this critical period can impede language development milestones. This research serves to reinforce the notion that parents and caregivers play a vital role in guiding children's language experiences, thus enhancing their readiness for school.

Richard Warner (2017) develops the theme of interaction by examining the concept of intersubjectivity as a precursor to language and literacy development. The article presents the findings of a longitudinal investigation which highlights the significance of both the quantity and quality of child-directed speech in the acquisition of vocabulary. The same author adds that socially contingent interactions, which respond to a child's verbal and non-verbal cues, are instrumental in promoting language learning. Furthermore, the research addresses the influence of storybook reading and parental involvement on children's reading abilities, underscoring the complex and multifaceted nature of language development that encompasses diverse forms of interaction and engagement. On this regard, we must underline the transactional nature of parent-child interaction (Tomasello, 2003; Barker, M.,2008; Owens, 2014) hence communication skills develop within social interactions, indicating that the environment and context in which these interactions occur are crucial for fostering language development.

Thurman (2017) provides further contextualization of the importance of early parental interactions by asserting that parents are a child's first teachers, laying the groundwork for language and literacy skills. The research demonstrates that by 18 months of age, there are notable differences in vocabulary acquisition and language processing abilities, particularly in the context of a six-month gap observed between toddlers from higher and lower socio-economic backgrounds by the age of 24 months. This discrepancy places children from low-income households at a disadvantage, as they may lack the requisite support and stimulation to develop robust language skills. Thurman's work draws attention to the pivotal role of socio-economic factors in language acquisition, thereby underscoring the vital importance of cultivating positive parent-child interactions during the crucial early years.

Pierce Moye Skuban (2010) conducted further research into the relationship between language impairment and child adjustment in high-risk, low-income toddlers. The study demonstrates that mothers' ability to attune to their children's emotional expressivity can significantly contribute to the attainment of language milestones. The study foregrounds the pivotal function of maternal responsiveness in promoting vocabulary growth and elucidates the profiles of toddlers exhibiting delayed expressive language development. This research indicates that effective emotional and communicative parenting can serve as a protective factor for children at risk of language delays, thereby reinforcing the need for targeted interventions in low-income settings.

The collective findings of these studies underline the complex and multifaceted nature of communication and language development in young children, particularly those from disadvantaged backgrounds. These studies demonstrate the pivotal role of caregiver engagement and responsiveness in influencing children's language development. They also underscore the necessity for interventions that equip parents with the skills to become more effective communicators.

LANGUAGE AND COMMUNICATION DISORDERS

The research on communication and early language development indicates that there is considerable individual variability in the skills exhibited by the subjects. In this regard, a significant challenge for researchers in the field of early communication and language development in children is to identify the cut-off points and/or linguistic markers that enable a clear distinction between typical and atypical language development.

The exploration of language and communication disorders in children has attracted considerable attention in recent years, revealing a complex interplay of various factors that contribute to these challenges. The existing literature provides valuable insights into the nature, prevalence, and treatment of communication disorders, emphasizing the multifaceted impact these have on children's academic and social lives.

Expressive language delays are a common occurrence, with prevalence rates ranging from 13.5% to 17.5% in children aged 18-36 months (Horwitz et al., 2003). Such delays are associated with a number of factors, including low levels of education, poverty, parenting stress and parental concerns about language development. It would appear that poor social competence, rather than behavioral problems, is a critical early correlate of low expressive language development (Horwitz et al., 2003). It is of the utmost importance to identify language delays at an early stage, as they may act as a risk factor for social and emotional problems.

Language and communication disorders are a heterogeneous group of conditions that affect an individual's ability to communicate verbally and non-verbally. Such disorders have the potential to exert a considerable influence on language development, social interaction, and the overall efficacy of communication (Cui et al., 2023). The aetiology of said disorders may be multifactorial, including, but not limited to, autism spectrum disorders, hearing loss and diverse genetic syndromes (Ravid et al., 2013). Alternatively, it can manifest as a primary disorder, that is to say, not as a consequence of an associated clinical diagnosis. When such a condition is observed, the term "Developmental Language Disorder" (formerly referred to as "Specific Language Disorder") is employed (Bishop et al., 2016, 2017).

As posited by Black et al. (2015), communication disorders encompass articulation errors, language delays, or a combination of expressive and receptive language difficulties. These disorders affect approximately 8% of children aged 3-17 years in the United States, with a higher prevalence observed among younger children, males, and non-Hispanic Black children.

The DSM-V TR (APA, 2022) identifies social (pragmatic) communication disorder (SPCD) as a distinct dimension affecting language use in social exchanges. Childhood language disorders affect 7.4% of kindergarteners, with long-term effects on academic and social-emotional development (Simms & Jin, 2015). Differential diagnosis of autism and language disorders often necessitates a multidisciplinary evaluation and monitoring of developmental trajectories (Simms & Jin, 2015).

Children with communication difficulties display a range of symptoms that impede their ability to follow instructions, express ideas, and comprehend spoken or written material (Zebron et al., 2015). There is a high degree of comorbidity between communication and language problems and other problems, including learning, behavioral and mental health problems (Triska, 2016), which puts forth the proposition that a transactional model provides a plausible explanation for the overlap between these disorders, underscoring the intertwined nature of environmental factors and individual experiences.

It is therefore crucial to highlight the importance of comprehensive diagnostic approaches that consider not only language but also behavioral, emotional and environmental issues in children with language impairments. In order to achieve this, it is necessary to underline the importance of collaboration among clinicians, parents and educators to facilitate effective evaluation and treatment, particularly in addressing pragmatic issues that may arise. The findings indicate that a holistic approach that encompasses all contributing factors is essential for optimal outcomes (Owens, 2014).

As mentioned, children with a developmental language disorder (DLD) are at an elevated risk for encountering a range of future challenges. A greater propensity towards mental health issues is observed during adolescence, with parent-child conflict identified as a pivotal early risk factor (Fradley et al., 2024). DLD is associated with a greater number of cumulative risk factors than other mental disorders, which can impede early detection and intervention (Valade et al., 2023). Children with DLD frequently display a broader spectrum of impairments, including difficulties with executive and motor tasks, in comparison to those with dyslexia alone (Snowling et al., 2019). The relationship between language proficiency and social, emotional, and behavioral problems is not linear; rather, it is characterized by a stronger association at disordered language levels (Goh et al., 2021). These findings emphasis the necessity of early identification and provision of support for children with DLD in order to mitigate potential long-term consequences and improve developmental outcomes.

A review of the literature on developmental language disorder (DLD) reveals a troubling pattern of risk factors that extend beyond language difficulties, affecting various aspects of social and emotional development in affected children.

Conti-Ramsden and collegues (2018) provide a comprehensive examination of the emotional and behavioural challenges faced by children with DLD. The findings indicate that these children are particularly susceptible to elevated levels of emotional challenges, frequently exceeding those observed in typically developing peers. The authors highlight the persistence of these emotional difficulties from childhood into young adulthood, indicating a chronic risk that necessitates early intervention and support. Furthermore, the study highlights the necessity of acknowledging the variability in developmental trajectories among children with DLD, indicating that some may experience more pronounced difficulties than others.

Building upon this foundation, Sansavini et al. (2021) examine the diagnostic landscape of DLD, reinforcing the importance of early identification and intervention. The authors posit that while DLD is typified by language difficulties that are not attributed to known biomedical causes, affected children often exhibit co-occurring cognitive weaknesses that can compound their challenges. They foreground the prevalence of long-term learning difficulties and social adaptation issues in children with DLD, which may manifest more acutely during the transition to written language. This underscores the critical need for timely diagnosis and targeted rehabilitation strategies to mitigate the risk of enduring sequelae.

The literature suggests that children with DLD face a complex set of challenges that may persist throughout their development, requiring a holistic approach to intervention that addresses both linguistic and psychosocial needs.

THE IMPORTANCE OF EARLY DETECTION AND INTERVENTION

The early detection of Developmental Language Disorder (DLD) and other neurodeveplopmental Communication Disorders is of paramount importance for the mitigation of long-term consequences on cognitive, social, and emotional development (Van der Schuit, 2011; Fricke et al, 2013; Hulme et al, 2020; Rinaldi et al., 2021; Pak et al, 2023). Although identifying DLD before the age of two is challenging, late talkers can be identified by the end of the second year, with more reliable detection possible by the age of three (van der Schuit, 2011; Fricke et al, 2013; Sansavini et al., 2021). Early predictors of DLD include delayed production of gestures, vocabulary development, and the combination of words (Sansavini et al., 2021). A family history of language delay, maternal immigration, and the occurrence of first sentences at a later age are significant risk factors for DLD (Valade et al., 2022). The use of multiple linguistic measures and standardised tests has been demonstrated to enhance the accuracy of DLD diagnosis (Sansavini et al., 2021).

The importance of early detection of Developmental Language Disorder (DLD) is reinforced by an increasing body of literature that emphasizes the complex nature of this condition and its implications for children's overall development.

Law and colleagues (2019) highlight the necessity for bespoke interventions, designed to address the specific needs of children with DLD. It is imperative that key adults, particularly parents, are engaged in understanding DLD in order to ensure the success of these interventions. The authors posit that enhanced public awareness of DLD is imperative, underscoring the necessity for a more nuanced comprehension of the interrelationship between oral language abilities and social-emotional growth. Such awareness could facilitate more efficacious identification and support strategies within educational contexts, particularly for children facing social disadvantages.

Building on this foundation, Sansavini et al. (2021) conduct a more detailed examination of the characteristics of DLD. They observe that while some late talkers may eventually achieve catch-up growth, a significant proportion will not and will receive a diagnosis after the age of three. The author's scoping review reveals the considerable heterogeneity of DLD, which can manifest in a range of degrees of severity and co-occur with cognitive weaknesses. The authors emphasize the importance of early identification, as timely inclusion in rehabilitation programs can significantly improve language skills and mitigate long-term learning difficulties. This appeal for early detection is consistent with the broader public health implications presented by Law et al. (2019), which reinforce the idea that DLD screening should be a priority.

In order to further expand the discourse, Valade et al. (2023) present a case-control study that identifies specific risk factors associated with DLD. The findings indicate that the occurrence of specific milestones, such as the production of first sentences after 24 months, a family history of language delay, and maternal immigration status, can serve to distinguish DLD from other developmental disorders. The authors recommend that pediatricians and developmental nurses systematically document these milestones, emphasizing that early referral for assessment could facilitate timely intervention. It is of concern that children with DLD frequently remain undiagnosed until they are nearly five years old, thereby enduring years of language difficulties that could have been addressed at an earlier stage.

EFFECTIVENESS OF EARLY INTERVENTION FOR COMMUNICATION AND LANGUAGE DISORDERS

The effectiveness of early intervention for developmental language disorders has received considerable attention in recent years, as research continues to explore the impact of timely and appropriate therapeutic strategies on children's language development. The implementation of early intervention strategies for communication and language disorders, particularly developmental language disorders and communication disorders associated with autism spectrum disorders, has yielded encouraging results. The available evidence suggests that intensive treatment of preschool children can improve communication and language skills and facilitate the maintenance of these gains over time (Rinaldi et al., 2021). Both contextualized and decontextualized language interventions have been shown to be effective in improving sentence-level and discourse-level language skills in school-aged children (Gillam et al., 2012). In the case of children with intellectual disabilities, early language intervention based on neurocognitive principles has been shown to facilitate language development, particularly in children who are nonverbal. However, ongoing support is needed to maintain progress (van der Schuit et al., 2011). In autism spectrum disorders, early intervention is beneficial for young children and assists parents in implementing responsive engagement strategies. The combination of parent-mediated and clinician-implemented approaches has been shown to result in the greatest developmental gains (Landa, 2018). It is particularly important to implement early interventions for children with communication and language challenges, reinforcing the importance of responsive interactions within mother-child and caregiver-child dyads during the crucial formative years.

Wake et al. (2012) evaluated the efficacy of community-based interventions for preschoolers with language delays, highlighting the need for well-structured, protocol-driven studies to assess the effectiveness of interventions delivered by therapists.

However, when discussing the efficacy of interventions for communication and language disorders, it is imperative to acknowledge the difficulties in conducting well-designed studies with paired and significant samples. In addition, existing studies lack comprehensive follow-up and economic analysis, which limits understanding of the cost-effectiveness of such interventions. This highlights the complexity of language development and the need for targeted approaches that take into account individual developmental trajectories.

In addition, the review by Rinaldi and colleagues (2021) highlights the considerable heterogeneity in intervention approaches, delivery, and evaluation outcomes, and suggests that these factors have a significant impact on the overall effectiveness of treatment. They spotlight the need for continued research to refine intervention strategies, particularly regarding the nuances of language production versus comprehension. In summary, these studies emphasize the importance of early, intensive, and targeted interventions for children with developmental language disorders. Evidence supports the effectiveness of a variety of approaches tailored to specific populations and needs.

Collectively, these findings illustrate the evolving landscape of early intervention for developmental language disorders and highlight both the promise and the challenges associated with implementing effective strategies.

They draw attention to the necessity of evidence-based approaches that demonstrate nuance and responsiveness to children's individual needs - a framework that will advance both research and clinical practice in this crucial domain of developmental science.

EARLY SCREENING FOR COMMUNICATION AND LANGUAGE DISORDERS

The potential impact of early screening for communication and language disorders in young children on developmental outcomes has been a subject of research. The existing literature on the early detection places considerable emphasis on the urgency and complexity involved in identifying these conditions in young children.

Over the past decade, the American and Canadian pediatric societies have recommended the implementation of a routine surveillance and screening plan for young children with the objective of early detection of neurodevelopmental disorders, thereby facilitating appropriate referral for assessment and intervention. The term 'surveillance' is defined as the process of continuously monitoring a child's development. This should be conducted as part of the standard medical care provided from infancy through to adolescence. Such a program should include an inquiry into parental concerns, the procurement of a history of the child's development, an observation of the child during the visit, the identification of risk and protective factors, and the documentation of these observations (Council on Children With Disabilities, 2006). In the event that surveillance indicates a potential risk of a neurodevelopmental disorder, the clinician is advised to conduct a developmental screening in order to ascertain whether the child is indeed at risk. The term 'screening' is defined as the administration of a brief, standardized tool designed to identify children who may require a diagnostic assessment to ascertain whether they have a neurodevelopmental disorder. Universal screening involves the administration of a screening tool to all children, irrespective of whether they manifest symptoms or express parental concern. In contrast, targeted screening entails the utilization of a screening tool with children identified as being at risk of a specific condition. This risk may be determined by observing signs and symptoms, by parental concern, or by population characteristics associated with an increased likelihood of the condition's occurrence (US Preventive Services Task Force, 2015; US Preventive Services Task Force, 2024).

The early detection of communication disorders (CD) and developmental language disorders (DLD) is of paramount importance for the implementation of timely intervention measures. Building on this understanding, the scoping review by Sansavini et al. (2021) addresses the practical challenges faced in diagnosing DLD in preschoolers. The authors provide a comprehensive examination of the early predictors of DLD, the optimal timing for screening, and the effectiveness of various diagnostic tools. The findings indicate that there are significant obstacles that hinder accurate diagnosis during the preschool years, which is a critical period for intervention. The objective of the article is to enhance the accuracy of early detection efforts by identifying predictors and refining diagnostic processes. The insights provided by Sansavini et al. (2021) complement the foundational knowledge established by Rinaldi et al. (2021), collectively emphasizing the necessity for a systematic approach to identifying DLD at an early developmental stage.

Parent questionnaires seem to be reliable screening tools for the evaluation of communication and language abilities in children under the age of three (Suchodoletz, 2011; Cadime et al, 2018; Sapage & Cruz-Santos, 2021). Early predictors of DLD include delayed gesture production, vocabulary, and word combination up to 30 months, with family history being a significant risk factor (Sansavini et al., 2021). The optimal age for screening is between one and three years, with diagnosis occurring around age four in the case of DLD (Sansavini et al., 2021, De Santiago Herrero et al., 2017).

Nevertheless, a number of studies have explored the efficacy of different screening methods, including the use of parent questionnaires and specific communication and language-screening instruments (de Koning et al., 2004; van Agt et al, 2007; van Agt et al, 2008; Eriksson et al, 2010). It is of great importance to address the issue of early communication disorders in children, as numerous studies have demonstrated a discrepancy between parental reporting and professional identification (Spicer-Cain et al., 2023; Botting & Spicer-Cain, 2023). Parents frequently express a desire for more detailed information on infant communication development and often seek guidance from a range of professionals (Popich et al., 2006). Overall, the combination of a parental questionnaire and a direct screening test has been demonstrated to significantly enhance the identification of risk factors associated with communication and language disorders (Auza B et al., 2023).

It is recommended that multiple linguistic measures and clinical assessments be employed in order to increase diagnostic accuracy (Sansavini et al., 2021). Despite the feasibility of identifying communication and language disorders in their early stages, accurately predicting an individual's communication and language development remains a significant challenge (Suchodoletz, 2011). Universal screening approaches have been put forth as a means of addressing the critical need for early identification of language and social-emotional delays (Kaiser et al., 2022). However, a systematic review of screening tools revealed that only a small proportion achieved good accuracy, with notable variations in sensitivity and specificity (So & To, 2022). The accuracy of screening is influenced by a number of factors, including the proxy used to define communication and language disorders, the interval between screening and diagnosis, and the identity of the test administrator (So & To, 2022). Despite the potential benefits of early screening, large-scale implementation remains controversial due to the lack of evidence demonstrating short-term health benefits (de Koning et al., 2004; van Agt et al, 2007; van Agt et al, 2008; Eriksson et al, 2010).

In 2015 and 2016, the US Preventive Services Task Force (USPSTF) and the Canadian Task Force on Preventive Health Care issued recommendations that did not support universal screening for conditions related to developmental delay. Moreover, the Canadian Task Force on Preventive Health Care (2016) and Siu & US Preventive Services Task Force (2015) have also advised against the implementation of universal screening for autism spectrum disorder and language disorder (Siu, A. L., & US Preventive Services Task Force 2015; Siu, A. L., & US Preventive Services Task Force, 2016). These recommendations were based on the absence of evidence for the efficacy of the procedure, as well as the difficulty in demonstrating that the identification of false positives does not result in harm to children (Wallace et al., 2015; Jullien, 2021; US Preventive Services Task Force, 2024). These recommendations have been met with considerable criticism from professionals in the field (Dawson, 2016; LeBlanc et al., 2016; Marks & Glascoe, 2016), as the fundamental objective of screening is to enhance the developmental trajectory of children identified through the provision of early intervention. A number of studies have demonstrated that children who receive early intervention are able to make positive modifications to their developmental trajectory (Law et al., 2004; Cable & Domsch, 2011; Hebbeler et al., 2012; Bradshaw et al., 2015; Rinaldi et al., 2021).

In particular, with respect to communication and language disorders, it is essential to consider the following:

- the pervasiveness of communication and language development difficulties represents a significant concern, as they can potentially lead to future learning difficulties, school failure, and emotional and mental health problems (McLeod, S., & Harrison, 2009; Harrison & McLeod, 2010; Hammer et al., 2017). Furthermore, the prevalence of this type of problem is a matter of grave concern, particularly in Portugal, where Silva and Peixoto (2008) found a prevalence of 48%. In contrast, Aguiar (2014) identified a prevalence of

55.55% among four-year-olds with CD, while Lousada, Valente and Mendes (2016) reported a prevalence of 34.16% among children aged between three and five years and 11 months. Coutinho (2012) reported a prevalence of CD of 14.6% in children between 3 and 6 years of age, which is more in line with the figures reported in other international studies, which range between 6 and 8%. A prevalence of 10% has been reported in children aged 10 years (Norbury et al., 2016; Tomblin et al., 1997), while a figure of between 3 and 8% has been documented in children aged 30 months (Sim et al., 2013);

- the evidence indicates that early intervention is the most effective approach for children with atypical development in terms of communication (Rinaldi et al., 2021). There is a consensus among researchers that early detection is a crucial factor in the efficacy of intervention. However, the question of determining the most effective procedure for this detection remains unanswered.
- the variability that exists within the development of communication and language makes it challenging to identify clear-cut points that allow for the distinction between what we might consider typical and atypical development (Zambrana et al., 2014; Bishop et al., 2016; Armstrong et al., 2017; Borovsky et al. 2021), which makes it difficult to define clear criteria for identifying children with atypical communication development at an early stage (Borovsky et al., 2021; Wetherby et al., 2021).

It is therefore essential to ascertain which risk and protective factors are associated with communication disorders. This will enable us, in collaboration with families, to identify which children are at risk of developing atypical communication and to refer them for screening (Dockrell et al., 2022). The subsequent sub-chapter will examine the risk factors associated with the development of communication and language.

A knowledge base of the risk and protective factors associated with the development of communication and language in children enabled the identification of populations at risk in this area. This subsequently permitted the implementation of second-line screening, which is considered an effective preventive measure on these populations (Law, 2000; Linares-Orama 2005; Gardner et al., 2006; Rinaldi et al., 2021; Sansavini et al., 2021).

On the other hand, the USPSTF recommendations regarding the screening of communication and autism spectrum disorders highlight the limitations of existing research, particularly with regard to the characteristics of screening instruments. Existing international screening instruments for identifying children with communication disorders (CD) vary considerably in their design and construction, including the mode and age of administration and the skills assessed. Additionally, the type of validation employed varies, resulting in a significant range of accuracy in screening outcomes (Siu, A. L., & US Preventive Services Task Force, 2015; Wallace et al.,

2015; Donald et al., 2019; Dockrell et al., 2022). The USPSTF recommends the implementation of a study comprising a substantial sample of asymptomatic children, with the objective of evaluating the efficacy of the aforementioned tools (US Preventive Services Task Force, 2024).

In Portugal, as in many other countries, research has responded to the urgent need to identify instruments that facilitate the early assessment of children with communication disorders over the past decade. It is worth noting the parental inventory, the Language Use Inventory (LUI), which has been developed for children between 18 and 47 months and has been validated for the Portuguese population (Guimarães et al., 2013; Guimarães, 2016). Another valuable tool is the MacArthur-Bates Communicative Furthermore, Development Inventories for children between 8 and 30 months (Viana et al., 2017) and the translation and adaptation of the Early Communication Indicator for children between 6 and 41 months (Antunes & Cruz-Santos, 2017) have been developed. Nevertheless, there is currently no screening tool for children at risk of atypical communication development between 12 and 36 months that is rapid, straightforward to use and cost-effective, in line with the desired characteristics of a screening tool (Law et al., 1998).

In any case, there is still a lack of an early screening tool for children between 12 and 36 months of age, based on the knowledge currently available regarding the predictors of language development (i.e. joint attention, intentional use of gestures, symbolic play, understanding and expression of words), with highly reliable psychometric characteristics, such as sensitivity and specificity indices above at least 80 per cent.

Universal vs. At-Risk Population Screening

Universal screening for developmental language disorder (DLD) in schools is regarded as an efficacious method to enhance the identification of this underdiagnosed condition, which affects approximately 1 in 11 kindergarten-age children (Christopulos & Redmond, 2023). While educators are generally supportive of universal screening, there are several challenges to its implementation. These include concerns about the additional workload for educators and the need for increased awareness about language development (Christopulos & Redmond, 2023; Komesidou et al., 2022). The implementation of screening tools in primary care settings is a viable proposition, as evidenced by the promising diagnostic accuracy demonstrated by combined parent questionnaires and child observation tasks (Ebert et al., 2020). A number of tools are available for this purpose, where some of them have demonstrated high diagnostic accuracy (Dias et al., 2020). A review of 15 commercially available English language DLD screeners in North America revealed considerable variation in accessibility, usability, and technical standards. While the majority provided sufficient accessibility information, none included comprehensive usability features. Furthermore, only 67% of the screeners reported classification accuracy (Bao et al., 2024). It is recommended that future developments in DLD screening tools should focus on improving classification accuracy and providing clear follow-up instructions for at-risk children (Bao et al., 2024).

Although early screening can reliably estimate current language development, predicting future language abilities remains challenging prior to the age of three (van der Schuit, 2011).

The use of multiple screening tools may be necessary to identify children who are at risk, as different tools may detect various aspects of language impairment and dyslexia risk (Helland et al., 2017). It is recommended that screening for developmental language disorders (DLD) be conducted on the basis of evidence-based criteria by caregivers and healthcare providers in order to detect early risks and facilitate timely intervention and support.

Building upon this foundation, Sansavini et al. (2021) highlight the necessity of addressing several challenges, including the identification of early predictors, the optimal timing for screening, and the effectiveness of various screening tools, in order to enhance the accuracy of communication disorders and DLD identification, which is essential for the implementation of appropriate interventions. By focusing on early predictors and refining screening tools, the literature collectively advocates for a systematic approach to screening that can significantly improve outcomes for these children.

Law et al. (2019) accents the importance of training key adults, such as parents and educators, to gain an understanding of DLD and other communication disorders and to implement strategies that can facilitate language development. The authors highlight that children facing social and emotional challenges are particularly vulnerable to language difficulties, emphasizing the necessity for a comprehensive understanding of the ways in which social disadvantage intersects with language development. Their call for universal speech and language screening in the UK reflects a broader public health perspective, advocating for awareness and a life course approach to identify children in need of support.

RISK FACTORS ASSOCIATED WITH THE DEVELOPMENT OF COMMUNICATION AND LANGUAGE

As previously stated, the development of language in children is a complex process that is influenced by a multitude of factors. This has led to it becoming a prominent area of research, as investigators seek to identify risk factors and predictors associated with atypical communication and language outcomes. These factors can be broadly categorized into two main groups: biological and environmental influences. Each of these groups plays a significant role in shaping language outcomes.

Biological risk factors include premature birth, low birth weight, and neonatal health issues. For example, research has demonstrated that children born prematurely are at an elevated risk for language delays due to neurological vulnerabilities, which can result in auditory and motor impairments that subsequently impact language development (Carniel et al., 2017; Soares et al., 2017). Moreover, conditions such as respiratory distress syndrome (RDS) have been associated with an elevated risk of cognitive and language delays, particularly in receptive language skills (Abou-Elsaad et al., 2017).

Further risk factors have been identified, including male sex, family history of language delay (Valade et al., 2022; Chilosi et al., 2021; Hoque et al., 2021; Cronin & Goodhall, 2021), perinatal factors, including multiple birth, newborn conditions, and congenital abnormalities (Delgado et al., 2005; Bhadur, 2023). The findings of twin and family aggregation studies (Chilosi et al., 2021) suggest that genetic factors may contribute to the development of language abilities and disabilities.

It is similarly apparent that environmental factors exert a considerable influence on the process of language development. It is of the utmost importance that the home environment is stimulating. A substantial body of research has demonstrated that children from homes with limited cognitive and linguistic stimulation are at a significantly increased risk of language delays (Mondal et al., 2016; Kumar et al., 2022). The quality of parental interaction, including the quantity and richness of language exposure, is of vital importance for the fostering of language skills (Madya et al., 2019; Fradley et al., 2024). Moreover, a consistent association has been observed between socioeconomic status (SES) and language outcomes. A lower socioeconomic status (SES) is frequently linked to restricted access to educational resources and less parental involvement in activities that promote language development (Reilly et al., 2010; Mcnally & Quigley, 2014; So et al., 2021). Moreover, parental education levels and mental health status have been demonstrated to exert a significant influence on children's language development. Parents with lower educational attainment may, for instance, provide less stimulating environments (So et al., 2021) in contrast to children of educated mothers, and those attending daycare have higher vocabulary scores (Tulviste & Schults, 2020).

Pispati et al. (2019) discuss how children from lower socio-economic backgrounds are often exposed to a range of negative factors, including limited access to educational resources and less stimulating home environments, which can lead to developmental delays. This is further supported by Stansfeld et al. (2010), who indicate that repeated exposure to socio-economic disadvantage can have long-term effects on mental health and developmental outcomes, including language skills. Additionally, Luby et al. (2014) identify that early emotional and behavioral disorders can also serve as risk factors for later language impairments, suggesting a complex interplay between emotional well-being and language development.

Additionally, exposure to multiple languages at home may impact language development, with some studies suggesting that children exposed to a non-dominant language may face additional challenges in language acquisition (Sánchez et al., 2018).

A number of studies have identified children who are disadvantaged from a psychosocial perspective as a population at risk of communication and language disorders (Dockrell et al., 2022). The term "social disadvantage" is typically operationalized through the measurement of distal factors that influence child development, including family income, parental educational level, neighborhood, and other socio-economic indicators (Dockrell et al., 2022; Snow, 2021). The cumulative risk faced by socially disadvantaged children with communication and language disorders has been well documented (Alsford et al., 2017; Hoff, 2013). In light of the aforementioned evidence, there is a consensus that efforts must be made to reduce this inequality (Snow, 2021). One suggestion is that early identification and intervention for these children should be prioritized. It is therefore vital to implement an effective surveillance program to identify these children and refer them for support at the earliest opportunity (Law et al., 2017; Dobinson & Dockrell, 2021).

In particular, studies have indicated that children in residential care often experience difficulties in language development (Moreno Manso et al., 2010; Mor Moreno Manso et al., 2011; Moreno Manso et al., 2012; Krier & Kruger, 2018; Raby et al., 2019; Wade et al., 2020; Maguire et al., 2021).

The recent work of Valade et al. (2023) provides further elucidation of the individual and cumulative risk factors associated with DLD through the utilization of a case-control study. The findings indicate that specific factors, such as delayed speech and a family history of language delay, account for a notable percentage of the variance in language difficulties among preschoolers. This study underscores the importance of early detection, as many children experience significant language difficulties for years without a diagnosis. These findings have significant implications for the development of early detection programs, which must integrate cumulative risk measures to enhance early intervention efforts for children at risk for DLD. Furthermore, they highlight the necessity for public health policies to be informed by these findings in order to facilitate the implementation of effective early intervention strategies.

Regarding protective factors for language development, one of the primary protective factors is the quality of the home environment (Conti-Ramsden & Durkin, 2015; Cronin & Goodhall, 2021). Research indicates that children exposed to rich linguistic interactions at home, characterized by responsive communication and a variety of vocabulary, tend to develop stronger language skills. For instance, Hamzah emphasizes that interaction with caregivers significantly influences language acquisition, as children learn through engagement with their environment Hamzah (2023). Similarly, Fibla et al. (2022) highlight that the quantity and quality of language exposure in bilingual settings can enhance language development, suggesting that supportive environments are crucial for fostering linguistic skills. This aligns with findings from Aziz et al. (2021), who note that psychological and social factors, including the influence of peers and caregivers, are vital in acquiring a second language during early childhood. Sensitive parenting has been demonstrated to have a beneficial impact on language skills and social competence, with some gender-based differences observed (Barnett et al., 2012).

Moreover, the role of early childhood education and care (ECEC) cannot be overstated. Lim et al. (2022) found that ECEC attendance can mitigate the effects of social disadvantage on language outcomes, suggesting a protective factor that can enhance language development in vulnerable populations. This is consistent with the findings of Bishop et al. (2017) who found that high quality interactions in educational settings can support language development, particularly for vulnerable children. Programs that provide structured language-rich environments can serve as protective factors against the risks associated with socio-economic disadvantage (Levickis et al, 2022; Kittitongsophon et al, 2023). For instance, Gaffrey et al. (2010) discusses how early interventions can significantly improve language outcomes for children with a history of emotional difficulties, emphasizing the importance of timely support. Furthermore, the work of Arnold et al. (2011) illustrates how emotional regulation and reactivity can influence language development, indicating that interventions addressing these areas can be beneficial.

Overall, language development in early childhood is a multifaceted process influenced by a variety of risk and protective factors. Understanding these factors is essential for fostering positive language outcomes and for the early identification of potential communication disorders.

CONCLUSION

Language development in early childhood is influenced by a complex interplay of risk and protective factors that can significantly affect communication outcomes. Understanding these factors is critical for early identification and intervention of communication disorders. A number of factors, including parental involvement, socioeconomic status, and individual differences in temperament, have been shown to have a significant impact on the rate and success of language acquisition during these formative years (Duff et al., 2015; Das & Priya, 2017; Flensborg-Madsen et al., 2019). It is critical for parents and educators to understand these milestones in order to effectively support children's language development and identify potential delays early.

In addition, the role of early childhood education and care has been shown to mitigate some of the adverse effects associated with social disadvantage.

In terms of early identification of communication disorders, it is important to consider a range of early communication behaviors beyond vocabulary alone. Collisson et al. (2016) argue that behaviors such as eye gaze, comprehension of language, and use of gestures should be integrated into assessments to identify children who may require further evaluation and intervention. This holistic approach to assessment is echoed by McKean et al. (2017) who advocate for robust language surveillance and intervention pathways that monitor language development alongside other key domains such as literacy and psychosocial functioning.

A holistic understanding of the risk and protective factors that influence language development in early childhood highlights the importance of nurturing environments, socioeconomic contexts, and early educational interventions. By addressing these factors, caregivers and educators can promote better language outcomes and facilitate early identification of communication disorders.

The interaction of biological and environmental elements results in a complex risk profile for language development in children. Early identification and intervention of these risk factors is of paramount importance in promoting optimal language outcomes and mitigating potential delays.

In light of what has been reviewed here, and considering the prevalence of DLD and other communication disorders, as well as the consequences that these disorders have on the future of individuals (academic, social, employment and community participation, and mental health), it is imperative that we begin to view language problems as a public health issue.

Investing in prevention, i.e. effective early intervention, is an urgent, effective and efficient way to reduce future problems with learning difficulties, social inclusion, unemployment and mental health. The cost of investing in early identification and intervention would be rewarded by minimizing these problems, avoiding or reducing future expenditure on special education, unemployment and mental health costs. In addition to the economic benefits, we have a moral and ethical obligation to provide the best possible future for these children who already face great challenges in childhood.

In summary, a holistic perspective on risk and protective factors for language development underscores the importance of environmental influences, comprehensive screening strategies, and early educational interventions. By recognizing and addressing these factors, with a comprehensive understanding of risk factors and the integration of public awareness initiatives, practitioners can better support children at risk for communication disorders and ultimately promote improved language outcomes.

ACKNOWLEDGMENTS

This work was funded by National Funds through FCT - Foundation for Science and Technology under the CIEC (Research Centre in Child Studies from the University of Minho) projects with the references UIDB/00317/2020 and UIDP/00317/2020.

REFERENCES

Abou-Elsaad, T., Abdel-Hady, H., Baz, H., & ElShabrawi, D. (2017). Language and cognitive outcome for high-risk neonates at the age of 2-3 years - experience from an arab country. *World Journal of Clinical Pediatrics*, *6*(1), 24. DOI: 10.5409/wjcp.v6.i1.24 PMID: 28224092

Abrar-Ul-Hassan, S. (2011). Language Development Hinges on Communication: An Emergentist Perspective. *TESOL Journal*, *2*(4), 510–520. DOI: 10.5054/tj.2011.269749

Aguiar (2014) *Perturbações da Linguagem e da Fala em crianças dos 4:00A aos 4:11A do Concelho de Oeiras: Fatores de Risco e Necessidades de Encaminhamento para a Terapia da Fala.* Relatório de Investigação. https://repositorio-cientifico.essatla.pt/bitstream/20.500.12253/927/1/Artigo%20Cient%C3%ADfico_Tatiana%20Aguiar_vers%C3%A3o%20final%20corrigida.pdf

Alsford, E., Ralephata, A., Bolderson, S., Curtin, M., Parish, E., Klaber, V., Griffin, S., Nash, L., Cullen, R., Musoke, B., Bhalla, S., Walker, L., Duffer, L., O'Sullivan, S., Knowland, V., Cozens, S., McLaren, L., Camilleri, B., Halil, S., & Pring, T. (2017). The wrong side of the tracks: Starting school in a socially disadvantaged London borough. *Child Language Teaching and Therapy*, *33*(2), 145–156. DOI: 10.1177/0265659016654954

American Psychiatric Association. (2022). *Diagnostic and statistical manual of mental disorders* (5th ed., text rev.)., DOI: 10.1176/appi.books.9780890425787

Antunes, M., & Cruz-Santos, A. (2017). Avaliação da comunicação expressiva em crianças dos 6 aos 41 meses de idade na região norte de Portugal: Um estudo exploratório com o Early Communication Indicator. *Revista de Estudios e Investigación en Psicología y Educación*, *79*, 79–84. Advance online publication. DOI: 10.17979/reipe.2017.0.09.2847

Armstrong, R., Scott, J. G., Whitehouse, A. J. O., Copland, D. A., Mcmahon, K. L., & Arnott, W. (2017). Late talkers and later language outcomes: Predicting the different language trajectories. *International Journal of Speech-Language Pathology*, *19*(3), 237–250. DOI: 10.1080/17549507.2017.1296191 PMID: 28440674

Arnold, H. S., Conture, E. G., Key, A. P., & Walden, T. (2011). Emotional reactivity, regulation and childhood stuttering: A behavioral and electrophysiological study. *Journal of Communication Disorders*, *44*(3), 276–293. DOI: 10.1016/j.jcomdis.2010.12.003 PMID: 21276977

Auza, B. A., Murata, C., & Peñaloza, C. (2023). Early detection of Spanish-speaking children with developmental language disorders: Concurrent validity of a short questionnaire and a screening test. *Journal of Communication Disorders*, *104*, 106339. DOI: 10.1016/j.jcomdis.2023.106339 PMID: 37247522

Aziz, A. A., & Kashinathan, S. (2021). ESL Learners' Challenges in Speaking English in Malaysian Classroom. *International Journal of Academic Research in Progressive Education and Development*, *10*(2), 983–991.

Bahadur, E. (2023). Behavior problems of preschoolers with developmental language disorder. *Turkish Journal of Pediatric Disease*, 1-6. https://doi.org/DOI: 10.12956/tchd.1298463

Bao, X., Komesidou, R., & Hogan, T. P. (2024). A review of screeners to identify risk of developmental language disorder. *American Journal of Speech-Language Pathology*, *33*(3), 1548–1571. DOI: 10.1044/2023_AJSLP-23-00286 PMID: 38324341

Barker, R. (2008). *Predicting Oral Language Development in Toddlers with Significant Developmental Disabilities: The Role of Child and Parent Communication Characteristics*. Thesis, Georgia State University, https://doi.org/DOI: 10.57709/1061207

Barnett, M. A., Gustafsson, H., Deng, M., Mills-Koonce, W. R., & Cox, M. (2012). Bidirectional Associations Among Sensitive Parenting, Language Development, and Social Competence. *Infant and Child Development*, *21*(4), 374–393. DOI: 10.1002/icd.1750 PMID: 25126021

Barry, M. J., Nicholson, W. K., Silverstein, M., Chelmow, D., Coker, T. R., Davis, E. M., Donahue, K. E., Jaén, C. R., Li, L., Mangione, C. M., Ogedegbe, G., Rao, G., Ruiz, J. M., Stevermer, J., Tsevat, J., Underwood, S. M., & Wong, J. B.US Preventive Services Task Force. (2024). Screening for Speech and Language Delay and Disorders in Children: US Preventive Services Task Force Recommendation Statement. *Journal of the American Medical Association*, *331*(4), 329–334. DOI: 10.1001/jama.2023.26952 PMID: 38261037

Bishop, D., Snow, P., Thompson, P., & Greenhalgh, T. (2017). Phase 2 of catalise: A multinational and multidisciplinary delphi consensus study of problems with language development- terminology. *Journal of Child Psychology and Psychiatry, and Allied Disciplines*, *58*(10), 1068–1080. DOI: 10.1111/jcpp.12721 PMID: 28369935

Bishop, D. V., Snowling, M. J., Thompson, P. A., & Greenhalgh, T.CATALISE consortium. (2016). CATALISE: A Multinational and Multidisciplinary Delphi Consensus Study. Identifying Language Impairments in Children. *PLoS One*, *11*(7), e0158753. DOI: 10.1371/journal.pone.0158753 PMID: 27392128

Black, L. I., Vahratian, A. M., & Hoffman, H. J. (2015). Communication Disorders and Use of Intervention Services Among Children Aged 3-17 Years: United States, 2012. *NCHS Data Brief*, *205*, 1–8. PMID: 26079397

Bochane, M., Reijneveld, S., Krijnen, W., Schans, C., & Luinge, M. (2020). Identifying milestones in language development for young children ages 1 to 6 years. *Academic Pediatrics*, *20*(3), 421–429. DOI: 10.1016/j.acap.2019.07.003 PMID: 31306799

Borovsky, A., Thal, D., & Leonard, L. B. (2021). Moving towards accurate and early prediction of language delay with network science and machine learning approaches. *Scientific Reports*, *11*(1), 8136. DOI: 10.1038/s41598-021-85982-0 PMID: 33854086

Borovsky, A., Thal, D., & Leonard, L. B. (2021). Moving towards accurate and early prediction of language delay with network science and machine learning approaches. *Scientific Reports*, *11*(1), 8136. DOI: 10.1038/s41598-021-85982-0 PMID: 33854086

Botting, N., & Spicer-Cain, H. (2023). The importance and challenges of improving early identification of language abilities: A commentary on Gasparini et al. (2023). *Journal of Child Psychology and Psychiatry, and Allied Disciplines*, *64*(8), 1253–1255. DOI: 10.1111/jcpp.13810 PMID: 37185876

Bradshaw, J., Steiner, A. M., Gengoux, G., & Koegel, L. K. (2015). Feasibility and Effectiveness of Very Early Intervention for Infants At-Risk for Autism Spectrum Disorder: A Systematic Review. *Journal of Autism and Developmental Disorders*, *45*(3), 778–794. DOI: 10.1007/s10803-014-2235-2 PMID: 25218848

Cable, Amory & Domsch, Celeste. (2011). Systematic review of the literature on the treatment of children with late language emergence. *International journal of language & communication disorders / Royal College of Speech & Language Therapists*. 46. 138-54. DOI: 10.3109/13682822.2010.487883

Cadime, I., Silva, C., Ribeiro, I., & Viana, F. (2018). Early lexical development: Do day care attendance and maternal education matter? *First Language*, *38*(5), 503–519. Advance online publication. DOI: 10.1177/0142723718778916

Canadian Task Force on Preventive Health Care. (2016). Recommendations on screening for developmental dela. *Canadian Medical Association Journal, 188*(8), 579–587. https://www.cmaj.ca/content/188/8/579.full.pdf. DOI: 10.1503/cmaj.151437 PMID: 27026672

Carniel, C., Furtado, M., Vicente, J., Abreu, R., Tarozzo, R., Cardia, S., Massei, M. C. I., & Cerveira, R. (2017). Influência de fatores de risco sobre o desenvolvimento da linguagem e contribuições da estimulação precoce: Revisão integrativa da literatura. *Revista CEFAC, 19*(1), 109–118. DOI: 10.1590/1982-0216201719115616

Chilosi, A. M., Brovedani, P., Cipriani, P., & Casalini, C. (2023). Sex differences in early language delay and in developmental language disorder. *Journal of Neuroscience Research, 101*(5), 654–667. DOI: 10.1002/jnr.24976 PMID: 34822733

Christopulos, T. T., & Redmond, S. M. (2023). Factors Impacting Implementation of Universal Screening of Developmental Language Disorder in Public Schools. *Language, Speech, and Hearing Services in Schools, 54*(4), 1080–1102. DOI: 10.1044/2023_LSHSS-22-00169 PMID: 37459613

Clegg, J., & Ginsborg, J. (Eds.). (2006). *Language and Social Disadvantage: Theory into Practice* (1st ed.). Wiley.

Collisson, B., Graham, S., Preston, J., Rose, M., McDonald, S., & Tough, S. (2016). Risk and protective factors for late talking: An epidemiologic investigation. *The Journal of Pediatrics, 172*, 168–174.e1. DOI: 10.1016/j.jpeds.2016.02.020 PMID: 26968834

Conti-Ramsden, G., & Durkin, K. (2015). What factors influence language impairment considering resilience as well as risk. *Folia Phoniatrica et Logopaedica, 67*(6), 293–299. DOI: 10.1159/000444750 PMID: 27160319

Conti-Ramsden, G., Mok, P. L., Durkin, K., Pickles, A., Toseeb, U., & Botting, N. (2018). Do emotional difficulties and peer problems occur together from childhood to adolescence? The case of children with a history of developmental language disorder (DLD). *European Child & Adolescent Psychiatry, 28*(7), 993–1004. DOI: 10.1007/s00787-018-1261-6 PMID: 30519863

Council on Children With Disabilities, Section on Developmental Behavioral Pediatrics, Bright Futures Steering Committee, Medical Home Initiatives for Children With Special Needs Project Advisory Committee. (2006). Identifying Infants and Young Children With Developmental Disorders in the Medical Home: An Algorithm for Developmental Surveillance and Screening. *Pediatrics, 118*(1), 405–420. DOI: 10.1542/peds.2006-1231 PMID: 16818591

Cronin, P., & Goodall, S. (2021). Measuring the impact of genetic and environmental risk and protective factors on speech, language, and communication development-evidence from australia. *International Journal of Environmental Research and Public Health, 18*(8), 4112. DOI: 10.3390/ijerph18084112 PMID: 33924666

Cui, M., Ni, Q., & Wang, Q. (2023). Review of intervention methods for language and communication disorders in children with autism spectrum disorders. *PeerJ, 11*, e15735. DOI: 10.7717/peerj.15735 PMID: 37576502

Das, G., & Priya, D. (2017). Family history and its influence on infants' language development. *Universal Journal of Psychology, 5*(1), 8–16. DOI: 10.13189/ujp.2017.050102

Dawson, G. (2016). Why It's Important to Continue Universal Autism Screening While Research Fully Examines Its Impact. *JAMA Pediatrics, 170*(6), 527–528. DOI: 10.1001/jamapediatrics.2016.0163 PMID: 26882277

de Koning, H. J., de Ridder-Sluiter, J. G., van Agt, H. M., Reep-van den Bergh, C. M., van der Stege, H. A., Korfage, I. J., Polder, J. J., & van der Maas, P. J. (2004). A cluster-randomised trial of screening for language disorders in toddlers. *Journal of Medical Screening, 11*(3), 109–116. DOI: 10.1258/0969141041732229 PMID: 15333268

De Santiago Herrero, F., García-Mateos, D., Arconada Díez, I., Torres Delgado, C., & Trigo Bensusan, A. (2017). Significance of oral language delays and writing for early detection of developmental disorders. *European Psychiatry : the Journal of the Association of European Psychiatrists, 41*(S1), S435–S435. DOI: 10.1016/j.eurpsy.2017.01.426

Delgado, C. E. F., Vagi, S. J., & Scott, K. G. (2005). Early Risk Factors for Speech and Language Impairments. *Exceptionality, 13*(3), 173–191. DOI: 10.1207/s15327035ex1303_3

Dias, D. C., Rondon-Melo, S., & Molini-Avejonas, D. R. (2020). Sensitivity and specificity of a low-cost screening protocol for identifying children at risk for language disorders. *Clinics (São Paulo), 75*, e1426. DOI: 10.6061/clinics/2020/e1426 PMID: 32294668

Dobinson, K., & Dockrell, J. (2021). Universal strategies for the improvement of expressive language skills in the primary classroom: A systematic review. *First Language, 41*(5), 014272372198947. DOI: 10.1177/0142723721989471

Dockrell, J. E., Forrest, C. L., Law, J., Mathers, S., & Charlton, J. (2022). Screening for Language Difficulties in Disadvantaged Populations on Entry to Early Years Education: Challenges and Opportunities. *Frontiers in Pediatrics*, *10*, 833603. DOI: 10.3389/fped.2022.833603 PMID: 35601421

Donald, K. A., Wedderburn, C. J., Barnett, W., Nhapi, R. T., Rehman, A. M., Stadler, J. A. M., Hoffman, N., Koen, N., Zar, H. J., & Stein, D. J. (2019). Risk and protective factors for child development: An observational South African birth cohort. *PLoS Medicine*, *16*(9), e1002920. DOI: 10.1371/journal.pmed.1002920 PMID: 31560687

Duff, F., Reen, G., Plunkett, K., & Nation, K. (2015). Do infant vocabulary skills predict school-age language and literacy outcomes? *Journal of Child Psychology and Psychiatry, and Allied Disciplines*, *56*(8), 848–856. DOI: 10.1111/jcpp.12378 PMID: 25557322

Ebert, K. D., Ochoa-Lubinoff, C., & Holmes, M. P. (2020). Screening school-age children for developmental language disorder in primary care. *International Journal of Speech-Language Pathology*, *22*(2), 152–162. DOI: 10.1080/17549507.2019.1632931 PMID: 31262202

Eilan, N., & Associates. (Eds.). (2005) *Joint Attention: Communication and Other Minds: Issues in Philosophy and Psychology, Consciousness & Self-Consciousness Series*. Oxford, (online edn, Oxford Academic, 2010), DOI: 10.1093/acprof:oso/9780199245635.001.0001

Eriksson, M., Westerlund, M., & Miniscalco, C. (2010). Problems and limitations in studies on screening for language delay. *Research in Developmental Disabilities*, *31*(5), 943–950. DOI: 10.1016/j.ridd.2010.04.019 PMID: 20483561

Esseily, R., Somogyi, E., & Guellai, B. (2016). The Relative Importance of Language in Guiding Social Preferences Through Development. *Frontiers in Psychology*, *7*, 1645. DOI: 10.3389/fpsyg.2016.01645 PMID: 27812345

Fernald, A., Marchman, V., & Weisleder, A. (2012). SES differences in language processing skill and vocabulary are evident at 18 months. *Developmental Science*, *16*(2), 234–248. DOI: 10.1111/desc.12019 PMID: 23432833

Fibla, L., Kosie, J. E., Kircher, R., Lew-Williams, C., & Byers-Heinlein, K. (2022). Bilingual Language Development in Infancy: What Can We Do to Support Bilingual Families? *Policy Insights from the Behavioral and Brain Sciences*, *9*(1), 35–43. DOI: 10.1177/23727322211069312 PMID: 35224184

Flensborg-Madsen, T., Grønkjær, M., & Mortensen, E. (2019). Predictors of early life milestones: Results from the copenhagen perinatal cohort. *BMC Pediatrics, 19*(1), 420. Advance online publication. DOI: 10.1186/s12887-019-1778-y PMID: 31703689

Fradley, K., Oldfield, J., Marshall, J., & Toseeb, U. (2024). Early life risk factors for adolescent mental health difficulties for individuals at risk of developmental language disorder. *Journal of Research in Special Educational Needs, 24*(3), 713–728. DOI: 10.1111/1471-3802.12654

Fricke, S., Bowyer-Crane, C., Haley, A. J., Hulme, C., & Snowling, M. J. (2013). Efficacy of language intervention in the early years. *Journal of Child Psychology and Psychiatry, and Allied Disciplines, 54*(3), 280–290. DOI: 10.1111/jcpp.12010 PMID: 23176547

Gaffrey, M. S., Luby, J. L., & Barch, D. M. (2013). Towards the study of functional brain development in depression: An Interactive Specialization approach. *Neurobiology of Disease, 52*, 38–48. DOI: 10.1016/j.nbd.2012.06.012 PMID: 22750525

Gardner, H., Froud, K., McClelland, A., & van der Lely, H. K. (2006). Development of the Grammar and Phonology Screening (GAPS) test to assess key markers of specific language and literacy difficulties in young children. *International Journal of Language & Communication Disorders, 41*(5), 513–540. DOI: 10.1080/13682820500442644 PMID: 17050469

Gillam, S. L., Gillam, R. B., & Reece, K. (2012). Language outcomes of contextualized and decontextualized language intervention: Results of an early efficacy study. *Language, Speech, and Hearing Services in Schools, 43*(3), 276–291. DOI: 10.1044/0161-1461(2011/11-0022) PMID: 22269582

Goh, S. K. Y., Griffiths, S., & Norbury, C. F. (2021). Sources of variability in the prospective relation of language to social, emotional, and behavior problem symptoms: Implications for developmental language disorder. *Journal of Abnormal Psychology, 130*(6), 676–689. DOI: 10.1037/abn0000691 PMID: 34553962

Guédeney, A., Forhan, A., Larroque, B., Agostini, M., Pingault, J., & Heude, B. (2016). Social withdrawal behaviour at one year of age is associated with delays in reaching language milestones in the eden mother-child cohort study. *PLoS One, 11*(7), e0158426. DOI: 10.1371/journal.pone.0158426 PMID: 27391482

Guimarães, C., Cruz-Santos, A., & Almeida, L. (2013). Adaptação do Inventário Parental "Language Use Inventory (LUI)" para crianças entre 18 e 47 meses para o Português Europeu: Estudo Piloto. *Audiology - Communication Research, 18*(4), 332–338. DOI: 10.1590/S2317-64312013000400015

Hammer, C. S., Morgan, P., Farkas, G., Hillemeier, M., Bitetti, D., & Maczuga, S. (2017). Late Talkers: A Population-Based Study of Risk Factors and School Readiness Consequences. *Journal of Speech, Language, and Hearing Research: JSLHR*, *60*(3), 607–626. DOI: 10.1044/2016_JSLHR-L-15-0417 PMID: 28257586

Harrison, L. J., & McLeod, S. (2010). Risk and protective factors associated with speech and language impairment in a nationally representative sample of 4- to 5-year-old children. *Journal of Speech, Language, and Hearing Research: JSLHR*, *53*(2), 508–529. DOI: 10.1044/1092-4388(2009/08-0086) PMID: 19786704

He, M., Walle, E., & Campos, J. (2015). A cross-national investigation of the relationship between infant walking and language development. *Infancy*, *20*(3), 283–305. DOI: 10.1111/infa.12071

Hebbeler, K., Spiker, D., & Kahn, L. (2012). Individuals With Disabilities Education Act's Early Childhood Programs: Powerful Vision and Pesky Details. *Topics in Early Childhood Special Education*, *31*(4), 199–207. DOI: 10.1177/0271121411429077

Helland, T., Jones, L., & Helland, W. (2017). Detecting Preschool Language Impairment and Risk of Developmental Dyslexia. *Journal of Research in Childhood Education*, *31*(2), 295–311. Advance online publication. DOI: 10.1080/02568543.2016.1274928

Hoff, E. (2006). How social contexts support and shape language development. *Developmental Review*, *26*(1), 55–88. https://doi.org/doi:10.1016/j.dr.2005.11.002. DOI: 10.1016/j.dr.2005.11.002

Hoff, E. (2013). *Language Development* (5th ed.). Cengage Learning.

Hoque, F., Akhter, S., & Mannan, M. (2021). Risk factors identification of speech and language delay in children in a tertiary level hospital: A pilot study. *World Journal of Advanced Research and Reviews*, *11*(1), 103–112. DOI: 10.30574/wjarr.2021.11.1.0323

Horwitz, S. M., Irwin, J. R., Briggs-Gowan, M. J., Bosson Heenan, J. M., Mendoza, J., & Carter, A. S. (2003). Language delay in a community cohort of young children. *Journal of the American Academy of Child and Adolescent Psychiatry*, *42*(8), 932–940. DOI: 10.1097/01.CHI.0000046889.27264.5E PMID: 12874495

Hulme, C., Snowling, M. J., West, G., Lervåg, A., & Melby-Lervåg, M. (2020). Children's Language Skills Can Be Improved: Lessons From Psychological Science for Educational Policy. *Current Directions in Psychological Science*, *29*(4), 372–377. DOI: 10.1177/0963721420923684

Hamzah Idris, Ikhwan & Mustapha, Safinaz & Aljibori, Hakim & Al-tamimi, Adnan & Abdulrazaq Alshekhly, Mohammed & Alfiras, Mohanad. (2023). Enhancing Children's Communication Skills Through an Interactive *AR Board Game*. 1-6. .DOI: 10.1109/ICETAS59148.2023.10346447

Jethava, V., Kadish, J., Kakonge, L., & Wiseman-Hakes, C. (2022). Early Attachment and the Development of Social Communication: A Neuropsychological Approach. *Frontiers in Psychiatry*, *13*, 838950. DOI: 10.3389/fpsyt.2022.838950 PMID: 35463524

Jullien, S. (2021). Screening for language and speech delay in children under five years. *BMC Pediatrics*, *21*(S1, Suppl 1), 362. DOI: 10.1186/s12887-021-02817-7 PMID: 34496812

Kaiser, A., Chow, J., & Cunningham, J. (2022). A Case for Early Language and Behavior Screening: Implications for Policy and Child Development. *Policy Insights from the Behavioral and Brain Sciences*, *9*(1), 120–128. DOI: 10.1177/23727322211068886

Kittitongsophon, W., Wangwonsin, A., & Jariya, W. (2023). Factors influencing parents' behaviours to promote early childhood development of 1–3-year-old children with delayed language development in thailand. *Journal of Public Health Dentistry*, *21*(1), 150–160. DOI: 10.55131/jphd/2023/210111

Komesidou, R., Feller, M. J., Wolter, J. A., Ricketts, J., Rasner, M. G., Putman, C. A., & Hogan, T. P. (2022). Educators' Perceptions of Barriers and Facilitators to the Implementation of Screeners for Developmental Language Disorder and Dyslexia. *Journal of Research in Reading*, *45*(3), 277–298. DOI: 10.1111/1467-9817.12381 PMID: 36250042

Krier, J. C., Green, T. D., & Kruger, A. (2018). Youths in foster care with language delays: Prevalence, causes, and interventions. *Psychology in the Schools*, *55*(5), 523–538. DOI: 10.1002/pits.22129

Kumar, M., Sharan, S., Kishore, S., Gupta, A., & Kumar, A. (2022). Prevalence of speech and language delay in children (0-3 years) and its associated risk factors in a tertiary care teaching hospital of eastern india. *International Journal of Health Sciences*, •••, 1778–1784. DOI: 10.53730/ijhs.v6nS6.9917

Landa, R. J. (2018). Efficacy of early interventions for infants and young children with, and at risk for, autism spectrum disorders. *International Review of Psychiatry (Abingdon, England)*, *30*(1), 25–39. DOI: 10.1080/09540261.2018.1432574 PMID: 29537331

Law, James & Boyle, James & Harris, F & Harkness, A & Nye, C. (1998). Screening for Speech and Language Delay: A Systematic Review of the Literature. (Winchester, England). 2. 1-184. .DOI: 10.3310/hta2090

Law, J., Boyle, J., Harris, F., Harkness, A., & Nye, C. (2000). The feasibility of universal screening for primary speech and language delay: Findings from a systematic review of the literature. *Developmental Medicine and Child Neurology*, *42*(3), 190–200. DOI: 10.1111/j.1469-8749.2000.tb00069.x PMID: 10755459

Law, J., Garrett, Z., & Nye, C. (2004). The Efficacy of Treatment for Children With Developmental Speech and Language Delay/Disorder: A Meta-Analysis. *Journal of Speech, Language, and Hearing Research: JSLHR*, *47*(4), 924–943. DOI: 10.1044/1092-4388(2004/069) PMID: 15324296

Law, J., McCartney, E., & Roulstone, S. (2019). *The United Kingdom Vignette in McKean C, Murphy C & Thordardottir E (eds.) Managing children with developmental language disorder: theory and practice across Europe and beyond.* Abingdon: Routledge, pp. 497-509

LeBlanc, L., Belanger, S., & Andrews, D., & Charach. (2016). Take home message of Task Force report: NOT the strong recommendation against developmental screening, BUT the need for rigorous research and practice [letter]. *Canadian Medical Association Journal*, *20*(188).

Levickis, P., Conway, L., Smith, J., & Bennetts, S. (2022). *Parent–Child Interaction and Its Impact on Language Development.* In J. Law, S. Reilly, & C. McKean (Eds.), Language Development: Individual Differences in a Social Context (pp. 166–192). chapter, Cambridge: Cambridge University Press. DOI: 10.1017/9781108643719.010

Libertus, K., & Violi, D. (2016). Sit to talk: Relation between motor skills and language development in infancy. *Frontiers in Psychology*, *7*. Advance online publication. DOI: 10.3389/fpsyg.2016.00475 PMID: 27065934

Lim, S., Levickis, P., & Eadie, P. (2022). Associations between early childhood education and care (ecec) attendance, adversity and language outcomes of 2-year-olds. *Journal of Early Childhood Research*, *20*(4), 565–579. DOI: 10.1177/1476718X221087078

Linares-Orama, N. (2005). Language-learning disorders and youth incarceration. *Journal of Communication Disorders*, *38*(4), 311–319. DOI: 10.1016/j.jcomdis.2005.02.006 PMID: 15862813

Liszkowski, U. (2011). Three lines in the emergence of prelinguistic communication and social cognition. *Journal of Cognitive Education and Psychology, 10*(1), 32–43. DOI: 10.1891/1945-8959.10.1.32

Liu, X. L., Zahrt, D. M., & Simms, M. D. (2018). An Interprofessional Team Approach to the Differential Diagnosis of Children with Language Disorders. *Pediatric Clinics of North America, 65*(1), 73–90. DOI: 10.1016/j.pcl.2017.08.022 PMID: 29173721

Lousada, M., Valente, A., & Mendes, A. (2017). Validation of a Paediatric Speech and Language Screening (RALF). *Folia Phoniatrica et Logopaedica, 68*(6), 247–251. DOI: 10.1159/000479928 PMID: 29176312

Luby, J. L., Gaffrey, M. S., Tillman, R., April, L. M., & Belden, A. C. (2014). Trajectories of preschool disorders to full DSM depression at school age and early adolescence: Continuity of preschool depression. *The American Journal of Psychiatry, 171*(7), 768–776. DOI: 10.1176/appi.ajp.2014.13091198 PMID: 24700355

Madya, R., Malik, M., & Suparno, S. (2019). The impact of socioeconomic status (SES) on early childhood language development. *Advances in Social Science, Education and Humanities Research, 296*, 140–145. DOI: 10.2991/icsie-18.2019.26

Maguire, D., McCormack, D., Downes, C., Teggart, T., & Fosker, T. (2021). The impact of care-related factors on the language and communication needs of looked after and adopted children/young people. *Developmental Child Welfare, 3*(3), 235–255. DOI: 10.1177/25161032211021436

Manso, M. (2010). Pragmatic language development and educational style in neglected children. *Children and Youth Services Review, 32*(7), 1028–1034. DOI: 10.1016/j.childyouth.2010.04.008

Manso, M. (2012). Morphosyntactic development and educational style of parents in neglected children. *Children and Youth Services Review, 34*(1), 311–315. DOI: 10.1016/j.childyouth.2011.10.028

Manso, M., García-Baamonde, M. E., & Alonso, M. B. (2011). Design of a language stimulation program for children suffering abuse. *Children and Youth Services Review, 33*(7), 1325–1331. DOI: 10.1016/j.childyouth.2011.03.003

Marks, K. P., & Glascoe, F. P. (2016, February 1). USPSTF did not "connect the dots" between early detection and intervention. Pediatrics. *American Academy of Pediatrics*. DOI: 10.1542/peds.2015-4039A

McKean, C., Reilly, S., Bavin, E., Bretherton, L., Cini, E., Conway, L., Cook, F., Eadie, P., Prior, M., Wake, M., & Mensah, F. (2017). Language outcomes at 7 years: Early predictors and co-occurring difficulties. *Pediatrics*, *139*(3), e20161684. Advance online publication. DOI: 10.1542/peds.2016-1684 PMID: 28179482

McLeod, S., & Harrison, L. J. (2009). Epidemiology of speech and language impairment in a nationally representative sample of 4- to 5-year-old children. *Journal of Speech, Language, and Hearing Research: JSLHR*, *52*(5), 1213–1229. DOI: 10.1044/1092-4388(2009/08-0085) PMID: 19403947

Mcnally, S., & Quigley, J. (2014). An irish cohort study of risk and protective factors for infant language development at 9 months. *Infant and Child Development*, *23*(6), 634–649. DOI: 10.1002/icd.1861

Mondal, N., Bhat, B., Plakkal, N., Thulasingam, M., Ajayan, P., & Poorna, D. (2016). Prevalence and risk factors of speech and language delay in children less than three years of age. *Journal of Comprehensive Pediatrics*, *7*(2). Advance online publication. DOI: 10.17795/compreped-33173

Norbury, C. F., Gooch, D., Wray, C., Baird, G., Charman, T., Simonoff, E., Vamvakas, G., & Pickles, A. (2016). The impact of nonverbal ability on prevalence and clinical presentation of language disorder: Evidence from a population study. *Journal of Child Psychology and Psychiatry, and Allied Disciplines*, *57*(11), 1247–1257. DOI: 10.1111/jcpp.12573 PMID: 27184709

Owens, R. (2014). *Language disorders: a functional approach to assessment and intervention* (6th ed.). Pearson.

Owens, R. (2016). *Language development: An introduction* (8th ed.). Pearson.

Pak, N. S., Chow, J. C., Dillehay, K. M., & Kaiser, A. P. (2023). Long-Term Effects of Early Communication Interventions: A Systematic Review and Meta-Analysis. *Journal of Speech, Language, and Hearing Research: JSLHR*, *66*(8), 2884–2899. DOI: 10.1044/2023_JSLHR-22-00711 PMID: 37418755

Pispati, V., Africawala, A. N., & Varghese, S. (2019). Developmental Screening of Children of Migrant Construction Workers in Mumbai. *Indian Journal of Human Development*, *13*(1), 109–114. DOI: 10.1177/0973703019839820

Popich, E., Louw, B., & Eloff, I. (2006). The need for collaboration in early communication intervention: Whom do parents consult regarding the prevention of communication disorders? *Early Child Development and Care*, *176*(7), 675–692. DOI: 10.1080/03004430500206395

Raby, K. L., Freedman, E., Yarger, H. A., Lind, T., & Dozier, M. (2019). Enhancing the language development of toddlers in foster care by promoting foster parents' sensitivity: Results from a randomized controlled trial. *Developmental Science, 22*(2), e12753. DOI: 10.1111/desc.12753 PMID: 30230658

Ravid, D., Bar-On, A., & Dattner, E. (2013). Linguistics in the service of communication disorders: *New frontiers. AILA Review, 26*, 79–99. Advance online publication. DOI: 10.1075/aila.26.06rav

Reilly, S., Wake, M., Ukoumunne, O., Bavin, E., Prior, M., Cini, E., Conway, L., Eadie, P., & Bretherton, L. (2010). Predicting language outcomes at 4 years of age: Findings from early language in victoria study. *Pediatrics, 126*(6), e1530–e1537. DOI: 10.1542/peds.2010-0254 PMID: 21059719

Rinaldi, S., Caselli, M. C., Cofelice, V., D'Amico, S., De Cagno, A. G., Della Corte, G., Di Martino, M. V., Di Costanzo, B., Levorato, M. C., Penge, R., Rossetto, T., Sansavini, A., Vecchi, S., & Zoccolotti, P. (2021). Efficacy of the Treatment of Developmental Language Disorder: A Systematic Review. *Brain Sciences, 11*(3), 407. DOI: 10.3390/brainsci11030407 PMID: 33806938

Sánchez, K., Spittle, A., Cheong, J., Thompson, D., Doyle, L., Anderson, P., & Morgan, A. (2018). Language in 2-year-old children born preterm and term: A cohort study. *Archives of Disease in Childhood, 104*(7), 647–652. DOI: 10.1136/archdischild-2018-315843 PMID: 30470685

Sansavini, A., Favilla, M. E., Guasti, M. T., Marini, A., Millepiedi, S., Di Martino, M. V., Vecchi, S., Battajon, N., Bertolo, L., Capirci, O., Carretti, B., Colatei, M. P., Frioni, C., Marotta, L., Massa, S., Michelazzo, L., Pecini, C., Piazzalunga, S., Pieretti, M., & Lorusso, M. L. (2021). Developmental Language Disorder: Early Predictors, Age for the Diagnosis, and Diagnostic Tools. A Scoping Review. *Brain Sciences, 11*(5), 654. DOI: 10.3390/brainsci11050654 PMID: 34067874

Sapage, S., & Cruz-Santos, A. (2021). Portuguese Early Literacy Screening Tool-RaLEPE: Pilot Study. *Revista de Investigación en Logopedia, 11*(2), e71711. DOI: 10.5209/rlog.71711

Scribner, E. (2013) Exploring Different Factors of Language Development. Awards for Excellence in Student Research & Creative Activity - Documents. 1. https://thekeep.eiu.edu/lib_awards_2013_docs/1

Sheldrick, R. C., & Perrin, E. C. (2013). Evidence-Based Milestones for Surveillance of Cognitive, Language, and Motor Development. *Academic Pediatrics, 13*(6), 577–586. DOI: 10.1016/j.acap.2013.07.001 PMID: 24238685

Silva & Peixoto. (2008) Rastreio e prevalência das perturbações da comunicação num agrupamento de escolas. *Revista da Faculdade de Ciências da Saúde*. Porto. ISSN 1646-0480. 5 (2008) 272-282.

Sim, F., O'Dowd, J., Thompson, L., Law, J., Macmillan, S., Affleck, M., Gillberg, C., & Wilson, P. (2013). Language and social/emotional problems identified at a universal developmental assessment at 30 months. *BMC Pediatrics, 13*(1), 206. DOI: 10.1186/1471-2431-13-206 PMID: 24330767

Simms, M. D., & Jin, X. (2015). (in review). Autism, Language Disorder, and Social (Pragmatic) Communication Disorder: DSM-V and Differential Diagnoses. *Pediatrics, 36*(8), 355–362. PMID: 26232465

Siu, A. L. (2015). Screening for Speech and Language Delay and Disorders in Children Aged 5 Years or Younger: US Preventive Services Task Force Recommendation Statement. *Pediatrics, 136*(2), e474–e481. DOI: 10.1542/peds.2015-1711 PMID: 26152670

Siu, A. L.US Preventive Services Task Force. (2015, August). Screening for Speech and Language Delay and Disorders in Children Aged 5 Years or Younger: US Preventive Services Task Force Recommendation Statement. *Pediatrics, 136*(2), e474–e481. DOI: 10.1542/peds.2015-1711 PMID: 26152670

Skuban, E. (2010) *Language impairment and child adjustment in high-risk, low-income toddlers: moderating influences of parenting and emotion regulation.* Doctoral Dissertation, University of Pittsburgh. https://d-scholarship.pitt.edu/8134/

Snow, P. (2021) Psychosocial Adversity in Early Childhood and Language and Literacy Skills in Adolescence: The Role of Speech Language Pathology in Prevention, Policy, and Practice. *Perspectives of the ASHA Special Interest Groups,* 6, 253–261. https://pubs.asha.org 37.189.29.156

Snowling, M. J., Nash, H. M., Gooch, D. C., Hayiou-Thomas, M. E., & Hulme, C. (2019). Developmental Outcomes for Children at High Risk of Dyslexia and Children With Developmental Language Disorder. *Child Development, 90*(5), e548–e564. DOI: 10.1111/cdev.13216 PMID: 30676649

So, K. K. H., & To, C. (2022). Systematic Review and Meta-Analysis of Screening Tools for Language Disorder. *Frontiers in Pediatrics, 10*, 801220. Advance online publication. DOI: 10.3389/fped.2022.801220 PMID: 35281230

So, L., Miller, E., & Eastwood, J. (2021). Exploring mothers' experience of a linguistic feedback technology for children at risk of poor language development: Qualitative pilot study. *JMIR Pediatrics and Parenting*, *4*(3), e27049. DOI: 10.2196/27049 PMID: 34463633

Soares, A., Silva, K., & Zuanetti, P. (2017). Variáveis de risco para o desenvolvimento da linguagem associadas à prematuridade. *Audiology - Communication Research*, *22*(0). Advance online publication. DOI: 10.1590/2317-6431-2016-1745

Spicer-Cain, H., Camilleri, B., Hasson, N., & Botting, N. (2023). Early Identification of Children at Risk of Communication Disorders: Introducing a Novel Battery of Dynamic Assessments for Infants. *American Journal of Speech-Language Pathology*, *32*(2), 523–544. DOI: 10.1044/2022_AJSLP-22-00040 PMID: 36787149

Stansfeld, S. A., Clark, C., Rodgers, B., Caldwell, T., & Power, C. (2011). Repeated exposure to socioeconomic disadvantage and health selection as life course pathways to mid-life depressive and anxiety disorders. *Social Psychiatry and Psychiatric Epidemiology*, *46*(7), 549–558. DOI: 10.1007/s00127-010-0221-3 PMID: 20383489

Suchodoletz, Waldemar. (2011). Early identification of children with developmental language disorders - When and how?. *Zeitschrift für Kinder- und Jugendpsychiatrie und Psychotherapie*. 39. 377-84; 384. .DOI: 10.1024/1422-4917/a000136

Thurman, A. (2017). *Parent-child interaction: how it impacts language and literacy skills*, Graduate Research Papers. 617. https://scholarworks.uni.edu/grp/617

Tomasello, M. (2003). *Constructing a language: A usage-based theory of language acquisition*. Harvard University Press.

Tomblin, J. B., Smith, E., & Zhang, X. (1997). Epidemiology of specific language impairment: Prenatal and perinatal risk factors. *Journal of Communication Disorders*, *30*(4), 325–344. DOI: 10.1016/S0021-9924(97)00015-4 PMID: 9208366

Triska, V. L. (2016) *The Comorbidity of Communication and Psychological Disorders: An analysis of the origin and prevalence of children presenting with comorbid language, speech, and psychological disorders*. Student Research Submissions. 139. https://scholar.umw.edu/student_research/139

Tulviste, T., & Schults, A. (2020). Parental reports of communicative development at the age of 36 months: The Estonian CDI-III. *First Language*, *40*(1), 64–83. DOI: 10.1177/0142723719887313

Turnbull, K., & Justice, M. (2016). *Language Development From Theory to Practice* (3rd ed.). Pearson.

Valade, F., Béliveau, M.-J., Breault, C., Chabot, B., & Labelle, F. (2023). Individual and cumulative risk factors in developmental language disorder: A case-control study. *Clinical Child Psychology and Psychiatry*, *28*(1), 398–414. DOI: 10.1177/13591045221113389 PMID: 35797616

van Agt, H. M., van der Stege, H. A., de Ridder-Sluiter, H., Verhoeven, L. T., & de Koning, H. J. (2007). A cluster-randomized trial of screening for language delay in toddlers: Effects on school performance and language development at age 8. *Pediatrics*, *120*(6), 1317–1325. DOI: 10.1542/peds.2006-3145 PMID: 18055682

van Agt, H. M., van der Stege, H. A., de Ridder-Sluiter, J. G., & de Koning, H. J. (2007). Detecting language problems: Accuracy of five language screening instruments in preschool children. *Developmental Medicine and Child Neurology*, *49*(2), 117–184. DOI: 10.1111/j.1469-8749.2007.00117.x PMID: 17253998

van der Schuit, M., Segers, E., van Balkom, H., & Verhoeven, L. (2011). Early language intervention for children with intellectual disabilities: A neurocognitive perspective. *Research in Developmental Disabilities*, *32*(2), 705–712. DOI: 10.1016/j.ridd.2010.11.010 PMID: 21159487

Viana, F.; Cadime, I.; Silva, C. (…) Monteiro, J. (2017*) MacArthut-Bates inventários de desenvolvimento comunicativo.* Luso info Edutora.

Visser-Bochane, M. I., Reijneveld, S. A., Krijnen, W. P., van der Schans, C. P., & Luinge, M. R. (2019). Identifying Milestones in Language Development for Young Children Ages 1-6 Years. *Academic Pediatrics*. Advance online publication. DOI: 10.1016/j.acap.2019.07.003 PMID: 31306799

Wade, M., Zeanah, C. H., Fox, N. A., & Nelson, C. A. (2020). Social communication deficits following early-life deprivation and relation to psychopathology: A randomized clinical trial of foster care. *Journal of Child Psychology and Psychiatry, and Allied Disciplines*, *61*(12), 1360–1369. DOI: 10.1111/jcpp.13222 PMID: 32222079

Wake, M., Levickis, P., Tobin, S., Zens, N., Law, J., Gold, L., Ukoumunne, O. C., Goldfeld, S., Le, H. N., Skeat, J., & Reilly, S. (2012). Improving outcomes of preschool language delay in the community: Protocol for the Language for Learning randomised controlled trial. *BMC Pediatrics*, *12*(1), 96. DOI: 10.1186/1471-2431-12-96 PMID: 22776103

Wallace, I. F., Berkman, N. D., Watson, L. R., Coyne-Beasley, T., Wood, C. T., Cullen, K., & Lohr, K. N. (2015). Screening for Speech and Language Delay in Children 5 Years Old and Younger: A Systematic Review. *Pediatrics*, *136*(2), e448–e462. DOI: 10.1542/peds.2014-3889 PMID: 26152671

Walle, E., & Campos, J. (2014). Infant language development is related to the acquisition of walking. *Developmental Psychology*, *50*(2), 336–348. DOI: 10.1037/a0033238 PMID: 23750505

Warner, R. (2017). *Intersubjectivity as a precursor to literacy: revisiting the home-school study of language and literacy development.* Thesis in Doctor of Philosophy The University of Texas at Austin. https://repositories.lib.utexas.edu/server/api/core/bitstreams/457c869a-d1db-4e84-a211-7f8d99ee05e4/content

Wells, G. (2007). Semiotic mediation, dialogue and the construction of knowledge. *Human Development*, *50*(5), 244–247. DOI: 10.1159/000106414

Wetherby, A., Warren, S., & Reichle, J. (1998) *Transitions in Prelinguistic Communication.* Volume 7 de Communication and language intervention series. Brookes Publishing

Wetherby, A. M., Guthrie, W., Hooker, J. L., Delehanty, A., Day, T. N., Woods, J., Pierce, K., Manwaring, S. S., Thurm, A., Ozonoff, S., Petkova, E., & Lord, C. (2021). The Early Screening for Autism and Communication Disorders: Field-testing an autism-specific screening tool for children 12 to 36 months of age. *Autism*, *25*(7), 2112–2123. DOI: 10.1177/13623613211012526 PMID: 33962531

Zambrana, I. M., Pons, F., Eadie, P., & Ystrom, E. (2014). Trajectories of language delay from age 3 to 5: Persistence, recovery and late onset. *International Journal of Language & Communication Disorders*, *49*(3), 304–316. DOI: 10.1111/1460-6984.12073 PMID: 24382196

Zebron, S., Mhute, I., & Constantine Chando Musingafi, M. (2015). Classroom Challenges: Working with Pupils with Communication Disorders.*Journal of Education and Practice*, v6 n9 p181\11

Chapter 3

Assessment of Patient Perception in Clinical Practice in Mechanical Dysphagia

Rita Alegria
Escola Superior Fernando Pessoa, Portugal

Daniela Vieira
https://orcid.org/0000-0001-8263-0927
Escola Superior Fernando Pessoa, Portugal

ABSTRACT

Head and neck cancer treatment is closely associated with functional changes, such as dysphagia, which have a negative impact on quality of life. This study aims to compare the clinical assessment, intervention of the speech therapist and patient's perception. This chapter reports to a retrospective, quantitative, and descriptive study, based on a series of five participants, according to inclusion and exclusion criteria. Of the five cases included in this study, most were males aged between 50 and 65 years, and all had undergone radiotherapy. Most of them (60%) had oropharyngeal cancer and performed between 24 and 36 speech therapy sessions. A clinical evaluation of the swallow at initial and final moments was performed. Results show agreement between patient's perception, through SWAL-QOL-PT and FOIS results. This study shows the interception between patient perception and physiological findings; thus, we can increase the effectiveness of intervention results and therapeutic adherence, with real health gains.

DOI: 10.4018/979-8-3693-6432-1.ch003

INTRODUCTION

Head and neck cancer is the fifth most common cancer worldwide (Chapuy et al., 2013; Manikantan et al., 2009; Ward & Van As-Brooks, 2007). In Portugal, according to GLOBOCAN data, 58199 new cases appeared in 2018, with 0.63% in the oropharynx, 0.77% in the hypopharynx, 1.08% in the larynx and 1.65% in the lips and oral cavity (Cancer & Organization, 2019). Currently, treatments are focused on an "organ preservation" strategy using radiotherapy (RT) and chemotherapy (CT), which translate into profound and prolonged side effects (Lafer et al., 2013). These changes result from sensory alterations, motor denervation, and fibrosis of the upper aerodigestive tract and mucous membranes6, compromising orofacial functions. The speech language pathologist is a critical element, from the moment of diagnosis or at least soon after the start of treatments, maximizing functional results (Starmer & Edwards, 2019).

In recent decades, there has been increased focus on the investigation of physiological objective measures of swallowing (Simental & Carrau, 2004). However, the patient's perspective is increasingly being valued. An approach focusing on both concepts may improve the understanding of the experience of living with dysphagia (Nekhlyudov et al., 2017; Simental & Carrau, 2004). This bimodal approach may allow the effectiveness of treatment outcomes to be evaluated and controlled (Balaguer et al., 2020; Fung et al., 2005; Jones et al., 2018; Soldatova & Mirza, 2019; Su, 1997).

Swallowing disorders translate into functional limitations and complications, such as aspiration, pneumonia, and malnutrition, impacting quality of life (QoL) (Chen et al., 2001; McHorney, Bricker, Kramer, et al., 2000; Perry et al., 2016), as well as with limitations or restrictions in activity and participation (Perry et al., 2016; Threats, 2007). Dysphagia is present in 39-64% of patients (Arrese et al., 2017; Jones et al., 2018), especially in cases of advanced oral and oropharyngeal cancer (Ward & Van As-Brooks, 2007). At the Portuguese Institute of Oncology of Porto, between 2005 and 2008, the most frequent functional change after surgical treatment was dysphagia, in 82.68% of patients (Vieira & Monteiro, 2010).

The speech language pathologist (SLP) should be present from an early stage of treatment (Starmer & Edwards, 2019), achieving better health outcomes, with functional gains and better practices. The SLP intervention in patients with head and neck cancer aims to rehabilitate orofacial functions, namely swallowing, as well as to contribute to social integration, improving QoL. The patient perception assessment (QoL) specifically related to dysphagia allows for a broader understanding of the experience of living with dysphagia. It can be used to assess and monitor the therapeutic process and develop a more individualized intervention plan (Bandeira, 2004; McHorney, Bricker, Robbins, et al., 2000; Vieira & Antunes, 2017). It is important to acknowledge that the successful management of dysphagia in head and neck cancer patients is fundamentally a multidisciplinary effort. While this chapter focuses on the role of the Speech-Language Pathologist in relating clinical assessment to patient perception, optimal patient care involves close collaboration with oncologists, surgeons, radiation oncologists, dietitians, nurses, and psychologists to address the multifaceted needs of these individuals throughout their treatment and survivorship journey.

While existing research highlights the significant impact of dysphagia on the quality of life for head and neck cancer patients and increasingly values the patient's perspective, there remains a gap in studies that specifically correlate patient-reported outcome measures (PROMs). Prior work often examines these measures separately or in different populations. This chapter aims to address this gap by retrospectively analysing the relationship between SWAL-QOL-PT results, FOIS scores, and clinical swallowing assessment findings in Portuguese head and neck cancer patients undergoing speech-language pathology intervention. By doing so, it seeks to demonstrate the practical utility and synergy of using both subjective patient perceptions and objective functional measures to guide clinical practice and enhance therapeutic adherence.

BACKGROUND

Overview of SLP Dysphagia Interventions in HNC

Speech-language pathology intervention for mechanical dysphagia following head and neck cancer treatment typically involves a combination of approaches tailored to the individual's specific deficits and needs identified during assessment. Common intervention categories include rehabilitative exercises aimed at improving the range of motion, strength, and coordination of swallowing musculature; compensatory strategies designed to modify bolus flow and improve swallowing safety (e.g., postural adjustments, swallowing manoeuvres); recommendations for dietary texture modification to ensure safety and efficiency; and patient/caregiver education regarding safe swallowing practices and strategies. The specific techniques and protocols are selected based on comprehensive clinical and instrumental evaluations (when available) and patient goals, emphasizing a personalized approach to maximize functional outcomes and quality of life.

This study was granted with ethics approval by the HE-UFP Research Ethics Committee (CES-HE-FFP - 68) and was carried out in accordance with the guidelines of the Declaration of Helsinki on human studies. Participants' confidentiality and privacy of personal data were ensured.

A total of 5 patients with mechanical dysphagia were involved in this retrospective study.

Data were collected from the participants' clinical notes. From 2019 to y 2020, 13 patients diagnosed with mechanical dysphagia by the consultant were referred for speech language pathologist (SLP).

Patients were included in this study if they met the following criteria:

(1) were aged 18 or over
(2) were male or female
(3) had no neurological pathology (self-reported or following medical evaluation)
(4) had no medical conditions or medications that alter motor and sensory performance of the oropharynx or which contribute to salivary gland hypofunction
(5) had undergone treatment (surgical, RT and/or CT) for head and neck cancer with oropharyngeal dysphagia (self-reported and confirmed by SLP evaluation)

Exclusion criteria included participants who had:

(1) undergone previous speech therapy
(2) cognitive and/or behavioral alterations (according to clinical notes)
(3) alterations in the waking state that prevent them from completing the questionnaire
(4) difficulties reading or writing in Portuguese
(5) refused to participate or were unable to give informed consent

A SLP performed a comprehensive initial clinical history and assessment of patient swallow. Details of the overall procedure are outlined below.

While various instruments exist to assess swallowing function and related quality of life in head and neck cancer patients, such as the Eating Assessment Tool (EAT-10) and the M.D. Anderson Dysphagia Inventory (MDADI), this study utilized the Swallowing Quality of Life Questionnaire - Portuguese Version (SWAL-QOL-PT) and the Functional Oral Intake Scale (FOIS). The SWAL-QOL-PT was chosen for its comprehensive assessment of dysphagia's impact across multiple quality-of-life domains and its validation for the European Portuguese population. The FOIS was selected due to its specific focus on quantifying the functional level of safe oral intake on a simple, validated 7-point scale, its demonstrated sensitivity to change, ease of administration, and its validation in European Portuguese.

The clinical evaluation of the swallow included the collection of information through the following actions: clinical interview, Swallow Quality-of-Life Questionnaire the outcome tool for adults with oropharyngeal dysphagia (SWAL-QOL-PT), Functional Oral Intake Scale (FOIS) and a clinical assessment of swallowing.

The SWAL-QOL-PT is comprised of 10 dimensions (eating, burden, duration, desire, food selection, communication, fear, mental health, social impact, fatigue, and sleep), as well as a symptom scale, with a total of 44 items. Responses are made using a five-point Likert scale, with scores ranging from 0-100, after linear conversion. The lower the score, the worse the dysphagia related QoL. The result is the score value in each domain (McHorney et al., 2002).

In addition to these, the final part of this instrument includes four questions: 1) related to enteral feeding (nasogastric tube or gastrostomy); 2) the consistency of solid food; 3) the most frequent liquids ingested over the past week; and 4) the individual's perception of his/her general health. All these also have a Likert-type scale response model, except for the one referring to the use of enteral feeding (dichotomous). The questionnaire may be completed by the patient themself, through an interview with a technician or by the caregiver (McHorney et al., 2002).

The FOIS is a validated instrument to measure and document the amount and type of food that the user can safely ingest orally. This scale consists of seven levels from 1 (no oral intake) to 7 (oral diet with no restrictions). From levels 1 to 3 the user is dependent on an enteric route - nasogastric tube and levels 4-7, there is capacity for oral intake in modified degrees. This scale has demonstrated validity and reliability, content, and criterion validity, as well as sensitivity to changes in oral intake. These features, along with ease and short administration (about five minutes) (Chen et al., 2001; Crary et al., 2005; Lazarus et al., 2014; Sinn et al., 2020). This is the only scale for rating oral intake that has been translated and validated into European Portuguese (Queirós et al., 2013).

The clinical swallow assessment in the clinical practice of the HE-UFP is composed of two parts: 1) clinical evaluation; and 2) functional evaluation - during a small meal. In the first part, we performed anamnesis with collection of the clinical history related to swallowing, as well as the evaluation of the oromotor functions (cranial pairs V (trigeminal), VII (facial), XII (hypoglossal), orosensory (cranial pair trigeminal - V), inspection of the oral cavity, oropharynx, and evaluation of the pharyngo-laryngeal function (cranial pairs glossopharyngeal - IX and vagus - X). In the second part, functional evaluation, an evaluation of the performance during swallowing with thickened liquid and other foods brought by the patient, which are used in their daily diet, in cases with an oral route, was performed.

Descriptive statistical analysis of the quantitative variables included both average and standard deviation and median and interquartile range (IQR: 1st and 3rd quartiles), while the categorical variables were depicted by counts and percentages (n and %). In the analysis of the SWAL-QOL-PT results, a linear transformation from a Likert scale of 1 to 5 to 0-100 was performed for all items. At the end, for the classification of severity, a division by quartile was performed, with results between 0-25 being considered as severe change, between 26-50 as moderate change, between 51-75 as mild change and between 76-100 as no change (McHorney et al., 2002; Vieira et al., 2020).

MAIN FOCUS OF THE CHAPTER

Only 5 out of the 13 participants completed the swallow program and were re-assessed at the end of therapy (62% dropout). Eight participants were unable to complete the swallow program due to health problems. Participants' group characteristics according to sex, age, location, treatment, and number of sessions are presented in the Table 1. The average age of participants was 57 years (range 35-81 years), revealing a great variability. 80% were male and undergone radiotherapy. 60% of the participants had oncologic pathology of the oropharynx. Patients, on average, had 30 sessions, ranging from 24 to 36 sessions in total.

Table 2 are the complaints/reasons for starting therapy for each patient, as well as the results considered most relevant in the pre- and post-therapy clinical evaluation of swallowing.

In this series of five cases, it was possible to verify that the SWAL-QOL-PT total score was higher, showing better QoL related to dysphagia, i.e., improvement of the condition through the patient's perception. A more detailed analysis by domain also shows a positive evolution. These results translated into decreased severity of dysphagia, with better functionality and less impact on QoL (Table 3).

In this study, the application of the SWAL-QOL-PT allowed the importance of using instruments that measure the patient's perception in the context of assessment and intervention in patients with head and neck cancer, in speech therapy to be highlighted. Therefore, it shows the impact that dysphagia has on QoL 39. However, this is not yet a recurrent practice in the reality of SLP' interventions (Caçador et al., 2004; Pimentel, 2006). Nevertheless, there have been more studies that focus on the use of these instruments with physiological findings (Jones et al., 2018; Kendall et al., 2014; Pauloski et al., 2009; Pauloski et al., 2002; Rogers, 2016; Rogus-Pulia et al., 2015), allowing the effectiveness of intervention outcomes to be assessed and monitored (Balaguer et al., 2020; Fung et al., 2005; Jones et al., 2018; Soldatova & Mirza, 2019; Su, 1997).

Regarding the 1st case, there was an improvement in all domains of the SWAL-QOL-PT and in the FOIS scale. In more detail, the patient's complaints regarding the variety of consistencies/foods and residues, may be related to the findings of the clinical evaluation, namely the safety and efficacy only for the consistency of thin liquid; the increase in oral transit time, with the presence of residues in the oral cavity, which is probably associated with the limitation in the range of motion of the hyolaryngeal complex. Thus, in the SWAL-QOL-PT, the domains that showed the most significant changes from the functional point of view, with changes in the degree of severity were "burden", "oral symptoms" and "food selection", which is related to the change from an FOIS score of 4 to 5, as well as to the decrease in oral transit time and the greater variability of food options (soft and wet solids), according to the clinical evaluation.

In the 2nd case, the main complaints were related to the range of movement of the orofacial structures, which conditioned the oral and consequently the pharyngeal phase. In terms of the patient's perception, improvements were obtained, with positive progression of the degree of severity for the following domains: burden, food selection, mental health, fears, social functioning, fatigue, sleep, and total score. These changes led to dietary modification throughout the intervention, with a change from level 4 to 6 in the FOIS. At the clinical level, the improvement of about 5mm in the mouth opening amplitude allowed for more efficient chewing and consequently a decrease in the oral transit time and diet diversification; and it was even possible to introduce fibrous foods.

The 3rd case essentially presented a fear of swallowing, pain, and increased meal duration, which was verified in the assessment of the patient's perception with lower scores for domains such as "duration of eating" and "fears", and the clinical findings pointed to decreased elevation and support of the hyolaryngeal complex and the need for multiple swallowing, showing poor efficiency of the swallowing mechanism. At the global level, it was possible to observe improvements in the following domains: burden, desire to eat, duration of eating, oral symptoms, fears, sleep, and SWAL-QOL-PT total score, with a change in the severity of dysphagia from level 5 to 7 in the FOIS. In terms of clinical evaluation, the changes are compatible, with no pain, transition to an unrestricted diet, effective ejection movement, as well as elevation and support of the hyolaryngeal complex.

According to the clinical assessment, the complaint in case 4 was related to choking on thin liquid and saliva, which was justified by the change in orofacial movement speed and oral control deficit, as well as an ineffective lower airway protection mechanism at the glottal level. In terms of patient perception, the domains related to saliva, fears and food selection may be related to the complaint and clinical assessment. At discharge, it was possible to observe an evolution of the FOIS from level 6 to 7, i.e., for an unrestricted diet and for a total SWAL-QOL-PT score that showed no impairment. Thus, the main domains with changes in severity were: burden, duration of eating, symptoms - saliva, food selection and fears.

In the 5th and final case, the patient had difficulty chewing solid food and in the progression of the bolus along the aerodigestive tract. According to the clinical evaluation, a decrease in the amplitude of orofacial and pharyngolaryngeal movements was observed, compatible with the complaints presented. Regarding the patient's perception, the initial assessment showed severe to moderate deficits in the domains: burden, feeding duration, pharyngeal symptoms, and oral symptoms, which agrees with the patient's complaints and the clinical evaluation findings. At the end of the therapy, an improvement was noticed in functionality with progression to a more varied diet, from level 3 to level 5 of the FOIS. In addition, the patient's perception of the impact of dysphagia on his QoL showed improvements in the domains mentioned above as well as the following: desire to eat, symptoms - saliva, food selection, communication, fears, social functioning, fatigue, sleep, and SWAL-QOL-PT total score.

According to the results of the case series, it was possible to verify an agreement between the results of the assessment of patient perception, through the SWAL-QOL-PT, and the severity of dysphagia, through the FOIS, and the findings of the clinical evaluation. Thus, the importance of implementing a comprehensive assessment becomes evident, with increased knowledge and awareness on the part of the patient, increasing therapeutic adherence. It can be suggested that good efficacy of the intervention was obtained in the cases presented, with gains in health. The intervention of the SLP in patients with head and neck cancer in the team is urgently needed for effective recovery, in both time and quality. This professional should participate in assessment, guidance, rehabilitation, and research from a biopsychophysical and social perspective.

Despite the demonstrated value of integrating patient perception using PROMs like SWAL-QOL-PT, their routine implementation in clinical practice faces several potential challenges. Barriers can exist at the patient level, including factors such as health literacy, the time required for completion, and motivation or willingness to engage with questionnaires regularly. Clinician and healthcare system factors also play a role, such as limited consultation time, the need for staff training on administering and interpreting PROMs, difficulties integrating PROM data into existing clinical workflows or electronic health records, and the administrative burden associated with data collection and management. Furthermore, resource limitations in certain healthcare settings may pose additional obstacles to the widespread adoption of these valuable tools.

FUTURE RESEARCH DIRECTIONS

The successful management of dysphagia in head and neck cancer patients hinges on a comprehensive assessment. One promising direction is developing tools to predict dysphagia risk. This would allow for early intervention through exercises, dietary changes, and compensatory strategies, potentially minimizing dysphagia development altogether.

Future research should explore the integration of emerging technologies into dysphagia management for this population. Investigating the feasibility, validity, and effectiveness of telehealth platforms for delivering remote dysphagia assessments and interventions could improve access to care, particularly for patients in remote areas or with mobility limitations. Additionally, exploring the potential application of artificial intelligence and machine learning techniques to analyze complex datasets—including imaging studies, clinical assessments, and PROM data—could lead to improved diagnostic accuracy, better prediction of treatment outcomes, and the development of more highly personalized rehabilitation programs. Finally, investigating long-term management strategies and integrating dysphagia care into survivorship plans will ensure ongoing support for patients. By focusing on these areas, research can contribute to a more holistic and patient-centered approach to dysphagia management in head and neck cancer.

CONCLUSION

The findings from the 5-case report show that the intervention and management of head and neck cancer patients is challenging and depends on a multidisciplinary approach and patient involvement. Knowing the baseline and risk stratification, in addition to knowing the different types of dysphagia that may occur in this population, as well as the patient's goals, allow for increased therapeutic compliance and positive outcomes. In this regard, the SLP should make a comprehensive and holistic assessment, relating physiological findings with the patient's perception, making his or her intervention focused/centered on the person with dysphagia.

ACKNOWLEDGMENT

This research received no specific grant from any funding agency in the public, commercial, or not-for-profit sectors.

REFERENCES

Arrese, L. C., Carrau, R., & Plowman, E. K. (2017). Relationship Between the Eating Assessment Tool-10 and Objective Clinical Ratings of Swallowing Function in Individuals with Head and Neck Cancer. *Dysphagia*, *32*(1), 83–89. DOI: 10.1007/s00455-016-9741-7 PMID: 27538876

Balaguer, M., Pommée, T., Farinas, J., Pinquier, J., Woisard, V., & Speyer, R. (2020). Effects of oral and oropharyngeal cancer on speech intelligibility using acoustic analysis: Systematic review. *Head & Neck*, *42*(1), 111–130. DOI: 10.1002/hed.25949 PMID: 31571334

Bandeira, A. K. C. (2004). *Qualidade de vida relacionada à voz e à deglutição após tratamento para câncer de língua* Fundação Antônio Prudente]. http://livros01.livrosgratis.com.br/cp005138.pdf

Chapuy, C. I., Annino, D. J., Tishler, R. B., Haddad, R. I., Snavely, A., & Goguen, L. A. (2013). Success of endoscopic pharyngoesophageal dilation after head and neck cancer treatment. *The Laryngoscope*, *123*(12), 3066–3073. DOI: 10.1002/lary.24268 PMID: 23775806

Chen, A. Y., Frankowski, R., Bishop-Leone, J., Hebert, T., Leyk, S., Lewin, J., & Goepfert, H. (2001). The development and validation of a dysphagia-specific quality-of-life questionnaire for patients with head and neck cancer: The M. D. Anderson dysphagia inventory. *Archives of Otolaryngology—Head & Neck Surgery*, *127*(7), 870–876. PMID: 11448365

Crary, M. A., Mann, G. D., & Groher, M. E. (2005). Initial psychometric assessment of a functional oral intake scale for dysphagia in stroke patients. *Archives of Physical Medicine and Rehabilitation*, *86*(8), 1516–1520. DOI: 10.1016/j.apmr.2004.11.049 PMID: 16084801

Fung, K., Lyden, T. H., Lee, J., Urba, S. G., Worden, F., Eisbruch, A., Tsien, C., Bradford, C. R., Chepeha, D. B., Hogikyan, N. D., Prince, M. E. P., Teknos, T. N., & Wolf, G. T. (2005). Voice and swallowing outcomes of an organ-preservation trial for advanced laryngeal cancer. *International Journal of Radiation Oncology, Biology, Physics*, *63*(5), 1395–1399. DOI: 10.1016/j.ijrobp.2005.05.004 PMID: 16087298

Jones, E., Speyer, R., Kertscher, B., Denman, D., Swan, K., & Cordier, R. (2018). Health-Related Quality of Life and Oropharyngeal Dysphagia: A Systematic Review. *Dysphagia*, *33*(2), 141–172. DOI: 10.1007/s00455-017-9844-9 PMID: 28866854

Kendall, K. A., Kosek, S. R., & Tanner, K. (2014). Quality-of-life scores compared to objective measures of swallowing after oropharyngeal chemoradiation. *The Laryngoscope*, *124*(3), 682–687. DOI: 10.1002/lary.24344 PMID: 23929736

Lafer, M., Achlatis, S., Lazarus, C., Fang, Y., Branski, R. C., & Amin, M. R. (2013). Temporal measurements of deglutition in dynamic magnetic resonance imaging versus videofluoroscopy. *The Annals of Otology, Rhinology, and Laryngology*, *122*(12), 748–753. DOI: 10.1177/000348941312201204 PMID: 24592577

Lazarus, C. L., Husaini, H., Jacobson, A. S., Mojica, J. K., Buchbinder, D., Okay, D., & Urken, M. L. (2014). Development of a new lingual range-of-motion assessment scale: Normative data in surgically treated oral cancer patients. *Dysphagia*, *29*(4), 489–499. DOI: 10.1007/s00455-014-9534-9 PMID: 24810704

Manikantan, K., Khode, S., Sayed, S. I., Roe, J., Nutting, C. M., Rhys-Evans, P., Harrington, K. J., & Kazi, R. (2009). Dysphagia in head and neck cancer. *Cancer Treatment Reviews*, *35*(8), 724–732. DOI: 10.1016/j.ctrv.2009.08.008 PMID: 19751966

McHorney, C. A., Bricker, D. E., Kramer, A. E., Rosenbek, J. C., Robbins, J., Chignell, K. A., Logemann, J. A., & Clarke, C.Conceptual Foundation and Item Development. (2000). The SWAL-QOL outcomes tool for oropharyngeal dysphagia in adults: I. Conceptual foundation and item development. *Dysphagia*, *15*(3), 115–121. DOI: 10.1007/s004550010012 PMID: 10839823

McHorney, C. A., Bricker, D. E., Robbins, J., Kramer, A. E., Rosenbek, J. C., & Chignell, K. A. (2000). The SWAL-QOL outcomes tool for oropharyngeal dysphagia in adults: II. Item reduction and preliminary scaling. *Dysphagia*, *15*(3), 122–133. DOI: 10.1007/s004550010013 PMID: 10839824

McHorney, C. A., Robbins, J., Lomax, K., Rosenbek, J. C., Chignell, K., Kramer, A. E., & Bricker, D. E. (2002). The SWAL-QOL and SWAL-CARE outcomes tool for oropharyngeal dysphagia in adults: III. Documentation of reliability and validity. *Dysphagia*, *17*(2), 97–114. DOI: 10.1007/s00455-001-0109-1 PMID: 11956835

Nekhlyudov, L., Lacchetti, C., Davis, N. B., Garvey, T. Q., Goldstein, D. P., Nunnink, J. C., Ninfea, J. I. R., Salner, A. L., Salz, T., & Siu, L. L. (2017). Head and Neck Cancer Survivorship Care Guideline: American Society of Clinical Oncology Clinical Practice Guideline Endorsement of the American Cancer Society Guideline. *Journal of Clinical Oncology*, *35*(14), 1606–1621. DOI: 10.1200/JCO.2016.71.8478 PMID: 28240970

Pauloski, B. R., Rademaker, A. W., Lazarus, C., Boeckxstaens, G., Kahrilas, P. J., & Logemann, J. A. (2009). Relationship between manometric and videofluoroscopic measures of swallow function in healthy adults and patients treated for head and neck cancer with various modalities. *Dysphagia*, *24*(2), 196–203. DOI: 10.1007/s00455-008-9192-x PMID: 18956228

Pauloski, B. R., Rademaker, A. W., Logemann, J. A., Lazarus, C. L., Newman, L., Hamner, A., MacCracken, E., Gaziano, J., & Stachowiak, L. (2002). Swallow function and perception of dysphagia in patients with head and neck cancer. *Head & Neck*, *24*(6), 555–565. DOI: 10.1002/hed.10092 PMID: 12112553

Perry, A., Lee, S. H., Cotton, S., & Kennedy, C. (2016). Therapeutic exercises for affecting post-treatment swallowing in people treated for advanced-stage head and neck cancers. *Cochrane Database of Systematic Reviews*, *2016*(8), CD011112. Advance online publication. DOI: 10.1002/14651858.CD011112.pub2 PMID: 27562477

Pimentel, F. (2006). *Qualidade de vida e Oncologia*. Almedina.

Queirós, A., Moreira, S., Silva, A., Costa, R., & Lains, J. (2013). Contributo para a Adaptação e Validação da Eat Assessment Tool (EAT-10) e da Functional Oral Intake Scale (FOIS). *Revista da Sociedade Portuguesa de Medicina de Reabilitação*, *2*(24), 25–30.

Rogers, S. N. (2016). Improving quality-of-life questionnaires in head and neck cancer. *Expert Review of Quality of Life in Cancer Care*, *1*(1), 61–71. DOI: 10.1080/23809000.2016.1142357

Rogus-Pulia, N. M., Pierce, M., Mittal, B. B., Zecker, S. G., & Logemann, J. (2015). Bolus effects on patient awareness of swallowing difficulty and swallow physiology after chemoradiation for head and neck cancer. *Head & Neck*, *37*(8), 1122–1129. DOI: 10.1002/hed.23720 PMID: 24841209

Simental, A. A.Jr, & Carrau, R. L. (2004). Assessment of swallowing function in patients with head and neck cancer. *Current Oncology Reports*, *6*(2), 162–165. DOI: 10.1007/s11912-004-0028-z PMID: 14751094

Sinn, F. S., Charters, E., Stone, D., Janabi, M., & Bogaardt, H. (2020). Responsiveness of the EAT-10 to Clinical Change in Head and Neck Cancer Patients with Dysphagia. *International Journal of Speech-Language Pathology*, *22*(1), 78–85. DOI: 10.1080/17549507.2019.1596312 PMID: 31032643

Soldatova, L., & Mirza, N. (2019). Long-Term Voice and Swallowing Outcomes for Oral and Oropharyngeal Cancer Following Primary or Adjuvant Chemoradiation. *The Annals of Otology, Rhinology, and Laryngology*, *3489419842256*(9), 802–810. Advance online publication. DOI: 10.1177/0003489419842256 PMID: 31007044

Starmer, H., & Edwards, J. (2019). Clinical Decision Making with Head and Neck Cancer Patients with Dysphagia. *Seminars in Speech and Language*, *40*(3), 213–226. DOI: 10.1055/s-0039-1688979 PMID: 31158905

Su, C. Y. (1997). Aspiration and speech shunt stenosis in near-total laryngectomy patients. *European Archives of Oto-Rhino-Laryngology*, *254*(8), 401–404. DOI: 10.1007/BF01642559 PMID: 9332898

Threats, T. T. (2007). Use of the ICF in dysphagia management. *Seminars in Speech and Language*, *28*(4), 323–333. DOI: 10.1055/s-2007-986529 PMID: 17935017

Vieira, D., & Antunes, B. E. (2017). Clinical characteristics of dysphagia-related quality of life questionnaires. *Revista de Investigación en Logopedia*, *2*, 157–188.

Vieira, D., & Monteiro, E. (2010). Head and neck cancer: contribution for the analysis of the rehabilitation needs. *Revista da Faculdade de Ciências da Saúde*, *7*, 108-121. http://hdl.handle.net/10284/2984

Vieira, D. O., Antunes, E. B., Dinis-Ribeiro, M., & Monteiro, E. (2020). Psychometric validity of the Portuguese version of SWAL-QOL for head and neck cancer. *Revista de Logopedia, Foniatría y Audiología*.

Ward, E., & Van As-Brooks, C. (2007). *Head and Neck Cancer: Treatment, Rehabiliation, and Outcomes*. Plural Publishing Inc.

KEY TERMS AND DEFINITIONS

Head and Neck Cancer: Soft tissue tumors or cancer arising from the mucosal surfaces of the lip; oral cavity; pharynx; larynx; and cervical esophagus. other sites included are the nose and paranasal sinuses; salivary glands; thyroid gland and parathyroid glands; and melanoma and non-melanoma skin cancers of the head and neck.

Speech Language Pathology: The study of speech or language disorders and their diagnosis and correction.

Patient Reported Outcome Measures: Assessment of the quality and effectiveness of health care as measured and directly reported by the patient.

Oropharyngeal Dysphagia: Difficulty in swallowing which may result from neuromuscular disorder or mechanical obstruction. dysphagia is classified into two distinct types: oropharyngeal dysphagia due to malfunction of the pharynx and upper esophageal sphincter; and esophageal dysphagia due to malfunction of the esophagus.

Quality of Life: A generic concept reflecting concern with the modification and enhancement of life attributes, e.g., physical, political, moral, social environment as well as health and disease.

Chapter 4
Bibliometric and Visual Analysis of the Use of Complementary and Alternative Medicine in the Mental Health of Older Adults

Francisco Tiago de Vasconcelos
https://orcid.org/0009-0001-9374-7538
Universiy of Fortaleza, Brazil

Christina César Praça Brasil
https://orcid.org/0000-0002-7741-5349
Universiy of Fortaleza, Brazil

Ana Paula Vasconcellos Abdon
https://orcid.org/0000-0002-1597-1817
Universiy of Fortaleza, Brazil

Francisco Aquiles de Oliveira Caetano
https://orcid.org/0000-0002-1033-9855
Federal University of Ceará, Brazil

Thiago Medeiros da Costa Daniele
https://orcid.org/0000-0003-1241-7068
Universidade de Fortaleza, Brazil

DOI: 10.4018/979-8-3693-6432-1.ch004

ABSTRACT

This chapter explores the growing interest in Complementary and Alternative Medicine (CAM) for managing mental health issues among elderly individuals. The bibliographic search was conducted in the Web of Science Core Collection (WoSCC) database in March 2024. We included studies published in English from January 1, 2003, to December 31, 2023. This chapter investigates CAM's contribution to the mental well-being of older adults. Despite increasing research on CAM, findings reveal that the global integration of these practices remains limited and undervalued. The analysis identified the main trends, including the concentration of studies in the USA, China, and the UK, and highlighted gaps in Brazilian research and international collaboration. The chapter underscored the need for broader recognition of CAM in public health, emphasizing its potential as a low-cost, effective strategy to enhance mental health in aging populations.

1. INTRODUCTION

The global population is aging rapidly, with the proportion of individuals over 60 years old projected to double by 2050. This demographic shift presents significant challenges and opportunities in healthcare, especially regarding the mental health of older adults. Depression, anxiety, cognitive decline, and emotional well-being are key aspects that shape the quality of life in later years.

Primary Health Care (PHC), understood as the first level of contact in the health system, plays a central role in integrating ICPs and addressing the comprehensive needs of the aging population. To address these challenges, Integrative and Complementary Practices (ICPs) — such as mindfulness, meditation, Tai Chi, acupuncture, and herbal therapies — have been increasingly studied and adopted worldwide. They are gaining global recognition for their potential to enhance mental health, reduce psychological distress, and promote holistic well-being among older adults.

Although the Brazilian context provides important insights into the incorporation of ICPs into national healthcare strategies, including initiatives within the Unified Health System (SUS), it is crucial to frame this discussion within a broader, international context. Research from countries such as China, the United States, and various European nations highlights diverse approaches and varying levels of integration of ICPs into primary care and mental health programs for the older adults. This global perspective allows for richer comparisons and a more comprehensive understanding of how cultural, political, and healthcare systems shape the adoption of ICPs.

For example, Tai Chi has been shown not only to improve physical balance and postural control but also to significantly reduce symptoms of anxiety and depression in older adults, underscoring its mental health benefits (Cui et al., 2023). Likewise, interventions combining physical exercise, relaxation, meditation, and social interaction have demonstrated positive effects on stress reduction and overall emotional health among older adults at risk for neurodegenerative diseases (Kim et al., 2019; Tricco et al., 2015). It is important to note that memory is a specific dimension within broader cognitive functions, and references to improvements in memory should be understood as part of general cognitive health enhancement.

Mental health problems in older adults frequently coexist with chronic physical conditions such as diabetes, hypertension, fibromyalgia, insomnia, and obesity (Daniele et al., 2013; Luo et al., 2018). These overlapping conditions intensify the complexity of care required, emphasizing the importance of multidisciplinary strategies like ICPs to address both physical and psychological needs. Despite the promising potential, the widespread implementation of ICPs faces persistent barriers, including societal skepticism, insufficient professional training, lack of infrastructure, and, importantly, limited robust scientific evidence supporting their efficacy. Addressing this gap is crucial for enhancing the credibility and acceptance of ICPs in healthcare settings.

Objectives and Research Question

This chapter seeks to conduct a comprehensive bibliometric and visual analysis of the global scientific literature regarding the use and implementation of ICPs in the mental health of older adults. Specifically, the chapter aims to: (1) examine how ICPs are adopted by older adults in primary care across different countries and healthcare systems; and (2) explore the challenges, outcomes, and conditions influencing the use of ICPs in supporting mental health in this population. To guide this investigation, the following research question is posed: **How is the scientific production concerning Integrative ICPs in the mental health of older adults presented and characterized at a global level?**

2. METHODS

Study Design

This quantitative, exploratory, and descriptive study conducts a bibliometric literature review. Initially, a theoretical and documentary survey was performed to contextualize the theme and the object of study (Speckemeier et al., 2022). The review was organized into three main stages: 1) data collection, 2) screening, and 3) data analysis.

Bibliometric Review

Bibliometrics was initially introduced by Pritchard (1969) and consists of the quantitative and qualitative analysis of academic production, monitoring the development of a research field over time. This method can provide information about a specific area by investigating characteristics such as authorship, sources, institutions, journals, citations, authors' countries of origin, and co-citation networks.

The bibliometric review in this study uses a quantitative approach with qualitative elements to analyze the collected data. It is characterized by its exploratory nature, as it investigates the global scientific production on a topic, including production rates, scientific cooperation between authors and countries, and methods of disseminating knowledge and their gaps (Mugnaini, Fujino, & Kobashi, 2017).

Analyzing the consolidated literature on the use and implementation of ICPs in the mental health of older adults, this study aims to highlight, in more detail, the following issues: 1) the understanding and how ICPs are adopted by older adults in primary care worldwide; and 2) the challenges, effects, and conditions for using ICPs in the mental health of older adults (Kim et al., 2019; Tricco et al., 2015). This bibliometric analysis seeks to answer the following guiding question: How is the scientific production of ICPs in the mental health of older adults presented?

Bibliometric Review Procedures

Search Strategy

The literature search was conducted in the Web of Science Core Collection (WoSCC) database on March 20, 2024. Ethical approval for this review was not required, as the research uses previously published secondary data. The following combinations of keywords and Boolean operators were employed to integrate the search strategies: Complementary Therap* OR Integrative Therap* OR Holistic Therap* OR Chinese Medicine Therap* OR Integrative Care (All Fields) AND Elderly OR Aging OR Older People OR Senior (All Fields) AND NOT Children OR Adolescent* (All Fields) AND Primary Health Care (All Fields) AND Mental Health (All Fields).

Eligibility Criteria

We included studies published in English from January 1, 2003, to December 31, 2023, that used PNPIC practices in older adults, focused on mental health, and with approval from a Human Research Ethics Committee. We excluded articles that used non-validated assessment instruments, were outside the scope of the study, or had methodological bias.

Methodological bias was assessed based on the absence of appropriate control groups, lack of randomization, incomplete or missing data reporting, and the use of statistical analyses that did not align with the stated objectives.

Specifically, methodological bias was defined based on the absence of appropriate control groups, lack of randomization in trials, incomplete or missing data reporting, or statistical analyses that did not align with the stated objectives.

Study Selection and Data Extraction

Two independent reviewers selected eligible articles initially based on the titles and then by reading the abstracts. Then, they extracted data such as author, year of publication, country, study design, number of participants, age, gender, groups, study objectives, tasks, procedures, and results. Finally, they reviewed full articles.

A strict data quality control protocol was adopted during all the study's stages to ensure the robustness of the findings.

This protocol involved multiple stages: verification of inclusion and exclusion criteria, double-checking of data extraction by two independent reviewers, cross-validation of bibliometric parameters, and periodic reconciliation meetings to resolve discrepancies. Additionally, adherence to PRISMA guidelines was ensured throughout the review process.

During the screening, the studies were evaluated for methodological consistency and adherence to the proposed theme, using tools such as the Kappa agreement index, which ensured a 96% agreement rate, minimizing possible interpretation biases among the reviewers (Casagrande, Fabris, & Girometti, 2020).

Furthermore, the impact factors of the journals from which the selected articles originated were analyzed using the Journal Citation Reports (JCR) database, ensuring that the sources used were of high scientific relevance. Another critical aspect was using a source triangulation approach to validate the data collected and cross-reference information between different databases, strengthening the conclusions' consistency.

In addition to impact factors, the quartile rankings of the journals were assessed using the JCR classification system, providing further insight into the distribution and quality of the selected publications within the global research landscape.

Any disagreement would be referred to a third researcher, who would decide whether to include or exclude studies. Finally, a complete critical analysis of the studies was conducted.

Bibliometric Analysis of Findings

Lotka's Law (Authors)

Lotka's Law (1926) establishes that author productivity follows an inverse squared relationship, whereby few authors produce much, and many authors produce little (Silva & Mayworm, 2020). This indicator allows us to identify the primary authors and those with sporadic production (Gregorio-Chaviano, Limaymanta, & López-Mesa, 2020).

Bradford's Law (Sources)

Bradford's Law (1934) assesses the thematic dispersion of journals, identifying the core of the most productive journals on a given subject (Silva et al., 2020). The Law categorizes sources into productivity zones, distinguishing between scientific production's core, center, and periphery (Gregorio-Chaviano, Limaymanta, & López-Mesa, 2020).

Zipf's Law (Keywords)

Zipf's Law studies the frequency of co-occurrence of keywords in publications, observing a pattern of low dispersion when a theme is consolidated (Silva et al., 2020). The Law's equation is represented by $y = f(1/x)$, where y is the expected value, f is the word's frequency, and x is its position in the descriptor ranking.

Data Processing and Presentation

After selecting the studies, the results were scientifically mapped using the R (version 2022.07.0) and VOSviewer (version 1.6.17) software. The R software (*Bibliometrix* package) was used for thematic evolution analysis and to build a global distribution network of publications on ICPs in older adults (Aria, 2017). VOSviewer was adopted to extract information on collaboration, co-citation, and co-occurrence of keywords, creating network maps of countries, institutions, and authors (Pan, 2018; Zhang et al., 2020). The findings related to using ICPs in the mental health of older adults in PHC were analyzed in depth. All references were managed by My Endnote Web (McKinney, 2013).

Ethical and Legal Aspects

This study follows the guidelines of the Committee on Publication Ethics (COPE) (Ethics, 2000), which establishes good practices in research ethics. The review did not directly involve human participants, as the data were in the public domain. However, all studies analyzed underwent peer review, ensuring the reliability of the results and the necessary methodological rigor.

3. RESULTS

In this section, we present the results regarding the research objectives, followed by a detailed discussion of the interpretation and its implications for primary care practice and future research. To this end, the findings will be divided into four categories: 1. Theoretical survey; 2. Bibliometric and general performance analysis of the findings; 3. Scientific mapping analysis; and 4. Quantitative and qualitative description of the studies.

Public Policies and Using Integrative Practices in Aging

Population aging also raises questions about the adequacy of public policies to ensure the quality of life of the older adults population. In Brazil, the National Policy for Older Adults (Brazil, 1994) and the Statute for Older Adults (Brazil, 2003) are milestones that ensure the right to comprehensive health, including in the SUS. However, the National Policy on Integrative and Complementary Practices (PNPIC), established in 2006 and expanded in 2017 and 2018, offers an innovative approach by including alternative therapies as part of health care, reflecting the global guidelines of the World Health Organization (WHO) on traditional and complementary practices (Brazil, 2006; WHO, 2013).

Although ICPs bring a more holistic approach to healthcare, focusing on the physical, emotional, and spiritual aspects of individuals, implementing them is challenging. Some studies (Habimorad et al., 2020; Magalhães et al., 2018) indicate that, although they are included in public health policies, ICPs still face resistance concerning acceptance and scientific validation, both among health professionals and managers, and difficulties in the infrastructure necessary for their effective implementation.

At an international level, countries such as China and the United States of America (USA) have already advanced in integrating practices such as acupuncture and meditation into the mental health of older adults (Amonkar et al., 2021; Basso et al., 2019).

The United States, where complementary therapies are increasingly integrated into chronic disease management; and Canada, where integrative approaches are being implemented in primary care settings.

In contrast, although some efforts to expand the use of ICPs are observed, improvements are still needed in Brazil to train professionals and in the infrastructure of health units (Carvalho & Nóbrega, 2017). This complement highlights the relevance of ICPs in promoting healthy aging, as established by the WHO Decade of Healthy Aging (2021-2030), which proposes global strategies to improve the quality of life of older adults (PAHO/WHO, 2020).

Bibliometric Analysis of the General Results of the Publications

One hundred thirty-eight documents were identified, and after the initial analyses, duplicates were manually eliminated and the selected filters applied, excluding 97 articles. Three hundred eighty authors, 175 institutions, 28 countries, and 144 keywords cited by the authors were identified from the 41 studies included (30 full-text articles and 11 review articles). Among the full-text articles analyzed, the majority (73.17%, n=30) were quantitative studies, indicating a notable predominance of quantitative approaches in the field. All studies included in this review were read in full.

Table 1 analyzes the research results, presenting the temporal breakdown and the number of sources (journals) that addressed topics in the area in the specific period (2003-2023), the total number of articles, and the growth rate of publications. Growth percentages were calculated using averages and percentage values when necessary. Also, an average of 20.34 references was observed in the studies included in this review.

Table 1. Summary of the main characteristics of the included studies.

Classification	Results
Time bracket	2003 – 2023
Sources	31
Articles	41
Number of authors	379
Average age of the article	3,95
Average of citations per article	20,34
Author's keywords (DE)	144

continued on following page

Table 1. Continued

Classification	Results
International Co-authorship (%)	34.15
Annual growth rate (%)	23.11
Type of articles Scientific articles Review articles	30 11

Bibliometrix/R-Studio (2024).

Figure 1 analyzes the total scientific production from 2003 to 2023. The total number of publications increased significantly, especially after 2019 (Figure 1), and the number of citations increased in 2022 (Figure 2).

Among the studies analyzed, the most cited ICPs were yoga, acupuncture, phytotherapy, homeopathy, meditation, biodance, music therapy, reiki, and art therapy. Other practices such as relaxation, outdoor physical activity, Tai Chi Chuan, active listening, and senior dance were identified in the articles.

Figure 1. Global trends in the number of publications on the topic from 2013 to 2023

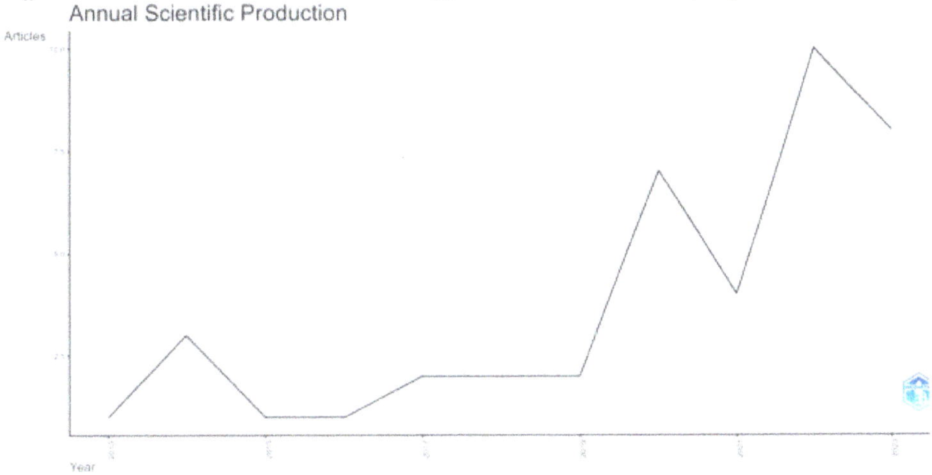

Source: Biblionshiny bibliometrix (2024)

Figure 2. Average number of publications/citations of articles per year

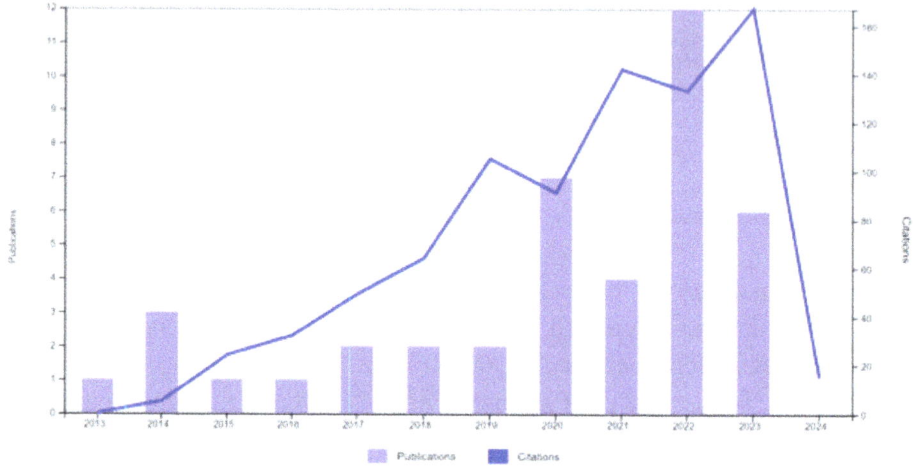

Source: Biblionshiny bibliometrix (2024)

Figure 3. Contribution map between countries on using ICPs in the mental health of older adults.

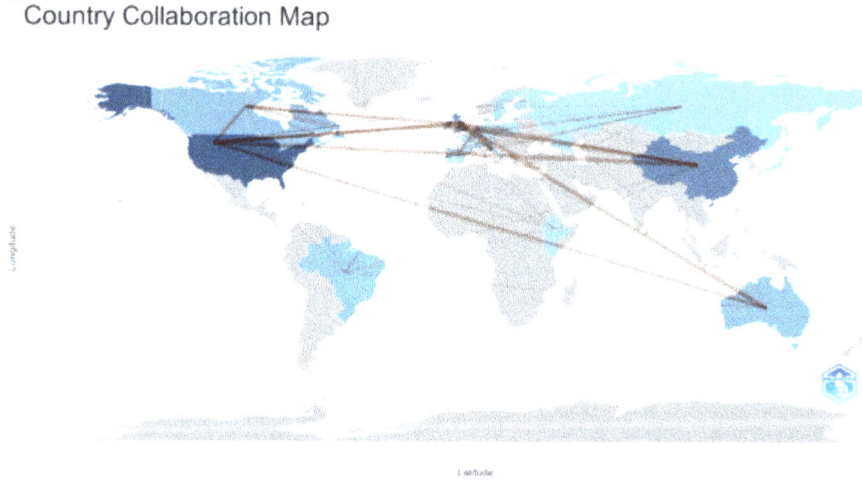

Source: Biblionshiny bibliometrix (2024)

Figure 3 presents the map of collaboration between countries on ICPs in the mental health of older adults. A worldwide map of collaboration between authors visually represents the collaborative relationships between researchers from different countries. These maps are constructed based on bibliometric analyses of scientific publications, which examine the co-authorship of articles and identify patterns of collaboration on a global scale.

An author collaboration map visually represents the collaborative relationships between researchers from different countries. These maps are constructed based on bibliometric analyses of scientific publications, which examine the co-authorship of articles and identify patterns of collaboration on a global scale. As noted, we observed an effective collaboration between countries and the institutions involved.

Each point on the map represents a country/region, institution, or author; the greater the radius of the point, the more articles are published. After identifying and analyzing relevant articles, we collected information about the authors and their institutional affiliations, including each author's country of origin.

By analyzing the map, we identified clusters of countries with solid collaboration relationships between some countries and patterns of collaboration in different regions of the world. This review identified a strong relationship between the USA, China, Canada, Australia, and the United Kingdom. In this context, a weak collaboration was found between Brazil and several other countries (Figure 3).

Collaborating Countries/Regions and Institutions Worldwide

One hundred seventy-five institutions in 28 countries/regions produced publications on ICPs in the mental health of older adults. Figure 2 provides additional information on the central countries and institutions related to productivity.

The five-most productive countries over time were the USA, China, the United Kingdom, Canada, and Australia. The USA had the most considerable amount of published literature. The USA's speed is relatively faster than other countries that study the subject (Figure 4). The USA emerged as the primary contributor in the number of authors, with 64 authors with published articles, followed by China (45), the United Kingdom (25), Canada (18), and Australia (16). In the case of Brazil, 10 authors were registered in the established period.

The top three institutions with the most significant scientific output on the topic (Figure 5) were the University of Toronto, the University of California, and Harvard University. This information can help one understand research trends in the area and identify potential collaborators or institutional partnerships.

Figure 6 shows the fourteen primary affiliations. By analyzing productions and affiliations over time, we can identify collaboration patterns between institutions and monitor the field's development over the years. In 2015, we identified an increase in the number of studies on the topic. In 2021, institutions increased their publications on ICPs in the mental health of older adults.

The findings indicate that North America is a leader in research on ICPs in the mental health of older adults. However, studies conducted in China and Oceania are growing over time. Identifying the most relevant countries and institutions in studies on ICPs in older adults' mental health provides a comprehensive overview of research in this field. It underscores the relevance of global collaboration to address the challenges and opportunities associated with aging.

Figure 4. Countries' production over time from 2013 to 2023

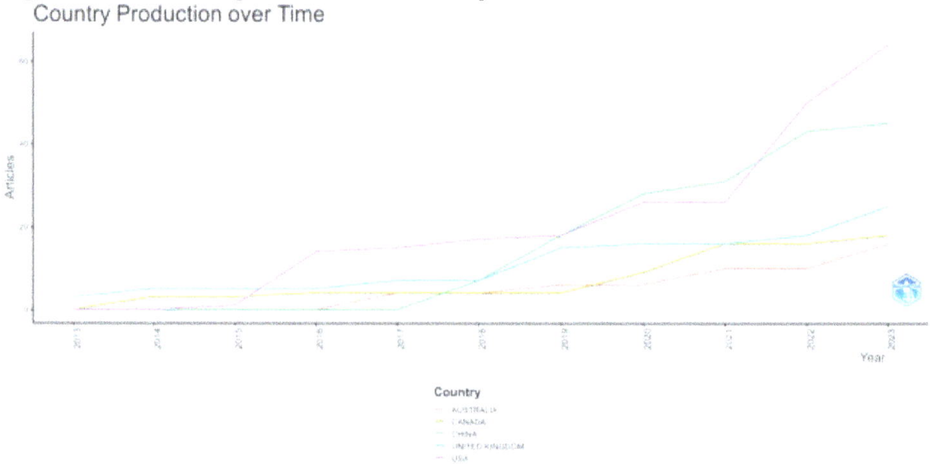

Capital Medical University (red), Fudan University (orange), Harvard Medical School (yellow), Harvard University (light green), King's College London (cyan), Peking University (dark green), Shanghai University of Traditional Chinese Medicine (light brown), Tianjin University of Traditional Chinese Medicine (light olive), University of Brasilia (dark green), University of California San Diego (blue), University of California System (purple), University of Toronto (violet), US Department of Veterans Affairs (pink), Veterans Health Administration (light red).

Figure 5. Most relevant institutions on the topic studied.

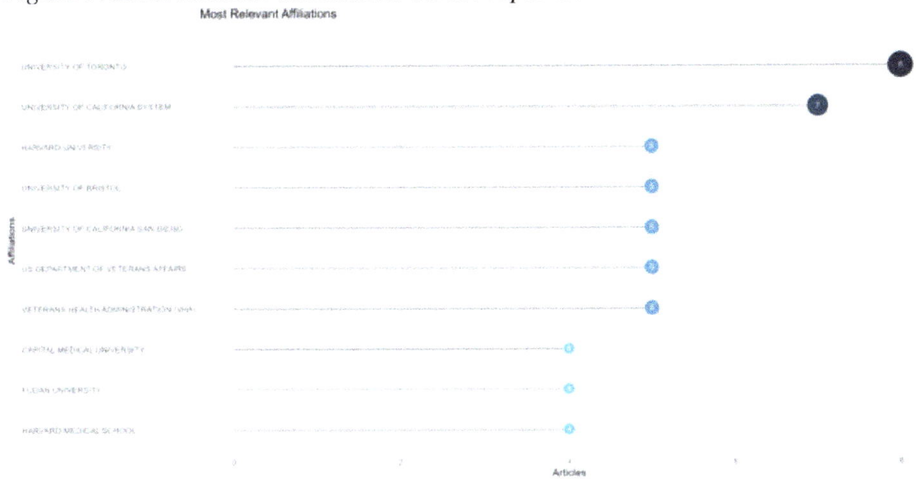

Source: Biblionshiny bibliometrix (2024)

Figure 6. Production and affiliations over time.

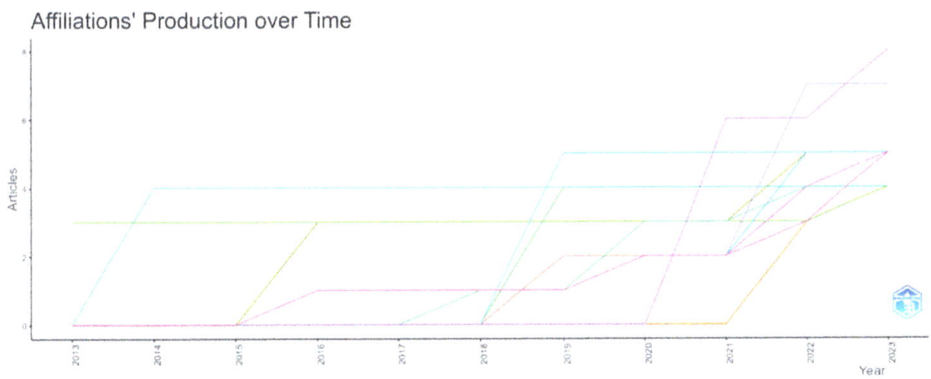

Note: *Colors represent the number of publications per country, with darker shades indicating higher publication counts.*

Most Cited Journals and Authors

The countries and journals mentioned are those whose researchers have contributed to the field, whether through publications, international collaborations, or scientific advances, expressed in quantitative citation values.

The present study identified 31 academic journals actively researching ICPs in the mental health of older adults worldwide. The quantitative data of the prominent journals (Figure 7) and the most relevant authors (Figure 8) were highlighted. The five most cited journals were Lancet (n=48) and J. Affect Disorders (n=39), Cochrane DB Syst Rev. (n=36), BMJ-Brit Med J. (n=33), and Jama Journal (n=32). New Zealand was the country with the highest number of citations (n=235), followed by the USA (n=192) and China (n=120).

Figure 7. Most cited journals from 2013 to 2023

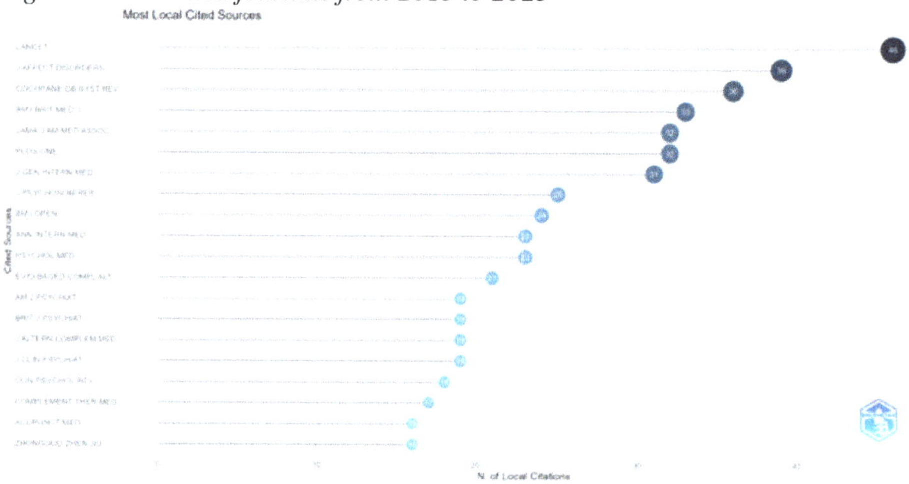

Source: Biblionshiny bibliometrix (2024)

Figure 8. Most relevant authors.

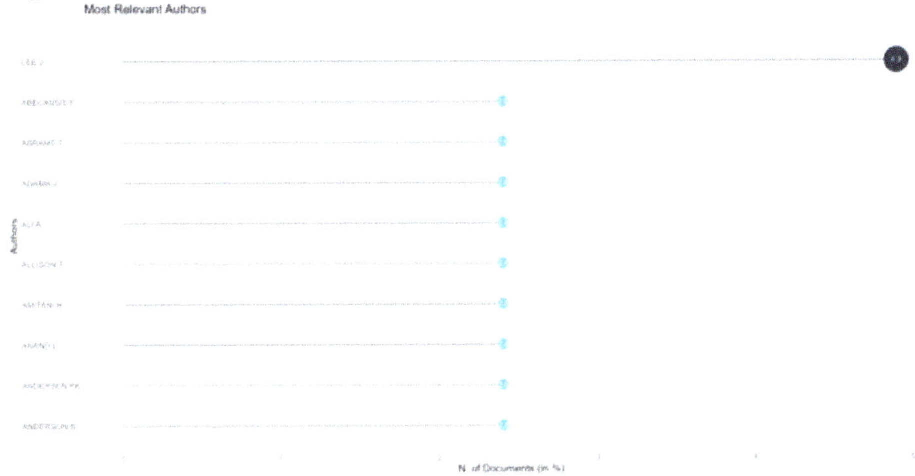

Note: *Circle sizes indicate the number of citations (larger circles = more citations).*

Number of Citations and Keywords

The global number of citations represents the total number of citations received by a document in all publications indexed in a source. In contrast, local citation refers to the number of citations a document received from other documents in the specific search performed (Figure 4).

Regarding the 2,644 references cited in the period analyzed (quantitative data), the Cochrane Database of Systematic Reviews was the most relevant source (n=232), followed by Lancet Psychiatry (n=98), Jama Internal Medicine (n=98), and Age and Ageing Journal (n=61). Thus, the three journals had the highest number of citations (Figure 11).

Regarding local impact per author, using the H-index, the Cochrane Database of Systematic Reviews and Frontiers in Psychiatry were the most relevant. In Table 2, it is possible to find the analysis of the G and M indices and their relationships with the total number of citations per author.

Figure 9. Local impact source by total citation index (TC)

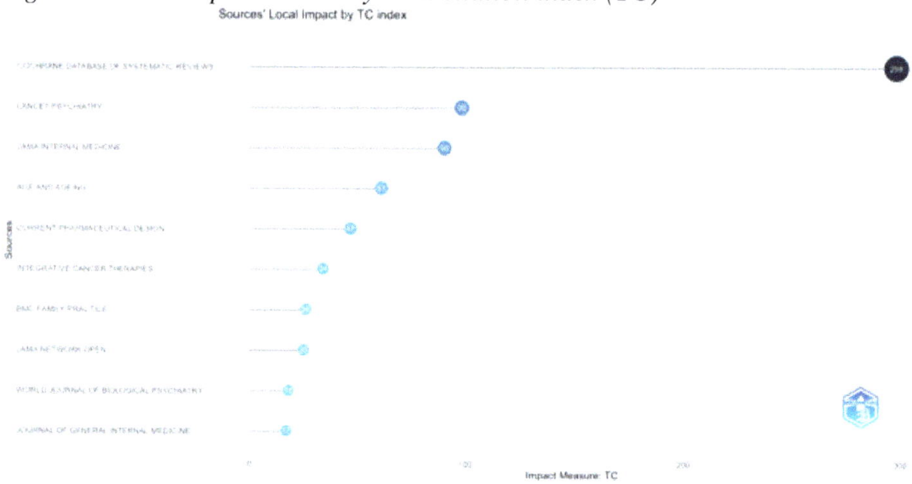

Source: Biblionshiny bibliometrix (2024)

Figure 10. Local impact of the author by H-index

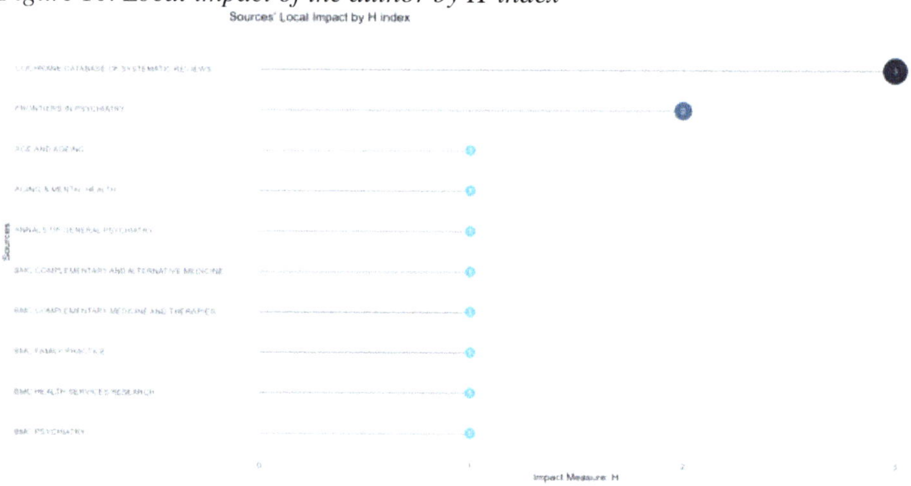

Figure 11. Most relevant keywords

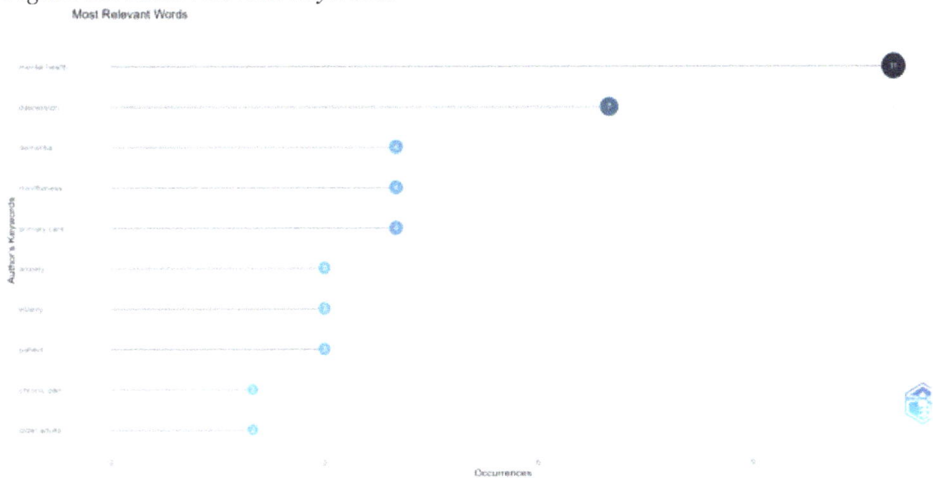

Figure 12. Cloud of keywords on ICPs in the mental health of older adults.

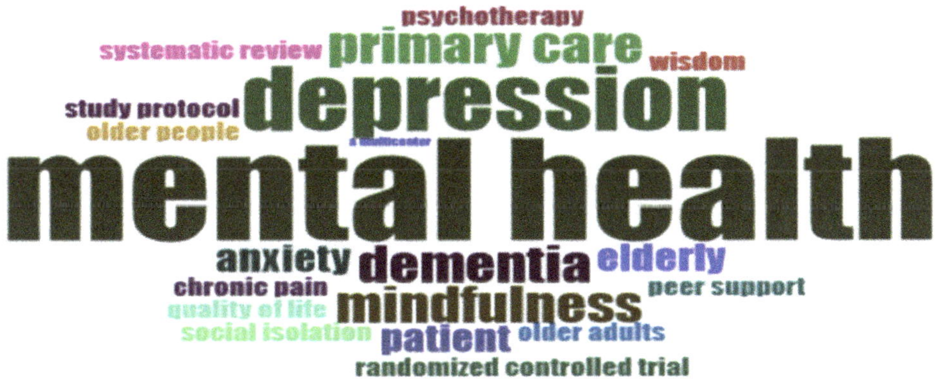

Note: *Circle sizes indicate the number of citations (larger circles = more citations).*

Table 2. Analysis of the G and M indexes and their relationships with the total number of citations

JOURNAL/DATABASE	G-INDEX	M-INDEX	TC	YEAR
Cochrane Database of Systematic Reviews	3	0.273	298	2014
Frontiers in Psychiatry	3	0.400	10	2020
Age and Ageing	1	0.143	61	2018
Aging & Mental Health	1	0.500	3	2023
Annals of General Psychiatry	1	0.200	13	2020
BMC Complementary and Alternative Medicine	1	0.091	13	2014
BMC Complementary Medicine and Therapies	2	0.333	7	2022
BMC Family Practice	1	0.083	26	2013
BMC Health Services Research	1	0.250	5	2021
BMC Psychiatry	1	0.167	10	2019

Bibliometrix/R-Studio (2024).

Keywords are crucial in indexing and efficiently searching for studies and scientific research. The present study identified 144 keywords, and the authors cited the most relevant ones as mental health (12%), depression (8%), and dementia (4%), which represent the central themes and concepts addressed (Figures 4C and 4D).

Figure 4E analyzes the cloud of keywords on ICPs in the mental health of older adults from 2003 to 2023. Terms "Integrative and Complementary Practices", "Mental Health", "Depression", and "Primary Care" are more prominent, reflecting the relevance of these concepts in the context of ICPs regarding the mental health of older adults.

We conducted a cluster analysis using appropriate processing techniques and clustering algorithms to identify similar groups of keywords based on their co-occurrence in the articles selected for this review. To this end, we adopted specialized software for bibliometric analysis and data visualization, VOSviewer version 1.6.2 (Figure 13).

Figure 13. Clusters formed from the authors' keywords

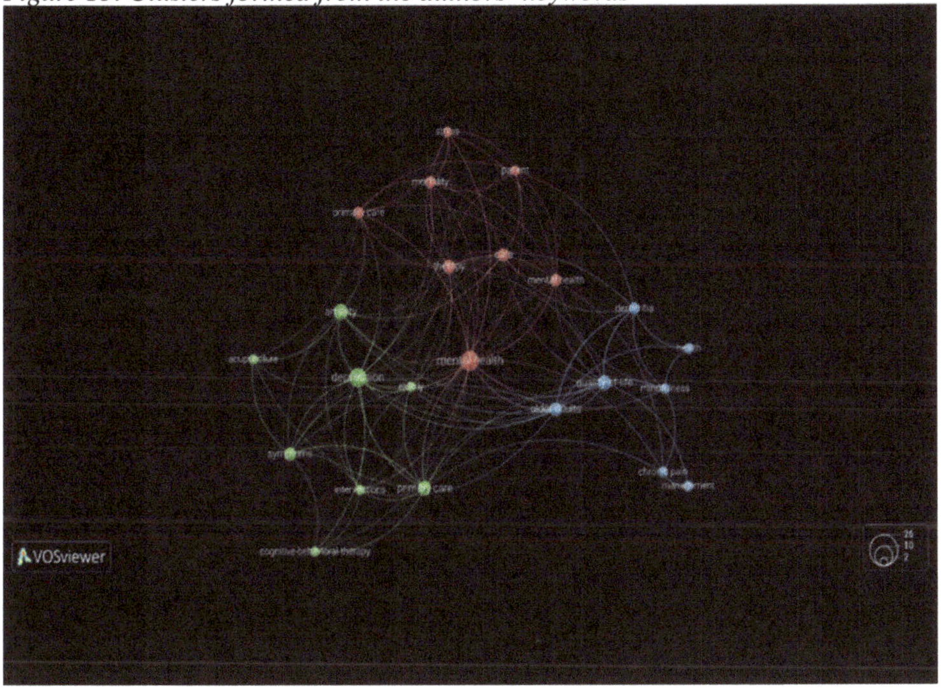

Source: *VosViewer (2024)*

4. DISCUSSION

We identified research trends, the leading countries, institutions, authors, and collaboration networks when analyzing the characteristics of global scientific production on the use of ICPs in the mental health of older adults treated in primary care. The results of this bibliometric review indicated that scientific production on the subject is still limited, especially in the WoS database, which underscores the need for a more in-depth debate and the promotion of additional research to better understand the use of ICPs in public health, especially regarding the mental health of older adults.

This bibliometric review highlights the increasing academic and policy interest in integrating ICPs into the mental health care of older adults, aligning with the global challenges highlighted by the Decade of Healthy Aging (2021–2030) proposed by the World Health Organization (WHO).

This growing need is driven by demographic shifts, such as global population aging, the increasing prevalence of chronic mental health conditions in older adults, and the limited effectiveness of current biomedical approaches to address the multifaceted needs of this population.

However, it is important to note that bibliometric findings reflect trends in scientific production and collaboration, not necessarily evidence of clinical effectiveness or an urgent need for widespread adoption.

Including ICPs in the mental healthcare of older adults reflects a paradigm shift towards a more integrative and patient-centered approach, aligning with global trends to promote healthy and holistic aging (Agarwal et al., 2016). As supported by previous studies, the biomedical model often overlooks psychological, social, and cultural dimensions of care, highlighting the need for integrative approaches like ICPs (Lindström and Eriksson, 2020; Smith et al., 2019).

As discussed in the literature review, population aging and the increased prevalence of chronic diseases and mental health problems require broader interventions considering individuals' physical, emotional, social, and spiritual aspects (Murniati et al., 2022).

Including ICPs in this context diversifies care, exceeding the traditional biomedical model, which is often insufficient to address the complex needs of this population.

We identified significant gaps in the literature on ICPs applied to the mental health of older adults throughout this study. These gaps include the scarcity of longitudinal studies examining long-term effects, heterogeneity in study designs and outcome measures, and the limited number of randomized controlled trials assessing the clinical efficacy of ICPs.

The bibliometric analysis revealed that, despite the progressive increase in scientific production since 2013, the topic remains underexplored, particularly in countries such as Brazil, where international collaboration is weak.

Although the United States and China have emerged as principal contributors in this field, Brazilian scientific production on the subject remains scarce, with few research initiatives in collaboration with other countries.

This contrast highlights the need to strengthen national research efforts, especially regarding implementing ICPs in the Unified Health System (SUS) and their inclusion in mental healthcare for older adults.

General Characteristics of the Bibliometric Analysis

The evolution of scientific production has revealed a gradual increase in the number of publications, especially since 2022, which may reflect the growing interest in ICPs due to the global population aging and the increasing challenges in the mental health of older adults (UN, 2021).

This growth is also related to strengthened public policies that encourage complementary practices in the SUS, as seen in the literature review. In Brazil, the National Policy on Integrative and Complementary Practices (PNPIC) was a milestone in including alternative therapies as an integral part of healthcare, following recommendations from the World Health Organization (Brazil, 2006).

The analysis revealed that 31 academic journals/databse are actively engaged in research on ICPs in the mental health of older adults, and the Lancet and Cochrane Database of Systematic Reviews had the highest citation numbers. These journals reflect the topic's relevance in global discussions on mental health and integrative practices.

However, as observed in the literature, ICPs still face challenges regarding their scientific validation and social acceptance (Magalhães et al., 2018). Despite recognizing their benefits, many health professionals and researchers still lack robust data proving their efficacy and safety.

Furthermore, one of the main barriers to broader adoption of ICPs is the limited availability of high-quality scientific evidence supporting their clinical efficacy. While there is growing enthusiasm, the absence of large-scale, rigorous clinical trials limits the credibility and acceptance of these practices among health professionals and policymakers.

Institutions, Countries, and Authors Involved

The analysis of institutional collaborations revealed that US universities, the University of Toronto, the University of California, and Harvard University are at the forefront of research on ICPs and the mental health of older adults. The strong presence of these institutions highlights the global impact of research conducted in these fields.

The literature review also underscores the relevance of academic institutions in developing innovative health policies and practices, especially in aging and chronic diseases (WHO, 2021).

The research also indicated that, although the USA and China lead the field of ICPs in the mental health of older adults, Brazil has negligible participation, with few publications and international collaborations. In the United States, research has focused largely on randomized controlled trials and pragmatic trials assessing the effectiveness of integrative approaches, while in China, numerous studies have examined the incorporation of Traditional Chinese Medicine within community health settings.

The literature review highlighted the role of the Family Health Strategy (ESF) and Primary Health Care (APS) in integrating ICPs into the comprehensive care of older adults but adopting these practices still needs to be expanded and better investigated (Azevedo et al., 2020).

Analysis of Co-Occurrence of Keywords and Journals

The keyword co-occurrence analysis indicated that "mental health", "depression", and "dementia" are the most frequent terms associated with ICPs in the mental health of older adults. These findings suggest that despite increasing academic activity, significant challenges remain in translating research into effective mental health interventions for older adults (World Health Organization/WHO, 2013; Andrade et al., 2010).

By complementing traditional pharmacological approaches, ICPs offer a viable and less invasive alternative for managing these conditions, improving the quality of life of older adults, as pointed out by studies such as that of Aguiar, Kanan, and Masiero (2019).

Relevant Points and Significant Topics of the Studies

The main topics addressed in the analyzed publications are related to reducing the prevalence of mental disorders in older adults and promoting well-being through ICPs. As previously discussed, these practices do not replace conventional treatment but complement care by offering interventions focused on self-care, stress reduction, and promoting comprehensive health (Magalhães et al., 2018; Habimorad et al., 2020).

Demystifying ICPs and their broader acceptance among health professionals are central issues that need to be addressed in future studies. The literature review showed that, while many studies recognize ICPs as safe and effective, their implementation in the SUS still faces barriers regarding infrastructure and professional training (Brazil, 2018).

The analysis of the most productive countries in the field of ICPs, such as the USA and China, reflects the greater acceptance of these practices in these contexts, which can be explained by the strong tradition of using Traditional Chinese Medicine and complementary therapies, such as acupuncture, widely adopted in the health systems of these countries.

On the other hand, Brazil still faces challenges in implementing these practices, as evidenced by the low scientific production on the subject and the weak international collaboration identified in our findings.

This study has some limitations. Notably, the bibliometric review was based on a single database (WoS), which may have excluded relevant publications from other sources. Moreover, the analysis was restricted to articles in English, which may limit the scope of the findings, especially considering the Brazilian backdrop, where scientific production on ICPs may be more developed in publications in Portuguese.

Additionally, it is important to acknowledge that the broader field of ICPs in mental health research still faces limitations in the strength and consistency of available evidence. Previous studies in this area present heterogeneous methodologies, small sample sizes, or limited generalizability, which underscores the need for future research focused on rigorous clinical evaluation (Wang et al., 2020; Zhang et al., 2010; Lindström; Erikisson, 2020).

These findings suggest that despite a growing academic interest, there remains a disconnect between research production and practical implementation, especially in low- and middle-income countries.

Future research should prioritize randomized controlled trials, long-term follow-up studies, and systematic reviews to evaluate the clinical efficacy, safety, and cost-effectiveness of ICPs in older adults' mental health care. Additionally, studies focusing on health system integration and policy implementation will be essential to bridge the gap between evidence and practice.

5. CONCLUSION

This study conducted a comprehensive bibliometric analysis of global research on Integrative and Complementary Practices (ICPs) in the mental health care of older adults. It identified publication trends, key contributing countries and institutions, research gaps, and methodological patterns, providing valuable insights into the current state of the field.

The bibliometric analysis conducted in this study revealed that, although the number of studies on ICPs has gradually increased in recent years, their global dissemination and effective integration into healthcare systems—especially within the domain of mental health—remain limited. Implementation of ICPs is still underexplored and undervalued in many national contexts, including Brazil, where there is a noticeable lack of international collaborations and applied research efforts.

Therefore, this study highlights the importance of continuing to disseminate, investigate, and critically analyze ICPs—not only as a research focus but also as a promising area with potential applicability for the mental healthcare of older adults, while recognizing the need for further scientific validation.

However, it is essential to recognize that the broader acceptance and integration of ICPs depend on strengthening the evidence base supporting their clinical efficacy, safety, and long-term outcomes.

Advancing this knowledge may contribute to the informed development of public policies, encourage greater acceptance among health professionals and decision-makers, and, in the future, support the thoughtful expansion of ICPs within the Unified Health System (SUS), fostering more humanized and effective care for the older adult population.

REFERENCES

Agarwal, A., Durairajanayagam, D., Tatagari, S., Esteves, S. C., Harlev, A., Henkel, R., Roychoudhury, S., Homa, S., Puchalt, N. G., Ramasamy, R., Majzoub, A., Ly, K. D., Tvrda, E., Assidi, M., Kesari, K., Sharma, R., Banihani, S., Ko, E., Abu-Elmagd, M., & Bashiri, A. (2016). Bibliometrics: Tracking research impact by selecting the appropriate metrics. *Asian Journal of Andrology*, *18*(2), 296–309. DOI: 10.4103/1008-682X.171582 PMID: 26806079

Aguiar, J., Kanan, L. A., & Masiero, A. V. (2019). Práticas integrativas e complementares na atenção básica em saúde: Um estudo bibliométrico da produção brasileira. *Saúde em Debate*, *43*(123), 1205–1218. DOI: 10.1590/0103-1104201912318

Amonkar, N., Su, W. C., Bhat, A. N., & Srinivasan, S. M. (2021). Effects of creative movement therapies on social communication, behavioral-affective, sensorimotor, cognitive, and functional participation skills of individuals with autism spectrum disorder: A systematic review. *Frontiers in Psychiatry*, *12*, 722874. DOI: 10.3389/fpsyt.2021.722874 PMID: 34867515

Andrade, F. B. D., & Ferreira Filho, M. de O., Dias, M. D., Silva, A. O., Costa, I. do C. C., De Lima, É. A. R., & Mendes, C. K. T. (2010). Promoção da saúde mental do idoso na atenção básica: As contribuições da Terapia Comunitária. *Texto & Contexto - Enfermagem*, *19*(1), 129–136. https://doi.org/DOI: 10.1590/S0104-07072010000100015

Azevedo e Silva, G., Giovanella, L., & De Camargo, K. R.Jr. (2020). Brazil's National Health Care System at risk for losing its universal character. *American Journal of Public Health*, *110*(6), 811–812. DOI: 10.2105/AJPH.2020.305649 PMID: 32374681

Básica. Política Nacional de Práticas Integrativas e Complementares no SUS - PNPIC- SUS, 1ª Ed. Brasília; 2006. 92 p. Available: < https://bvsms.saude.gov.br/bvs/saudelegis/gm/2006/prt0971_03_05_2006.html >

Basso, J. C., McHale, A., Ende, V., Oberlin, D. J., & Suzuki, W. A. (2019). Brief, daily meditation enhances attention, memory, mood, and emotional regulation in non-experienced meditators. *Behavioural Brain Research*, *356*, 208–220. DOI: 10.1016/j.bbr.2018.08.023 PMID: 30153464

Bitta, M. A., Kariuki, S. M., Gona, J., Abubakar, A., Newton, C. R., & Alcock, K. (2019). Priority mental, neurological and substance use disorders in rural Kenya: Traditional health practitioners' and primary health care workers' perspectives. *PLoS One*, *14*(7), e0220034. DOI: 10.1371/journal.pone.0220034 PMID: 31335915

Cano-López, I., Aliño, M., Duque, A., Martínez, P., & Meléndez, J. C. (2021). Educational level as a protective factor against the influence of depressive symptoms on cognition in older adults: Implications for functional independence during a 10-year follow-up. *International Psychogeriatrics*, *33*(8), 813–825. DOI: 10.1017/S1041610221000272 PMID: 33762060

Carvalho, J. L. D. S., & Nóbrega, M. D. P. S. (2017). Complementary therapies as resources for mental health in Primary Health Care. *Revista Gaúcha de Enfermagem*, *38*(4), e2017–e2014. DOI: 10.1590/1983-1447.2017.04.2017-2014 PMID: 29791533

Casagrande, A., Fabris, F., & Girometti, R. (2020). Beyond kappa: An informational index for diagnostic agreement in dichotomous and multivalue ordered-categorical ratings. *Medical & Biological Engineering & Computing*, *58*(12), 3089–3099. DOI: 10.1007/s11517-020-02261-2 PMID: 33145661

Chang, Y. K., Erickson, K. I., Aghjayan, S. L., Chen, F. T., & Lin, S. (2022). The multi-domain exercise intervention for memory and brain function in late middle-aged and older adults at risk for Alzheimer's disease: A protocol for Western-Eastern Brain Fitness Integration Training trial. *Frontiers in Aging Neuroscience*, *14*, 929789. DOI: 10.3389/fnagi.2022.929789 PMID: 36062144

Cui, R., Liu, H., Li, M., Wang, J., Wang, L., & Han, L. (2023). Effects of "Taking the Waist as the Axis" Therapy on trunk postural control disorder after stroke: A randomized controlled trial. *Frontiers in Aging Neuroscience*, *15*, 1040277. DOI: 10.3389/fnagi.2023.1040277 PMID: 36819714

Daniele, T. M., Bruin, V. M., Oliveira, D. S., Pompeu, C. M., & Forti, A. C. (2013). Associations among physical activity, comorbidities, depressive symptoms and health-related quality of life in type 2 diabetes. *Arquivos Brasileiros de Endocrinologia & Metabologia*, *57*(1), 44–50. DOI: 10.1590/S0004-27302013000100006 PMID: 23440098

Habimorad, P. H. L., Catarucci, F. M., Bruno, V. H. T., Silva, I. B. D., & Bernardes, L. C. (2020). Implementation of Brazil's National Policy on Complementary and Integrative Practices: Strengths and weaknesses. *Ciencia & Saude Coletiva*, *25*(2), 395–405. DOI: 10.1590/1413-81232020252.11332018 PMID: 32022181

Lindström, B., & Eriksson, M. (2020). Complexity, Reductionism and the Biomedical Model. In *Health Promotion in Health Care – Vital Theories and Research* (pp. 57–70). Springer., DOI: 10.1007/978-3-030-63135-2

Luo, H., Li, J., Zhang, Q., Cao, P., Ren, X., Fang, A., Liao, H., & Liu, L. (2018). Obesity and the onset of depressive symptoms among middle-aged and older adults in China: Evidence from the CHARLS. *BMC Public Health*, *18*(1), 909. DOI: 10.1186/s12889-018-5834-6 PMID: 30041632

Murniati, N., Al Aufa, B., Kusuma, D., & Kamso, S. (2022). A scoping review on biopsychosocial predictors of mental health among older adults. *International Journal of Environmental Research and Public Health*, *19*(17), 10789. DOI: 10.3390/ijerph191710909 PMID: 36078627

Padilha, C. O. S., & De Oliveira, W. F. (2013). Representação social do terapeuta comunitário no Sistema Único de Saúde. *Ciencia & Saude Coletiva*, *18*(8), 2211–2220. DOI: 10.1590/S1413-81232013000800005 PMID: 23896903

Pritchard, A. (1969). Statistical bibliography or bibliometrics? *The Journal of Documentation*, *25*(4), 348–349.

Zhang, A.. (2010). Clinical Studies with Traditional Chinese Medicine in the Past Decade: A Review. *Chinese Journal of Integrative Medicine*, *16*(1), 1–7.

Chapter 5
Communication-Enabling Materials in Healthcare: Narrative Review

Stefanie Azeredo Tomás
https://orcid.org/0000-0002-7293-4860
Escola Superior de Saúde Fernando Pessoa, Portugal

Maria Conceição Manso
https://orcid.org/0000-0002-1774-1337
Universidade Fernando Pessoa, RISE-Health, Portugal

Fátima Maia
https://orcid.org/0000-0003-4698-2284
Escola Superior de Saúde Fernando Pessoa, RISE-Health, Portugal

ABSTRACT

The effectiveness of communication in the context of health care delivery is increasingly emphasized and discussed, not only because of the importance of the relationship established between the health care professional and the patient, but also because it increases the overall quality of care. Ineffective communication is the consequence of the existence of communicative barriers resulting from the patient's own health/emergency situation and/or pre-existing communicative conditions. The mission of this chapter is to present materials that facilitate communication in the provision of health care in different contexts and to identify some related needs. Communication Facilitating Materials were searched on different databases, books and several reference sites. The authors identified (n=79) and grouped into three categories: communication support, information to professionals and to preparation/ anticipation of situations. The results highlight the need to develop more materials to enhance communication in health care services as an integral component of

DOI: 10.4018/979-8-3693-6432-1.ch005

population health promotion.

INTRODUCTION

It is through communication that human beings are able to learn, interact with others and develop at a personal level. It assumes a fundamental role in the provision of health care services (Beukelman & Mirenda, 2013; Naughton, 2018), both relationally and in terms of intervention and patient satisfaction (Blackstone et. al., 2011; The Joint Commission, 2022), and even in terms of cost reduction for the entities involved (Blackstone et. al., 2011; Hurtig et al., 2019). According to The Joint Commission (USA) (2022), effective communication in the context of health care services is when professionals and their patients exchange information, so that the patients can participate in their own intervention. This becomes especially relevant in virtual or telehealth settings, where communication challenges can be amplified for patients using AAC (Beneteau et al., 2022). Since communication is a human right health care professionals, by giving importance to the concerns and wishes of patients and/or their caregivers/family members, are able to achieve greater confidence in the treatment (Ahmed, 2020; Benson, 2014; Blackstone, 2018; Naughton, 2018; Khan et al., 2018; Topia & Hocking, 2012). Thus, effective communication also positively influences the patient's quality of life and safety (Blackstone et al., 2011; Blackstone, 2015; Khan et al., 2018; Naughton, 2018) and is fundamental to understanding the patient holistically and knowing his/her needs (Alcântara et al., 2016; Khan et al., 2018). It is then important that health professionals let the patients state their wills/opinions so that this exchange of information allows both (health professionals and patients) to be understood (Benson, 2014; Beukelman e Mirenda, 2013; Levinson et al., 1997; Naughton, 2018). It is therefore essential to adopt an equity-centered approach to inclusive communication — in which the terminology and narratives used are consistent with how the target audience sees and understands themselves, as well as their characteristics, and can thus reaching more people and, therefore, being more effective (Boston University Medical Group, Office of Equity, Vitality, and Inclusion, and BUMC Faculty Development and Diversity, 2022). These aspects, among others, are highlighted in the Health Equity Guiding Principles for Inclusive Communication (Centers for Disease Control and Prevention, 2024).

However, communication is not always effective in the provision of health care services, since the patient cannot always adequately understand the health professional and/or the health professional does not understand the patient, and this situation may be associated with different types of communication barriers (Zubow & Hurtig, 2013). A communicative barrier is any situation in which the transmitted message is not decoded by the receiver (Blackstone, 2015), that is, when there is difficulty in transmission, processing and/or understanding of verbal and/or nonverbal concepts (ASHA, 1993; Blackstone, 2015; Holm et al., 2021).

Therefore, communication in health interventions should not only focus on oral verbal communication but also be focused on other signs/forms of communication, so that the therapeutic plan, the intervention and the results can be more appropriate and effective, as is the responsibility of health professionals (Araújo et al., 2007; Greenslade, 2021). For this, it is essential that health care professionals use communicative tools to be able to communicate effectively with all their patients, so that the quality of care increases significantly (Finke et al., 2008; Greenslade, 2021). Therefore, it is essential to give importance to communication and to instruct all healthcare professionals in the area of communication, so that they can more easily implement communicative strategies, involve the patient and family members in the intervention, and provide more time to respond to patients (Hemsley & Baladin, 2014; Holm et al., 2021; Hopf & White, 2021). In this process, the use of materials specifically for this purpose can be of extreme importance (Hanberg & Voss, 2018; Holm et al., 2021; Thunberg et al., 2016).

The aim of this article was to present materials that facilitate communication in the provision of health care and to identify some related needs in a narrative review form. It is considered that this compilation of information could be useful for the international context, in addition to analysing the Portuguese reality in particular.

BACKGROUND

For the development of this work, facilitating communication materials were searched on different databases (B-on, SciELO, PubMed and Cochrane) and books. The search terms and strategy are given in Box 1. To complement the results that were found, additional research was conducted including several reference sites.

Database search strategy listing database search terms used:

1. AAC AND tools
2. AAC AND instrument
3. AAC OR augmentative and alternative communication AND instruments OR tools OR scales
4. Communication healthcare AND tools
5. Healthcare AND ambulance OR paramedic OR emergency medical service
6. Communication tools AND ambulance OR paramedic OR emergency medical service
7. AAC AND ambulance OR paramedic OR emergency medical service

8. Without language restriction and time limitation

Data collected were treated through thematic and content analysis techniques, based on the purpose of each material. The data analysis followed three steps: 1) Reading and comprehension of the materials; 2) Identification of the base units; 3) Clipping (data was grouped into units and categories). The unit of analysis adopted was the usefulness/function of the material, which allowed to obtain categories and subcategories, checked by two evaluators. There are some communication-facilitating materials that have more than one utility/function, and for this reason are referenced in more than one category. The categories are presented with an indication of the number of materials that meet the purpose associated with them, so the total number of references in categories and subcategories is higher than the total number of materials examined.

A total of 79 health care communication facilitators were identified. From the data analysis, three distinct categories emerged, based on the purpose of each material, each with subcategories, as shown in Figure 1.

Figure 1. Categories of the 79 communication-facilitating materials identified in the Health Care Delivery Context, and subcategories according to the function of the materials (their accounting (no.) in parentheses)

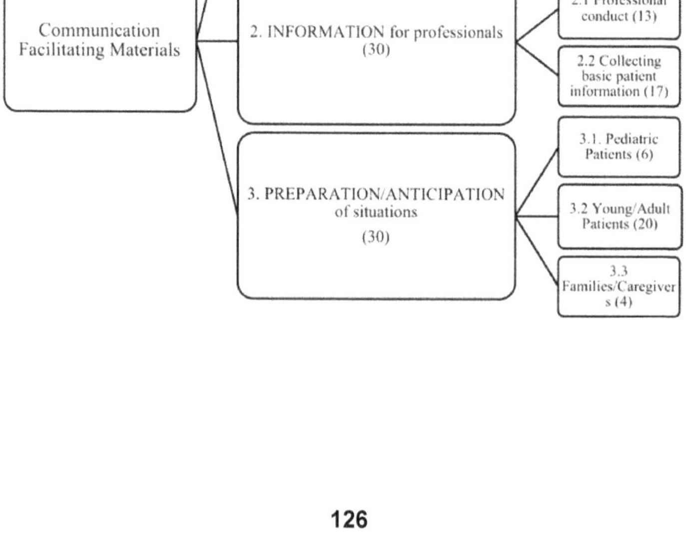

The category "Communication SUPPORT" refers to material that supports communication in health care delivery, either to support health care professionals or to support the patients themselves. This category is divided into three subcategories, concerning the specific context in which the communication support material is used, namely: Health care services in different contexts (12 materials); Health care services in pre-hospital emergencies (13 materials) and health care services in hospital environment (6 materials).

The second category "INFORMATION for Professionals" includes specific material for health professionals, with the purpose of providing important information about the patient, such as: general patient information, the patient's preferred form of communication (when necessary), how to behave in certain situations, among others. This category is subdivided into two subcategories related to Professional Conduct (13 materials) and Gathering basic information from the patient (17 materials).

The third category "PREPARATION/ANTECIPATION of Situations" refers to materials to prepare the professional and/or the patient for a future health care situation by, for example, filling out a checklist, emergency plans, among others. It focuses on materials that belong to the subcategories: Paediatric Patients (6 materials); Young/Adult Patients (20 materials); Families/Caregivers (4 materials).

The results of each category and corresponding subcategories are presented in Tables 1 to 3 in a detailed and systematized way for the support for communication, Tables 4 to 5 regarding information for professionals and Tables 6 to 8 for the preparation/anticipation of situations. These tables compile information about the sites where more information about the materials can be found, their format (digital/paper), recipients (who will use the material), whether the material considers the provision of health care services to people with Disability/Special Needs (SN), the context of action (where the material can be used - this information concerns only Categories 2 and 3), the existing material resources in Portuguese and also which materials are mentioned in another category.

1. Communication SUPPORT

Table 1 summarizes the existing communication SUPPORT materials in the provision of health care services in different contexts and shows that most of them are in paper format (there are only 3 materials in digital format). All of them were created to be used by health professionals and, mostly, to assist people with SN. With respect to language, few materials are adapted to the Portuguese language.

Table 1. Results from Category 1 "communication support" in the provision of health care services (12 materials)

Subcategory: 1.1. Provision of health care services in a variety of contexts (12)	More information	Material format	Users	People with SN	Material in Portuguese**
Vidatalk	https://www.vidatak.com/vidatalk.ml	Digital [Android e IPAD]	Professionals	√	
EZ Board (communication board)	https://www.vidatak.com/ezboards.html	Digital + Paper [Android e IPAD]	Professionals	√	(just the words board)
Basic Medical Signs Language*	https://www.slideshare.net/kratzkek/basic -medical-sign-language	Paper	Professionals	√	
The Hospital Communication Book *- various forms of communication	http://www.surreyhealthaction.org/downloads/ Hospital%20Communication%20Book%20 -%20version%202%20-%20web.pdf	Paper (Book)	Professionals	√	
Home & Health set	http://www.greenhousepub.com/homehealthset .html	Paper (Cards/ images)	Professionals	√	
Patient Communication Board	https://widgit-health.com/	Paper	Professionals	√	
Medical Encounters Board	https://widgit-health.com/download-files/ medical-encounter-board/MEB-grid-A4.pdf	Paper	Professionals	√	
Health Care Communication Board	https://www.amazon.com/EZ-Board-Vidatak -Patient-Communication/dp/B01A72VXV0	Paper	Professionals	√	
Communication Board Medical (Tobiidynavox)	https://www.tobiidynavox.com/globalassets/ downloads/special-events/communication -board-hurricane-harvey1.pdf	Digital	Professionals	√	
Refugee Communication Boards	https://www.tobiidynavox.com/support -training/downloads/boardmaker/refugee -communication-boards/	Paper	Professionals		Multiple Languages
I Speak...	https://www.dhs.gov/xlibrary/assets/crcl/crcl-i -speak-booklet.pdf	Paper	Professionals		Multiple Languages
Critical Communicator	https://www.alimed.com/the-critical -communicator.html?refSrc=82431&nosto= productpage-nosto-1	Paper	Professionals	√	Multiple Languages

*These materials are also referenced in Category 2. INFORMATION for professionals; SN - Special Needs; **English, if nothing is mentioned.

With regard to the SUPPORT materials for communication in the Providing of Health Care in Pre-Hospital Emergency (Table 2), it is again perceptible that there are more materials in paper format than digital (there is only one digital). However, regarding the recipients, in this subcategory, it is possible to verify that the materials are not only addressed to health professionals, but also to other users, such as patients and caregivers. Most of these materials are adapted for people with SN, with only one in Portuguese language.

Table 2. Results from Category 1 "communication support" in the Providing of Health Care in Pre-Hospital Emergency (13 materials)

Subcategory: 1.2. Pre-Hospital Emergency (13)	**More information**	**Material format**	**Users**	**People with SN**	**Material in Portuguese****
Paramedic & EMS Symbol Board	https://widgit-health.com/downloads/paramedic-board.htm	Paper	Professionals	√	
First Aid Communication Book	https://widgit-health.com/first-aid-communication-booklet.htm	Paper (Book A5)	Professionals	√	
First Response Communication Book	https://widgit-health.com/first-response-communication-book.htm	Paper	Professionals	√	
Emergency Multilingual Phrasebook (for those who don't speak the language)	https://health.wyo.gov/wp-content/uploads/2016/04/43-5873_DH_4073282.pdf	Paper (Book)	Professionals		√ (Adaptation for children required; written only)
Communication Book (British RedCross)	https://www.widgit.com/success-stories/health-emergency-justice/british-red-cross.htm	Paper (Book)	Professionals	√	
Emergencia! Emergency Translation Manual (for those who are not fluent in Spanish)	https://www.amazon.com/Emergencia-Translation-Lisa-Maitland-Hernandez/dp/0766836266	Paper (Book)	Professionals		
Emergency Medical Services Visual Language Translator – considers different languages	https://www.kwikpoint.com/products-page/fire-and-ems-prodcat/emergency-medical-services-visual-language-translator-2009-health-information-awards-gold-winner/	Paper (Compact and small (pocket size))	Professionals		
First Responder Communication Boards *	http://www.greenhousepub.com/fireco.html	Paper	Professionals, Patients and Caregivers	√	
Emergency communication 4all *	https://rems.ed.gov/docs/TempleUniv_FeelingSafe.pdf	Paper	Professionals, Patients and Caregivers	√	
ICE Communication Cards*	https://widgit-health.com/ICE-communication-cards.htm	Paper (the size of an unfolded credit card)	Professionals, Patients and Caregivers	√	
Pre-Hospital Communication APP	https://apkpure.com/br/pre-hospital-communication-app/com.wast.prehospitalcommunication	Digital	Professionals, Patients and Caregivers	√	
Communication Picture Boards	https://www.eadassociates.com	Paper	Professionals, Patients and Caregivers	√	
EC4all – APP	https://play.google.com/store/apps/details?id=com.createabilityinc.EC4All&hl=en	Digital	Professionals, Patients and Caregivers	√	

*These materials are also referenced in Category 2. INFORMATION for professionals; SN - Special Needs; **English, if nothing is mentioned.

When it comes to communication SUPPORT materials oriented for use in Health Care Delivery in Hospitals (Table 3), it is possible to understand that there are no materials in digital format, and that all of them are addressed to multiple recipients (Professionals, Patients and Caregivers). Also in this subcategory, it is possible to verify that almost all materials are adjusted for people with SN, with only two in Portuguese language.

Table 3. Results from Category 1 "communication support" materials oriented for use in Health Care Delivery in Hospitals (6 materials)

Subcategory: 1.3. Hospital (6)	More information	Material format	Users	People with SN	Material in Portuguese**
Patient Communication Sheet	https://widgit-health.com/patient-communication-sheet.htm	Paper (communication board)	Professionals, Patients and Caregivers	√	
Discomforts and Requests…	https://www.yumpu.com/en/desmaiar	Paper (writing)	Professionals, Patients and Caregivers		√
Bedside Messages (also for pediatrics)	https://widgit-health.com/downloads/bedside-messages.htm	Paper	Professionals, Patients and Caregivers	√	√
Health Care Communication APP	https://greenhousepublications.stores.yahoo.net/index.html	Digital	Professionals, Patients and Caregivers	√ It has a pediatric part	
General Questions	https://widgit-health.com/download-files/medical-encounter-board/MEB-grid-A4.pdf	Paper	Professionals, Patients and Caregivers	√	
The Hospital Communication Book section downloads *	http://www.surreyhealthaction.org/downloads/Hospital%20Communication%20Book%20-%20version%202%20-%20web.pdf	Paper (board)	Professionals, Patients and Caregivers	√	

*These materials are also referenced in Category 2. INFORMATION for professionals; SN - Special Needs; **English, if nothing is mentioned.

2. INFORMATION to professionals

In this second category on the subcategory Professional Conduct (Table 4), there is only one material in digital format in a total of 13 materials, to be used practically in Emergency and Hospital contexts. It is also remarkable the existence of only one material to be used in the context of Pre-hospital emergency, not having found any material in Portuguese language.

Table 4. Category 2 Results: Information to professionals (13 materials)

Subcategory: 2.1. professional conduct (13)	More information	Material format	Users	People with SN	Material in Portuguese**
Tips for Emergency Responders	http://cdd.unm.edu/dhpd/tips/tipsenglish.html	Paper	Emergency	√	
Advancing Effective Communication, Cultural Competence, and Family-Centered Care (A roadmap for Hospitals)	https://www.jointcommission.org/-/media/tjc/documents/resources/patient-safety-topics/health-equity/aroadmapforhospitalsfinalversion727pdf.pdf	Paper (Book)	Hospital	√	
Have we supported you during emergency? [satisfaction survey British Red Cross]	https://feedback.redcross.org.uk/s/CR-CRWB/	Digital	Pre-hospital emergency		
Your stay in hospital [satisfaction survey]	http://www.surreyhealthaction.org/going-to-hospital-section/the-hospital-questionnaires.html	Paper	Hospital	√	
Basic Medical Signs Language	https://www.slideshare.net/kratzkek/basic-medical-sign-language	Paper	Hospital	√	
The Hospital Communication Book*	http://www.surreyhealthaction.org/downloads/Hospital%20Communication%20Book%20-%20version%202%20-%20web.pdf	Paper (Book)	Hospital	√	
Improving Communication with Patients who have Intellectual and Developmental Disabilities	http://flfcic.fmhi.usf.edu/docs/FCIC_PhysicianFactSheet_1_Improving_Communication.pdf	Paper	Hospital	√	
Access and Functional Needs (AFN) Checklist	https://disabilities.temple.edu/programs/eprep/docs/afn-checklist-interactive-2017-1221.pdf	Paper	Emergency	√	
Durable Medical Equipment (DME) and Assistive Technology (AT) Emergency planning Guide	https://disabilities.temple.edu/programs/eprep/docs/PA-DOH-DME-GUIDE-2017-12.pdf	Paper	Emergency	√	
Checklist for integrating people with disabilities and others with access and Functional Needs into Emergency Preparedness, Planning, Response & Recovery	http://www.jik.com/planckl st.pdf	Paper	Emergency	√	
Be real, Specific and current: emergency preparedness information for people with disabilities and others with access and functional needs	http://www.jik.com/pubs/RealEPtips.pdf	Paper	Emergency	√	

continued on following page

Table 4. Continued

Subcategory: 2.1. professional conduct (13)	More information	Material format	Users	People with SN	Material in Portuguese**
Disaster Preparedness tips for emergency Management Personnel	https://aac-rerc.psu.edu/_userfiles/file/TipsForEMP.pdf	Paper	Emergency	√	
Emergency Checklist for People with communication Access and Functional Needs	https://disabilities.temple.edu/programs/eprep/docs/afn-checklist-interactive-2017-1221.pdf	Paper	Emergency	√	

*This material is also referenced in Category 1. communication SUPPORTs; SN - Special Needs; **English, if nothing is mentioned.

The subcategory Collecting Basic Patient Information (Table 5), refers to material that gathers information about patients, that could be useful for health professionals. They can be used by different users, according to their age group, i.e.: paediatric users, senior users and/or users without age specification. They can also be used by Caregivers. All the materials identified are in paper format. The context of application of the materials is mostly for use in the Emergency Department, followed by the Hospital environment, with reference to only one material which can also be used at home by family members.

Table 5. Category 2 Results: Information to professionals regarding their patients (17 materials)

Subcategory: 2.2. gathering basic information from the user (17)	More information	Material format	Users	Operating context	People with SN	Material in Portuguese***
Emergency Information Form for Children with Special Needs	https://www.survival-goods.com/Emergency-Information-Form-For-Children-With-Special-Needs-s/371.htm	Paper	Paediatric Patients	Emergency	√	
Emergency Readiness Wheel for Seniors **	http://www.eadassociates.com/seniors.html	Paper	Senior Patients	Emergency		
Emergency Communication 4all *	https://rems.ed.gov/docs/TempleUniv_FeelingSafe.pdf	Paper	Patients without age specification	Emergency	√	
ICE Communication Cards*	https://widgit-health.com/ICE-communication-cards.htm	Paper (size of 1 folding credit card)	Patients without age specification	Emergency	√	
Cartão de Emergêncial Emergency ID Card [INEM+ police +GNR]	https://www.inem.pt/wp-content/uploads/2018/11/Emergency-ID-Card-2018-v2.pdf	Paper (size of 1 folding credit card)	Patients without age specification	Emergency		√

continued on following page

Table 5. Continued

Subcategory: 2.2. gathering basic information from the user (17)	More information	Material format	Users	Operating context	People with SN	Material in Portuguese***
Communication Passport_Accident and Emergency	https://widgit-health.com/downloads/A-and-E-passport.htm	Paper	Patients without age specification	Emergency	√	
Emergency Readiness Wheel for families	https://www.eadassociates.com/families.html	Paper	Caregivers	Emergency		
Emergency Readiness Wheel for people with disabilities	https://www.eadassociates.com/disabil.html	Paper	Patients without age specification	Emergency	√	
Feeling save, being safe - My Personal Safety in an Emergency **	https://mn.gov/mnddc/emergency-planning/docs/feelingSafe-CA.pdf	Paper	Patients without age specification	Emergency	√	
Premise alert request form person specific information for first responders	https://www.uwchlan.com/DocumentCenter/View/70/Premise-Alert-Form-PDF?bidId=	Paper	Patients without age specification	Emergency	√	
First Responder Communication Boards *	http://www.greenhousepub.com/firecobd4ta2.html	Paper	Patients without age specification	Pre-hospital emergency	√	
My Health Passport	http://flfcic.fmhi.usf.edu/docs/FCIC_Health_Passport_Form_Typeable_English.pdf	Paper	Patients without age specification	Hospital	√	
My Health Report	http://flfcic.fmhi.usf.edu/docs/FCIC_My_Health_Report_Fillable.pdf	Paper	Patients without age specification	Hospital	√	
My Hospital Passport (Surrey County Council)	http://www.surreyhealthaction.org/downloads/hospital%20passport%20surrey.pdf	Paper	Patients without age specification	Hospital	√	
This is me My Care Passport	https://www.sunderlandactionforhealth.co.uk/wp-content/uploads/2019/06/This-is-me-my-care-passport-enabled-2019.pdf	Paper	Patients without age specification	Hospital	√	
This is My Hospital Passport	https://www.nhs.uk/Livewell/Childrenwithalearningdisability/Documents/Hospital%20Passport%20Template%20example%20from%20South%20West%20London%20Access%20to%20Acute%20Group.doc	Paper	Patients without age specification	Hospital	√	
My Hospital Passport - for people on the autism spectrum	https://carersmatternorfolk.org.uk/wp-content/uploads/2019/05/3327_Hospital-passport_A4_6pp_4C_FINAL-ARTWORK_120917-1.pdf	Paper	Patients without age specification	Hospital	√	

*This material is also referenced in Category 1. communication SUPPORT; **This material is also referenced in Category 3. PREPARATION/ANTICIPATION of situations; SN - Special Needs; ***English, if nothing is mentioned.

3. PREPARATION/ANTECIPATION of situations

Finally, when analysing the Category 3 "PREPARATION/ANTECIPATION of situations", regarding the resources directed to paediatric patients (Table 6), it is possible to understand that the format of this material is still mostly paper-based (there is only one digital). The use of these materials is designed for Hospital, Pre-Hospital Emergency and Emergency contexts. Only two are designed to be used with children with SE, and only one is in Portuguese.

Table 6. Results from Category 3: Situation preparation/anticipation of situations, regarding the resources directed to paediatric patients (6 materials)

Subcategory: 3.1. Pediatric users (6)	**More information**	**Material format**	**Operating context**	**People with SN**	**Material in Portuguese****
What do you need to know? Pupils (prepare children to act in emergency situations)	https://lifeliveit.redcross.org.uk/~/media/BritishRedCross/Documents/What%20we%20do/LLI/pdf/001_What_you_need_to_know_pupils_2016.pdf	Paper	Pre-hospital emergency		
Baby and Child First Aid APP	https://play.google.com/store/apps/details?id=com.cube.rca.bcfa&hl=pt	Digital	Emergency		
My Daycase Operation + flashcards – Child	https://widgit-health.com/download-files/hospital-procedures/Child_Daycase_Operation_Booklet.pdf	Paper	Hospital		
Going to the Hospital*	https://widgit-health.com/easy-read-sheets/pdfs/Going%20to%20Hospital%20-%20key%20symbols.pdf	Paper	Hospital	√	
Leaving Hospital Checklist *	https://widgit-health.com/easy-read-sheets/pdfs/Leaving%20Hospital%20-%20checklist.pdf	Paper	Hospital	√	
A Estrelinha (INEM)	https://www.inem.pt/2017/06/07/a-estrelinha-mascote-do-inem/	Paper (Information Flyer)	Pre-hospital emergency		√

*These materials are also directed to Young/Adult Patients; SN - Special Needs; **English, if nothing is mentioned.

With regard to the subcategory Young/Adult Patients (Table 7), we can see that, once again, most of the materials are in paper format (there is only one in digital format). As for the context of action, most of the materials are to be used in Emergency and Hospital contexts, although there is material to be used in Disaster and Pre-Hospital Emergency situations. About half of the material can be used by people with SN and no material of this type was identified in the Portuguese language.

Table 7. Results from Category 3: Situation preparation/anticipation of situations, regarding the resources directed to young/adult patients (20 materials)

Subcategory: 3.2. young/adult users (20)	More information	Material format	Operating context	People with SN	Material in Portuguese****
My Daycase Operation + flashcards	https://widgit-health.com/downloads/hospital-procedures.htm#dayadult	Paper	Hospital		
Emergency Readiness Wheel for Seniors **	http://www.eadassociates.com/seniors.html	Paper	Emergency		
British Red Cross Emergency App	https://www.redcross.org.uk/get-help/prepare-for-emergencies/free-emergency-apps	Digital	Pre-hospital emergency		
Tips for Emergency use of mobile devices	http://www.jik.com/Mobile%20Devices.pdf	Paper	Emergency	√	
My Emergency readines plan	https://disabilities.temple.edu/programs/eprep/docs/EmergencyPlanForm2015-07.pdf	Paper	Emergency	√	
Emergency Power Planning for People who use electricity and battery dependent	https://adata.org/sites/adata.org/files/files/Emergency%20Power%20Planning_final2018.pdf	Paper	Emergency	√	
Going to Hospital*	https://widgit-health.com/easy-read-sheets/pdfs/Going%20to%20Hospital%20-%20key%20symbols.pdf	Paper	Hospital		
Leaving Hospital Checklist *	https://widgit-health.com/easy-read-sheets/pdfs/Leaving%20Hospital%20-%20checklist.pdf	Paper	Hospital	√	
Nobody Left Behind	http://www2.ku.edu/~rrtcpbs/resources/pdf/a_individual_preparedness.pdf	Paper	Catastrophes		
Disaster Preparedness for People who have limited speech: taking responsibility for your safety ***	https://aac-rerc.psu.edu/index-41568.php.html	Paper	Catastrophes	√	
How to call an ambulance?	https://widgit-health.com/easy-read-sheets/pdfs/How%20to%20call%20an%20ambulance.pdf	Paper	Emergency		
Emergency Readiness Wheel for people with Disabilities	https://www.eadassociates.com/disabil.html	Paper	Emergency	√	
Disability specific supplies for emergency kits	http://www.jik.com/Supply_checklist.pdf	Papel	Emergency	√	
Feeling save, being safe – My Personal Safety in Emergency **	https://mn.gov/mnddc/emergency-planning/docs/feelingSafe-CA.pdf	Paper	Emergency		

continued on following page

Table 7. Continued

Subcategory: 3.2. young/adult users (20)	More information	Material format	Operating context	People with SN	Material in Portuguese****
Beyond Words [Empowering people]	https://booksbeyondwords.co.uk/	Paper (Book)	Hospital	√	
What to bring to a visit - autism	https://autismandhealth.org/inc/forms/hc_prep_checklist.pdf	Paper	Hospital	√	
Symptoms Worksheet - autism	https://autismandhealth.org/inc/forms/hc_symptoms_worksheet.pdf	Paper	Hospital	√	
Making an Appointment – autism	https://autismandhealth.org/inc/forms/hc_appointment_worksheet.pdf	Paper	Hospital	√	
Things to Know Before you go worksheet- autism	https://autismandhealth.org/inc/forms/hc_aftervisit_worksheet.pdf	Paper	Hospital	√	
Emergency Kit Checklist **	https://www.archives-pmr.org/article/S0003-9993(11)00833-1/pdf	Paper	Emergency	√	

*These materials are also directed to Pediatric Patients; ** These materials are also referenced in Category 2. INFORMATION for Professionals; ***Material also directed to Caregivers; SN - Special Needs; ****English, if nothing is mentioned.

Table 8 shows the results for the third subcategory (Families/Caregivers). In this subcategory, all the materials are in paper format and are aimed at different contexts (Pre-Hospital Emergency, Emergency, Hospital and Disaster). Most of them are adapted for people with SN and there is no material in Portuguese language.

Table 8. Results from Category 3: Situation preparation/anticipation of situations, regarding the resources directed to families/caregivers (4 materials)

Subcategory: 3.3. Families/ Caregivers (4)	More information	Material format	Operating context	People with SN	Material in Portuguese***
What do you need to know? parents (teaching parents how to teach emergency to their children)	https://lifeliveit.redcross.org.uk/~/media/BritishRedCross/Documents/What%20we%20do/LLI/pdf/101What_you_need_to_know_parents_2003.pdf	Paper	Pre-hospital emergency		
Emergency Preparedness for Personal Assistant	http://www.jik.com/pubs/PAS-EP.pdf	Paper	Emergency	√	
Emergency Readiness Wheel for Families*	https://www.eadassociates.com/families.html	Paper	Hospital	√	
Disaster Preparedness for People who have limited speech: taking responsibility for your safety**	https://aac-rerc.psu.edu/images/file/EmergencyChecklist(2).pdf	Paper	Catastrophes	√	

*This material is also referenced in Category 2. INFORMATION for Professionals; **Material also directed to Young/Adult Patients; SN - Special Needs; ***English, if nothing is mentioned.

MAIN FOCUS OF THE CHAPTER

After the overall analysis of the data and according to the categories that emerged from this review (1. SUPPORT for communication; 2. INFORMATION for professionals and 3. PREPARATION/ ANTICIPATION of situations), the results highlight the need to develop more communication-facilitating materials, to be used in different health care contexts (Hospital, Pre-Hospital, Emergency Medicine and Disasters). This factor is also highlighted in the literature, since the patient and the entire surrounding population should be aware of the need to use communication facilitators in health care services (Baylor et al., 2019; Blackstone, 2015; Hanberg & Voss, 2018; Thunberg et al., 2016), since communication is a human right (Moreira, 2020) and improves the overall quality of care (Blackstone & Pressman, 2016; Turner et al., 2016; Centers for Disease Control and Prevention, 2024).

In general, it was possible to verify that the materials directed specifically for the adult population (20 materials) are more numerous than those directed specifically for thc paediatric population (10 materials), and most of the material identified does not specify a target population. The smaller number of materials for the paediatric population may be related to the lack of instruction and knowledge of health professionals in this area (Gormley & Light, 2019; Hanberg & Voss, 2018; Mesko et al., 2011; Stans et al., 2018; Thunberg et al., 2016). This is particulary relevant for children with motor impairments, where the use of AAC technologies has been shown to significantly enhance both communication and participation (Bianquin et al., 2022), as well as for children with autism spectrum disorder, for whom recent advances in AAC highlight the need for more individualized approaches (Schlosser & Koul, 2023). It is known that family members or caregivers play a key role in supporting patients with communicative difficulties in the delivery of health care, as indicated in the study by McFadd and Hustad (2020). This also reflected in studies on individuals with neurodegenerative conditions, such as ALS, where access to AAC and ongoing support are essential to maintain communication (Peters et al., 2022). However, it was possible to observe that the existing materials for this subcategory (Families/Caregivers), are also reduced in number, being important to enable health professionals to incorporate communicative facilitators to integrate, not only patients, but also family members in their interventions (Gormley & Light, 2021).

Another important aspect to highlight is the fact that there are several materials adapted to people with SN, reinforcing that communication should be seen as a human right and that it is essential to give importance to the needs of patients with communication difficulties, as highlighted by relatives in Thunberg's study (2016) and in several other studies (Berenguer et al., 2022; Taveira et al., 2023).

Regarding the format of the materials, there was a clear predominance of materials in paper format (83 materials) over digital format (8 materials). It would be important, in view of the increasing use of the Internet and advances in technology to access health information, to have materials that facilitate communication in digital format to improve communication in health care services, as pointed out by different authors who outline advances in AAC access methods tailored to clinical and rehabilitation contexts (Brumberg et al., 2021; Davidoff, 2017; Reed, 2021; Xu et al., 2025). This recommendation is reinforced by recent technological reviews that highlight the growing role of digital and AI-driven AAC tools to personalize and enhance communication in healthcare (Draffan & Banes, 2022; Evangeline & Anitha, 2024; Land et al., 2023). Murray and Hopf (2022) verified that the particular context of healthcare provision can also influence the choice of high-tech or low-tech communication resources used, considering the usefulness recognized by professionals and family members in that context, as well as negative attitudes towards AAC related to the lack of initial training and ongoing support, the perception of impersonal content, limited functionality and the lack of consistent availability. They also found that positive attitudes towards low-tech AAC seem to be more prevalent when training and support are offered, when the effectiveness of low-tech AAC is demonstrated and when organizational, financial and procedural commitments are made.

With regard to language, it was possible to verify that there is only a total of 7 materials in Portuguese. Clearly most of the materials found are written in English, although the use of communicative facilitators is equally sought worldwide (Hutchins, 2020). The fact that there are not so many resources in the Portuguese language may possibly be justified by the instruction and access of health professionals to the use of these materials in the different contexts in which they operate (Gormley & Light, 2019; Handberg & Voss, 2018; Thunberg et al., 2016).

This review presents an important contribution in the sense of clearly highlighting existing weaknesses related to communicative facilitator materials, as well as increasing awareness of the need for further research related to the area of communication in the health care delivery process. Recent initiatives such as those described by Araújo et al. (2023), show that implementing communication tools in healthcare-validated by users with disabilities and supported by staff training, can reduce communication barriers. Communication is a basic need and right of all human beings (Mulcair et al., 2018; Taveira et al., 2023; UN, 2008). Specifically with regard to the context of health care provision, it is indeed important to look at the intervention process, to support the development of best practices and effective strategies in this area, in order to improve health education, especially for population groups with difficult access, investing in the construction of communication facilitator materials and in the instruction of those same materials to health professionals and the patient's surrounding community (Baylor et al., 2019; Gormley & Light, 2019, 2021; Hurtig et al., 2018).

SOLUTIONS AND RECOMMENDATIONS

It is recommended that materials to facilitate communication be created in different languages (in addition to English), for use in different health contexts, with different intervention objectives (communication support, information for professionals and preparation/anticipation of situations). It will also be important to create these materials adapted to foreign children and children with SN, as the quantity of materials for these specific populations is very low.

FUTURE RESEARCH DIRECTIONS

The mixing of different cultures, and consequently with different languages, has been increasingly felt in recent years, and is expected to increase in the coming years. Therefore, efficient communication between healthcare professionals and their patients is an increasingly important topic in the days to come.

As the scenario of the relevance of communication in hospital contexts has changed abruptly, it is important that professional skills and technological strategies (communicative facilitators), are acquired by future professionals, to overcome the challenges that these professions face in their daily lives.

It is expected that in the future there will not be so many communication failures in the provision of healthcare, and that any citizen will have the right to the same quality of care regardless of their limitations in terms of communication. Therefore, it is increasingly feasible to implement measures to include this type of material in the clinical practice of these professionals. It would be interesting to include studies to test the effectiveness of communication facilitating materials that could be developed for different health care contexts.

CONCLUSION

Research demonstrates that:

- Communication is a human right, and it assumes a fundamental role in the provision of health care services.
- Communication is not always effective in the provision of health care services.
- Communicative barrier is any situation in which the transmitted message is not decoded by the receiver, which may result in the patient not adequately understanding the health professional and/or the opposite.
- The use of materials specifically for this purpose can be of extreme relevance in order to improve communication in health care services as an integral component of population health promotion.
- It is important and necessary to produce more communication-facilitators materials in different languages.Special attention should be given to groups where communication may be more difficult (e.g., people with special needs, paediatrics, people with different mother tongues/cultures,) or in emergencies, to make these services less demanding and complex.There are still barriers that need to be addressed, such as: training and recognition/acceptance by health professionals about the benefits of using these materials (Zubow & Hurtig, 2021).

In summary, the studies described in the literature provide evidence supporting the use of communication facilitating materials in different health care contexts.

ACKNOWLEDGMENT

This research received no specific grant from any funding agency in the public, commercial, or not-for-profit sectors.

REFERENCES

Ahmed, H. M. (2020). Role of verbal and non-verbal communication of health care providers in general satisfaction with birth care: A cross-sectional study in government health settings of Erbil City. *Reproductive Health, 17*(1), 35–44. DOI: 10.1186/s12978-020-0894-3 PMID: 32151284

Alcântara, P., Zonho, A. W., Lobo, M. I. R., Rodrigues, I. N., & Llonch, A. S. (2016). Efeito da interação com palhaços nos sinais vitais e na comunicação não verbal de crianças hospitalizadas. *Revista Paulista de Pediatria : Orgao Oficial da Sociedade de Pediatria de Sao Paulo, 34*, 432–438. DOI: 10.1016/j.rpped.2016.02.001 PMID: 27080219

American Speech-Language-Hearing Association. (n.d.). *Augmentative and alternative communication* (Practice portal). Retrieved November, 20, 2024, from www.asha.org/Practice-Portal/Professional-Issues/Augmentative-and-Alternative-Communication/

Araujo, M. M. T., da Silva, L. F., & Souza, R. C. (2023). Comunicação aumentativa e alternativa na saúde –tecnologia assistiva reduzindo barreiras comunicacionais. *Revista ISAAC, 15*(2), 125–138. https://publicacoes.softaliza.com.br/isaac2023/article/view/7892?utm_source=chatgpt.com

Araújo, M. M. T., Silva, M. J. P., & Puggina, A.C. G. (2007). A comunicação não-verbal enquanto fator iatrogênico. *Revista da Escola de Enfermagem da USP, 41*, 419-425. 07 https://doi.org/DOI: 10.1590/S0080-62342007000300011

ASHA. (1993). *Definitions of communication disorders and variations*. Accessed November 20, 2024. https://www.asha.org/policy/rp1993-00208/

Baylor, C., Burns, M., McDonough, K., Mach, H., & Yorkston, K. (2019). Teaching medical students skills for effective communication with patients who have communication disorders. *American Journal of Speech-Language Pathology, 28*(1), 155–164. DOI: 10.1044/2018_AJSLP-18-0130 PMID: 31072161

Beneteau, E., Paradiso, A., & Pratt, W. (2022). Telehealth experiences of providers and patients who use augmentative and alternative communication. *Journal of the American Medical Informatics Association : JAMIA, 29*(3), 462–470. DOI: 10.1093/jamia/ocab273 PMID: 34897460

Benson, B. J. (2014). Domain of competence: Interpersonal and communication skills. *Academic Pediatrics, 14*(2), 55–65. DOI: 10.1016/j.acap.2013.11.016 PMID: 24602649

Berenguer, C., Martínez, E.R., De Stasio, S., & Baixauli, I. (2022). Parents' perceptions and experiences with their children's use of augmentative/alternative communication: a systematic review and qualitative meta-synthesis. *International Journal of Environmental Research and Public Health,19*, 809.n DOI: 10.3390/ijerph19138091

Beukelman, D., & Mirenda, P. (2013). *Augmentative & alternative communication - supporting children & adults with complex communication needs.* Baltimore, Maryland, Ed. Paul H Brookes.

Bianquin, N., Sacchi, F., & Besio, S. (2022). Enhancing communication and participation using AAC technologies for children with motor impairments: A systematic review. *Educational Sciences and Society, 13*(1), 49–71.

Blackstone, S. (2015). Issues and challenges in advancing effective patient-provider communication. In Blackstone, S., Beukelman, D., & Yorkston, K. (Eds.), *Patient-Provider Communication - Roles for Speech-Language Pathologists and Other Health Care Professionals* (pp. 9–35). Plural Publishing.

Blackstone, S., Ruschke, K., Wilson-Stronks, A., & Lee, C. (2011). Converging communication vulnerabilities in health care: An emerging role for speech-language pathologists and audiologists. *Perspectives on Communication Disorders and Sciences in Culturally and Linguistically Diverse, 18*(1), 3–11. DOI: 10.1044/cds18.1.3

Blackstone, S. W. (2018). What does the patient want? *ASHA Leader, 21*(3), 38–44. https://leader.pubs.asha.org/doi/10.1044/leader.FTR1.21032016.38. DOI: 10.1044/leader.FTR1.21032016.38

Blackstone, S. W., & Pressman, H. (2016). Patient communication in health care settings: New opportunities for augmentative and alternative communication. *Augmentative and Alternative Communication, 32*(1), 69–79. DOI: 10.3109/07434618.2015.1125947 PMID: 26694249

Boston University Medical Group, Office of Equity, Vitality, and Inclusion, and BUMC Faculty Development and Diversity. *Inclusive language practices*. (2022). Accessed November 20, 2024. https://www.bumc.bu.edu/bumg/files/2021/10/Inclusive-Language-Practices_101821.pdf

Brumberg, J. S., Pitt, K. M., & Burnison, J. D. (2021). Emerging trends in augmentative and alternative communication access methods. *Current Physical Medicine and Rehabilitation Reports*, *9*(1), 8–17. DOI: 10.1007/s40141-021-00281-w

Burke, J. P., & Tsiouris, J. A. (2022). Communication supports in emergency healthcare settings: A review of tools and applications. *Journal of Communication in Healthcare*, *15*(3), 223–232. DOI: 10.1080/17538068.2022.2023991

Centers for Disease Control and Prevention. *Health equity guiding principles for inclusive communication*. 2024. Accessed November 20, 2024. https://www.cdc.gov/healthcommunication/Health_Equity.html

Davidoff, B. E. (2017). AAC with energy-earlier. *ASHA Leader*, *22*(1), 48–53. DOI: 10.1044/leader.FTR2.22012017.48

Draffan, E. A., & Banes, D. (2022). Augmentative and alternative communication: Emerging trends, opportunities and innovations. In Miesenberger, K., Kouroupetroglou, G., Mavrou, K., & Manduchi, R. (Eds.), *Recent Advances in Technologies for Inclusive Well-Being* (pp. 469–485). Springer., https://www.researchgate.net/publication/361677133

Evangeline, B., & Anitha, D. (2024). A comprehensive review on augmentative and alternative communication tools for speech-impaired individuals. In *Lecture Notes in Networks and Systems* (pp. 321–331). Springer., DOI: 10.1007/978-981-97-3973-8_20

Finke, E. H., Light, J., & Kitko, L. (2008). A systematic review of the effectiveness of nurse communication with patients with complex communication needs with a focus on the use of augmentative and alternative communication. *Journal of Clinical Nursing*, *17*(16), 2102–2115. DOI: 10.1111/j.1365-2702.2008.02373.x PMID: 18705734

Gomes, N. A. C., & Gibson, M. Q. (2023). A comunicação aumentativa e alternativa para desenvolvimento da linguagem e comunicação no autismo. *Revista ISAAC, 15*(2), 150–162. https://publicacoes.softaliza.com.br/isaac2023/article/view/7904

Gormley, J., & Light, J. (2019). Providing services to individuals with complex communication needs in the inpatient rehabilitation setting: The experiences and perspectives of speech-language pathologists. *American Journal of Speech-Language Pathology*, *28*(2), 456–468. DOI: 10.1044/2018_AJSLP-18-0076 PMID: 31136227

Gormley, J., & Light, J. (2021). Child-parent-provider interactions of a child with complex communication needs in an inpatient rehabilitation facility: A pilot study. *American Journal of Speech-Language Pathology*, *30*(1), 105–118. DOI: 10.1044/2020_AJSLP-20-00031 PMID: 33316177

Greenslade, K. J. (2021). Using analog tasks to assess children's social communication skills. *Perspectives of the ASHA Special Interest Groups*, *6*(1), 39–54. DOI: 10.1044/2020_PERSP-20-00155

Handberg, C., & Voss, A. K. (2018). Implementing augmentative and alternative communication in critical care settings: Perspectives of healthcare professionals. *Journal of Clinical Nursing*, *27*(1–2), 102–114. DOI: 10.1111/jocn.13851 PMID: 28401613

Hemsley, B., & Balandin, S. (2014). A metasynthesis of patient-provider communication in hospital for patients with severe communication disabilities: Informing new translational research. *Augmentative and Alternative Communication*, *30*(4), 329–343. DOI: 10.3109/07434618.2014.955614 PMID: 25229213

Holm, A., Karlsson, V., Nikolajsen, L., & Dreyer, P. (2021). Strengthening and supporting nurses' communication with mechanically ventilated patients in the intensive care unit: Development of a communication intervention. *International Journal of Nursing Studies Advances*, *3*, 100025. DOI: 10.1016/j.ijnsa.2021.100025 PMID: 38746735

Hopf, S. C., & White, D. (2021). Supporting communication access in healthcare: An interprofessional approach to training. *Perspectives of the ASHA Special Interest Groups*, *6*(4), 838–847. DOI: 10.1044/2021_PERSP-21-00120

Hurtig, R., Alper, R. M., Bryant, K. N. T., Davidson, K. R., & Bilskemper, C. (2019). Improving patient safety and patient-provider communication. *Perspectives of the ASHA Special Interest Groups*, *4*(5), 1017–1027. DOI: 10.1044/2019_PERS-SIG12-2019-0021 PMID: 34113718

Hutchins, S. D. (2020). SLP Brings AAC to COVID-19 Patients. *Leader Live*, https://leader.pubs.asha.org/do/10.1044/leader.LML.25062020.26/full/

Khan, A., Spector, N. D., Baird, J. D., Ashland, M., Starmer, A. J., Rosenbluth, G., Garcia, B. M., Litterer, K. R., Rogers, J. E., Dalal, A. K., Lipsitz, S., Yoon, C. S., Zigmont, K. R., Guiot, A., O'Toole, J. K., Patel, A., Bismilla, Z., Coffey, M., Langrish, K., & Landrigan, C. P. (2018). Patient safety after implementation of a coproduced family centered communication programme: Multicenter before and after intervention study. *BMJ (Clinical Research Ed.)*, *363*, k4764. Advance online publication. DOI: 10.1136/bmj.k4764 PMID: 30518517

Lang, R., McLay, L., & Rispoli, M. (2023). Advanced language models: Potential to improve augmentative and alternative communication for individuals with intellectual and developmental disabilities. *Advances in Neurodevelopmental Disorders*, *7*(3), 481–484. DOI: 10.1007/s41252-023-00350-5

Levinson, W., Roter, D. L., Mullooly, J. P., Dull, V. T., & Frankel, R. M. (1997). Physician-patient communication. The relationship with malpractice claims among primary care physicians and surgeons. *Journal of the American Medical Association*, *277*(7), 553–559. DOI: 10.1001/jama.1997.03540310051034 PMID: 9032162

McFadd, E. D., & Hustad, K. C. (2020). Communication modes and functions in children with cerebral palsy. *Journal of Speech, Language, and Hearing Research: JSLHR*, *63*(6), 1776–1792. DOI: 10.1044/2020_JSLHR-19-00228 PMID: 32459163

Mesko, P. J., Eliades, A. B., Christ-Libertin, C., & Shelestak, D. (2011). Use of picture communication aids to assess pain location in pediatric postoperative patients. *Journal of Perianesthesia Nursing*, *26*(6), 395–404. DOI: 10.1016/j.jopan.2011.09.006 PMID: 22099132

Moreira, M. O. (2020). A Comunicação como um direito humano. *Revista Científica Multidisciplinar Núcleo do Conhecimento, 4*(6), 17-35. https://www.nucleodoconhecimento.com.br/comunicacao/direito-humano

Mulcair, G., Pietranton, A. A., & Williams, C. (2018). The international communication project: Raising global awareness of communication as a human right. *International Journal of Speech-Language Pathology*, *20*(1), 34–38. DOI: 10.1080/17549507.2018.1422023 PMID: 29355390

Murray, S., & Hopf, S. C. (2022). Attitudes toward the use of low-tech AAC in acute settings: A systematized review. *Augmentative and Alternative Communication*, *38*(3), 184–195. DOI: 10.1080/07434618.2022.2122870 PMID: 36128661

Naughton, C. A. (2018). Patient-centered communication. *Pharmacy (Basel, Switzerland)*, *6*(1), 18–25. DOI: 10.3390/pharmacy6010018 PMID: 29438295

Peters, B., O'Brien, K., & Fried-Oken, M. (2022). AAC use and service delivery experiences of people with ALS in the United States. *Disability and Rehabilitation. Assistive Technology*, *17*(7), 762–771. DOI: 10.1080/17483107.2022.2149866 PMID: 36448513

Reed, B. R. (2021). What are key considerations when selecting high-tech AAC? *Leader Live*, https://leader.pubs.asha.org/do/10.1044/2021-high-tech-aac/full/

Schlosser, R., & Koul, K. (2023). Advances in augmentative and alternative communication research for individuals with autism spectrum disorder: Moving research and practice forward. *Augmentative and Alternative Communication*, *39*(1), 2–6. DOI: 10.1080/07434618.2023.2181214 PMID: 36994996

Stans, S. E. A., Dalemans, R. J. P., Roentgen, U. R., Smeets, H. W. H., & Beurskens, A. J. H. M. (2018). Who said dialogue conversations are easy? The communication between communication vulnerable people and health-care professionals: A qualitative study. *Health Expectations*, *21*(5), 848–857. DOI: 10.1111/hex.12679 PMID: 29671920

Taveira, L., Gaspar, A. C., Pinto, M., Dias, J. C., Mendes, J., Martins, A. L., & Prata, J. (2023). Intervenção em Comunicação Aumentativa. In Alves, D. C., Correia, P., Cruz, S., Fonseca, J., Ibrahim, S., Lopes, I., Lousada, M., Oliveira, P., & Pinto, C. (Eds.), *Compendium de Terapia da Fala – Avaliar e intervir com evidência* (pp. 933–1024). Sociedade Portuguesa de Terapia da Fala.

The Joint Comission. (2022). *National Patient Safety Goals| The Joint Commission.* https://www.jointcommission.org/standards/national-patient-safety-goals/

Thunberg, G., Buchholz, M., & Nilsson, S. (2016). Strategies that assist children with communicative disability during hospital stay: Parents' perceptions and ideas. *Journal of Child Health Care*, *20*(2), 224–233. DOI: 10.1177/1367493514568298 PMID: 25676537

Topia, M., & Hocking, C. (2012). Enabling development and participation through early provision of augmentative and alternative communication. *New Zealand Journal of Occupational Therapy*, *59*(1), 24–30.

Turner, J. S., Pettit, K. E., Buente, B. B., Humbert, A. J., Perkins, A. J., & Kline, J. A. (2016). Medical student use of communication elements and association with patient satisfaction: A prospective observational pilot study. *BMC Medical Education*, *16*(1), 150–158. DOI: 10.1186/s12909-016-0671-8 PMID: 27209065

United Nations. (2008). *Final report of the Ad Hoc Committee on a Comprehensive and Integral International Convention on the Protection and Promotion of the Rights and Dignity of Persons with Disabilities | United Nations Enable*. Accessed November 20, 2024.https://www.un.org/development/desa/disabilities/final-report-of-the-ad-hoc-committee-on-a-comprehensive-and-integral-international-convention-on-the-protection-and-promotion-of-the-rights-and-dignity-of-persons-with-disabilities.html

World Health Organization. (2024). *Disability*. Accessed November 20, 2024. https://www.who.int/news-room/fact-sheets/detail/disability-and-health

Xu, Y., Chakraborti, M., Zhang, T., Eng, K., Mohan, A., & Prpa, M. (2025). Your voice is your voice: supporting self-expression through speech generation and LLMs in AAC. arXiv preprint arXiv:2503.17479. https://arxiv.org/abs/2503.17479

Zubow, L., & Hurtig, R. (2013). A demographic study of AAC/AT needs in hospitalized patients. *Perspectives on Augmentative and Alternative Communication, 22*(2), 79–90. DOI: 10.1044/aac22.2.79

Zubow, L., & Hurtig, R. (2021). The role of speech-language pathologists in improving communication access in healthcare settings. *Communication Disorders Quarterly, 42*(4), 215–225. DOI: 10.1177/1525740120975805

KEY TERMS AND DEFINITIONS

Augmentative and Alternative Communication (AAC): supplements or compensates for impairments in speech-language production and/or comprehension, including spoken and written modes of communication. AAC falls under the broader umbrella of assistive technology, or the use of any equipment, tool, or strategy to improve functional daily living in individuals with disabilities or limitations (ASHA, n.d.). Is when communication can take many forms, such as: speech, a shared look, text, gestures, facial expressions, touch, sign language, symbols, images, devices that generate speech, etc.

Communication Aids: any type of aid that facilitates communication between two or more people, healthcare professionals and patients (in healthcare contexts) such as physical materials that facilitate communication.

Communicative Facilitators: Communicative facilitators encompass any procedures and/or material that facilitates communication between two or more people.

Disability: It is part of being human and an integral part of the human experience. It results from the interaction between health problems and a series of environmental and personal factors. Factors such as gender, age, gender identity, sexual orientation, religion, race, ethnicity and economic status affect the life experiences and health needs of people with disabilities. They die earlier, have poorer health and suffer more limitations in their daily functioning than other people (WHO, 2024). These people often have special needs in order to participate fully in various life contexts (including healthcare).

Emergency Medical Service: The provision of urgent health services.

Health Communication: Communication used in the provision of healthcare.

Patient-Provider Communication: When the exchange of information shared between healthcare professionals and patients is mutually understood.

Quality Health Care: When patients and their families are satisfied with the work provided in healthcare contexts, and their needs are met with all ethical issues and respect for their condition covered

Chapter 6
Complementary Approaches for Autism Spectrum Disorder Intervention:
A Holistic View

Vânia Peixoto
https://orcid.org/0000-0002-8212-2137
Escola Superior de Saúde Fernando Pessoa, Portugal

Inês Cadório
Escola Superior de Saúde Fernando Pessoa, Portugal

Rita Alegria
https://orcid.org/0000-0001-6327-6088
Escola Superior de Saúde Fernando Pessoa, Portugal

Pedro Pestana
Escola Superior de Saúde Fernando Pessoa, Portugal

ABSTRACT

Autism Spectrum Disorder (ASD) is a neurodevelopmental condition marked by deficits in social interaction, communication, and repetitive behaviors or interests. The prevalence of ASD has risen in recent years, with an estimated one in 36 children in the US affected. This has led to increased research into effective interventions. Today, many individuals with ASD have better outcomes than in the past, with more becoming verbal, reading, and living in the community. This progress is due in part to improved knowledge and evidence-based treatments. Alongside traditional ther-

DOI: 10.4018/979-8-3693-6432-1.ch006

apies, complementary therapies—used alongside conventional treatments—have gained attention. This chapter provides an overview of ASD's defining traits and explores innovative interventions, including water-based speech therapy, music therapy, and animal-assisted therapy. These approaches not only enhance speech, sensory integration, and social skills but also support relaxation and inclusion, empowering individuals with ASD to achieve their full potential and contributing to a more inclusive future.

INTRODUCTION

Autism Spectrum Disorders (ASD) encompasses a spectrum of neurodevelopmental lifelong conditions characterized by diverse symptoms and varying levels of disability (Brondino eta al, 2015, Hume et al, 2021).

Symptoms typically manifest in early childhood and can significantly impact social functioning, educational engagement, and occupational performance, overall with a significant impact on the quality of life of child and family (Levy et al, 2015, Steinbrenner, 2020).

Background

The revisions made in the DSM-5 (APA, 2013) refined the diagnostic criteria to include two core symptoms: persistent deficits in social communication and the presence of restricted, repetitive behaviors. The acknowledgment of varying severity levels among individuals with ASD underscores the complexity of the disorder, as it can range from mild to profound impairment, further complicating both diagnosis and treatment.

Research on ASD reflects a growing understanding of its prevalence and multifactorial causes, which have significant implications for early diagnosis and intervention strategies.

In this regard, we must highlight the increasing prevalence of ASD diagnoses, with the Centers for Disease Control and Prevention (CDC, 2014) reporting that 1 in 68 children are identified as having some form of ASD, in 2020, the same organization reports an even higher prevalence of 1 in 44 children (Maenner et al., 2021, CDC 2020) and in 2024 refer that about 1 in 36 children has been identified with ASD according to estimates from CDC's Autism and Developmental Disabilities Monitoring (ADDM) Network (Maenner et al., 2023). This increase in prevalence raises critical questions regarding whether it is attributable to a true increase in cases or simply improved diagnostic practices (Elder et al., 2017).

The etiology of ASD is a subject that has been the focus of much research, however, despite several recent findings, there is still no single answer to the question. Masini et al., (2020) explores into the intricate interplay of genetic, epigenetic, and environmental factors that contribute to the etiology of ASD. The findings suggest a strong genetic component, as ASD is often familial, while also recognizing the role of environmental influences, such as parental health and perinatal conditions. The authors explore how epigenetic mechanisms, including DNA methylation and microRNA alterations, may further elucidate the biological underpinnings of ASD. This comprehensive overview of the factors involved in ASD pathogenesis is crucial for understanding the disorder's complexity. The emphasis on early diagnosis and intensive therapeutic interventions reinforces the notion that timely identification of ASD can lead to better outcomes for individuals.

Knowledge on ASD has evolved significantly, particularly in understanding the critical impact of early diagnosis and intervention. In their recent work (Okoye et al., 2023), the authors examine the concept of "sensitive periods" in brain development, emphasising the importance of early intervention during these critical phases. They argue that during early childhood, the brain exhibits heightened neuroplasticity, allowing for the formation of new neural connections that can be positively influenced by tailored learning experiences. This insight highlights the potential of early interventions to shape neural pathways, ultimately improving outcomes for children with autism.

However, the same authors also address the complexities surrounding the early diagnosis of ASD. The heterogeneous nature of autism symptoms poses a significant challenge in creating a universally applicable diagnostic tool. Cultural and social factors further complicate the landscape of ASD diagnosis, as these elements can influence both the recognition of symptoms and the response to interventions. Understanding these challenges is crucial for developing effective diagnostic strategies and interventions, thereby underscoring the need for a nuanced approach to ASD that accounts for individual differences and contextual factors (Okoye et al., 2023).

The rise in the amount of autistic children identified, has resulted in an augmented demand for the provision of high-quality services. The literature surrounding evidence-based practice (EBP) in ASD has undergone a significant evolution over the past decade. This reflects a growing recognition of the necessity for effective strategies that are tailored to this unique population (Stahmer et al., 2023; Sandham et al., 2021). The implementation of evidence-based practices (EBPs) in the context of early intervention for ASD has the possibility to facilitate positive developmental outcomes for children and to address the needs of their families. Nevertheless, the effective implementation of EBPs in community-based early intervention programmes necessitates a nuanced consideration of the contextual factors influencing their delivery (Stahmer et al., 2019; Melgarejo et al., 2020; Aranbarri et al., 2021; Locke et al., 2019).

The crucial role that educators and therapists play in the successful implementation of EBP must be highlighted, emphasizing that the increasing demand for ASD programming necessitates a robust understanding of effective teaching methods (Young Carson, 2014; Merle et al 2023; Steinbrenner et al., 2020; Hume et al., 2020). There is a pressing need to train the professionals who are part of the intervention teams, noting that training programs must incorporate evidence-based principles to equip them with the necessary skills to support students with ASD (Young Carson, 2014). Among the many different aspects considered necessary for an intervention to be effective, we must emphasize the fundamental role of early intervention, team work family involvement, and program evaluation (Steinbrenner et al., 2020; Hume et al., 2020, Bond et al., 2016).

Complementary Approaches and Chapter Focus

As noted, the practices used in the educational and treatment processes of individuals with ASD have increased, direct a range of approaches, from EBPs such as behavioural and educational interventions to complementary and alternative medicine (CAM) treatments (Hyman & Levy, 2011; Saral et al., 2023; Steinbrenner et al., 2020; Hume et al., 2020)

The exploration of complementary therapies for ASD has gained significant attention in recent years, reflecting a growing interest in alternative treatment modalities beyond conventional pharmacological approaches (Brondino et al, 2015).

Over the course of the last 40 years, a wide-ranging of intervention strategies have been proposed for children diagnosed with ASD. These strategies include the frequently used Applied Behavioral Analysis, the TEACCH program, peer-mediated and parent-assisted programs, alternative/augmentative communication programs, computer-based programs, as well as somewhat new strategies like music and animal-assisted therapy (Sourvinos et al., 2021).

Since numerous studies have demonstrated the vital significance of early intervention in ASD, numerous of these emphasis on children at an early age. According to research, a child's age at which they begin an intervention is thought to be one of the most significant elements affecting its effectiveness. If the child starts a program before the age of five, they may make more progress (Kodak & Bergmann, 2020).

Since many preschool-aged children with ASD have severe language deficiencies, many of which are nonverbal, SLP is particularly relevant in the early intervention of this population (Maksimović et al., 2023).

The term "complementary and alternative medicine" (CAM) encompasses a range of medical and philosophical systems that are both conventional and unconventional in nature. CAM treatments encompass a diverse range of healthcare protocols that are not integrated into the conventional healthcare system. Despite the existence of various categorisations and meanings of CAM proposed by researchers and organisations, the treatments employed in conjunction with traditional medicine are defined as complementary treatments. In contrast, alternative treatments are used as a substitute for conventional medicine or treatments such as applied behavioural analytic practices (i.e., a non-mainstream approach used in place of conventional medicine) (Saral et al., 2023; Mortada, 2024).

More recently, another term has come to be used to refer to this type of approach is integrative medicine (IM), which is comprised of a diverse range of conventional and complementary therapies that involve the incorporation of CAM into biomedicine within the context of conventional care. The objective of IM is to combine traditional medicine with alternative therapies in order to create a more efficient and cost-effective healthcare delivery system. Traditional medicine relies on methods that have been proven to be safe and effective through the implementation of carefully designed trials and research. IM is characterised as being patient-centred, taking into consideration the whole person, that is to say, the body, mind, and spirit (Mortada, 2024, Vandana et al, 2023).

The utilisation of CAM treatments in children and adolescents with ASD is prevalent, with over half of parents attempting at least one of these treatments at some point following their child's diagnosis (DeFilippis M., 2018).

Despite the plethora of therapeutic modalities, four principal domains of CAM treatments for autism can be identified: "mind-body medicine interventions, biology-based treatments, manipulative and body-based practices, and energy medicine". The former category encompasses approaches that seek to modulate the intricate interplay between the brain and behaviour, whereas the latter three domains represent a diverse array of techniques that employ natural substances, body manipulation, and the directing of energy, respectively, to endorse healing. Common CAM procedures for treating ASD include "dietary supplements, vitamins, hyperbaric oxygen, hormone injections, swimming with dolphins, horseback riding, yoga, and massage". These appear appealing and pose minimal risk, however, not all of these treatments have been the subject of well-designed and reliable research, so the results of their application are still undetermined, there is insufficient evidence to suggest that they are effective (Singer & Ravi, 2015).

Despite the above, studies show that 50-88 percent of children with autism use some CAM in an effort to improve symptoms (Lee at al, 2023; Singer & Ravi, 2015, Vogal et al, 2024) . Approximately half of these children use biology-based therapies, 30 percent use mind-body therapies, and 25 percent use manipulation or body-based therapies (Singer & Ravi, 2015). This places greater urgency on the need to design research studies that answer the question "what CAM therapies are effective in intervening with children with autism?"

In 2017, Bang et al. conducted a systematic review that highlighted the potential effectiveness of Chinese herbal medicine in treating children with ASD. The analysis of randomised controlled trials (RCTs) indicated that herbal medicines, particularly when combined with integrative therapy, led to improvements. The authors emphasised the holistic approach of Traditional Chinese Medicine (TCM), which encompasses not only pharmacological treatment but also comprehensive care strategies. This study underscores the promise of herbal therapies as adjunctive treatments for ASD, suggesting that they may enhance the overall treatment efficacy when integrated with conventional methods.

In a recent contribution to the discourse on non-pharmacological approaches, Mondal et al. (2023) examined a range of complementary and alternative therapies for managing ASD. The authors' review encompassed a range of interventions, including dietary supplements, antioxidants, and herbal remedies, as well as emerging treatments such as camel milk and cannabidiol. They argued for the significance of these alternative therapies in light of the rising prevalence of ASD and the limitations of existing behavioural and pharmacological treatments. They proposed that integrating such therapies could provide new avenues for effectively managing symptoms associated with ASD, thereby enriching the therapeutic landscape available to patients and caregivers.

In the same year (Lee et al., 2023), a six-month integrative treatment programme, comprising herbal medicine (HM), Floortime and sensory enrichment therapy (SET), was employed in the treatment of children with ASD. The results demonstrated that this integrative treatment program may offer a theoretically effective, safe and viable option for children with ASD.

Other alternative therapies for ASD with a growing evidence base include animal-assisted therapy (Brondino et al., 2015; Rehn et al., 2023) and music, dance and drama therapies (Brondino et al., 2015).

These findings collectively elucidate the intricacies and prospective efficacy of complementary therapies in the context of ASD, thereby underscoring the necessity for further research to establish robust evidence and elucidate the underlying therapeutic mechanisms. The evolving comprehension of these interventions reflects a broader transition towards a more integrative approach to autism treatment, emphasising the imperative for personalised care strategies that consider the distinctive needs of each patient.

The National Center for Complementary and Alternative Medicine (NCCAM) categorizes nonbiological CAM therapies into three principal groups: mind-body medicine (encompassing practices such as prayer, yoga, meditation, music, dance, and art in general), manipulative and body-based practices (including massage, chiropractic care, and acupuncture), and energy medicine (such as Reiki or homeopathy) (Govindaraju et al, 2020, Brondino et al, 2015).

The objective of this review is to concentrate on non-biological CAM therapies, specifically music therapy, aquatic therapy and animal therapy. The following section will present a description of the aforementioned three types of therapy and will also include a review of the studies that have been conducted on them, with a view to establishing the evidence base for each.

MUSIC THERAPY

Music therapy has been conceptualized in numerous ways across countries and institutions. Though all definitions share the premise that music therapy is an intervention approach that relies on the professional use of music and its elements to induce gains on physical, social, communicative, emotional, cognitive, and spiritual health (WHMT, 2011). Individuals, dyads, groups, families, or communities who aim to improve their quality of life have their strengths and needs assessed, and proceed with creating, singing, moving to, and/or listening to music (AMTA, 2024). In fact, music therapists use music properties to establish a relationship with the client, access emotions and memories, structure behavior, and prompt social experiences while targeting clinical goals (Wheeler, 2015). Experts believe that musical engagement might underpin gains in socialization in children with ASD (Lagasse, 2017).

Over the years, studies have been establishing that music therapy plays a relevant role in the assessment, diagnosis, and treatment of ASD (Wigram & Gold, 2005). Whether music therapy is used as the only form of clinical assessment or as a complement of formal standardized tests, the strengths and weaknesses are evaluated and a baseline is determined (Moller, Odell-Miller & Wigram, 2002). In a less procedural way, music therapy assessment not only allows to accurately characterize many areas of development, but also provides the opportunity to explore child's creative potential (Wigram & Gold, 2005).

Following the clinical assessment and diagnosis, an individualized intervention plan is developed based on the goals to achieve. Like in any other intervention, target skills must be tailored to the individual and respective family. Examples of outcome variables could be: decreasing undesirable behaviour; prompting social interaction and social communication; strengthen independent everyday functioning; improving emotions recognition; promoting cognitive and motor skills; and increasing verbal communication (James et al., 2015; Lagasse, 2017).

The question one poses is: how does music therapy lead to the expected outputs?

Overall, two main methods have been extensively reported: active and receptive music therapy. While active methods imply an active participation of the individual with the music (i.e., the client makes music), receptive methods imply a passive participation of the individual (i.e., the client receives music) (Wheeler, 2015). When active methods are employed, individuals are encouraged to re-create, improvise, or compose music. On the other hand, when receptive methods are implemented, individuals are exposed to music, which means the client is a recipient of the music experience, rather than a music maker (Grocke, & Wigram, 2006). Music listening seems to stand out in ASD therapy sessions when compared to other techniques (Gold, Wigram, & Elefant, 2006). Regardless the approach (active vs. receptive), children and young adults seem to respond positively to music therapy interventions (Hillier, Greher, Poto, & Dougherty, 2012).

Within the methods described, music therapy can branch out into different techniques: i) free improvisation (i.e., no music restrictions associated); ii) structured improvisation (i.e., implementation of some constraints to the music); iii) performing or recreating pre-composed music, songs, and related activities; iv) composing songs and instrumental music; and/or v) engaging in listening experiences (Wheeler, Shultis, & Polen, 2005).

The majority of music therapy interventions feature the use of songs with lyrics carefully selected to target specific skills. Other music therapy interventions use pre-composed songs aligned with the treatment goals, adapted lyrics set to familiar melodies, or original songs, both in terms of melody and lyrics (James et al., 2015).

Music therapy is usually delivered in a one-to-one basis within the ASD population. Nevertheless, group-based and peer-mediated interventions have been reported (Boso, Emanuele, Minazzi, Abbamonte, & Politi, 2007; Kern, 2007).

Based on different reviews, most studies seem to outline the positive effects of music therapy on children diagnosed with ASD (Gold, Wigram, & Elefant, 2006; James et al., 2015; Marquez-Garcia et al., 2021). Significant effects favoring music therapy over placebo or control conditions have been found for verbal and non-verbal communication, as well as social interaction (Gold, Wigram, & Elefant, 2006; Lagasse, 2017). In adults diagnosed with severe ASD, combined dance/movement and music therapy seemed to be beneficial by reducing behavioural symptoms, particularly when used regularly (Mateos-Moreno & Atencia-Dona, 2013). However, a number of studies also revealed no significant improvements (Marquez-Garcia et al., 2021). For example, no main differences were found in speech production, when comparing speech training and music training (Lim, 2010; Lim & Draper, 2011). In a randomized controlled study, music-based social stories were considered ineffective for targeted social skills in children with ASD (Schwartzberg & Silverman, 2013). When music therapy unfolds successful, ideally the new skills become a stable part of a child's repertoire. Generalization occurs when gains are transferred to other natural environments, when performance of the learned skills is observed with the use of different materials, and/or when improved interaction occurs with multiple people (Rogers & Dawson, 2010). Parental reports might inform the music therapist about the generalization of target skills, as parents provide input on the treatment's relevance to the family unit, despite the potential for bias (LaGasse, 2017). A study comprising both children and adults with ASD analyzed music therapy interventions and concluded that clients seen in The Cleveland Music School Settlement were able to generalize responses acquired in music therapy to nonmusic therapy environments (Kaplan & Steele, 2005). Contrary, another study showed that children with ASD failed to generalize targeted social skills through music-based social stories training (Schwartzberg & Silverman, 2013).

Another important aspect that accounts for treatment effectiveness is the capacity to maintain trained skills for a period of time. Off-treatment periods, such as vacation periods, are part of ASD individuals' life. In a study where children received music therapy for three months, the improvement in social skills was relatively maintained at follow-up, three months after treatment active-phase (Bharathi, Venugopal & Vellingiri, 2019).

Despite the variability of treatment methods/techniques, the decision to measure generalization and maintenance of outcomes or not, ASD quality of life appears to be optimized, which aligns with the increasing demand for music therapy services in ASD population.

Overall, a greater body of literature is available on the use of music therapy in childhood ASD, compared to adolescence or adulthood. Noteworthy is the need to gain a lifespan perspective on the symptoms management through music therapy. Furthermore, additional research is needed to investigate whether the effects of music therapy are enduring (Gold, Wigram, & Elefant, 2006), and to what extent might they transfer to contexts other than the clinical setting. Regardless the intervention outcomes are positive, negative, mixed or neutral, the generalization of research findings to clinical practice is limited (Wigram & Gold, 2005).

While music therapy utilizes auditory and creative engagement, another approach influences the unique properties of water.

WATER-BASED THERAPY

Water-based treatments appear to be a promising approach among the several types of interventions. Children with ASD are fond of engaging in water-related activities as a form of exercise (Faraji et al., 2022).

Using the natural stress-relieving and therapeutic efficacious qualities of water, as well as the positive effects of the aquatic environment, occupational therapists have already started incorporating water into their sessions with children diagnosed with ASD (Güeita-Rodríguez et al., 2021). Water-based activities have been shown to help with language development, sensory development, and maintaining eye contact and attention, for these children's. The potential advantages of aquatic interventions can be summed up in four main ways, according to the above succinct review of the literature:

(a) Favorable effects on mental health and cognition
(b) Stress reduction
(c) Facilitation of maintaining attention and eye contact
(d) Improvement of language and general communication skills

Consequently, there are enough signs to warrant more research into the potential advantages of a water-based treatment environment for ASD (Zanobini, 2019).

Children with ASDs may, for instance, display stereotyped behaviors that impede their ability to develop motor skills. Nonetheless, engaging in water-based activities can decrease stereotyped behaviors. From the standpoint of dynamic systems, children with ASDs may benefit more from the water-based setting because of its special qualities in terms of the development of their motor skills (Shariat et al., 2024). Water-based activities have been shown to help with language development, sensory development, and maintaining eye contact and attention, for these children's. Only in a swimming pool context can the special qualities of water be utilized. These characteristics are resistance, turbulence, and buoyancy. As noted by Becker (2024), by promoting upward motions and lowering joint loadings, buoyancy and cushioning shield swimmers from injuries caused by falling. As a result, activities that require upward motion, like jumping or bobbing, are easier in water. The unpredictable velocity of water caused by human movement is known as "water turbulence," and it presents a balancing and coordination problem that is unusual for land-based situations. Water resistance is produced by turbulence, water's inherent viscosity, and movements that are counter to the buoyancy of the water (downward movement) (Lee & Porretta, 2013).

The resistance of water reduces movement speed and demands more energy to accomplish the same movement than it does on land. Further, health and motor skill profits of buoyancy, turbulence, and resistance include enhanced "cardiorespiratory endurance, balance, coordination, flexibility, and muscle strength". These advantages are significant because physical activity is predicted by both fitness and motor skill competence and because fitness and motor skill competence are connected with each other. People can practice basic motor skills in ways that suit their ability levels and help them become independent mover because to the special qualities of water (Ruggeri et al., 2020).

According to several studies, children with ASDs typically love the water, and it can even improve their performance and learning. The findings of those studies demonstrate improvements in motor and health-related fitness, decreased stereotypical behaviors, and increased social interactions. They also show improvements in aquatic play skills, basic swimming skills, and water-orientation skills. Water-based activities can help children with ASDs develop their movement abilities and encourage good responses in addition to eliciting a positive response (Alaniz et al., 2017).

Water temperature and depth are two examples of aquatic environmental elements, as are buoyancy and other distinct characteristics. Movements performed in water-based setting can have an impact on motor skill development due to their interplay with environmental and individual aspects. Experts can alter learners' movement patterns by adjusting movement goals, task difficulties, and equipment. According to Newell (1986), children have internal and external forces known as limitations that can either support or improve movement. The utilization of a water-based setting can impact ambient and task elements, hence reducing individual inhibiting factors that decrease movement in children with ASD (Pendergast et al., 2015).

A scoping review (Ogonowska-Slodownik et al., 2024) suggest that aquatic interventions, including structured exercise and swimming programs, can positively impact individuals with ASD. Improvements are frequently reported in motor skills (gross motor functions, aquatic skills, balance, coordination) and water competency/safety. Some evidence also points towards benefits in social functioning (social competence, interaction skills), reduced stereotypical behaviors, and potentially enhanced attention, communication skills, and overall well-being (relaxation, enjoyment). Programs lasting 8-10 weeks or longer seem effective for skill development.

However, the quality of evidence supporting these benefits needs careful consideration. Many reviews highlight significant limitations in the existing research, including a prevalence of studies with small sample sizes, lack of adequate control groups, non-standardized outcome measures, and potential methodological biases. This makes it difficult to definitively conclude the extent of the effects and generalize findings. While promising, there is a clear need for more high-quality RCTs with rigorous designs to solidify the evidence base for aquatic therapy in ASD.

Furthermore, practical challenges such as limited access to appropriate facilities and qualified therapists, as well as cost, can be barriers to implementation.

In summary, the unique properties of the aquatic environment offer a valuable and often motivating setting for therapeutic intervention in ASD. Current evidence suggests potential benefits for motor and social skills, as well as behavioral aspects, but is constrained by methodological limitations in the research. Consistent participation, often facilitated by family support, is likely key to achieving gains. Further high-quality research is needed, but aquatic therapy presents a promising complementary approach for many individuals with ASD.

Beyond structured physical environments like water, interaction with animals offers another avenue for complementary intervention.

ANIMAL-ASSISTED INTERVENTIONS

Animal-assisted interventions (AAIs) have emerged as a promising therapeutic modality for children with autism spectrum disorder (ASD), addressing various challenges associated with this neurodevelopmental condition. These interventions typically involve the incorporation of animals, such as dogs or horses, into therapeutic settings to enhance social interaction, emotional regulation, and overall well-being among individuals with autism. The growing body of research indicates that AAIs can facilitate engagement and improve social behaviors in children with ASD, as they often relate better to animals than to humans, thus creating a unique therapeutic dynamic that can foster communication and social skills development (O'Haire et al., 2013; Ang & MacDougall, 2022).

Research has shown that AAIs can lead to significant improvements in social functioning and emotional well-being among children with autism. The presence of animals can serve as a motivational tool, encouraging children to participate more actively in therapeutic activities (Hill et al., 2020; Hill et al., 2020).

Systematic reviews have highlighted the effectiveness of AAIs in various settings, including schools and therapy farms, where structured interactions with animals can provide a supportive environment for children with ASD (Brelsford et al., 2017; Barnhart et al., 2023; Sissons et al., 2022). However, while the evidence supporting the efficacy of AAIs is growing, there remains a need for further high-quality research to establish standardized protocols and guidelines for their implementation (Harris & Williams, 2017; Sissons et al., 2022).

Dogs serve as effective therapeutic tools for children with ASD by enhancing social interaction, emotional regulation, and family functioning. Research indicates that dog assisted therapy can facilitate therapeutic engagement, allowing autistic children to respond more effectively to treatment demands (Silva et al., 2011; Kilmer,

2024). The presence of therapy dogs has been shown to improve prosocial behaviors and reduce anxiety in children, which can lead to better participation in therapeutic activities (Wright et al., 2015; Morgan, 2023). Additionally, the companionship of dogs can alleviate stress for caregivers, thereby fostering a more supportive family environment (Wright et al., 2015; Appleby et al., 2022). Studies suggest that interactions with dogs can provide multisensory stimulation, which may be more engaging for autistic children than interactions with humans (Grigore & Rusu, 2014; Marszałek et al., 2022). Therefore, the integration of dogs into therapeutic practices not only benefits the children but also enhances the overall family dynamics (Leighton et al., 2023; Hellings et al., 2022).

Equine-assisted interventions (EAIs) have emerged as a promising therapeutic tool for children with ASD, facilitating improvements in social functioning, emotional well-being, and adaptive behaviors. Studies indicate that interactions with horses can enhance engagement and reduce social withdrawal, which are common challenges faced by individuals with ASD (Llambias et al., 2016; Borgi et al., 2015; Warner et al., 2022). The presence of horses during therapy sessions encourages non-verbal communication and fosters emotional connections, leading to increased eye contact and social interactions (Malcolm et al., 2017; Collacchi et al., 2023). Research highlights the effectiveness of structured programs, such as therapeutic horseback riding, in promoting self-regulation and communication skills among children with ASD (Gabriels et al., 2015; Xiao et al., 2023). Furthermore, systematic reviews have shown that EAIs can significantly improve adaptive behaviors and motor functions, underscoring their potential as a complementary approach in autism therapy (Zoccante et al., 2021; Sissons et al., 2022). Overall, the integration of horses into therapeutic practices offers a unique and beneficial avenue for enhancing the quality of life for children with autism.

Table 1. Summarizes the effectiveness of the above-mentioned complementary approaches in ASD population and includes additional approaches that were not the focus of this chapter (Zhukova et al., 2020).

Approach	Results	Safety	Effectiveness	Recommendation
Melatonin (Parker et al., 2019; Rossignol & Frye, 2011)	Significant improvements of sleep quality (sleep duration, sleep onset latency)	Safe	Effective	Melatonin should be implemented in the face of comorbid sleep problems.
Music therapy (Geretsegger et al., 2014)	Positive effects on social interaction, communicative skills, initiating behavior and social-emotional reciprocity	Safe	Inconclusive due to small sample sizes	Music therapy should be implemented when it does not interfere with front line treatment.
Neuromodulation (Barahona-Corrêa et al, 2018; Finisguerra et al., 2019)	Small to moderate effects on stereotyped behaviors, social behaviors and executive functioning.	Safe	Inconclusive	Neurostimulation techniques should be combined with cognitive training.
Physical activity (Yang et al., 2015)	Beneficial for physical and mental health.	Safe	Inconclusive due to heterogeneous outcomes across studies	Physical activity programs should be delivered by a qualified specialist.
Dance therapy (Koch et al., 2019)	Medium effect on mental health.	Safe	Inconsistent and limited to adult samples	Not recommended as alternative treatment, only recommended as complimentary.
Animal assisted interventions (Charry-Sánchez et al., 2018; Nimer & Lundahl, 2007)	Low to moderate effect size in decreasing ASD symptoms and problem behaviors. Social skills improvement.	Unknown	Inconclusive due to heterogeneity of samples and different animals used	Animal assisted interventions should be implemented when it does not interfere with front line treatment.
Sensory integration therapy (Schoen et al., 2019)	Ayres sensory integration showed positive effects on children with ASD while sensory-based interventions were less conclusive.	Unknown	Inconclusive	Not recommended as alternative treatment, only recommended as complimentary.
Holding therapy (Mercer, 2013)	Positive effects associated with severe side effects were reported including lethal cases.	Harmful	Inconclusive due to flawed methods	Not recommended
Hyperbaric Oxygen Therapy (Xiong et al., 2016)	No improvements in ASD symptoms. Adverse effects were found.	Harmful	No efficacy	Not recommended

CONCLUSION AND FUTURE RESEARCH DIRECTIONS

The combination of traditional practice and complementary techniques is now a common practice that cannot be ignored. An amount of studies have demonstrated the success of this approach, and it is also evident that families are willing to adhere to this type of practice.

It is noteworthy that there is a notable discrepancy among the prevalent use of CAM by families and the dearth of scientific evidence supporting the efficacy of alternative treatments. One potential explanation for this discrepancy is that CAM therapies are typically regarded as "natural," with an enhanced safety profile and fewer adverse effects than traditional pharmaceuticals.

Consequently, there is an urgent need to conduct further studies to prove which CAM therapies are effective.

Neverthless, in recent years, there has been a notable growth in interest from the scientific community in the field of CAM therapies. This has led to a number of studies being conducted with the aim of investigating the efficacy and safety of these therapies in the context of ASD.

Among biologically based CAMs, only the gluten/casein-free diet, omega 3, vitamin supplementation (vitB6, vitB12, and tetrahydrobiopterin), and hyperbaric oxygen therapy have been the subject of more extensive study. All the other biological therapies were tested in single trials and therefore provided insufficient data to determine their usefulness in clinical practice (Brondino, 2015).

Although the most widely used and studied complementary therapies focus on biological complementary and alternative medicine (such as vitamins and minerals) (Saral et al 2023, Simith et al, 2020, An et al, 2020), non-biological complementary therapies are gaining ground in EBP.

The evidence base regarding the efficacy of CAM treatments in ASD is currently limited. One possible justification for these inconclusive results is that well-designed studies have only recently been developed and typically have a limited sample size. Furthermore, the heterogeneous nature of ASD and the potential presence of comorbidities could have resulted in several trials being negatively impacted by an inadequate participant stratification (Locke et al., 2019; Brondino, 2015; Melgarejo et al., 2020; Aranbarri et al., 2021). It is noteworthy that the majority of the reviewed trials were conducted with children diagnosed with ASD. As the prevalence of ASD continues to rise, it is becoming increasingly important to extend research to include adults with autism, who are also facing significant challenges. It would therefore be of interest to test the efficacy of CAM therapies in an adult population. It is recommended that healthcare professionals encourage their patients and their families to debate the efficiency and safety of all CAMs.

It is recommended that clinicians permit families or patients to utilise CAMs that have restricted clinical evidence, provided that they are safe, cost-effective and do not impede patients from accessing evidence-based treatments, such as behavioural therapies. It is noteworthy that numerous CAMs can be readily integrated with traditional clinical care. In particular, non-biologically based CAMs, such as music therapy and animal therapy, can be incorporated into existing treatment plans, not as a substitute but as a complement to typical therapies. It is recommended that practitioners advise patients to try one CAM at a time and to monitor clinical changes and adverse events on an ongoing basis.

In conclusion, the potential efficacy of CAM in autism remains poorly understood and, to gain further insight into the efficacy of CAM in ASD, it is essential to conduct larger-scale randomised controlled trials that provide a more detailed characterisation of the patient population (Brondino, 2015).

Parents are frequently confronted with the challenge of selecting from a myriad of intervention options, which vary considerably in their efficacy for their children with ASD. A multitude of factors influence parental decision-making regarding the initiation, continuation, rejection, and cessation of specific treatments for their children with ASD (Saral et al., 2023).

Our narrative review of the literature reveals that there is a substantial evidence supporting the use of music therapy, water-based therapy, and animal-assisted therapy in conjunction with traditional therapeutic modalities.

REFERENCES

Alaniz, M. L., Rosenberg, S. S., Beard, N. R., & Rosario, E. R. (2017). The Effectiveness of Aquatic Group Therapy for Improving Water Safety and Social Interactions in Children with Autism Spectrum Disorder: A Pilot Program. *Journal of Autism and Developmental Disorders*, *47*(12), 4006–4017. DOI: 10.1007/s10803-017-3264-4 PMID: 28864911

American Music Therapy Association. (2024, July 30th). About music therapy and AMTA. Retrieved from https://www.musictherapy.org/about/

American Psychiatric Association. (2013). *Diagnostic and statistical manual of mental disorders* (5th ed.)., DOI: 10.1176/appi.books.9780890425596

An, S., Kanderzhanova, A., Akhmetova, A., Foster, F., & Chan, C. K. (2020). "Chasing hope": Parents' perspectives on complementary and alternative interventions for children with autism in Kazakhstan. *Autism*, *24*(7), 1817–1828. DOI: 10.1177/1362361320923494 PMID: 32498539

Ang, C., & MacDougall, F. (2022). An evaluation of animal-assisted therapy for autism spectrum disorders: Therapist and parent perspectives. *Psychological Studies*, *67*(1), 72–81. DOI: 10.1007/s12646-022-00647-w PMID: 35287312

Appleby, R., Wright, S., Williams, L., & Stanley, M. (2022). Australian parents' experiences of owning an autism assistance dog. *Health & Social Care in the Community*, *30*(6), e4113–e4121. DOI: 10.1111/hsc.13805 PMID: 35352418

Aranbarri, A., Stahmer, A. C., Talbott, M. R., Miller, M. E., Drahota, A., Pellecchia, M., Barber, A. B., Griffith, E. M., Morgan, E. H., & Rogers, S. J. (2021). Examining US Public Early Intervention for Toddlers With Autism: Characterizing Services and Readiness for Evidence-Based Practice Implementation. *Frontiers in Psychiatry*, *12*, 786138. DOI: 10.3389/fpsyt.2021.786138 PMID: 34975582

Bang, M., Haeng Lee, S., Cho, S. H., Yu, S. A., Kim, K., & Lu, Y. H., Tae Chang, G., & Yeon Min, S. (2017). Herbal Medicine Treatment for Children with Autism Spectrum Disorder: A Systematic Review. ncbi.nlm.nih.gov

Barahona-Corrêa, J. B., Velosa, A., Chainho, A., Lopes, R., & Oliveira-Maia, A. J. (2018). Repetitive transcranial magnetic stimulation for treatment of autism spectrum disorder: A systematic review and meta-analysis. *Frontiers in Integrative Neuroscience*, *12*, 27. DOI: 10.3389/fnint.2018.00027 PMID: 30038561

Barnhart, G., Silverwood, A., Efird, W., & Wells, K. (2023). Animal assisted interventions on therapy farms for those with autism. *The Humanistic Psychologist, 51*(2), 160–172. DOI: 10.1037/hum0000217

Becker, B. E. (2024). Aquatic Therapy: History, Theory, and Applications. In The Use of Aquatics in Orthopedics and Sports Medicine Rehabilitation and Physical Conditioning (pp. 3-16). Routledge.

Bharathi, G., Venugopal, A., & Vellingiri, B. (2019). Music therapy as a therapeutic tool in improving the social skills of autistic children. *The Egyptian Journal of Neurology, Psychiatry and Neurosurgery, 55*(44), 1–6. DOI: 10.1186/s41983-019-0091-x

Bond, C., Symes, W., Hebron, J., Humphrey, N., Morewood, G., & Woods, K. (2016). Educational interventions for children with ASD: A systematic literature review 2008-2013. [PDF]

Borgi, M., Loliva, D., Cerino, S., Chiarotti, F., Venerosi, A., Bramini, M., Nonnis, E., Marcelli, M., Vinti, C., De Santis, C., Bisacco, F., Fagerlie, M., Frascarelli, M., & Cirulli, F. (2015). Effectiveness of a standardized equine-assisted therapy program for children with autism spectrum disorder. *Journal of Autism and Developmental Disorders, 46*(1), 1–9. DOI: 10.1007/s10803-015-2530-6 PMID: 26210515

Boso, M., Emanuele, E., Minazzi, V., Abbamonte, M., & Politi, P. (2007). Effect of long-term interactive music therapy on behavior profile and musical skills in young adults with severe autism. *Journal of Alternative and Complementary Medicine (New York, N.Y.), 13*(7), 709–712. DOI: 10.1089/acm.2006.6334 PMID: 17931062

Brelsford, V., Meints, K., Gee, N., & Pfeffer, K. (2017). Animal-assisted interventions in the classroom—A systematic review. *International Journal of Environmental Research and Public Health, 14*(7), 669. DOI: 10.3390/ijerph14070669 PMID: 28640200

CDC. (2014, March 28). - Developmental Disabilities Monitoring Network Surveillance Year 2010 Principal Investigators; Centers for Disease Control and Prevention (CDC). Prevalence of autism spectrum disorder among children aged 8 years - autism and developmental disabilities monitoring network, 11 sites, United States, 2010. *MMWR. Surveillance Summaries, 63*(2), 1–21.

Centers for Disease Control and Prevention. (2020). National diabetes statistics report, 2020. Atlanta, GA: Centers for Disease Control and Prevention, US Department of Health and Human Services, https://www.cdc.gov/diabetes/pdfs/data/statistics/national-diabetes-statisticsreport.pdf

Charry-Sánchez, J. D., Pradilla, I., & Talero-Gutiérrez, C. (2018). Animal-assisted therapy in adults: A systematic review. *Complementary Therapies in Clinical Practice*, *32*, 169–180. DOI: 10.1016/j.ctcp.2018.06.011 PMID: 30057046

Collacchi, B., Pinchaud, N., Borgi, M., & Cirulli, F. (2023). Equine-Assisted Activities (EAAs) for Children with Autism Spectrum Disorder (ASD): Positive Effects Revealed Using an Ethological Approach. *Applied Sciences (Basel, Switzerland)*, *13*(13), 7417. DOI: 10.3390/app13137417

DeFilippis, M. (2018). The Use of Complementary Alternative Medicine in Children and Adolescents with Autism Spectrum Disorder. *Psychopharmacology Bulletin*, *48*(1), 40–63. PMID: 29382959

Disorder, S. (•••).. . *Children (Basel, Switzerland)*, *10*(1), 122. DOI: 10.3390/children10010122

Elder, J. H., Kreider, C. M., Brasher, S. N., & Ansell, M. (2017, August 24). Clinical impact of early diagnosis of autism on the prognosis and parent-child relationships. *Psychology Research and Behavior Management*, *10*, 283–292. DOI: 10.2147/PRBM.S117499 PMID: 28883746

Faraji, S., Najafabadi, M. G., Zandi, H. G., & Parent-Nichols, J. (2022). Water-based exercise therapy and improvement in the motor skills and cognitive function of children with autism spectrum disorder: A commentary. *Russian Open Medical Journal*, *11*(1), 112. DOI: 10.15275/rusomj.2022.0112

Finisguerra, A., Borgatti, R., & Urgesi, C. (2019). Non-invasive brain stimulation for the rehabilitation of children and adolescents with neurodevelopmental disorders: A systematic review. *Frontiers in Psychology*, *10*, 135. DOI: 10.3389/fpsyg.2019.00135 PMID: 30787895

Gabriels, R., Pan, Z., Dechant, B., Agnew, J., Brim, N., & Mesibov, G. (2015). Randomized controlled trial of therapeutic horseback riding in children and adolescents with autism spectrum disorder. *Journal of the American Academy of Child and Adolescent Psychiatry*, *54*(7), 541–549. DOI: 10.1016/j.jaac.2015.04.007 PMID: 26088658

Geretsegger, M., Elefant, C., Mössler, K. A., & Gold, C. (2014). Music therapy for people with autism spectrum disorder. *Cochrane Database of Systematic Reviews*, *2016*(3), 6. DOI: 10.1002/14651858.CD004381.pub3 PMID: 24936966

Gold, C., Wigram, T., & Elefant, C. (2006). Music therapy for autistic spectrum disorder. *Cochrane Database of Systematic Reviews*, (2), CD004381. PMID: 16625601

Govindaraju, A., Lakshminarayanan, P., Sabarathinam, S., & Meganathan, H. (2020). Alternative therapies for children's with autism spectrum disorder. *International Journal of Contemporary Pediatrics, 7*(12), 2421. DOI: 10.18203/2349-3291.ijcp20205111

Grocke, D., & Wigram, T. (2006). *Receptive methods in music therapy: Techniques and clinical applications for music therapy clinicians, educators and students.* Jessica Kingsley Publishers.

Güeita-Rodríguez, J., Ogonowska-Slodownik, A., Morgulec-Adamowicz, N., Martín-Prades, M. L., Cuenca-Zaldívar, J. N., & Palacios-Ceña, D. (2021). Effects of Aquatic Therapy for Children with Autism Spectrum Disorder on Social Competence and Quality of Life: A Mixed Methods Study. *International Journal of Environmental Research and Public Health, 18*(6), 3126. DOI: 10.3390/ijerph18063126 PMID: 33803581

Harris, A., & Williams, J. (2017). The impact of a horse riding intervention on the social functioning of children with autism spectrum disorder. *International Journal of Environmental Research and Public Health, 14*(7), 776. DOI: 10.3390/ijerph14070776 PMID: 28708075

Hellings, D., Joosten, A., Hatfield, M., & Netto, J. (2022). Benefits and Challenges of Assistance Dogs for Families of Children on the Autism Spectrum: Mothers' Perspectives. *Qualitative Health Research, 32*(11), 1648–1656. DOI: 10.1177/10497323221111247 PMID: 35772944

Hill, J., Ziviani, J., & Driscoll, C. (2020). "the connection just happens": Therapists' perspectives of canine-assisted occupational therapy for children on the autism spectrum. *Australian Occupational Therapy Journal, 67*(6), 550–562. DOI: 10.1111/1440-1630.12680 PMID: 32510649

Hill, J., Ziviani, J., & Driscoll, C. (2020). Canine-assisted occupational therapy for children on the autism spectrum: Parents' perspectives. *Australian Occupational Therapy Journal, 67*(5), 427–436. DOI: 10.1111/1440-1630.12659 PMID: 32201966

Hillier, A., Greher, G., Poto, N., & Dougherty, M. (2012). Positive outcomes following participation in a music intervention for adolescents and young adults on the autism spectrum. *Psychology of Music, 40*(2), 201–215. DOI: 10.1177/0305735610386837

Hume, K., Steinbrenner, J., Odom, S., Morin, K., Nowell, S., Tomaszewski, B., Szendrey, S., McIntyre, N., Yücesoy-Özkan, S., & Savage, M. (2021). Evidence-Based Practices for Children, Youth, and Young Adults with Autism: Third Generation Review. *Journal of Autism and Developmental Disorders, 51*(11), 4013–4032. DOI: 10.1007/s10803-020-04844-2 PMID: 33449225

James, R., Sigafoos, J., Green, V. A., Lancioni, G. E., O'Reilly, M. F., Lang, R., Davis, T., Carnett, A., Achmadi, D., Gevarter, C., & Marschik, P. B. (2015). Music therapy for individuals with autism spectrum disorder: A systematic review. *Review Journal of Autism and Developmental Disorders*, *2*(1), 39–54. DOI: 10.1007/s40489-014-0035-4

Kern, P., Wolery, M., & Aldridge, D. (2007). Use of songs to promote independence in morning greeting routines for young children with autism. *Journal of Autism and Developmental Disorders*, *37*(7), 1264–1271. DOI: 10.1007/s10803-006-0272-1 PMID: 17120150

Kilmer, M., Hong, M., Randolph, D., Reichel, A., Huetter, S., Bowden, M., & Kilmer, C. (2024). Animal-assisted therapy in pediatric autism spectrum disorder: A case report. *The Nurse Practitioner*, *49*(3), 31–39. DOI: 10.1097/01.NPR.0000000000000151 PMID: 38386471

Koch, S. C., Riege, R. F., Tisborn, K., Biondo, J., Martin, L., & Beelmann, A. (2019). Effects of dance movement therapy and dance on health-related psychological outcomes. A meta-analysis update. *Frontiers in Psychology*, *10*, 1806. DOI: 10.3389/fpsyg.2019.01806 PMID: 31481910

Kodak, T., & Bergmann, S. (2020). Autism Spectrum Disorder: Characteristics, Associated Behaviors, and Early Intervention. *Pediatric Clinics of North America*, *67*(3), 525–535. DOI: 10.1016/j.pcl.2020.02.007 PMID: 32443991

LaGasse, A. B. (2017). Social outcomes in children with autism spectrum disorder: A review of music therapy outcomes. *Patient Related Outcome Measures*, *8*, 23–32. DOI: 10.2147/PROM.S106267 PMID: 28260959

Lee, B., Park, S., Kwon, H. J., Hwang, G. S., & Kim, M. (2023, January 4). Integrative treatment program for the treatment of children with autism spectrum disorder: A prospective observational case series. *Frontiers in Neurology*, *13*, 1017005. DOI: 10.3389/fneur.2022.1017005 PMID: 36686506

Lee, J., & Porretta, D. L. (2013). Enhancing the motor skills of children with autism spectrum disorders: A pool-based approach. *Journal of Physical Education, Recreation & Dance*, *84*(1), 41–45. DOI: 10.1080/07303084.2013.746154

Leighton, S., Rodriguez, K., Nieforth, L., & O'Haire, M. (2023). Service dogs for autistic children and family system functioning: A constant comparative analysis. *Frontiers in Psychiatry*, *14*, 1210095. Advance online publication. DOI: 10.3389/fpsyt.2023.1210095 PMID: 37520226

Levy, S., & Hyman, S. (2015). Complementary and Alternative Medicine Treatments for Children with Autism Spectrum Disorders. *Child and Adolescent Psychiatric Clinics of North America, 24*(1), 117–143. DOI: 10.1016/j.chc.2014.09.004 PMID: 25455579

Lim, H., & Draper, E. (2011). The effects of music therapy incorporated with applied behavior analysis verbal behavior approach for children with autism spectrum disorders. *Journal of Music Therapy, 48*(4), 532–550. DOI: 10.1093/jmt/48.4.532 PMID: 22506303

Lim, H. A. (2010). Effect of "developmental speech and language training through music" on speech production in children with autism spectrum disorders. *Journal of Music Therapy, 47*(1), 2–26. DOI: 10.1093/jmt/47.1.2 PMID: 20635521

Llambias, C., Magill-Evans, J., Smith, V., & Warren, S. (2016). Equine-assisted occupational therapy: Increasing engagement for children with autism spectrum disorder. The American journal of occupational therapy, 70(6), 7006220040p1-7006220040p9. DOI: 10.5014/ajot.2016.020701

Locke, J., Lawson, G., Beidas, R., Aarons, G., Xie, M., Lyon, A., Stahmer, A., Seidman, M., Frederick, L., Oh, C., Spaulding, C., Dorsey, S., & Mandell, D. (2019). Individual and organizational factors that affect implementation of evidence-based practices for children with autism in public schools: A cross-sectional observational study. *Implementation Science : IS, 14*(1), 29. DOI: 10.1186/s13012-019-0877-3 PMID: 30866976

Maenner, M. J., Shaw, K. A., Bakian, A. V., Bilder, D. A., Durkin, M. S., Esler, A., Furnier, S. M., Hallas, L., Hall-Lande, J., Hudson, A., Hughes, M. M., Patrick, M., Pierce, K., Poynter, J. N., Salinas, A., Shenouda, J., Vehorn, A., Warren, Z., Constantino, J. N., & Cogswell, M. E. (2021, December 3). Prevalence and Characteristics of Autism Spectrum Disorder Among Children Aged 8 Years - Autism and Developmental Disabilities Monitoring Network, 11 Sites, United States, 2018. *MMWR. Surveillance Summaries, 70*(11), 1–16. DOI: 10.15585/mmwr.ss7011a1 PMID: 34855725

Maenner MJ, Warren Z, Williams AR, Amoakohene E, Bakian AV, Bilder DA, Durkin MS, Fitzgerald RT, Furnier SM, Hughes MM, Ladd-Acosta CM, McArthur D, Pas ET, Salinas A, Vehorn A, Williams S, Esler A, Grzybowski A, Hall-Lande J, Nguyen RHN, Pierce K, Zahorodny W, Hudson A, Hallas L, Mancilla KC, Patrick M, Shenouda J, Sidwell K, DiRienzo M, Gutierrez J, Spivey MH, Lopez M, Pettygrove S, Schwenk YD, Washington A, Shaw KA. (2023) Prevalence and Characteristics of Autism Spectrum Disorder Among Children Aged 8 Years - Autism and Developmental Disabilities Monitoring Network, 11 Sites, United States, 2020. MMWR Surveill Summ. 24;72(2):1-14. . PMID: 36952288; PMCID: PMC10042614.DOI: 10.15585/mmwr.ss7202a1

Maksimović, S., Marisavljević, M., Stanojević, N., Ćirović, M., Punišić, S., Adamović, T., Đorđević, J., Krgović, I., & Subotić, M. (2023). Importance of Early Intervention in Reducing Autistic Symptoms and Speech-Language Deficits in Children with Autism

Malcolm, R., Ecks, S., & Pickersgill, M. (2017). 'it just opens up their world': Autism, empathy, and the therapeutic effects of equine interactions. *Anthropology & Medicine*, *25*(2), 220–234. DOI: 10.1080/13648470.2017.1291115 PMID: 28513182

Marquez-Garcia, A. V., Magnuson, J., Morris, J., Iarocci, G., Doesburg, S., & Moreno, S. (2021). Music therapy in autism spectrum disorder: A systematic review. *Review Journal of Autism and Developmental Disorders*, *9*(2), 1–17.

Masini E, Loi E, Vega-Benedetti AF, Carta M, Doneddu G, Fadda R, Zavattari P. (2020) An Overview of the Main Genetic, Epigenetic and Environmental Factors Involved in Autism Spectrum Disorder Focusing on Synaptic Activity. Int J Mol Sci. 5;21(21):8290. . PMID: 33167418; PMCID: PMC7663950.DOI: 10.3390/ijms21218290

Mateos-Moreno, D., & Atencia-Doña, L. (2013). Effect of a combined dance/movement and music therapy on young adults diagnosed with severe autism. *The Arts in Psychotherapy*, *40*(5), 465–472. DOI: 10.1016/j.aip.2013.09.004

Melgarejo, M., Lind, T., Stadnick, N., Helm, J., & Locke, J. (2020). Strengthening Capacity for Implementation of Evidence-Based Practices for Autism in Schools: The Roles of Implementation Climate, School Leadership and Fidelity. *The American Psychologist*, *75*(8), 1105–1115. DOI: 10.1037/amp0000649 PMID: 33252948

Mercer, J. (2013). Holding therapy: A harmful mental health intervention. *Focus on Alternative and Complementary Therapies*, *18*(2), 70–76. DOI: 10.1111/fct.12024

Merle, J. L., Cook, C. R., Locke, J. J., Ehrhart, M. G., Brown, E. C., Davis, C. J., & Lyon, A. R. (2023). Teacher attitudes toward evidence-based practices: Exploratory and confirmatory analyses of the school-adapted evidence-based practice attitude scale. *Implementation Research and Practice*, *4*, 26334895221151026. Advance online publication. DOI: 10.1177/26334895221151026 PMID: 37091537

Moller, A. S., Odell-Miller, H., & Wigram, T. (2002). Indications in music therapy: Evidence from assessment that can identify the expectations of music therapy as a treatment for autistic spectrum disorder (ASD); meeting the challenge of evidence based practice. *British Journal of Music Therapy*, *16*(1), 11–28. DOI: 10.1177/135945750201600104

Mondal, A., Sharma, R., Abiha, U., Ahmad, F., Karan, A. L., Jayaraj, R., & Sundar, V. (2023). A Spectrum of Solutions: Unveiling Non-Pharmacological Approaches to Manage Autism Spectrum Disorder. ncbi.nlm.nih.gov

Morgan, S., & O'Byrne, D. A. (2023). How Autism Assistance Canines Enhance the Lives of Autistic Children. INQUIRY. *Inquiry : a Journal of Medical Care Organization, Provision and Financing*, *60*, 00469580231195029. Advance online publication. DOI: 10.1177/00469580231195029 PMID: 37615078

Mortada (2024) Evidence-Based Complementary and Alternative Medicine in Current Medical Practice. Cureus 16(1): e52041. DOI DOI: 10.7759/cureus.52041

Music Therapy Handbook. https://books.google.pt/books?hl=pt-PT&lr=&id=mfnhBQAAQBAJ&oi=fnd&pg=PP1&dq=music+therapy&ots=0l7lwb413X&sig=y6-8hXKsOXS9OVzKMYrPO4YasKM&redir_esc=y#v=onepage&q=music%20therapy&f=false

Nimer, J., & Lundahl, B. (2007). Animal-assisted therapy: A meta-analysis. *Anthrozoos*, *20*(3), 225–238. DOI: 10.2752/089279307X224773

O'Haire, M., McKenzie, S., Beck, A., & Slaughter, V. (2013). Social behaviors increase in children with autism in the presence of animals compared to toys. *PLoS One*, *8*(2), e57010. DOI: 10.1371/journal.pone.0057010 PMID: 23468902

Ogonowska-Slodownik, A., Jakobowicz, O., Alexander, L., Marinho-Buzelli, A. R., Devion, C., & Morgulec-Adamowicz, N. (2024). Aquatic Therapy in Children and Adolescents with Disabilities: A Scoping Review. *Children (Basel, Switzerland)*, *11*(11), 1404. DOI: 10.3390/children11111404 PMID: 39594979

Okoye, C., M Obialo-Ibeawuchi, C., A Obajeun, O., Sarwar, S., Tawfik, C., Subhan Waleed, M., Ullah Wasim, A., Mohamoud, I., Y Afolayan, A., & N Mbaezue, R. (2023). Early Diagnosis of Autism Spectrum Disorder: A Review and Analysis of the Risks and Benefits.

Parker, A., Beresford, B., Dawson, V., Elphick, H., Fairhurst, C., Hewitt, C., Scantlebury, A., Spiers, G., Thomas, M., Wright, K., & McDaid, C. (2019). Oral melatonin for non-respiratory sleep disturbance in children with neurodisabilities: Systematic review and meta-analyses. *Developmental Medicine and Child Neurology*, *61*(8), 880–890. DOI: 10.1111/dmcn.14157 PMID: 30710339

Pendergast, D. R., Moon, R. E., Krasney, J. J., Held, H. E., & Zamparo, P. (2015). Human Physiology in an Aquatic Environment. *Comprehensive Physiology*, *5*(4), 1705–1750. DOI: 10.1002/j.2040-4603.2015.tb00655.x PMID: 26426465

Rehn, A. K., Caruso, V. R., & Kumar, S. (2023). The effectiveness of animal assisted therapy for children and adolescents with autism spectrum disorder: A systematic review. *Complementary Therapies in Clinical Practice*, *50*, 101719. DOI: 10.1016/j.ctcp.2022.101719 PMID: 36599281

Rogers, S., & Dawson, G. (2010). *Early start denver model for young children with autism: Promoting language, learning, and engagement*. The Guilford Press.

Rossignol, D. A., & Frye, R. E. (2011). Melatonin in autism spectrum disorders: A systematic review and meta-analysis. *Developmental Medicine and Child Neurology*, *53*(9), 783–792. DOI: 10.1111/j.1469-8749.2011.03980.x PMID: 21518346

Ruggeri, A., Dancel, A., Johnson, R., & Sargent, B. (2020). The effect of motor and physical activity intervention on motor outcomes of children with autism spectrum disorder: A systematic review. *Autism*, *24*(3), 544–568. DOI: 10.1177/1362361319885215 PMID: 31782658

Victoria Sandham, Anne E. Hill & Fiona Hinchliffe (2021): The current practices of Australian speech-language pathologists in providing communication services to children with autism spectrum disorder, International Journal of Speech-Language Pathology, DOI: To link to this article: https://doi.org/DOI: 10.1080/17549507.2021.1923800

Saral, D., Olcay, S., & Ozturk, H. (2023). Spectrum Disorder: When There is no Cure, There are Countless of Treatments. *Journal of Autism and Developmental Disorders*, *53*(12), 4901–4916. DOI: 10.1007/s10803-022-05745-2 PMID: 36222992

Schoen, S. A., Lane, S. J., Mailloux, Z., May-Benson, T., Parham, L. D., Smith Roley, S., & Schaaf, R. C. (2019). A systematic review of ayres sensory integration intervention for children with autism. *Autism Research, 12*(1), 6–19. DOI: 10.1002/aur.2046 PMID: 30548827

Schwartzberg, E., & Silverman, M. (2013). Effects of music-based social stories on comprehension and generalization of social skills in children with autism spectrum disorders: A randomized effectiveness study. *The Arts in Psychotherapy, 40*(3), 331–337. DOI: 10.1016/j.aip.2013.06.001

Shariat, A., Najafabadi, M. G., Dos Santos, I. K., Anastasio, A. T., Milajerdi, H. R., Hassanzadeh, G., & Nouri, E. (2024). The Effectiveness of Aquatic Therapy on Motor and Social Skill as Well as Executive Function in Children With Neurodevelopmental Disorder: A Systematic Review and Meta-analysis. *Archives of Physical Medicine and Rehabilitation, 105*(5), 1000–1007. DOI: 10.1016/j.apmr.2023.08.025 PMID: 37690741

Silva, K., Correia, R., Lima, M., Magalhães, A., & Sousa, L. (2011). Can dogs prime autistic children for therapy? evidence from a single case study. *Journal of Alternative and Complementary Medicine (New York, N.Y.), 17*(7), 655–659. DOI: 10.1089/acm.2010.0436 PMID: 21689015

Singer, A., & Ravi, R. (2015). Complementary and alternative treatments for autism part 2: Identifying and avoiding non-evidence-based treatments. *AMA Journal of Ethics, 17*(4), 375–380. DOI: 10.1001/journalofethics.2015.17.4.sect2-1504 PMID: 25901708

Sissons, J., Blakemore, E., Shafi, H., Skotny, N., & Lloyd, D. (2022). calm with horses? a systematic review of animal-assisted interventions for improving social functioning in children with autism. *Autism, 26*(6), 1320–1340. DOI: 10.1177/13623613221085338 PMID: 35403450

Smith, C. A., Parton, C., King, M., & Gallego, G. (2020). Parents' experiences of information-seeking and decision-making regarding complementary medicine for children with autism spectrum disorder: A qualitative study. *BMC Complementary Medicine and Therapies, 20*(1), 1–13. DOI: 10.1186/s12906-019-2805-0 PMID: 32020887

Sourvinos, S., Mavropoulos, A., Kasselimis, D. S., Korasidi, A., Voukouni, A. L., Papadopoulos, P., Vlaseros, S., Damianos, G., Potagas, C., & Damianos, D. (2021). Brief Report: Speech and Language Therapy in Children with ASD in an Aquatic Environment: the ASLT (Aquatic Speech and Language Therapy) Program. *Journal of Autism and Developmental Disorders, 51*(4), 1406–1416. DOI: 10.1007/s10803-020-04629-7 PMID: 32748193

Stahmer, A., Dababnah, S. & Rieth, S. (2019) Considerations in implementing evidence-based early autism spectrum disorder interventions in community settings. Pediatr Med;2:18 | DOI: 10.21037/pm.2019.05.01

Steinbrenner, J. R., Hume, K., Odom, S. L., Morin, K. L., Nowell, S. W., Tomaszewski, B., Szendrey, S., & McIntyre, N. S. YücesoyÖzkan, S., & Savage, M. N. (2020). Evidence-Based Practices for Children, Youth, and Young Adults with Autism. FPG Child Development Institute.

Vandana, P., Simkin, D. R., Hendren, R. L., & Arnold, L. E. (2023). Autism Spectrum Disorder and Complementary-Integrative Medicine. *Child and Adolescent Psychiatric Clinics of North America, 32*(2), 469–494. DOI: 10.1016/j.chc.2022.08.004 PMID: 37147047

Vogel, S.W., Mullins, K.L., & Kumar, S. (2024). Art therapy for children and adolescents with autism: a systematic review. *International Journal of Art Therapy.*

Warner, K., Keville, S., Hockley, J., & Ludlow, A. (2023). Experiences of equine assisted therapy for females with autism spectrum disorders. *Advances in Autism, 9*(2), 150–164. DOI: 10.1108/AIA-10-2021-0040

Wheeler, B. (2015). Music therapy as a profession. In Wheeler, B. (Ed.), *Music therapy handbook* (pp. 5–16). The Guilford Press.

Wheeler, B. L., Shultis, C. L., & Polen, D. W. (2005). Clinical training guide for the student music therapist. Barcelona: Gilsum.

Wigram, T., & Gold, C. (2006). Music therapy in the assessment and treatment of autistic spectrum disorder: Clinical application and research evidence. *Child: Care, Health and Development, 32*(5), 535–542. DOI: 10.1111/j.1365-2214.2006.00615.x PMID: 16919132

World Federation of Music Therapy. (2024, July 30th). About WFMT. Retrieved from https://www.wfmt.info/about

Wright, H., Hall, S., Hames, A., Hardiman, J., Mills, R., & Mills, D.PAWS Project Team. (2015). Pet dogs improve family functioning and reduce anxiety in children with autism spectrum disorder. *Anthrozoos*, *28*(4), 611–624. DOI: 10.1080/08927936.2015.1070003

Xiao, N., Shinwari, K., Kiselev, S., Huang, X., Li, B., & Qi, J. (2023). Effects of Equine-Assisted Activities and Therapies for Individuals with Autism Spectrum Disorder: Systematic Review and Meta-Analysis. *International Journal of Environmental Research and Public Health*, *20*(3), 2630. DOI: 10.3390/ijerph20032630 PMID: 36767996

Xiong, T., Chen, H., Luo, R., & Mu, D. (2016). Hyperbaric oxygen therapy for people with autism spectrum disorder (ASD). *Cochrane Database of Systematic Reviews*, *2016*(11), 10. DOI: 10.1002/14651858.CD010922.pub2 PMID: 27737490

Yang, Y. J., Siao, M. R., Tsai, F. T., & Luo, H. J. (2015). Effect of physical activity interventions on children and adolescents with autism spectrum disorder: A systematic review and meta-analysis. *Physiotherapy*, *101*, e1685–e1686. DOI: 10.1016/j.physio.2015.03.091

Young Carson, B. (2014). An Evaluation of the Attitudes Teachers Have Towards Adopting Evidence-Based Practices for Students with Autism in Preschool Classrooms.

Zanobini, M., & Solari, S. (2019). Effectiveness of the Program "Acqua Mediatrice di Comunicazione" (Water as a Mediator of Communication) on Social Skills, Autistic Behaviors and Aquatic Skills in ASD Children. *Journal of Autism and Developmental Disorders*, *49*(10), 4134–4146. DOI: 10.1007/s10803-019-04128-4 PMID: 31267291

Zoccante, L., Marconi, M., Ciceri, M. L., Gagliardoni, S., Gozzi, L. A., Sabaini, S., Di Gennaro, G., & Colizzi, M. (2021). Effectiveness of equine-assisted activities and therapies for improving adaptive behavior and motor function in autism spectrum disorder. *Journal of Clinical Medicine*, *10*(8), 1726. DOI: 10.3390/jcm10081726 PMID: 33923582

ADDITIONAL READING

Ansari, S., Hosseinkhanzadeh, A. A., AdibSaber, F., Shojaei, M., & Daneshfar, A. (2021). The Effects of Aquatic Versus Kata Techniques Training on Static and Dynamic Balance in Children with Autism Spectrum Disorder. *Journal of Autism and Developmental Disorders*, *51*(9), 3180–3186. DOI: 10.1007/s10803-020-04785-w PMID: 33206268

Caputo, G., Ippolito, G., Mazzotta, M., Sentenza, L., Muzio, M. R., Salzano, S., & Conson, M. (2018). Effectiveness of a Multisystem Aquatic Therapy for Children with Autism Spectrum Disorders. *Journal of Autism and Developmental Disorders*, *48*(6), 1945–1956. DOI: 10.1007/s10803-017-3456-y PMID: 29313176

Kolachahi, S. A. (2020). Water-based training in combined with vitamin D supplementation improves lipid profile in children with ASD. *Research in Autism Spectrum Disorders*, *76*, 101603. DOI: 10.1016/j.rasd.2020.101603

Marzouki, H., Soussi, B., Selmi, O., Hajji, Y., Marsigliante, S., Bouhlel, E., Muscella, A., Weiss, K., & Knechtle, B. (2022). Effects of Aquatic Training in Children with Autism Spectrum Disorder. *Biology (Basel)*, *11*(5), 657. DOI: 10.3390/biology11050657 PMID: 35625385

Pan, C. Y. (2010). Effects of water exercise swimming program on aquatic skills and social behaviors in children with autism spectrum disorders. *Autism*, *14*(1), 9–28. DOI: 10.1177/1362361309339496 PMID: 20124502

Yanardag, M., Akmanoglu, N., & Yilmaz, I. (2013). The effectiveness of video prompting on teaching aquatic play skills for children with autism. *Disability and Rehabilitation*, *35*(1), 47–56. DOI: 10.3109/09638288.2012.687030 PMID: 22624856

KEY TERMS AND DEFINITIONS

Autism Spectrum Disorder: Is a complex neurodevelopmental condition characterized by persistent deficits in social communication and interaction, alongside restricted and repetitive patterns of behavior, interests, or activities. The Diagnostic and Statistical Manual of Mental Disorders, Fifth Edition (DSM-5), outlines these core features, emphasizing the variability in symptom presentation and severity across individuals, which is why it is referred to as a "spectrum" disorder.

Complementary Approcahes: Complementary approaches refer to a range of therapeutic practices that are used alongside conventional medical treatments to enhance patient care and promote overall well-being.

Speech-Language Pathology: Speech-Language Pathology (SLP) is a specialized field within healthcare focused on the assessment, diagnosis, treatment, and prevention of communication disorders, including speech, language, voice, and swallowing difficulties.

Intervention: Intervention is a multifaceted term used across various fields, including healthcare, psychology, education, and social services. In a broad sense, an intervention refers to a deliberate action or set of actions designed to bring about a change in a specific situation, behavior, or health condition. The goal of an intervention is typically to improve outcomes for individuals or groups by addressing identified needs or problems.

Outcomes: Outcomes refer to the measurable results or effects that arise from specific interventions, treatments, or programs. In healthcare and social sciences, outcomes are critical for evaluating the effectiveness of various interventions, as they provide insights into the impact on patients' health, well-being, and quality of life.

Chapter 7
Emerging Strategies for Food Allergen Management: Innovation and Potential

Sachi Dubey
University Institute of Chemical Technology, Kavayitri Bahinabai Chaudhari North Maharashtra University, India

Sunil Jayant Kulkarni
https://orcid.org/0000-0002-5988-3448
Gharda Institute of Technology, Lavel, India

Ajaygiri K. Goswami
University Institute of Chemical Technology, Kavayitri Bahinabai Chaudhari North Maharashtra University, India

ABSTRACT

Food allergies are a major global health concern that affect millions of people. The intricacy of the food supply chain and the range of allergens cannot be fully accommodated by traditional methods, such as labeling laws and manufacturing procedures. In response, new approaches and cutting-edge technologies are being developed to improve the management of food allergies. By enhancing the identification, management, and dissemination of allergen risks, these strategies hope to boost consumer confidence and safety. This review examines recent developments in food allergen management, such as innovative food processing techniques, state-of-the-art detection methods, and regulatory advancements. In order to address the changing issues surrounding food allergies and safeguard the public's health, the review highlights how crucial it is for stakeholders to keep coming up with new

DOI: 10.4018/979-8-3693-6432-1.ch007

ideas and working together.

1. INTRODUCTION

Food allergies are a significant and growing public health concern, affecting millions worldwide and impacting families, communities, and healthcare systems (News-Medical, 2024). The worldwide data indicates about 1 to 10% of the population is affected by food allergies (Food and agricultural organization of united nations, 2024). It is estimated that about 220 million people worldwide have food allergies (Food and agricultural organization of united nations, 2024). With increasing prevalence, particularly in children and adults in developed nations, effective management strategies are essential to ensure consumer safety. Traditional allergen control methods, such as avoidance, ingredient labeling, and food processing interventions, have proven insufficient in addressing the complexities of modern food production and globalized supply chains (Sathe & Sharma, 2009). Additionally, the introduction of novel protein sources, including plant-based and lab-grown proteins, presents new challenges in allergen risk assessment and mitigation (Lehrer et al., 2002). Therefore, innovative approaches and advanced technologies are required to enhance allergen detection, food safety monitoring, and consumer confidence.

Recent advancements in food technology are revolutionizing allergen management. Cutting-edge analytical tools, such as mass spectrometry, polymerase chain reaction (PCR)-based DNA detection, and biosensors, enable highly sensitive and rapid identification of allergens in food products, minimizing the risk of accidental exposure (Rejeb et al., 2020). Machine learning algorithms and artificial intelligence (AI)-driven predictive models are also being developed to assess allergen risks in food processing and supply chains, allowing for proactive intervention strategies (Papadopoulos et al., 2012). Furthermore, emerging food processing techniques, including enzymatic hydrolysis and genetic modification, are being explored to reduce allergenicity in food ingredients, offering safer alternatives for allergic individuals (Sampath et al., 2021).

Beyond detection and processing innovations, improvements in allergen traceability and consumer communication are gaining momentum. Blockchain technology and smart labeling systems, such as near-field communication (NFC) and QR code-enabled packaging, provide real-time allergen information, empowering consumers to make informed choices (Papadopoulos et al., 2012). The integration of these digital solutions with wearable health monitoring devices and mobile applications allows allergic individuals to track exposure, receive alerts, and manage their dietary restrictions more effectively (Rejeb et al., 2020). These advancements not only improve consumer safety but also drive regulatory compliance and industry-wide adoption of best practices in allergen management.

Despite these promising developments, challenges remain in implementing and standardizing new allergen control technologies across global food industries. Regulatory agencies, food manufacturers, and researchers must collaborate to establish uniform guidelines and safety assessment protocols for emerging food products and processing techniques (Ortolani & Pastorello, 2006). Investment in research and development is crucial to refining allergen risk assessment tools, improving food labeling accuracy, and enhancing public awareness initiatives (De Blok et al., 2007).

Voluntary Incidental Trace Allergen Labelling (VITAL) is one of the evolving tools for food allergen risk management (Liu et al., 2025). Algorithm based diagnostic tools are being developed for diagnosis and response to the food allergen (Santos et al., 2025). According to Li et al. (2025), with increasing use of alternative protein options, the concern about their allergen character needs to be studied in depth. The simple measures like cross contact prevention and cleaning efficacy can improve the food safety to a large extent (Lopez-Calvo et al., 2025). Various fruits and food supplements have specific allergen effects on mankind and various researchers have reported their effects (Satnarine et al., 2025; Edpuganti et al., 2025; Ma et al., 2025; Konstantinou al., 2025; Parrinello et al., 2025).

This chapter provides an in-depth review of the latest innovations in food allergy management, emphasizing the role of advanced detection methods, food processing techniques, and digital solutions in mitigating allergen-related risks. By integrating these technologies into food safety frameworks, the industry can enhance consumer confidence, reduce health risks, and address the growing challenges associated with food allergies in an evolving dietary landscape. Continued research, collaboration, and innovation will be essential to advancing food allergen management and ensuring public health protection in the years to come.

Understanding Food Allergies

Food allergies, resulting from unusual immune reactions to proteins, can cause moderate to severe symptoms and potentially be fatal, necessitating understanding for the food industry, medical professionals, and consumer safety (Institute for Quality and Efficiency in Health Care (IQWiG), 2023).

Millions of people worldwide suffer from food allergies, ranging from small hives to severe symptoms like anaphylaxis. Preventative and therapy options are being studied, with early identification and education about managing allergies critical for preventing catastrophic health effects. The FDA requires companies to declare ingredients on packaged foods and beverages in order to safeguard people with food allergies and hypersensitivity reactions. The FDA offers advice to stakeholders, the food industry, and consumers on how to manage food allergen hazards, carry out sampling and inspections to guarantee accurate labeling, and avoid cross-contact and undeclared allergens during the manufacturing and packaging process (*Food Allergies*, 2024).

Food Allergy and Food Intolerance

Food Allergy

Food allergies and intolerances are two different conditions with different underlying causes and mechanisms that result in adverse reactions to particular foods. They are immune system responses to specific proteins in food, causing the body to mistakenly recognize harmful substances and release antibodies, specifically IgE (Nettleton et al., 2009)

Food Intolerance

Food intolerance is a non-immune response to certain foods or components, causing adverse reactions like bloating, gas, diarrhea, abdominal pain, and headaches. Food intolerance, encompassing lactose, gluten, and sulfites, is a prevalent ailment that is typified by heterogeneous symptoms contingent on the quantity of food ingested and personal sensitivity (Muthukumar et al., 2020).

The following are among the primary differences between food intolerance and food allergy (T C, 2024):

> *Food intolerance and food allergies differ significantly in their mechanisms and effects on the body. Unlike food allergies, which involve the immune system reacting to specific amino acids in food, food intolerance does not trigger an immune response. The onset of symptoms also varies; food allergies can cause reactions within minutes to hours of consuming the allergenic food, whereas food intolerance symptoms may take hours or even days to appear. The severity of symptoms further distinguishes the two conditions—food allergies can lead to severe and potentially fatal reactions, while food intolerance generally results in mild to moderate discomfort. Additionally, the amount of food required to trigger symptoms differs; even trace amounts of an allergenic food can cause severe allergic reactions, whereas food intolerance typically requires larger quantities of the offending food to produce symptoms. In terms of treatment, avoiding the allergenic food is the primary strategy for managing food allergies, whereas dietary modifications, such as reducing or eliminating the problematic food, can help manage food intolerance.*

Common Food Allergens

The "big eight" allergens, including milk, eggs, peanuts, tree nuts, fish, shellfish, wheat, and soy, cause over 90% of all food allergies. These common allergens pose a significant health risk, causing symptoms ranging from minor hives to severe reactions like anaphylaxis. Recognizing and controlling these allergens is crucial for safeguarding individuals and maintaining food safety (Rd, 2024). Common allergens, like peanuts, milk, and egg allergies, trigger distinct immune responses, with peanut allergies causing severe reactions, milk and egg allergies causing outgrown reactions, and seafood allergies persisting into adulthood (Secord, 2021). Figure 1 depicts major types of food allergen sources.

Figure 1. Major types of food allergens

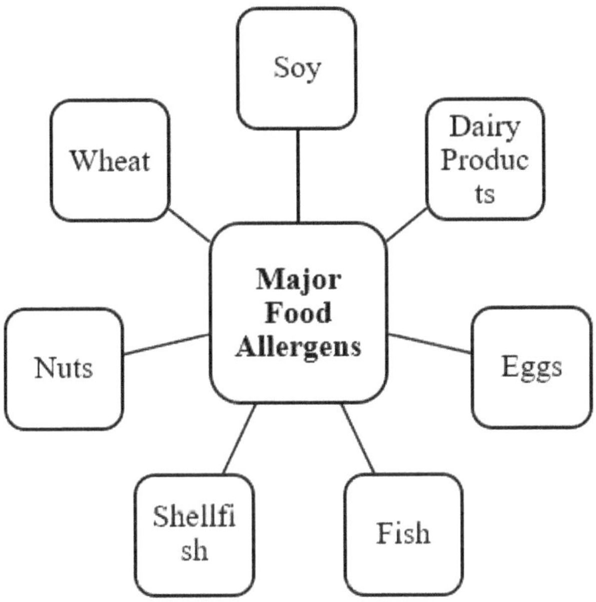

Source: (J. C. M. Rd, 2024)

Common Food Allergens

Peanuts and Tree Nuts

- One of the most common and dangerous food allergies.
- May result in potentially fatal anaphylactic reactions.

- Present in a large range of dishes, including baked products, sauces, and peanut butter.
- Add a variety of nuts, such as hazelnuts, cashews, pecans, and walnuts.
- frequently cross-reactive, which means a person with an allergy to one tree nut might react to others.
- Additionally, frequently present in a variety of processed foods (*Food Allergies Symptoms, Diagnosis & Treatment | AAAAI*, 2018).

Shellfish

Shellfish, aquatic animals with shells, are classified as crustaceans and mollusks, with crustaceans including shrimp, crab, lobster, and crayfish, and mollusks including clams, oysters, mussels, and scallops.

Comprises crustaceans such as lobster, crab, and shrimp.

May result in acute, instantaneous allergic responses.

Allergies can worsen with repeated exposure and are frequently lifelong (Professional, 2024).

Fish

Fish allergy, affecting up to 1% of the adult population, is a prevalent food allergen that can cause severe reactions in some individuals.

Fish fall into two categories: shellfish and finfish. Shrimp, crab, and lobster are examples of shellfish, whereas salmon, tuna, cod, and halibut are examples of finfish.

Allergy can manifest in any age group, including adults.

Can be found submerged in foods like Worcestershire sauce and Caesar dressing (*Food Allergies*, 2024).

Eggs

Egg allergy, a prevalent food allergen, affects up to 2% of children, causing severe allergic reactions in some individuals.

A typical allergy in children that many outgrow over time.

Found in baked goods, pastas, and other foods in addition to the obvious egg dishes (*Major Allergens: The Big Nine – School Nutrition Association*, 2022).

Dairy Products

Dairy products are a common food allergen, causing severe reactions in newborns and early childhood, impacting up to 3% of children under three.

Children frequently have allergies to milk proteins including casein and whey.

Reactions can range from severe anaphylaxis to digestive problems (*Food Allergy*, 2023).

Soy

Soy allergy, a common food allergen, affects up to 0.5% of children and can cause severe allergic reactions in some individuals.

Soy protein allergies are rather common, especially in young children.

May be found concealed in many processed foods and Asian dishes (*Common Allergens - Peanut, Egg, and Sesame Allergies | FARE*, 2023).

Wheat

Wheat allergy, a prevalent food allergen, affects up to 1% of children, causing severe allergic reactions in some individuals.

Some people may experience allergic reactions to the wheat protein gluten.

Distinct from celiac disease, an autoimmune illness (Lyons et al., 2019).

Mechanisms of Food Allergic Reactions

Food allergies occur when the immune system mistakenly perceives a food protein as dangerous, resulting in the production of antibodies to neutralize the perceived threat (Yu et al., 2016). Food allergies occur when the immune system misinterprets a food or component as harmful, leading to the secretion of immunoglobulin E (IgE), an antibody that neutralizes the allergen. Despite oral tolerance being the body's normal physiological reaction, there has been a breakdown in this process in the last 20 years, increasing the frequency of sensitization to food allergens. Research is ongoing to understand the function of gut microbiota, immunologic mechanisms behind desensitization, and factors influencing tissue and immunological responses to dietary antigens (Sicherer, 2011).

Sensitization Phase

The immune system responds to food allergens by producing IgE antibodies that bind to mast cells and basophils, causing allergic reactions. Upon first exposure to allergens like peanuts or shellfish, the immune system may identify them as harmful (Van Wijk & Knippels, 2007). Antigen-presenting cells introduce these allergens to naive T lymphocytes in the gut, leading to Th2 cell differentiation and the release of cytokines like IL-4, IL-5, and IL-13. These cytokines stimulate B cells to produce allergen-specific IgE antibodies, which bind to mast cells and basophils, increasing sensitivity and the risk of allergic reactions upon future exposure (Van Bilsen et al., 2017).

Allergic Reaction Phase

Upon repeated exposure to a food allergen, it binds to IgE antibodies on mast cells and basophils, triggering histamine release. Initially, the immune system identifies the allergen as foreign, producing IgE antibodies that sensitize the individual. On subsequent exposures, the allergen binds to IgE on sensitized cells, causing cross-linking and degranulation (Sampson, 2016). This releases mediators like histamine, proteases, prostaglandins, and leukotrienes, along with cytokines and chemokines that recruit inflammatory cells. Symptoms vary by exposure route and may include hives, angioedema, nausea, vomiting, diarrhea, wheezing, and hypotension (Turnbull et al., 2014).

Severe Reactions

Anaphylaxis is a severe, life-threatening allergic reaction that can occur due to food allergies (Anderson, 1996). It involves the rapid release of chemical mediators from mast cells and basophils, leading to systemic responses such as vasodilation, reduced blood pressure, and airway constriction. Symptoms include difficulty breathing, swelling of the face and throat, and potential cardiovascular complications. Immune cells like T cells and eosinophils contribute to inflammation and tissue damage. The severity of reactions depends on allergen consumption, sensitivity, and exposure route. Immediate medical attention, including epinephrine, is crucial for managing anaphylaxis (Turnbull et al., 2014).

2. DIAGNOSIS AND TESTING OF FOOD ALLERGIES

A physical examination, a medical history review, and specialized testing are used to diagnose food allergies and determine whether an allergic response to a specific food is present (Lieberman & Sicherer, 2010).

To diagnose food allergies, follow these essential procedures and techniques:

Diagnostic Approaches

Medical History

- The healthcare provider will take a detailed medical history, including symptoms, reaction timing, and suspected trigger foods. They will also gather data on family allergy history, other allergic conditions like eczema or asthma, and previous food-related reactions (Gupta et al., 2018).

Physical Examination

- Patients may be advised to keep a food diary to track potential food triggers and symptoms. During a physical exam, the physician will look for signs of allergic reactions, such as swelling or hives, to rule out other causes and confirm an allergy (Gupta et al., 2018).

Allergy Testing

Skin Prick Tests

A common diagnostic test involves placing a small amount of suspected food allergen on the skin and observing for a raised, itchy bump within 15-20 minutes, indicating a positive result. Conducted in an allergist's office, this skin prick test is reliable for identifying IgE-mediated food allergies but is not recommended for those using antihistamines or with certain skin conditions due to potential false results (Urisu et al., 2011).

Blood Test (IgE Test)

Food allergies can be diagnosed using a blood test that measures the concentration of specific IgE antibodies. This test determines food-specific IgE levels but cannot predict reaction severity. Elevated IgE levels suggest a possible allergy, but results should be interpreted with the patient's medical history and other test outcomes.

Results are slower than skin prick tests and may yield false positives. Examples include RAST and ImmunoCAP (Asero et al., 2006).

Oral Food Challenge (OFC)

An oral food challenge is the "gold standard" for diagnosing food allergies. Under medical supervision, the suspected food is given in increasing doses while monitoring symptoms. This method provides the most definitive diagnosis by assessing the body's actual reaction to the food but requires medical care due to the risk of severe allergic reactions (Nowak-Węgrzyn & Albin, 2015).

Elimination Diet

An elimination diet helps identify food allergies and intolerances by temporarily removing suspected allergens from the diet and then reintroducing them. Symptom improvement during elimination and recurrence upon reintroduction suggest an allergy. This non-invasive method aids in identifying dietary triggers but requires strict adherence and may risk nutritional deficiencies (Fiocchi et al., 2021).

Component Resolved Diagnostic Testing (CRD)

Component-resolved diagnostic testing is a newer method for identifying food allergies by measuring IgE antibodies specific to certain food proteins (Bulanda et al., 2018). This test helps pinpoint the exact proteins causing allergic reactions and assesses the risk of severe responses. It provides detailed allergen component information, useful in complex cases, but is costly and less accessible than standard IgE tests (Figure 2).

No single test can definitively diagnose food allergies. Allergists consider medical history, physical exams, and test results for accurate diagnosis (Patel & Volcheck, 2015). Proper identification is crucial as food allergies can be life-threatening. Patients must avoid trigger foods and carry emergency epinephrine (Fleischer & Burks, 2015).

Figure 2. The clinical method for identifying food allergies mediated by IgE includes oral food challenge (OFC), mast cell activation test (MAT), and basophil activation test (BAT).

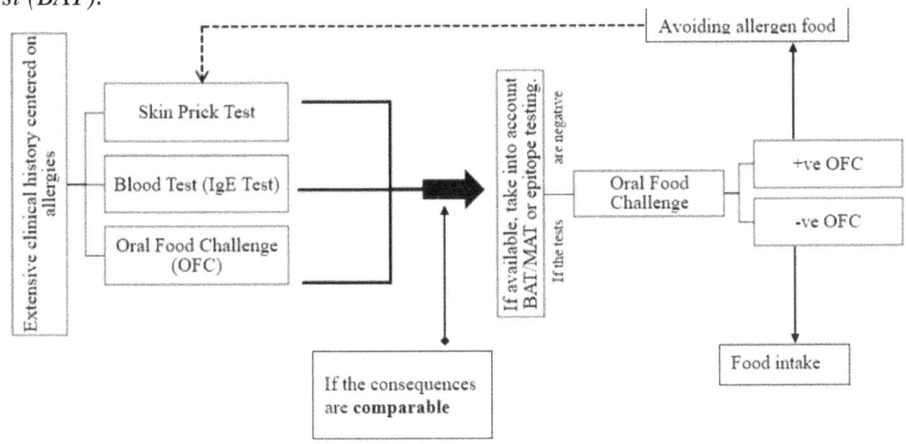

Source: (Foong et al., 2021)

Technological Innovations in Food Allergen Detection and Management

Innovation and Technological Advancements in Allergen Management

The management and treatment of food allergies have improved with technological advancements. Modern methods like mass spectrometry, immunoassays, and PCR enhance allergen detection sensitivity and accuracy (Ekezie et al., 2018). Food manufacturers are reducing allergen cross-contamination through new processing techniques. Promising treatments such as Oral Immunotherapy (OIT) are effective for peanut and milk allergies, and researchers are exploring desensitization vaccines. Personalized medicine approaches, including pharmacogenomics and precision nutrition, further enhance diagnosis and management.

Advancements in Allergen Detection Technologies

Technological advancements have transformed allergen detection, enhanced food safety and reducing cross-contamination risks. Techniques like ELISA, PCR, and mass spectrometry have improved detection accuracy (Picariello et al., 2011). Portable devices using microfluidic technology or lateral flow assays enable real-time on-site testing (Ross et al., 2018). Multiplex assays allow simultaneous detection of multiple allergens, streamlining testing processes (Kalita et al., 2019). Advances in antibody development, sample preparation, and allergen traceability via RFID and blockchain technologies further enhance food safety (Nath, 2024). Predictive modeling and data analytics help forecast allergen risks in food production (Zhou et al., 2021).

Improvements in Allergen Labeling

Recent improvements in allergen labeling have enhanced transparency and consumer safety. Measures like plain language labeling, precautionary allergen labeling (PAL), and mandatory allergen disclosure help consumers make informed choices (Linders et al., 2023). Digitalized labeling and traceability systems improve efficiency and accuracy, enabling effective recalls (Turnbull et al., 2014). Smart labeling and dynamic displays provide real-time allergen information tailored to individual needs (Curulli, 2022). Standardized formats, multilingual pictorial labeling, and allergen threshold labeling further ensure compliance and safety (Ippolito & Mathios, 1993; Allen et al., 2014). Advanced search filters and augmented reality applications enhance consumer interaction with allergen information (Temple & Fraser, 2014; Chen, 2022).

Challenges and Future Directions in Allergen Detection

Despite advancements, challenges persist in allergen detection methods. High equipment costs and specialized knowledge limit widespread adoption (Food Allergies, 2024). Regulatory inconsistencies across countries complicate compliance, necessitating harmonized standards (Bayen et al., 2024). Legacy system integration, lack of awareness, and adapting to emerging allergens remain barriers (Agrawal et al., 2013; Ortolani & Pastorello, 2006). Collaborative research, training, and investment in innovative detection methods are essential to enhance food safety and consumer confidence (Verhoeckx et al., 2015; Food Chain Allergen Management, 2009).

3. TRADITIONAL ALLERGEN MANAGEMENT STRATEGIES

Traditional allergy management techniques, such as label reading, avoidance, emergency preparations, education, allergen-free zones, cross-contamination prevention, and allergy alerts, are crucial for people with food allergies. Avoiding allergens involves reading food labels, asking about ingredients, and preventing cross-contamination by using separate utensils and cooking surfaces (Nio et al.,

2017). Education helps family members recognize allergies and warning signs, while allergy alerts notify of potential hazards. Establishing allergen-free zones reduces exposure risk, and having an emergency plan is vital in case of accidental ingestion. Despite their effectiveness, these methods are not foolproof, and individuals must be prepared to handle allergic reactions (Institute for Quality and Efficiency in Health Care (IQWiG), 2023).

Those with food allergies can prevent or minimize their exposure to allergenic foods by using traditional allergy management techniques. Some conventional methods for managing allergens are as follows:

Living With Food Allergies

Although having a food allergy might be difficult, those who have it can have active, healthy lives if they manage it well. Some coping mechanisms for managing food allergies include the following:

Understand Your Allergens

Eliminating allergenic foods is crucial for managing food allergies. This involves carefully reading food labels, asking about ingredients when dining out, and avoiding cross-contamination. Understanding specific allergens and their various forms is essential. For example, those with peanut or milk allergies must avoid products like peanut butter, oil, flour, cheese, yogurt, and butter. Similarly, individuals with shellfish allergies should avoid krill, crayfish, shrimp, and crab, while those with wheat allergies should avoid bread, pasta, and cereal (Barnett et al., 2018).

Cross-contamination can occur through shared utensils, cutting boards, or frying oil. Hidden allergens may be present in processed foods, so it's important to read labels and contact manufacturers with any ingredient questions. Effective management requires understanding specific allergens, their forms, potential cross-contamination sources, and hidden allergens to reduce the risk of allergic reactions (Renz et al., 2018).

Carry Emergency Medication

Food allergy sufferers must be prepared for unexpected reactions by carrying emergency medication, such as an epinephrine auto-injector, and ensuring it is current and not expired. Regular practice with the auto-injector is essential. In case of a severe allergic reaction, use the auto-injector immediately and seek emergency medical treatment, as delaying can worsen symptoms and lead to fatal outcomes. Educate family, friends, and caregivers about proper usage and recognize reaction signs. Have an emergency plan with hospital details and special instructions. Emergency preparedness, including immediate medication administration and seeking medical attention, is crucial for managing food allergies (Clark et al., 2004).

Develop an Emergency Plan and Educate Others

Managing food allergies requires proactive health management and emergency planning. This includes having procedures for allergic reactions, hospital details, emergency contacts, and special instructions. Individuals should keep a list of medications and allergies and educate family, friends, and caregivers about warning signs and emergency plans. Disclosing allergies to teachers, employers, and food service establishments is crucial. Inquire about ingredients and cross-contamination when dining out, and consider bringing safe food from home.

Regular follow-ups with healthcare providers, symptom monitoring, and treatment adjustments are essential. Food allergy sufferers should carry emergency medication, wear medical alert jewelry, and be prepared to administer treatment immediately. Creating an emergency plan and educating others about dietary restrictions can reduce reaction risks.

Effective management involves constant awareness of foods to avoid, having emergency supplies, and considering allergen immunotherapy. By taking these precautions, individuals with food allergies can lead active, healthy lives (Schauberger & Singh, 2020; Warren et al., 2017; Bacal, 2013).

Labeling Regulations

The Food Safety and Standards Authority of India (FSSAI) oversees food labeling laws, requiring manufacturers to list eight main allergens on packaged and processed foods: cereals containing gluten, peanuts, soybeans, milk, eggs, fish, crustaceans, and tree nuts. Even if these allergens are not primary ingredients, their presence must be disclosed. In 2020, the FSSAI proposed updates to labeling standards, including adding sesame and mustard as allergens and mandating more prominent allergy labeling (De et al., 2019). Figure 3 depicts allergen labelling regulations in India.

Figure 3. Allergen labelling regulations in India

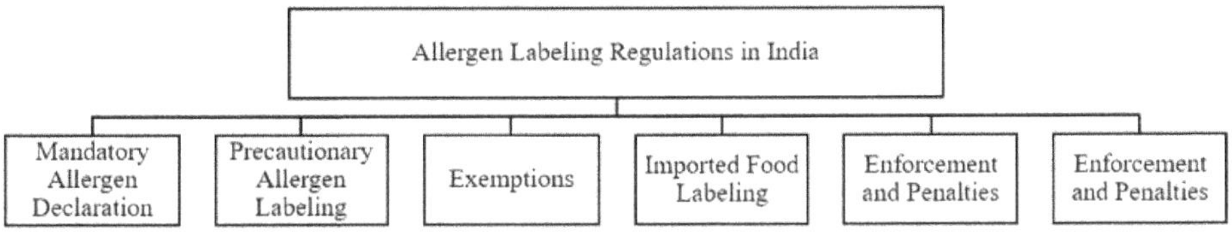

The following is an overview of conventional allergy management techniques that concentrate on food labeling laws in India (Varghese et al., 2022):

Mandatory Allergen Declaration

The FSSAI Food Labeling and Display Regulations 2020 mandate that certain allergies must be clearly and concisely disclosed on food labels:

a) Cereals containing gluten (wheat, rye, barley, oats, spelt)
b) Crustaceans and their products
c) Milk and milk products
d) Eggs and egg products
e) Fish and fish products
f) Peanuts, tree nuts and their products
g) Soybeans and soy products
h) Sulphites in concentrations of 10mg/kg or more

Specified names (e.g., “Contains: Milk, Wheat”) must be used when declaring allergies.

Precautionary Allergen Labeling

The FSSAI allows optional precautionary allergy labeling for potential cross-contamination, such as “May contain: Peanuts.” Exemptions apply to refined oils and proven-safe food components. Imported foods must display importer information and FSSAI license numbers. The FSSAI enforces these regulations through inspections, imposing penalties like fines and license suspensions for non-compliance.

Accurate and thorough labeling is crucial for allergy safety. The FSSAI regulates labeling for packaged foods and food service establishments, including allergen and cross-contamination information. Adherence to these guidelines helps ensure food safety in India. Continuous innovation and research are essential to enhance traditional allergy control methods (Meijer et al., 2021).

Manufacturing Practices

Conventional approaches to managing allergies in India center on keeping allergens accurately labeled and avoiding cross-contamination. Guidelines are provided by the Food Safety and Standards Authority of India (FSSAI) to assist producers in upholding safe practices for customers with food allergies (*Basic Food Safety Handbook/Manual for Food Manufacturers, Processors and Packers*, 2011). Figure 4 depicts manufacturing practices in India.

Figure 4. Manufacturing practices

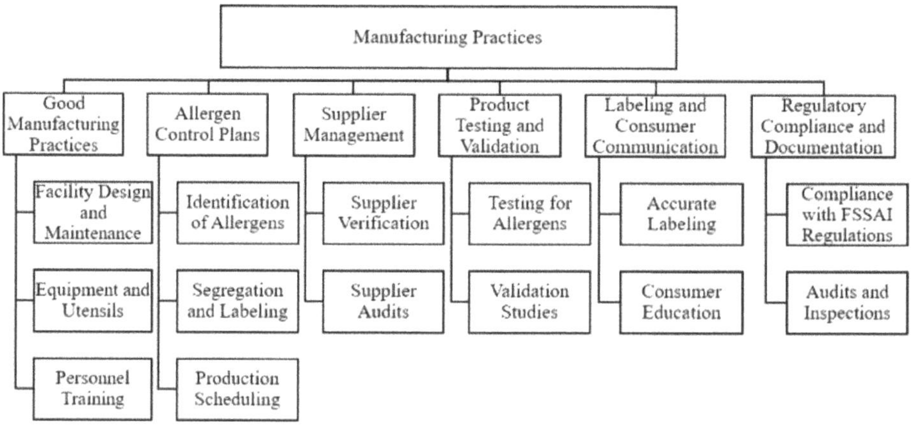

Good Manufacturing Practices (GMP)

Food producers must follow Good Manufacturing Practices (GMP) to ensure product quality and safety. GMPs cover all aspects of food manufacturing, from sourcing raw materials to packaging and shipping. They are crucial for reducing allergen cross-contamination and ensuring food safety for allergy sufferers. GMPs emphasize effective allergen management, including identifying and controlling allergenic ingredients, and having written procedures for handling, storage, use, and equipment cleaning.

Facility Design and Maintenance

Good Manufacturing Practices (GMPs) require manufacturers to prevent allergen cross-contamination by using dedicated equipment and implementing effective cleaning practices. This includes physically segregating production areas for allergenic and non-allergenic items, managing airflow to prevent allergen circulation, and designating specific storage areas for allergen-containing materials. Regular cleaning and sanitation protocols, along with periodic deep cleaning and validation, ensure allergen residues are removed. Effective pest control and equipment maintenance further reduce cross-contamination risks (Hasnan et al., 2022).

Equipment and Utensils

Good Manufacturing Practices (GMPs) require producers to establish quality control procedures, including regular testing and inspection of raw materials, finished products, and environmental samples to ensure product reliability and safety. This involves using distinct, labeled equipment for handling allergen-containing and allergen-free items, and designing equipment with smooth, non-porous surfaces like food-grade plastics or stainless steel to prevent allergen residue buildup. Validated cleaning and sanitization protocols, along with dedicated tools and thorough rinsing and drying, help remove allergen residues. Regular preventive maintenance and inspections, coupled with comprehensive staff training on equipment handling and allergen management, are crucial for compliance (Blanchfield, 2005).

Personnel Training

The Food Safety and Standards Authority of India (FSSAI) sets GMP guidelines for the Indian food sector, ensuring adherence through regular audits and inspections. This includes allergen awareness training to educate employees about food allergens, cross-contamination risks, and allergen-containing ingredients. Detailed standard operating procedures (SOPs) for allergen handling, along with training on cleaning, sanitation, and waste management, are crucial for preventing cross-contamination. Employees should also be trained on accurate allergen labeling and traceability systems, as well as emergency response and reporting procedures for allergen-related incidents. Encouraging employee feedback and regularly updating training programs are essential for continuous improvement in allergen management practices (Abou-El-Enein et al., 2013).

Allergen Control Plans

An allergy management plan is a crucial document in food manufacturing to ensure the safety of people with food allergies and prevent cross-contamination. It outlines the steps and protocols a food maker takes to control allergens in their establishment. The plan starts by identifying allergens in the production facility and products, and evaluating risks to determine the severity of allergic reactions.

- Identification of Allergens: An allergen control plan involves identifying and managing allergens in manufacturing facilities and products. This includes maintaining an allergen inventory, mapping allergen zones, and implementing strict ingredient and supplier management. Regularly reviewing and auditing labeling and packaging processes ensures accurate allergen declarations. Conducting a thorough risk assessment helps identify and address cross-contamination risks, with regular updates as processes or ingredients change (Hasnan et al., 2022).
- Segregation and Labeling: An allergen control plan should outline procedures for managing allergens, including segregation and labeling. Segregation involves storing allergenic ingredients separately and establishing dedicated production lines to prevent cross-contamination. Accurate labeling of allergens on product labels is essential for consumer safety. In India, manufacturers must declare eight major allergens on food labels. This includes implementing a traceability system for allergen-containing products and maintaining thorough records. Comprehensive employee training on allergen handling, cross-contamination risks, and incident reporting is crucial for effective allergen management (Mtewa et al., 2020).
- Production Scheduling: Production scheduling is crucial for preventing cross-contamination in allergen control plans. Strategies include scheduling allergen-free products before allergen-containing ones, using dedicated equipment, and implementing thorough cleaning and sanitization protocols. Allergen sequencing minimizes changeovers by grouping similar products and dedicating specific lines for allergen-containing items. Clear changeover procedures, strict inventory management, and detailed documentation ensure effective allergen control and safety for individuals with allergies (McKenna et al., 2007).

Supplier Management

Supplier management is crucial for allergen control in the food industry. It involves selecting and managing suppliers of raw materials, ingredients, and packaging to ensure they meet required standards. Strategies include thorough assessments, clear specifications, requiring certificates of analysis, implementing vendor approval programs, conducting regular audits, and maintaining accurate records. Regular review and updating of these strategies help minimize allergen cross-contamination risks and ensure the safety of individuals with food allergies.

Supplier Verification

Effective supplier management is crucial for allergen control in Indian food manufacturing. This involves rigorous supplier qualification, detailed allergen specifications, regular monitoring, and corrective actions. Implementing a supplier rating system, fostering collaboration, and providing training help mitigate allergen-related issues. Regular evaluations ensure suppliers align with industry standards and regulatory requirements (Karim et al., 2008).

Supplier Audits

Supplier audits are crucial in the food industry for evaluating allergen control measures and quality control procedures. This involves on-site inspections, reviewing documentation, and conducting interviews to assess allergen control practices. Audits identify non-conformities, provide detailed reports, and offer recommendations for improvement. Integrating audit findings and regularly reviewing supplier performance ensures effective evaluation and approval, minimizing cross-contamination risks (Ndubisi et al., 2005).

Product Testing and Validation

Product testing and validation are crucial for allergen management in the food industry. This involves developing a testing plan, conducting allergen testing and validation studies, implementing a monitoring program, and regularly reviewing and updating the plan. These strategies ensure products meet allergen control standards and minimize cross-contamination risks, safeguarding individuals with food allergies.

Validated methods and established protocols are crucial for allergen testing and validation in food products. Regular testing ensures accuracy and reliability, minimizing cross-contamination risks. Key techniques include ELISA, which uses antibodies to detect allergens by color change, PCR, which amplifies DNA to detect low allergen levels, Lateral Flow Devices (LFDs), which are quick, user-friendly tests indicating allergen presence with a line, and Mass Spectrometry (MS), which detects allergens by ionizing and analyzing food fragments (Ledezma & Correa, 2023).

Validation studies are essential in the food industry to ensure processes meet required specifications and quality attributes. They involve defining the process or product, developing a validation protocol, conducting a process qualification (PQ) to ensure consistent quality, and evaluating results. A validation report summarizes the study's objectives, methods, and conclusions, including any deviations and corrective actions. Regular review and updating of validation strategies minimize allergen cross-contamination risks and maintain product quality (Digalwar & Sangwan, 2007).

Labeling and Consumer Communication

Labeling and consumer communication are crucial for allergen management in the food industry. Best practices include complying with regulations, using clear language, using appropriate formats, providing complete information, educating consumers about allergens, and responding to inquiries. Regular review and updating of these strategies ensure effective allergen management and protects consumer health.

- Accurate Labeling: Labeling and consumer communication are vital for allergen management in the food industry. Best practices include clearly declaring allergens on product labels, adhering to FSSAI regulations, and standardizing allergen labeling across product lines. Allergen information should be prominently displayed using clear, unambiguous terminology and visual cues. Precautionary allergen labeling should be based on thorough risk assessments, and allergen information should be provided in multiple languages to cater to India's diverse consumer base. Increasing allergen transparency on digital platforms and implementing interactive tools can further enhance consumer access to up-to-date information (Agrahari & Hiremath, 2017).
- Consumer Education: Consumer education is crucial in the food industry for providing accurate information about allergens and control measures. Strategies include clear labeling with easy-to-understand language, offering allergen information resources through websites and educational materials, and issuing timely allergen alerts and recalls through various communication channels. Training food service workers and encouraging consumer feedback help enhance allergen control practices and communication strategies (Rustichelli et al., 2013).

Regulatory Compliance and Documentation

Regulatory compliance and documentation are crucial for food manufacturers in managing allergens. They include implementing control measures, maintaining accurate records, and being subject to inspections. Regular review and updating of these strategies ensure they meet allergen control standards and minimize cross-contamination risk. This ensures the safety of consumers.

- Compliance with FSSAI Regulations: India's food manufacturers must adhere to FSSAI regulations for product safety and quality. This includes obtaining necessary licenses and registrations, establishing a food safety management system (FSMS) with Hazard Analysis and Critical Control Points (HACCP), Good Manufacturing Practices (GMP), and Sanitation Standard Operating Procedure (SSOP) and ensuring accurate labeling and packaging. Regular product testing and validation, comprehensive record-keeping, and employee training on FSSAI standards and allergen management are also required to maintain compliance and product quality (K. Patel & Chotai, 2011).
- Audits and Inspections: Audits and inspections are vital in the food industry for ensuring regulatory compliance and reviewing allergen control measures. This involves planning the audit by identifying objectives and team members, conducting an opening meeting with management, reviewing documentation on allergen control and production processes, and conducting a facility tour to evaluate allergen control measures (Mtewa et al., 2020).

4. REVOLUTIONIZING FOOD ALLERGY DETECTION: INNOVATIONS IN DIAGNOSTIC TECHNOLOGIES

The identification of food allergies will continue to progress in 2024 as a result of cutting-edge testing methods that increase accessibility, speed, and accuracy. These days, traditional methods like skin prick testing and serum IgE measurement are integrated with molecular allergology, CRISPR-based diagnostics, and AI-powered prediction modeling (Khan et al., 2024). Next-generation sequencing (NGS) and multi-epitope allergen microarrays enable very accurate identification of allergenic proteins. Biosensors, such as nanotechnology-based wearables and diagnostic tools integrated into smartphones, provide real-time, non-invasive allergy testing. Mass spectrometry and sophisticated PCR techniques improve the tracking of food product allergens while ensuring compliance with stringent international regulations. Blockchain and RFID technology increase transparency in food supply chains and allergy labeling. Researchers are now better able to predict allergenicity and tailor dietary recommendations (B. Sharma & Deshmukh, 2023).

Current Challenges in Food Allergy Diagnosis

Conventional approaches to diagnosing food allergies, including the oral food challenge (OFC), skin prick testing (SPT), and specific IgE blood assays, exhibit considerable limitations (Wong & Santos, 2024). While the OFC is regarded as the gold standard, it is associated with high costs, extensive time requirements, and a risk of severe allergic responses. Additionally, both blood tests and SPT can yield inaccurate results, resulting in misdiagnoses and unwarranted dietary limitations (*New Test Improves Diagnosis of Allergies*, 2024).

Innovative Diagnostic Approaches

Innovative diagnostic methodologies are enhancing food allergy testing, improving patient safety and diagnostic accuracy. The Basophil Activation Test (BAT) offers high specificity and sensitivity for identifying allergies to peanuts and sesame seeds (Alcimed, 2024). Molecular allergology refines allergenic protein analysis by distinguishing true allergies from co-sensitization (EAACI, 2023). The Mast Cell Activation Test (MAT) assesses allergic reactions functionally, while the Bead-Based Epitope Assay (BBEA) detects IgE and IgG4 antibodies to predict allergic response severity. Advanced genetic testing identifies at-risk patients, enabling timely interventions. AI-driven diagnostics and exploratory approaches like immune response testing and microbiome analysis further enhance personalized and precise allergy management (Ben-Shoshan et al., 2014).

1. **Mast Cell Activation Test (MAT)** - Researchers at the University of Bern have created the Hoxb8 Mast Cell Activation Test (Hoxb8 MAT), which simulates allergic reactions in a lab. This test involves culturing mast cells and exposing them to serum from allergic patients to assess allergy severity. In clinical trials, the Hoxb8 MAT showed a diagnostic accuracy of 95%, surpassing traditional methods like IgE measurements and skin tests (Ebo et al., 2024).
2. **Basophil Activation Test (BAT)** - The Basophil Activation Test (BAT) is now included in clinical guidelines as a reliable method for diagnosing allergies, especially for peanuts and sesame seeds. It measures basophil activation in response to allergens, providing higher specificity and sensitivity compared to skin prick tests (SPT) and IgE tests. Additionally, BAT can help predict disease trajectories by monitoring changes in allergic responses over time (Okamura et al., 2017).

3. **Bead-Based Epitope Assay (BBEA)** - The Bead-Based Epitope Assay (BBEA) is a high-throughput method that detects IgE and IgG4 antibodies against multiple epitopes simultaneously. It has shown promising sensitivity and specificity for peanut allergies and could enable personalized treatment by identifying specific allergenic components that trigger (Banks & Andrews, 2022).
4. **GranulEye Test** - The GranulEye Test visualizes basophil degranulation upon allergen exposure, aiming to be a reliable and cost-effective diagnostic tool that avoids the need for oral food challenges (OFC). It is being optimized with AI technology to enhance its analytical capabilities (Vasilescu et al., 2016).

Artificial Intelligence Integration - AI is being explored to interpret complex diagnostic test panels more effectively. By integrating various data sources, AI could enhance diagnostic accuracy and assist clinicians in making better-informed decisions for patient management (Ferrante et al., 2020).

5. REGULATORY AND POLICY DEVELOPMENTS & CONSUMER AWARENESS EDUCATION ABOUT FOOD ALLERGENICITY

Food allergen management is crucial for ensuring food safety standards are met and Food allergen management is crucial for ensuring food safety and protecting individuals with allergies. Recent advancements include strengthening allergen labeling requirements and global harmonization of standards by bodies like the EU and ASEAN. Regulatory agencies are developing standardized testing methods for consistency and reliability, with regular updates based on the latest scientific research (DunnGalvin et al., 2019). Allergen-free zones are being established in public spaces, and food service regulations are enforcing strict allergen management practices (Hattersley et al., 2014).

Education campaigns by governments and NGOs raise awareness about food allergies, while schools teach allergen avoidance and emergency responses. Digital resources and tools, such as mobile apps, help manage food allergies. Training sessions focus on reading food labels and recognizing precautionary statements. First Aid programs train individuals on emergency treatment. Allergy support groups advocate for individuals with food allergies, providing platforms for shared experiences and support (Bronzwaer et al., 2019).

Regulatory and Policy Developments in the Area of Food Allergenicity

Regulatory and policy developments, along with consumer awareness education, are crucial for managing food allergens and ensuring safety for consumers with allergies. Key measures include allergen labeling regulations, which mandate food manufacturers to identify allergens, helping consumers make informed choices (DunnGalvin et al., 2019). Allergen thresholds set maximum allowable amounts of allergens, permitting minor unintentional contamination while ensuring safety. Precautionary allergen labeling (PAL) identifies potential allergens due to cross-contamination during production. Regulatory bodies are developing guidelines for consistent PAL use (Hattersley et al., 2014). Consumer education on allergens and labeling requirements further reduces the risk of allergic reactions. Collaboration among stakeholders can enhance food safety and quality for all consumers.

Consumer Awareness Education About Food Allergenicity

Consumer awareness education about food allergens is crucial for effective management and prevention. It helps consumers understand allergen labels, avoidance strategies, and symptoms of allergic reactions, emphasizing emergency preparedness and risk communication. By providing necessary information, consumers can make informed dietary decisions and take precautions, reducing allergic reaction risks and improving quality of life.

Key measures include allergen labeling regulations, which mandate food manufacturers to identify allergens, helping consumers make educated choices (DunnGalvin et al., 2019). Allergen thresholds set maximum allowable allergen levels, permitting minor unintentional contamination while ensuring safety. Precautionary allergen labeling (PAL) guidelines are being developed for consistent use (Hattersley et al., 2014). Regulatory agencies urge food manufacturers to create allergen management plans, including procedures for ingredient sourcing, storage, handling, and processing, along with employee training. Recall procedures ensure potentially dangerous products are quickly removed from the market.

Research funding by governments and academic institutions aims to advance knowledge on food allergies and develop new allergen identification techniques (Ayaz et al., 2020). Collaboration among stakeholders, along with educational programs and digital tools, promotes inclusivity and ensures robust food safety measures.

6. CONCLUSION

Technological advancements, increasing regulatory frameworks, and findings from science are all triggering a major revolution in food allergy management. Novel diagnostic techniques, gene editing technologies, tailored preventative plans, and sophisticated immunotherapies are examples of these emerging approaches that have the potential to significantly enhance the lives of people with food allergies. It takes a multidisciplinary strategy that incorporates research, policy creation, and education to handle the intricate problems that food allergies present. The convergence of these creative approaches offers hope for a safer, more inclusive food environment, even though there are still obstacles to overcome, such as guaranteeing fair access to new technologies and ethical considerations. Working together, scientists, legislators, business executives, and patient advocates can fully realize the promise of these advancements and enhance the lives of millions of people impacted by food insecurity.

With the power of innovation and technology, new approaches to managing food allergies have the potential to completely transform food safety. Modern methods of detection, improved regulatory policies, and thorough consumer education are essential for tackling the multifaceted problems that food allergies present. These methods seek to improve the quality of life for people with food allergies, decrease the frequency of allergic reactions, and promote a safer food environment by encouraging collaboration among scientists, policymakers, and industry stakeholders. These developments portend a time when controlling food allergies will be easier to do, more dependable, and available to everyone.

The Indian food industry is embracing innovative allergen detection technologies to manage food allergens more effectively. These technologies, combined with robust regulatory frameworks and increased consumer awareness, can transform the way food allergens are managed. By adopting this approach, food manufacturers can improve product safety, build consumer trust, streamline operations, and drive innovation. Despite challenges like technological limitations and implementation barriers, the long-term benefits of these solutions are undeniable. The Indian food industry can cultivate a more inclusive, transparent, and safe food ecosystem, empowering consumers to make informed choices. Advanced biosensors, rapid testing methods, and data-driven predictive analytics offer a glimpse into this future. Regulatory bodies and industry associations must continue to collaborate on harmonizing standards and incentivizing innovation to drive widespread adoption. Consumer awareness and education are also crucial. By partnering with patient organizations, implementing targeted information campaigns, and allergen-awareness initiatives, the industry can build trust and empower consumers to make informed choices.

In conclusion, the food sector places a high priority on managing food allergies, and new approaches are being developed to enhance allergy management, detection, and labeling. A complete strategy to food allergen control should include cutting edge technologies, viable tactics, new regulatory initiatives, and consumer education. We can increase the quality and safety of food items for all customers, including those who have food allergies, by cooperating to create and put into practice efficient solutions for managing food allergens. We must continue to be watchful in our efforts to control food allergies and guarantee the security and caliber of our food supply as the food business develops.

CONFLICT OF INTEREST STATEMENT

On behalf of the authors, the corresponding author states that there is no conflict of interest.

ACKNOWLEDGMENT

The authors are grateful to Gharda Institute of Technology and UICT, Jalgaon for their cooperation and support during preparation of this book chapter.

REFERENCES

Abou-El-Enein, M., Römhild, A., Kaiser, D., Beier, C., Bauer, G., Volk, H., & Reinke, P. (2013). Good Manufacturing Practices (GMP) manufacturing of advanced therapy medicinal products: A novel tailored model for optimizing performance and estimating costs. *Cytotherapy*, *15*(3), 362–383. DOI: 10.1016/j.jcyt.2012.09.006 PMID: 23579061

Agrahari, V., & Hiremath, P. (2017). Challenges associated and approaches for successful translation of nanomedicines into commercial products. *Nanomedicine (London)*, *12*(8), 819–823. DOI: 10.2217/nnm-2017-0039 PMID: 28338401

Agrawal, G. K., Sarkar, A., Righetti, P. G., Pedreschi, R., Carpentier, S., Wang, T., Barkla, B. J., Kohli, A., Ndimba, B. K., Bykova, N. V., Rampitsch, C., Zolla, L., Rafudeen, M. S., Cramer, R., Bindschedler, L. V., Tsakirpaloglou, N., Ndimba, R. J., Farrant, J. M., Renaut, J., & Rakwal, R. (2013). A decade of plant proteomics and mass spectrometry: Translation of technical advancements to food security and safety issues. *Mass Spectrometry Reviews*, *32*(5), 335–365. DOI: 10.1002/mas.21365 PMID: 23315723

Alcimed. (2024, April 23). *3 approaches to meet the challenges of food allergy management.* https://www.alcimed.com/en/insights/food-allergy-management/

Allen, K. J., Remington, B. C., Baumert, J. L., Crevel, R. W., Houben, G. F., Brooke-Taylor, S., Kruizinga, A. G., & Taylor, S. L. (2014). Allergen reference doses for precautionary labeling (VITAL 2.0): Clinical implications. ^the ‰Journal of Allergy and Clinical Immunology/Journal of Allergy and Clinical Immunology/ the œJournal of Allergy and Clinical Immunology, 133(1), 156–164. DOI: 10.1016/j.jaci.2013.06.042

Allen, K. J., Turner, P. J., Pawankar, R., Taylor, S., Sicherer, S., Lack, G., Rosario, N., Ebisawa, M., Wong, G., Mills, E. N. C., Beyer, K., Fiocchi, A., & Sampson, H. A. (2014). Precautionary labelling of foods for allergen content: are we ready for a global framework? the World Allergy Organization Journal, 7, 10. DOI: 10.1186/1939-4551-7-10

Anderson, J. A. (1996). Allergic reactions to foods. Critical Reviews in Food Science and Nutrition, 36(sup001), 19–38. DOI: 10.1080/10408399609527757

Asero, R., Ballmer-Weber, B. K., Beyer, K., Conti, A., Dubakiene, R., Fernandez-Rivas, M., Hoffmann-Sommergruber, K., Lidholm, J., Mustakov, T., Elberink, J. N. G. O., Pumphrey, R. S. H., Skov, P. S., Van Ree, R., Vlieg-Boerstra, B. J., Hiller, R., Hourihane, J. O., Kowalski, M., Papadopoulos, N. G., Wal, J., & Vieths, S. (2006). IgE-Mediated food allergy diagnosis: Current status and new perspectives. *Molecular Nutrition & Food Research, 51*(1), 135–147. DOI: 10.1002/mnfr.200600132 PMID: 17195271

Ayaz, A., Dedebayraktar, D., Inan-Eroglu, E., Besler, H. T., & Buyuktuncer, Z. (2020). How does nutrition education contribute to the consumers' use and attitudes towards food labels? *Nutrition & Food Science, 51*(3), 517–528. DOI: 10.1108/NFS-05-2020-0174

Bacal, L. R. (2013). The impact of food allergies on quality of life. *Pediatric Annals, 42*(7). Advance online publication. DOI: 10.3928/00904481-20130619-12 PMID: 23805962

Banks, J. R., & Andrews, T. (2022). Accurate and Reproducible Diagnosis of Peanut Allergy using Epitope Mapping. *Pediatrics, 150*(Supplement 3), S23. DOI: 10.1542/peds.2022-059346FF

Barnett, J., Begen, F. M., Gowland, M. H., & Lucas, J. S. (2018). Comparing the eating out experiences of consumers seeking to avoid different food allergens. *BMC Public Health, 18*(1), 1263. Advance online publication. DOI: 10.1186/s12889-018-6117-y PMID: 30442121

Bayen, S., Elliott, C., Arlorio, M., Ballins, N. Z., Birse, N., Brockmeyer, J., Chahal, S., Corradini, M. G., Hanner, R., Hann, S., Laursen, K. H., Mihailova, A., Steininger-Mairinger, T., Suman, M., Tian, L., Van Ruth, S., & Xia, J. (2024). Towards a harmonized approach for food authenticity marker validation and accreditation. *Trends in Food Science & Technology, 104550*, 104550. Advance online publication. DOI: 10.1016/j.tifs.2024.104550

Ben-Shoshan, M., DeSchryver, S., Dery, A., Mill, J., Mill, C., & O'Keefe, A. (2014). Diagnosis and management of food allergies: new and emerging options: a systematic review. *Journal of Asthma and Allergy, 141*, 141. Advance online publication. DOI: 10.2147/JAA.S49277

Blanchfield, J. (2005). Good manufacturing practice (GMP) in the food. Institute of Food Science & Technology. In Elsevier eBooks (pp. 324–347). DOI: 10.1533/9781845690533.3.324

Bronzwaer, S., Kass, G., Robinson, T., Tarazona, J., Verhagen, H., Verloo, D., Vrbos, D., & Hugas, M. (2019). Food Safety Regulatory Research Needs 2030. *EFSA Journal*, *17*(7). Advance online publication. DOI: 10.2903/j.efsa.2019.e170622 PMID: 32626400

Bulanda, M., Leśniak, M., Szałkowska, J., Madej, W., Wojtyna, A., Czarnobilska, M., Bulanda, D., & Czarnobilska, E. (2018). Component-resolved diagnosis (CRD) of food anaphylaxis. PubMed, 58(2), 89–102. DOI: 10.24425/fmc.2018.124661

Canonica, G. W., Bachert, C., Hellings, P., Ryan, D., Valovirta, E., Wickman, M., De Beaumont, O., & Bousquet, J. (2015). Allergen Immunotherapy (AIT): a prototype of Precision Medicine. the œWorld Allergy Organization Journal, 8, 31. DOI: 10.1186/s40413-015-0079-7

Chen, S. (2022). Analysis of cashew allergen in shared use of frying oil - ProQuest. https://search.proquest.com/openview/85432dc2a9662b6918c29e0100260054/1?pq-origsite=gscholar&cbl=18750&diss=y&casa_token=afrAn0hF1jAAAAAA:U1W_MiiuNMSyjhteUszXyVkxs71MIm4kQUTGzohFn9bbSv5zTbgyobdHINuFuDg6xB0j33mBalk

Clark, S., Bock, S., Gaeta, T. J., Brenner, B. E., Cydulka, R. K., & Camargo, C. A. (2004). Multicenter study of emergency department visits for food allergies☆. ^the ‰Journal of Allergy and Clinical Immunology/Journal of Allergy and Clinical Immunology/ the œJournal of Allergy and Clinical Immunology, 113(2), 347–352. DOI: 10.1016/j.jaci.2003.10.053

De, A., Rajagopalan, M., Godse, K., Shankar, D. K., Zawar, V., Sharma, N., Mukherjee, S., Sarda, A., & Dhar, S. (2019). Guidelines on management of atopic dermatitis in India: An evidence-based review and an expert consensus. Indian Journal of Dermatology. *Indian Journal of Dermatology*, *64*(3), 166. DOI: 10.4103/ijd.IJD_683_18 PMID: 31148854

De Blok, B. M. J., Vlieg-Boerstra, B. J., Elberink, J. N. G. O., & Duiverman, E. J. (2007). A framework for measuring the social impact of food allergy across Europe: A EuroPrevall state of the art paper. *Allergy*, *62*(7), 733–737. DOI: 10.1111/j.1398-9995.2006.01303.x PMID: 17484733

Digalwar, A. K., & Sangwan, K. S. (2007). Development And Validation of Performance Measures for World Class Manufacturing Practices in India. *Journal of Advanced Manufacturing Systems*, *06*(01), 21–38. DOI: 10.1142/S0219686707000887

EAACI. (2023, October 12). *EAACI - News: New Clinical Guidelines for the Diagnosis of Immediate-type Food Allergies are launched.* https://eaaci.org/news/new-clinical-guidelines-for-the-diagnosis-of-immediate-type-food-allergies-are-launched/

Ebo, D. G., Bahri, R., Tontini, C., Van Gasse, A. L., Mertens, C., Hagendorens, M. M., Sabato, V., & Elst, J. (2024). Mast cell versus basophil activation test in allergy: Current status. *Clinical and Experimental Allergy*, *54*(6), 378–387. DOI: 10.1111/cea.14487 PMID: 38686464

Edpuganti, S., Gaikwad, J. R., Maliyil, B. T., Koshy, R. R., Potdar, R., Latheef, S., & Korrapati, N. H. (2025). The not-so-sweet side of mango: Mango allergy. *Cosmoderma*, *5*, 18. Advance online publication. DOI: 10.25259/CSDM_212_2024

Ekezie, F. C., Cheng, J., & Sun, D. (2018). Effects of nonthermal food processing technologies on food allergens: A review of recent research advances. *Trends in Food Science & Technology*, *74*, 12–25. DOI: 10.1016/j.tifs.2018.01.007

Ferrante, G., Licari, A., Fasola, S., Marseglia, G. L., & La Grutta, S. (2020). Artificial intelligence in the diagnosis of pediatric allergic diseases. *Pediatric Allergy and Immunology*, *32*(3), 405–413. DOI: 10.1111/pai.13419 PMID: 33220121

Fiocchi, A., Vickery, B. P., & Wood, R. A. (2021). The use of biologics in food allergy. Clinical & Experimental Allergy. *Clinical and Experimental Allergy*, *51*(8), 1006–1018. DOI: 10.1111/cea.13897 PMID: 33966304

Fleischer, D. M., & Burks, A. W. (2015). Pitfalls in food allergy diagnosis: serum IGE testing. the Journal of Pediatrics/the Journal of Pediatrics, 166(1), 8–10. DOI: 10.1016/j.jpeds.2014.09.057

Food allergies. (2024, April 12). FDA. https://www.fda.gov/food/food-labeling-nutrition/food-allergies

Food Allergies Symptoms. Diagnosis & Treatment | AAAAI. (2018, April). American Academy of Allergy Asthma & Immunology. https://www.aaaai.org/conditions-treatments/allergies/food-allergy

Food allergy. (2023, August 16). www.nhs.ukNHS-UK. https://www.nhs.uk/conditions/food-allergy/

Food and agricultural organization of united nations(2023-24). Scintific advice. https://www.fao.org/food-safety/scientific-advice/food-allergens/en/

Food chain Allergen management. (2009). Google Books. https://books.google.com/books?hl=en&lr=&id=FHIoDwAAQBAJ&oi=fnd&pg=PR3&dq=Remaining+Challenges+Allergen+Detection+-+Collaboration+and+Knowledge+Sharing:&ots=xJkYxRSdmA&sig=Ie-vVVp_bdNRqlSao5TwBXElvr0

Food labelling. (2000). Google Books. https://books.google.com/books?hl=en&lr=&id=PwXnAgAAQBAJ&oi=fnd&pg=PP1&dq=Improvements+in+Allergen+Labeling+-+Multilingual+and+Pictorial+Labeling&ots=MQOIrcCzaE&sig=7sXeebe4zLDCFzNPwljNsBe-lbs

Foong, R., Dantzer, J. A., Wood, R. A., & Santos, A. F. (2021). Improving diagnostic accuracy in food allergy. Journal of Allergy and Clinical Immunology. In Practice/ the Journal of Allergy and Clinical Immunology. *In Practice*, *9*(1), 71–80. DOI: 10.1016/j.jaip.2020.09.037 PMID: 33429723

Goodwin, P. R. (2004). Food Allergen Detection Methods: A Coordinated approach. *Journal of AOAC International*, *87*(6), 1383–1390. DOI: 10.1093/jaoac/87.6.1383 PMID: 15675450

Gupta, M., Cox, A., Nowak-Węgrzyn, A., & Wang, J. (2018). Diagnosis of food allergy. *Immunology and Allergy Clinics of North America*, *38*(1), 39–52. DOI: 10.1016/j.iac.2017.09.004 PMID: 29132673

Hasnan, N. Z. N., Basha, R. K., Amin, N. M., Ramli, S. H. M., Tang, J. Y. H., & Aziz, N. A. (2022). Analysis of the most frequent nonconformance aspects related to Good Manufacturing Practices (GMP) among small and medium enterprises (SMEs) in the food industry and their main factors. *Food Control*, *141*, 109205. DOI: 10.1016/j.foodcont.2022.109205

Hattersley, S., Ward, R., Baka, A., & Crevel, R. W. (2014). Advances in the risk management of unintended presence of allergenic foods in manufactured food products – An overview. *Food and Chemical Toxicology*, *67*, 255–261. DOI: 10.1016/j.fct.2014.01.036 PMID: 24508586

Institute for Quality and Efficiency in Health Care (IQWiG). (2023, August 21). Overview: Food allergies. InformedHealth.org - NCBI Bookshelf. https://www.ncbi.nlm.nih.gov/books/NBK447107/

Kalita, J. J., Buragohain, P., Mosahari, P. V., & Bora, U. (2019). Food allergens: Detection and management. In Apple Academic Press eBooks (pp. 243–279). DOI: 10.1201/9780429242793-11

Karim, M., Smith, A., Halgamuge, S., & Islam, M. (2008). A comparative study of manufacturing practices and performance variables. *International Journal of Production Economics*, *112*(2), 841–859. DOI: 10.1016/j.ijpe.2007.07.005

Khan, M., Banerjee, S., Muskawad, S., Maity, R., Chowdhury, S. R., Ejaz, R., Kuuzie, E., & Satnarine, T. (2024). The impact of artificial intelligence on allergy diagnosis and treatment. *Current Allergy and Asthma Reports*, *24*(7), 361–372. DOI: 10.1007/s11882-024-01152-y PMID: 38954325

Konstantinou, G. N., Pampoukidou, O., Sergelidis, D., & Fotoulaki, M. (2025). Managing Food Allergies in Dining Establishments: Challenges and Innovative Solutions. *Nutrients*, *17*(10), 1737. DOI: 10.3390/nu17101737 PMID: 40431476

Ledezma, J. M., & Correa, J. C. P. (2023). Definition and evaluation of good manufacturing practices for plastic injection molding. *Energy Efficiency*, *16*(4), 24. Advance online publication. DOI: 10.1007/s12053-023-10103-x

Lehrer, S. B., Ayuso, R., & Reese, G. (2002). Current understanding of food allergens. *Annals of the New York Academy of Sciences*, *964*(1), 69–85. DOI: 10.1111/j.1749-6632.2002.tb04133.x PMID: 12023195

Li, P., Sheng, L., Ye, Y., Wang, J. S., Geng, S., Ning, D., & Sun, X. (2025). Allergenicity of alternative proteins: research hotspots, new findings, evaluation strategies, regulatory status, and future trends: a bibliometric analysis. *Critical Reviews in Food Science and Nutrition*, *65*(9), 1749–1760. DOI: 10.1080/10408398.2023.2299748 PMID: 38189352

Lieberman, J. A., & Sicherer, S. H. (2010). The diagnosis of food allergy. *American Journal of Rhinology & Allergy*, *24*(6), 439–443. DOI: 10.2500/ajra.2010.24.3515 PMID: 21144222

Linders, Y. F., Lentz, L. R., Blom, W. M., Michelsen-Huisman, A., Strikwerda, J., Van Dijk, L. M., Knulst, A. C., Houben, G. F., Van Os-Medendorp, H., & Holleman, B. C. (2023). Precautionary allergen labeling: Current communication problems and potential for future improvements. *Food Control*, *147*, 109561. DOI: 10.1016/j.foodcont.2022.109561

Liu, W., Yang, Q., Wang, Z., Wang, J., Min, F., Yuan, J., Tong, P., Li, X., Wu, Y., Gao, J., & Chen, H. (2025). Quantitative food allergen risk assessment: Evolving concepts, modern approaches, and industry implications. *Comprehensive Reviews in Food Science and Food Safety*, *24*(2), e70132. DOI: 10.1111/1541-4337.70132 PMID: 39929606

López-Calvo, R., Montero-Barrantes, M., González-Vargas, M., Henderson-García, M., & Víquez-Barrantes, D. (2025). Allergen Management in Costa Rican Food Industries: Challenges and Future Actions. *Food and Humanity*, *100502*, 100502. Advance online publication. DOI: 10.1016/j.foohum.2025.100502

Lyons, S. A., Burney, P. G., Ballmer-Weber, B. K., Fernandez-Rivas, M., Barreales, L., Clausen, M., Dubakiene, R., Fernandez-Perez, C., Fritsche, P., Jedrzejczak-Czechowicz, M., Kowalski, M. L., Kralimarkova, T., Kummeling, I., Mustakov, T. B., Lebens, A. F., Van Os-Medendorp, H., Papadopoulos, N. G., Popov, T. A., Sakellariou, A., & Le, T. (2019). Food allergy in adults: Substantial variation in prevalence and causative foods across Europe. Journal of Allergy and Clinical Immunology. In Practice/ the œJournal of Allergy and Clinical Immunology. *In Practice*, *7*(6), 1920–1928.e11. DOI: 10.1016/j.jaip.2019.02.044 PMID: 30898689

Ma, J., Yu, J., Jia, Y., Luo, Z., Yang, X., Li, H., & Long, F. (2025). Fermented Apple Juice Reduces the Susceptibility of Offspring Mice to Food Allergy Exacerbated by Maternal High-Fat Diet. *Nutrients*, *17*(11), 1927. DOI: 10.3390/nu17111927 PMID: 40507196

Major allergens: The Big Nine – School Nutrition Association. (2022). School Nutrition Association. https://schoolnutrition.org/resource/major-allergens-the-big-nine/

McKenna, D. H.Jr, Sumstad, D., Bostrom, N., Kadidlo, D. M., Fautsch, S., McNearney, S., DeWaard, R., McGlave, P. B., Weisdorf, D. J., Wagner, J. E., McCullough, J., & Miller, J. S. (2007). Good manufacturing practices production of natural killer cells for immunotherapy: A six-year single-institution experience. *Transfusion*, *47*(3), 520–528. DOI: 10.1111/j.1537-2995.2006.01145.x PMID: 17319835

Monaci, L., De Angelis, E., Montemurro, N., & Pilolli, R. (2018). Comprehensive overview and recent advances in proteomics MS based methods for food allergens analysis. *Trends in Analytical Chemistry*, *106*, 21–36. DOI: 10.1016/j.trac.2018.06.016

Mtewa, A. G., Chikowe, I., Kumar, S., Ngwira, K. J., & Lampiao, F. (2020). Good manufacturing practices and safety issues in functional food industries. In Springer eBooks (pp. 613–628). DOI: 10.1007/978-3-030-42319-3_27

Mtewa, A. G., Chikowe, I., Kumar, S., Ngwira, K. J., & Lampiao, F. (2020). Good manufacturing practices and safety issues in functional food industries. In Springer eBooks (pp. 613–628). DOI: 10.1007/978-3-030-42319-3_27

Muthukumar, J., Selvasekaran, P., Lokanadham, M., & Chidambaram, R. (2020). Food and food products associated with food allergy and food intolerance – An overview. *Food Research International*, *138*, 109780. DOI: 10.1016/j.foodres.2020.109780 PMID: 33288166

Nath, S. (2024, July 19). (2024). Advancements in food quality monitoring: Integrating biosensors for precision detection. [RSC Publishing]. *Sustainable Food Technology*, *2*(4), 976–992. Advance online publication. DOI: 10.1039/D4FB00094C

Ndubisi, N. O., Jantan, M., Hing, L. C., & Ayub, M. S. (2005). Supplier selection and management strategies and manufacturing flexibility. *Journal of Enterprise Information Management, 18*(3), 330–349. DOI: 10.1108/17410390510592003

Nettleton, S., Woods, B., Burrows, R., & Kerr, A. (2009). Food allergy and food intolerance: Towards a sociological agenda. *Health, 13*(6), 647–664. DOI: 10.1177/1363459308341433 PMID: 19841024

New test improves diagnosis of allergies. (2024, October 24). ScienceDaily. https://www.sciencedaily.com/releases/2024/10/241015141449.htm

News-Medical. (2024, February 23). The future of food allergy Management: New technologies and treatments. https://www.news-medical.net/health/The-Future-of-Food-Allergy-Management-New-Technologies-and-Treatments.aspx

Nio, R. A., Esteban, P. R., De Faria Catarina, T., & Conrado, C. (2017). Allergen management as a key issue in food safety. In CRC Press eBooks (pp. 195–241). DOI: 10.1201/9781315153414-6

Nowak-Węgrzyn, A., & Albin, S. (2015). Oral immunotherapy for food allergy: Mechanisms and role in management. Clinical & Experimental Allergy. *Clinical and Experimental Allergy, 45*(2), 368–383. DOI: 10.1111/cea.12382 PMID: 25077670

Okamura, I., Matsuyama, N., Yasui, K., Hirayama, F., & Ikeda, T. (2017). Clinical utility of the basophil activation test for analysis of allergic transfusion reactions: A pilot study. *Vox Sanguinis, 112*(2), 114–121. DOI: 10.1111/vox.12471 PMID: 28070919

Ortolani, C., & Pastorello, E. A. (2006). Food allergies and food intolerances. Baillière's Best Practice & Research. Clinical Gastroenterology/Baillière's. *Best Practice & Research. Clinical Gastroenterology, 20*(3), 467–483. DOI: 10.1016/j.bpg.2005.11.010 PMID: 16782524

Papadopoulos, N. G., Agache, I., Bavbek, S., Bilo, B. M., Braido, F., Cardona, V., Custovic, A., Demonchy, J., Demoly, P., Eigenmann, P., Gayraud, J., Grattan, C., Heffler, E., Hellings, P. W., Jutel, M., Knol, E., Lötvall, J., Muraro, A., Poulsen, L. K., & Akdis, C. A. (2012). Research needs in allergy: An EAACI position paper, in collaboration with EFA. *Clinical and Translational Allergy, 2*(1), 21. Advance online publication. DOI: 10.1186/2045-7022-2-21 PMID: 23121771

Parrinello, G., Fontana, D. E., & Villalta, D. (2025). An overview of hidden food allergens: Need for change to the priority food allergen lists? *European Annals of Allergy and Clinical Immunology, 57*(2), 51–67. DOI: 10.23822/EurAnnACI.1764-1489.370 PMID: 39450657

Patel, B. Y., & Volcheck, G. W. (2015). Food allergy: Common causes, diagnosis, and treatment. *Mayo Clinic Proceedings*, *90*(10), 1411–1419. DOI: 10.1016/j.mayocp.2015.07.012 PMID: 26434966

Patel, K., & Chotai, N. (2011). Documentation and records: Harmonized GMP requirements. *Journal of Young Pharmacists : JYP*, *3*(2), 138–150. DOI: 10.4103/0975-1483.80303 PMID: 21731360

Picariello, G., Mamone, G., Addeo, F., & Ferranti, P. (2011). The frontiers of mass spectrometry-based techniques in food allergenomics. Journal of Chromatography a. *Journal of Chromatography. A*, *1218*(42), 7386–7398. DOI: 10.1016/j.chroma.2011.06.033 PMID: 21737089

Poms, R. E., Klein, C. L., & Anklam, E. (2004). Methods for allergen analysis in food: A review. Food Additives & Contaminants. *Food Additives and Contaminants*, *21*(1), 1–31. DOI: 10.1080/02652030310001620423 PMID: 14744677

Professional, C. C. M. (2024, March). Food allergies. Cleveland Clinic. https://my.clevelandclinic.org/health/diseases/9196-food-allergies

Rd, H. W. (2024, March 7). The 9 most common food allergies. Healthline. https://www.healthline.com/nutrition/common-food-allergies

Rd, J. C. M. (2024, April 3). The 9 most common food allergies. Verywell Health. https://www.verywellhealth.com/the-most-common-food-allergies-1324134

Rejeb, A., Keogh, J. G., Zailani, S., Treiblmaier, H., & Rejeb, K. (2020). Blockchain Technology in the Food Industry: A review of potentials, challenges and future research directions. *Logistics (Basel)*, *4*(4), 27. DOI: 10.3390/logistics4040027

Renz, H., Allen, K. J., Sicherer, S. H., Sampson, H. A., Lack, G., Beyer, K., & Oettgen, H. C. (2018). Food allergy. *Nature Reviews. Disease Primers*, *4*(1), 17098. Advance online publication. DOI: 10.1038/nrdp.2017.98 PMID: 29300005

Ross, G. M. S., Bremer, M. G. E. G., & Nielen, M. W. F. (2018). Consumer-friendly food allergen detection: moving towards smartphone-based immunoassays. Analytical and Bioanalytical Chemistry/Analytical & Bioanalytical Chemistry, 410(22), 5353–5371. DOI: 10.1007/s00216-018-0989-7

Rustichelli, D., Castiglia, S., Gunetti, M., Mareschi, K., Signorino, E., Muraro, M., Castello, L., Sanavio, F., Leone, M., Ferrero, I., & Fagioli, F. (2013). Validation of analytical methods in compliance with good manufacturing practice: A practical approach. *Journal of Translational Medicine*, *11*(1), 197. DOI: 10.1186/1479-5876-11-197 PMID: 23981284

Sabaghi, M., & Jamali, S. N. (2024). Advancements, challenges, and future prospects of nanobiosensors in food packaging for allergen detection. *Journal of Food Measurement and Characterization, 18*(5), 3444–3457. Advance online publication. DOI: 10.1007/s11694-024-02416-x

Sampath, V., Abrams, E. M., Adlou, B., Akdis, C., Akdis, M., Brough, H. A., Chan, S., Chatchatee, P., Chinthrajah, R. S., Cocco, R. R., Deschildre, A., Eigenmann, P., Galvan, C., Gupta, R., Hossny, E., Koplin, J. J., Lack, G., Levin, M., Shek, L. P., . . . Renz, H. (2021). Food allergy across the globe. ^the ‰Journal of Allergy and Clinical Immunology/Journal of Allergy and Clinical Immunology/ the œJournal of Allergy and Clinical Immunology, 148(6), 1347–1364. DOI: 10.1016/j.jaci.2021.10.018

Sampson, H. A. (2016). Food allergy: Past, present and future. *Allergology International, 65*(4), 363–369. DOI: 10.1016/j.alit.2016.08.006 PMID: 27613366

Santos, A. F., Riggioni, C., Du Toit, G., & Skypala, I. (2025). An algorithm for the diagnosis and management of IgE-mediated food allergy, 2024 update. https://doi.org/DOI: 10.1111/all.16321

Sathe, S. K., & Sharma, G. M. (2009). Effects of food processing on food allergens. *Molecular Nutrition & Food Research, 53*(8), 970–978. DOI: 10.1002/mnfr.200800194 PMID: 19603400

Satnarine, T., Makkoukdji, N., Pundit, V., Vignau, A., Sharma, P., Warren, D., Kleiner, G., & Gans, M. (2025). Peanut Allergy Diagnosis: Current Practices, Emerging Technologies, and Future Directions. *Allergies, 5*(1), 4. DOI: 10.3390/allergies5010004

Schauberger, E. M., & Singh, A. M. (2020). Food allergy management. *Journal of Food Allergy, 2*(1), 59–63. DOI: 10.2500/jfa.2020.2.200021 PMID: 39022156

Secord, E. A. MD. (2021, May). Food Allergies: practice Essentials, background, pathophysiology. https://emedicine.medscape.com/article/135959-overview?form=fpf

Sharma, B., & Deshmukh, R. (2023). An overview of nanotechnological approaches for the diagnosis and treatment of allergic illness. *Current Pharmaceutical Design, 29*(26), 2050–2061. DOI: 10.2174/1381612829666230828104015 PMID: 37641985

Sicherer, S. H. (2011). Epidemiology of food allergy. The Journal of Allergy and Clinical Immunology/Journal of Allergy and Clinical Immunology. *The Journal of Allergy and Clinical Immunology, 127*(3), 594–602. DOI: 10.1016/j.jaci.2010.11.044 PMID: 21236480

Sindher, S., Long, A. J., Purington, N., Chollet, M., Slatkin, S., Andorf, S., Tupa, D., Kumar, D., Woch, M. A., O'Laughlin, K. L., Assaad, A., Pongracic, J., Spergel, J. M., Tam, J., Tilles, S., Wang, J., Galli, S. J., Nadeau, K. C., & Chinthrajah, R. S. (2018). Analysis of a large standardized food challenge data set to determine predictors of positive outcome across multiple allergens. *Frontiers in Immunology*, *9*, 2689. Advance online publication. DOI: 10.3389/fimmu.2018.02689 PMID: 30538699

T C. J. (2024, February 28). Food allergy vs. food intolerance: What's the difference? Mayo Clinic. https://www.mayoclinic.org/diseases-conditions/food-allergy/expert-answers/food-allergy/faq-20058538

Taylor, S. L., & Lehrer, S. B. (1996). Principles and characteristics of food allergens. Critical Reviews in Food Science and Nutrition, 36(sup001), 91–118. DOI: 10.1080/10408399609527761

Turnbull, J. L., Adams, H. N., & Gorard, D. A. (2014). Review article: The diagnosis and management of food allergy and food intolerances. *Alimentary Pharmacology & Therapeutics*, *41*(1), 3–25. DOI: 10.1111/apt.12984 PMID: 25316115

Urisu, A., Ebisawa, M., Mukoyama, T., Morikawa, A., & Kondo, N. (2011). Japanese guideline for food allergy. *Allergology International*, *60*(2), 221–236. DOI: 10.2332/allergolint.11-RAI-0329 PMID: 21636968

Van Bilsen, J., Szłapka, E. S., Ojalvo, D. L., Willemsen, L. E. M., Antunes, C. M., Molina, E., Smit, J. J., & Wróblewska, B. (2017). Application of the adverse outcome pathway (AOP) concept to structure the available in vivo and in vitro mechanistic data for allergic sensitization to food proteins. *Clinical and Translational Allergy*, *7*(1), 13. Advance online publication. DOI: 10.1186/s13601-017-0152-0 PMID: 28507730

Van Wijk, F., & Knippels, L. (2007). Initiating mechanisms of food allergy: Oral tolerance versus allergic sensitization. *Biomedicine and Pharmacotherapy*, *61*(1), 8–20. DOI: 10.1016/j.biopha.2006.11.003 PMID: 17218079

Varghese, S. M., Parisi, S., Singla, R. K., & Begum, A. S. A. (2022). Food safety and quality control in food industry. In Springer briefs in molecular science (pp. 31–44). DOI: 10.1007/978-3-031-06304-6_5

Vasilescu, A., Nunes, G., Hayat, A., Latif, U., & Marty, J. (2016). Electrochemical affinity biosensors based on disposable Screen-Printed electrodes for detection of food allergens. *Sensors (Basel)*, *16*(11), 1863. DOI: 10.3390/s16111863 PMID: 27827963

Verhoeckx, K. C., Vissers, Y. M., Baumert, J. L., Faludi, R., Feys, M., Flanagan, S., Herouet-Guicheney, C., Holzhauser, T., Shimojo, R., Van Der Bolt, N., Wichers, H., & Kimber, I. (2015). Food processing and allergenicity. *Food and Chemical Toxicology*, *80*, 223–240. DOI: 10.1016/j.fct.2015.03.005 PMID: 25778347

Warren, C. M., Dyer, A. A., Otto, A. K., Smith, B. M., Kauke, K., Dinakar, C., & Gupta, R. S. (2017). Food Allergy–Related Risk-Taking and Management Behaviors among Adolescents and Young Adults. Journal of Allergy and Clinical Immunology. In Practice/the Journal of Allergy and Clinical Immunology. *In Practice*, *5*(2), 381–390.e13. DOI: 10.1016/j.jaip.2016.12.012 PMID: 28132799

Wong, D. S. H., & Santos, A. F. (2024). The future of food allergy diagnosis. *Frontiers in Allergy*, *5*, 1456585. Advance online publication. DOI: 10.3389/falgy.2024.1456585 PMID: 39575109

Yu, W., Freeland, D. M. H., & Nadeau, K. C. (2016). Food allergy: Immune mechanisms, diagnosis and immunotherapy. *Nature Reviews. Immunology*, *16*(12), 751–765. DOI: 10.1038/nri.2016.111 PMID: 27795547

Zhou, F., He, S., Sun, H., Wang, Y., & Zhang, Y. (2021). Advances in epitope mapping technologies for food protein allergens: A review. *Trends in Food Science & Technology*, *107*, 226–239. DOI: 10.1016/j.tifs.2020.10.035

Chapter 8
Emotional Intelligence as a Strategy for Caregiver Health and Burnout Prevention in Geriatric Settings

Tiago Manuel Horta Reis da Silva
https://orcid.org/0000-0001-5220-1718
King's College, London, UK

ABSTRACT

This chapter investigates the role of Emotional Intelligence (EI) as a proactive strategy to enhance caregiver well-being and mitigate burnout in geriatric settings. As the ageing population grows globally, professional and informal caregivers face increasing emotional demands, stress, and moral fatigue. Through the lens of EI, the chapter explores how self-awareness, emotional regulation, empathy, and relationship management contribute to healthier caregiving environments. Practical models and case studies are presented to illustrate how EI training can reduce emotional exhaustion, improve communication, and foster resilience. The chapter also outlines institutional and educational approaches for embedding EI into caregiving practice, emphasizing the importance of systemic support for long-term sustainability.

DOI: 10.4018/979-8-3693-6432-1.ch008

1. INTRODUCTION

The increasing age of the global population has necessitated a critical examination of pain management strategies, particularly as they pertain to older adults. This population is frequently burdened with chronic pain due to degenerative diseases, comorbidities, and age-related physiological changes (Hackett et al., 2020). Pain perception and management in this demographic involve a complex interplay of biological, psychological, emotional, and social factors that must be integrated within holistic and person-centred care frameworks (Booker et al., 2021). The emerging body of literature underscores the urgent need to refine pain care strategies that are sensitive and responsive to the unique needs of this demographic.

The scope of this chapter expands upon the diverse modalities available for pain management in older adults, scrutinising pharmacological and non-pharmacological approaches, and emphasising a multidisciplinary care framework. Traditional reliance on opioids as a primary treatment for chronic pain in this population comes under scrutiny, as practitioners recognise potential adverse effects, including cognitive impairment and increased disability (Pask et al., 2020; Reis da Silva, 2025a). This prompts an exploration of complementary therapies, including behavioural interventions and integrative health modalities, that enhance the efficacy of pain management while minimising risks associated with pharmacotherapy (Tang et al., 2019; Reis da Silva, 2025a). This chapter offers an expanded discussion of evidence-based approaches to chronic pain management in older adults, incorporating interdisciplinary and integrative methods, with emphasis on emotional intelligence (EI), physiotherapy, coping strategies, environmental adaptations, and digital literacy. The content is grounded in a biopsychosocial model of care and aligns with current policy trends, ethical considerations, and Sustainable Development Goals (SDGs).

1.1 Emotional Intelligence and Pain: Theoretical Foundations and Interventions

Emotional intelligence (EI), as originally articulated by Salovey and Mayer in 1990, refers to the capacity to perceive, understand, regulate, and use emotions effectively (da Silva, 2022). This foundational definition is essential to understanding the multidimensional aspects of EI, which Goleman later expanded upon, identifying five critical domains: self-awareness, self-regulation, motivation, empathy, and social skills (Carragher & Gormley, 2016; Reis da Silva et al., 2025). These components of EI are crucial, especially within healthcare contexts, where they play a pivotal role in enhancing pain perception and coping mechanisms, particularly among older adults (Prezerakos, 2018). Research indicates that individuals with higher levels of EI exhibit greater resilience and adaptive coping strategies, leading to more effective engagement with healthcare providers (Jiménez-Picón et al., 2021). This highlights the necessity of implementing EI training within healthcare frameworks to improve patient outcomes, particularly in pain management scenarios.

In clinical settings, healthcare professionals, including nurses, equipped with advanced EI competencies, are significantly better at recognising patients' emotional distress and nurturing therapeutic alliances (da Silva, 2022). The work by Prezerakos (2018) underscores the importance of emotional intelligence in promoting effective healthcare leadership and patient-centred care. Similarly, the findings from the literature confirm that emotional intelligence fosters effective interpersonal interactions within healthcare environments (Carragher & Gormley, 2016). Through comprehensive training methodologies, such as Mindfulness-Based Emotional Intelligence Training (MBEIT) and Compassionate Mind Training (CMT), healthcare institutions can enhance their workforce's EI competencies, leading to improved care for older adults (Jiménez-Picón et al., 2021).

1.2 Non-Pharmacological Strategies

Non-pharmacological strategies, such as cognitive-behavioural therapy (CBT) and mindfulness-based stress reduction, are gaining traction in scholarly discourse as viable options for alleviating pain and improving function in older adults (Morone, 2019; Niknejad et al., 2018). These approaches promote self-management skills that empower older individuals to navigate their pain with greater agency while addressing underlying psychosocial factors contributing to their suffering (Niknejad et al., 2018). Intriguingly, the integration of technology, including mobile health applications and telehealth services, presents a contemporary avenue to bridge gaps in pain management accessibility, especially for older adults living in rural or underserved areas (Dunham et al., 2021; Suntai et al., 2020).

Chronic pain is a multifaceted challenge that often precipitates an emotional crisis characterised by fear, anxiety, and depression, which, in turn, compels maladaptive coping strategies and intensifies pain perception (Prezerakos, 2018). To address this emotional cycle, the Transactional Model of Stress and Coping, formulated by Lazarus and Folkman, offers a framework for understanding how older adults can employ both adaptive and maladaptive coping strategies (Kozlowski et al., 2017). Key mediators such as self-efficacy, health beliefs, and social support are pivotal in determining how individuals navigate their pain experiences (Prezerakos, 2018). Evidence-based strategies, including cognitive-behavioural therapy and group-based self-management education, have shown promise in ameliorating pain catastrophising and fostering agency, which is particularly vital for older adults facing cognitive challenges (Kozlowski et al., 2017).

1.3 Interdisciplinary in Pain Management

The role of interprofessional collaboration becomes imperative in fostering comprehensive care pathways tailored to meet the complexities of older adults' pain experiences. Effective pain management necessitates that various healthcare providers—physicians, nurses, psychologists, and allied health professionals—coalesce their expertise to deliver care that is holistic, addressing not merely the physiological aspects of pain but also its psychological and social dimensions (Golden et al., 2019). This collaborative model is reinforced by evidence indicating significant benefits in outcomes when care is coordinated across disciplines (Golden et al., 2019). Moving towards interdisciplinary and interprofessional collaboration, it is increasingly clear that effective pain management for older adults necessitates a coordinated approach involving a diverse array of health professionals, including nurses, physiotherapists, and psychologists, among others (Jiménez-Picón et al., 2021). The integrative process, as outlined in the Chronic Care Model, advocates for structured cooperation within teams informed by the biopsychosocial model (Reis da Silva, 2025b; Reis da Silva, 2025c). Implementing case conferencing and shared patient records furthers this collaboration, ensuring a cohesive service delivery model that can adapt to individual patient needs (Turton et al., 2017). By leveraging the diverse skillsets of each professional involved, healthcare can fundamentally improve care quality and patient satisfaction, ultimately leading to better health outcomes (Reis da Silva, 2025b).

Physiotherapy plays a crucial role in chronic pain management, addressing both the physical and emotional facets of pain. Physiotherapists engage in advanced therapies that promote emotional regulation through techniques like proprioceptive training and sensorimotor stimulation (Turton et al., 2017). Interventions specifically designed to combat kinesiophobia—the fear of movement—support autonomy and functional recovery (Turton et al., 2017). According to the literature, therapies focusing on movement through guided imagery not only reinforce physical resilience but also enhance emotional coping abilities, contributing to a holistic approach to pain management (Reis da Silva, 2025c). Research suggests that employing affect-laden movements can evoke emotional memories, thereby assisting patients in reprocessing their pain experiences more adaptively (Reis da Silva, 2025c).

Equally critical is the need for culturally competent pain assessment techniques that ensure older adults from diverse backgrounds receive equitable care. Challenges persist in the use of self-report pain scales, particularly among older adults with cognitive impairments or those from minority backgrounds (Booker & Herr, 2016; Zwakhalen et al., 2018). The development and validation of culturally sensitive pain assessment tools should be prioritised so that all individuals feel both understood and valued in their pain management journey (Booker & Herr, 2015; Rostad et al., 2017).

Considering the implications of healthcare inequities, it is essential to acknowledge the unique barriers faced by rural older adults in accessing pain management services, including transportation challenges and insufficient local healthcare resources (Suntai et al., 2020; Anderson et al., 2017). Addressing these barriers requires strategic public health interventions and an advocacy focus on ensuring that healthcare systems are responsive to geographic and demographic diversity. Of paramount importance is the recognition of the psychosocial dimensions of chronic pain. Literature highlights the correlation between chronic pain and increased incidences of depression and anxiety among older adults, indicating the need for a comprehensive approach to pain management that addresses mental health (Niknejad et al., 2018; Brant, 2018). Integrating psychological support into pain management paradigms not only enhances treatment efficacy but also attends to the holistic well-being of individuals.

Finally, the development of integrative care pathways that capitalise on both conventional and alternative treatment modalities showcases promise for improved health outcomes. Strategies such as physical therapy, acupuncture, and yoga—all documented to yield significant benefits in pain reduction—should be mainstreamed within the standard care provisions for older adults (Tang et al., 2019; Golden et al., 2019). Ensuring that older adults have access to these diverse approaches will be key to enhancing their pain management experiences and overall quality of life.

In summary, the intricate interplay among emotional intelligence, coping strategies, physiotherapy practices, and interdisciplinary collaboration underscores a profound need to incorporate these elements into the evolving landscape of healthcare. By prioritizing the development of EI among healthcare providers, integrating emotional regulation therapies, and fostering collaborative approaches, we create a healthcare environment that not only addresses the direct clinical needs of patients, particularly older adults, but also nurtures their emotional and psychological well-being, significantly enhancing their overall health outcomes.

2. UNDERSTANDING THE COMPLEXITY OF PAIN IN OLDER ADULTS

Understanding the complexity of pain in older adults requires an in-depth examination of the physiological and psychological factors that contribute to pain perception and management, as well as the sociocultural considerations that often exacerbate the challenges faced by this demographic.

2.1 Age-Related Physiological and Psychological Factors

As people age, both their physiological and psychological systems undergo significant changes that influence their pain experiences. Age-related physiological changes can affect pain perception; for instance, there is often a decline in endogenous pain modulation, meaning older adults may experience pain differently than younger populations (Hackett et al., 2020). Research indicates that this decline can lead to a heightened sensitivity to pain (hyperalgesia) and an increased prevalence of chronic pain conditions, which significantly impair the quality of life for older adults (Hackett et al., 2020). Chronic pain is not just a standalone condition in older adults; it is frequently accompanied by comorbidities such as dementia, which complicates both pain assessment and the overall management of pain (Zwakhalen et al., 2018).

Psychologically, older adults may also face unique challenges, including an increased incidence of depression and anxiety, which can both emerge as a response to chronic pain and further complicate the management of pain conditions (Niknejad et al., 2018; Reis da Silva, 2024a). Emotional distress often manifests through somatic complaints rather than through explicit expressions of psychological discomfort, leading to potential underdiagnosis and undertreatment of mood disorders in the context of chronic pain (Carley et al., 2015). Studies suggest that older adults frequently report pain without effectively communicating the psychological burden associated with their conditions, necessitating healthcare providers to employ nuanced assessment techniques sensitive to these issues (Booker & Herr, 2016; Booker & Herr, 2015).

Moreover, chronic pain in the older population affects their functional capabilities and independence. Those with chronic pain often face barriers to engaging in physical activity, which further exacerbates their pain conditions by promoting muscle atrophy and decreasing mobility (Reis da Silva, 2023a; Reis da Silva, 2024b). This creates a vicious cycle where reduced physical activity due to pain leads to worse psychological outcomes, including feelings of helplessness and loss of identity, reinforcing the need for integrated treatment approaches that address both the physical and psychological components of pain (Brant, 2018).

2.2 Sociocultural Considerations and Stigma

The context in which older adults experience pain is also shaped by sociocultural factors that influence their pain experiences and management options. Stigma surrounding pain, particularly among older adults, can hinder effective communication with healthcare providers. There is a pervasive cultural narrative that associates aging with diminished value and strength, which can lead to psychological resistance in older patients seeking help for their pain (McMaughan et al., 2020). Furthermore, among diverse populations, disparities in pain treatment can emerge due to historical marginalisation and discrimination, leading to differences in how pain is perceived and managed across different racial and ethnic groups (Reis da Silva, 2024c).

Cultural beliefs and attitudes toward pain significantly dictate how older adults report pain and engage with treatment options. For instance, in certain cultures, there may be a strong emphasis on stoicism in the face of pain, prompting individuals to underreport their pain experiences (Anderson et al., 2017). This dynamic is particularly pronounced in immigrant populations, where prior experiences and cultural norms can lead to a reluctance in discussing pain due to fears of not being understood or being dismissed by healthcare providers (Reis da Silva, 2024c).

The unique needs of LGBTQ+ older adults present another layer of complexity. Research indicates that these individuals often face compounded stigma related to their sexual orientation or gender identity, which can further complicate their access to appropriate pain management (Fredriksen-Goldsen et al., 2016). Fear of discrimination may lead to avoidance of healthcare settings, exacerbating unmet health needs and pain. Fostering an environment of cultural competence in healthcare is crucial for ensuring that all older adults, regardless of their background, receive the support and care necessary to manage their pain effectively (Jurček & Urek, 2021).

To mitigate these issues, it is essential that pain management approaches in older populations adopt a biopsychosocial model. This model integrates biological, psychological, and social factors into a comprehensive strategy for pain assessment and management. By addressing the multifaceted nature of pain, healthcare providers can better understand and respond to the unique challenges faced by older adults, thereby enhancing the effectiveness of pain management strategies (Golden et al., 2019). Furthermore, increased education for healthcare providers regarding the cultural contexts and expected norms within the populations they serve can foster a more empathetic approach to care. This involves not only recognising the sociocultural dimensions of pain but also actively working to dismantle the stigmas associated with aging and chronic pain conditions (McMaughan et al., 2020). Emphasising open communication and trust in patient-provider relationships can empower older adults to share their pain experiences more freely, leading to improved treatment outcomes.

3. TYPES OF PAIN AND THEIR CLINICAL PRESENTATION

The complexity of pain in older adults necessitates a thorough understanding of its various types, including the difference between acute and chronic pain, the distinction between nociceptive, neuropathic, and psychogenic pain, and the occurrence of mixed pain syndromes. Each of these types of pain presents unique clinical challenges and necessitates tailored treatment approaches.

3.1 Acute vs. Chronic Pain

Acute pain is typically defined as a transient sensation that occurs in response to tissue injury or damage, serving a protective function to alert individuals to harmful stimuli and facilitate avoidance behaviours (Yang & Chang, 2019; Cao et al., 2019). This type of pain is usually well-defined, lasts for a short duration, and resolves as the underlying injury heals. Examples of acute pain conditions often encountered in older adults include postoperative pain, acute fractures, or pain from acute conditions such as renal colic or acute pancreatitis. Research indicates that properly managed acute pain can significantly improve recovery outcomes and reduce the likelihood of subsequent chronic pain (Yang & Chang, 2019; Mallari et al., 2019).

Conversely, chronic pain is characterised by a persistent sensation that lasts longer than the expected time for healing, often extending beyond three to six months (Yang & Chang, 2019; Cao et al., 2019). Chronic pain can arise from various sources and is often associated with chronic conditions prevalent in older populations, such as arthritis, neuropathy, and fibromyalgia. The transition from acute to chronic pain can occur due to inadequate treatment of acute pain, leading to pain chronification that is complex and multifactorial in its aetiology (Yang & Chang, 2019; Vachon-Presseau et al., 2016). Chronic pain not only affects the physical function of older adults but also has profound psychological implications, contributing to depression, anxiety, and diminished quality of life (Yang & Chang, 2019; Cao et al., 2019).

3.2 Nociceptive, Neuropathic, and Psychogenic Pain

Understanding the types of pain related to their underlying mechanisms is critical in managing pain effectively. Nociceptive pain is the result of direct tissue damage that stimulates nociceptors—pain-sensing nerves—which send signals to the brain informing it of potential harm. This type of pain typically mirrors the injury and can include somatic pain (from the skin, muscles, or joints) and visceral pain (from internal organs) (Yang & Chang, 2019; Lauder, 2017). Nociceptive pain is generally responsive to conventional analgesics, such as nonsteroidal anti-inflammatory drugs (NSAIDs) or opioids, making it more straightforward to manage from a pharmacological perspective (Chary, 2021).

Neuropathic pain, on the other hand, results from damage or disease affecting the somatosensory nervous system, leading to altered pain processing (Khammissa et al., 2020; Vachon-Presseau et al., 2016). Conditions such as diabetic neuropathy, post-herpetic neuralgia, and trigeminal neuralgia are examples of neuropathic pain that older adults may experience. Neuropathic pain is often resistant to standard analgesics, necessitating the use of adjuvant medications like antiepileptics or certain antidepressants to achieve adequate pain control (Khammissa et al., 2020).

Moreover, neuropathic pain can present with unique sensations, including burning, tingling, or electric shock-like feelings, complicating the clinical picture and treatment approaches (Khammissa et al., 2020).

Psychogenic pain involves emotional, psychological, or behavioural factors and does not have an identifiable physical cause. This type of pain often complicates the pain management landscape in older adults, as they may have coexisting mental health conditions such as depression or anxiety (Vachon-Presseau et al., 2016; Lauder, 2017). The approach to managing psychogenic pain often requires a multidisciplinary strategy, incorporating psychological therapies alongside physical interventions, to ensure the holistic treatment of the patient (Chary, 2021).

3.3 Mixed Pain Syndromes in Older Adults

Mixed pain syndromes are increasingly recognised in older populations, where patients may present with overlapping characteristics of both nociceptive and neuropathic pain. For instance, an older adult with osteoarthritis may experience nociceptive pain due to joint degeneration alongside neuropathic pain from a coexisting condition like diabetic neuropathy. This mixed presentation complicates treatment plans, as healthcare providers must tailor strategies that address both components to mitigate the patients' suffering effectively (Johnson, 2019; Cravello et al., 2019).

Recent research indicates that a significant proportion of older adults may experience mixed pain presentations, which can further exacerbate challenges in assessment and management (Yang & Chang, 2019; Vachon-Presseau et al., 2016). A comprehensive approach that includes assessing for both types of pain is essential in developing an effective pain management plan. Therapeutic interventions should, therefore, include a combination of pharmacological and non-pharmacological treatments, emphasising the need for a personalised, patient-centred approach. Techniques such as cognitive-behavioural therapy, physical rehabilitation, and the use of neuropathic pain medications may all play key roles in managing these complex pain syndromes (Vachon-Presseau et al., 2016; Kemp et al., 2019).

4. ASSESSMENT CHALLENGES IN OLDER PEOPLE

Assessment of pain in older adults, particularly those with cognitive impairments, poses significant challenges. Cognitive impairment can hinder effective communication and the ability to self-report pain, complicating clinical assessment and management of pain. The review of validated tools and innovative methods for assessing pain is crucial to enhance the quality of care provided to this vulnerable population.

4.1 Cognitive Impairment and Communication Barriers

Cognitive impairment is prevalent among older adults, particularly those with dementia or other neurodegenerative disorders. Such impairments significantly impact their ability to communicate effectively, which is essential for pain assessment (Eldufani & Blaise, 2019; Cravello et al., 2019). For age-related cognitive decline, various factors contribute to these communication challenges. Cognitive impairment often encompasses deficits in memory, attention, language, and executive functions, all of which can limit older adults' capacity to articulate their pain experiences (Beswick et al., 2020; Cravello et al., 2019).

Research underscores that many patients with cognitive impairments may not be able to accurately describe their pain, leading to underassessment and inadequate pain management (Eldufani & Blaise, 2019; Cravello et al., 2019). For instance, when assessing pain in the emergency department setting, standard tools may fall short due to the patient's inability to respond adequately, resulting in a reliance on behavioural cues from caregivers or staff (Eldufani & Blaise, 2019).

Moreover, many assessment protocols traditionally relied upon self-reporting, which is typically the most reliable method for evaluating pain based on subjective experiences. However, as cognitive abilities decline, the utility of self-report diminishes, necessitating alternative approaches (D'Cruz et al., 2020). Consequently, clinicians may overlook or misinterpret pain expressions, resulting in untreated or undertreated pain, which can exacerbate functional decline and diminish quality of life (Scurrah et al., 2017; Cravello et al., 2019).

4.2 Validated Tools and Innovative Assessment Methods

To address these gaps in pain assessment, several validated tools and innovative methods have emerged. Pain management in older adults, particularly those with cognitive impairments, presents unique challenges that necessitate the use of validated assessment tools. Several pain assessment scales have been developed to cater to this demographic's needs, focusing on non-verbal cues and observational methods due to potential communication difficulties. Here, we discuss some widely accepted pain scales, namely the Doloplus-2, PAINAD, and Abbey Pain Scale, detailing their advantages and limitations.

For instance, the Doloplus-2 scale is a widely reported measurement tool that has proven effective in assessing pain in adults with cognitive impairments. Its design incorporates both observational methods and self-reported components, enabling a more comprehensive pain evaluation (Rostad et al., 2017). The tool recognises various pain indicators, including facial expressions, body movements, and vocalisations, which can signal pain even when a patient is unable to communicate verbally (Strand et al., 2018; Rostad et al., 2017). The scale includes somatic reactions (somatic complaints, protective body postures adopted at rest, protection of sore areas, expression and sleep pattern), psychomotor reactions (washing and/or dressing, mobility), and psychosocial reactions (communication, social life and problems of behaviour). The Doloplus-2 tool is effective in recognising pain indicators when patients cannot communicate verbally, thus bridging a significant gap in pain assessment for older adults with dementia or other cognitive issues (Rostad et al., 2017). Other characteristic is the comprehensive nature of the scale helps ensure a holistic view of the patient's pain experience. The disadvantages are that Implementing the Doloplus-2 scale necessitates training for staff, meaning the increasing demands on healthcare resources (Kang & Demiris, 2017). Also, it may not be suitable for very low-functioning patients who may demonstrate limited observable reactions, potentially leading to under-diagnosis of pain in these individuals (Rostad et al., 2017).

Furthermore, observational pain scales have been developed to allow caregivers and healthcare providers to infer pain based on non-verbal behaviours, such as facial grimacing or changes in body posture (Eldufani & Blaise, 2019; Strand et al., 2018). These approaches are particularly critical in settings where patients may be non-communicative or unable to articulate their pain due to cognitive decline. Training caregivers to recognise and document these non-verbal cues is essential for incorporating observational tools into routine pain management protocols (Kim et al., 2020).

Other important pain assessment tool is called PAINAD (Pain Assessment in Advanced Dementia). The PAINAD scale was developed specifically for patients with advanced dementia and relies on behavioural cues to assess pain. The PAINAD evaluates several observable behaviours: Breathing patterns (e.g., laboured breathing when in pain); vocalisation (e.g., moaning or whimpering), facial expressions (e.g., grimacing), body language (e.g., rigid posture or restlessness) and interactions (e.g., withdrawal from social contact). As benefits, this scale is simple to administer, allowing healthcare staff to quickly assess pain without the need for extensive training and it has been validated for use in non-verbal patients, making it suitable for the target population (McGuire et al., 2016). The negatives are the scale relies heavily on the subjective interpretation of behaviour, which can vary between observers, potentially leading to inconsistencies in pain evaluation (Kwon et al., 2018) and it may not sufficiently differentiate between various pain types or underlying issues, which could limit comprehensive treatment plans (Dillane & Doody, 2019).

The Abbey Pain Scale is another useful tool designed to assist nursing home staff in assessing pain levels in non-verbal older patients, particularly those with dementia. The components for this scale are the vocalisation (e.g., loud moans or whimpers), the facial expressions (e.g., grimaces indicating discomfort), the body language (e.g., tense or protective postures), the behavioural changes (e.g., aggression or restlessness), and the changes in physiological responses (e.g., signs of infection or fever). There are several benefits in using this scale, such as it was developed specifically for individuals with cognitive impairments, it has been validated for reliability and accuracy in pain detection in older adults (Cirillo et al., 2019), and the scale promotes a standardised framework for pain assessment across nursing staff, enhancing inter-rater reliability in various care settings. The negatives of this scale, similar to other observational scales, it may miss nuanced pain expressions in patients who have become accustomed to chronic pain and the reliance on subjective behaviours may not encompass an individual's full pain experience, leading to possible undertreatment (Scher et al., 2020).

Innovative assessment methods also include using technology and smart devices to monitor vital signs or detect physiological changes that may indicate pain (Scurrah et al., 2017; Reis da Silva, 2025a). For example, wearable devices can track changes in heart rates or movement patterns that suggest discomfort, providing an indirect measure of pain and allowing for timely interventions. This modality is particularly beneficial for older adults who may struggle to articulate their feelings but can still experience pain-related physiological responses (Reis da Silva, 2025b; D'Cruz et al., 2020; Cravello et al., 2019). Moreover, the introduction of integrated pain management interventions, which combine traditional pain assessment tools with behavioural health considerations, is becoming increasingly significant. This holistic approach can improve overall outcomes by simultaneously addressing pain and its psychosocial components, ensuring that interventions are tailored to individual needs and capabilities (D'Cruz et al., 2020; Rostad et al., 2017).

In their systematic reviews, researchers have emphasised the need of a biopsychosocial model of pain assessment, which considers the physiological, psychological, and social factors contributing to pain experiences in older adults (Kim et al., 2020; Rostad et al., 2017). Adapting existing tools to incorporate these elements can facilitate a more comprehensive understanding of the patient's pain narrative, leading to better-targeted interventions.

5. CONTRIBUTIONS TO PAIN RESEARCH

In the realm of pain management, particularly for older adults, recent research indicates a growing understanding of various factors contributing to pain perception, innovative assessment methods, and integrative care strategies. This section will explore three primary aspects: the role of emotional intelligence in pain perception, the implementation of integrative nursing strategies for effective pain relief, and illustrative case studies reflecting the nursing process in gerontological practice.

5.1 Emotional Intelligence and Pain Perception

Emotional intelligence (EI) refers to an individual's ability to recognise, understand, and manage emotions—both their own and those of others (da Silva, 2022; Reis da Silva et al., 2025). In nursing practice, high EI can profoundly shape interactions between nurses and older adults experiencing pain. Research indicates that nurses with developed emotional intelligence are often better equipped to recognise the emotional aspects of pain and manage the psychosocial factors that influence a patient's pain experience (Chatchumni et al., 2020; Reis da Silva, 2024d; Reis da Silva, 2025c). The nuances of pain perception are intricately linked to emotional states; for example, anxiety and fear can exacerbate pain experiences, while empathetic engagement by healthcare providers can facilitate pain relief (Yamanaka, 2018).

Studies suggest that improving nurses' emotional intelligence can correlate with enhanced pain outcomes by fostering a therapeutic environment where patients feel safe and valued (Chatchumni et al., 2020). By acknowledging the emotional components of pain, nurses can offer more personalised care tailored to individual needs (Reis da Silva, 2025d). This aligns with the biopsychosocial model of pain management, which incorporates psychological and social dimensions alongside physiological factors (Bruckenthal et al., 2016). Thus, further research on training programs designed to enhance emotional intelligence in nursing curricula is warranted, as they may significantly impact the quality of pain management provided to older adults (Chatchumni et al., 2020; Reis da Silva, 2025e).

5.2 Integrative Nursing Strategies for Pain Relief

Integrative nursing represents a holistic approach that combines conventional medical practices with complementary therapies to address pain management comprehensively (Reis da Silva, 2024d). Such strategies have become particularly relevant in gerontological nursing, where older adults often present with multiple comorbidities and complex pain syndromes (Bruckenthal et al., 2016). Integrative approaches can include various practices, such as promoting physical therapies, cognitive-behavioural strategies, and alternative treatments like acupuncture, which have shown effectiveness in reducing pain perception (Bruckenthal et al., 2016; Berger et al., 2021).

For instance, a recent systematic review highlighted the efficacy of techniques such as mindfulness and relaxation training in managing chronic pain, demonstrating that these strategies significantly improve patients' self-efficacy and pain outcomes (Yamanaka, 2018). By integrating these complementary therapies into routine care, nurses can empower older adults in self-management of pain, leading to a more active role for patients in their treatment plans (Bruckenthal et al., 2016). The outcomes of these initiatives not only enhance pain relief but also improve overall patient satisfaction and engagement with healthcare services (Berger et al., 2021). A systematic evaluation of such programs in nursing education may yield valuable insights into the preparedness of future nurses to deliver these integrative strategies effectively (Crawford et al., 2016).

5.3 Case Studies from Gerontological Practice and the Nursing Process

Case Study 1: Managing Chronic Pain in a 75-year-Old Female with Arthritis

An older woman diagnosed with osteoarthritis presented with severe joint pain in her knee, significantly impairing her mobility. The nursing assessment involved using the Doloplus-2 scale to evaluate her pain, complemented by discussions to gauge her emotional state. The nurse employed integrative strategies, including regular physical therapy and recommendations for participation in a local Tai Chi class—known for its benefits for arthritis. Through this comprehensive approach, the patient's pain levels reduced, and she reported improved well-being, illustrating the efficacy of a holistic pain management plan guided by thorough nursing assessment (Bruckenthal et al., 2016).

Case Study 2: Emotional Support for a Dementia Patient Experiencing Pain

A 70-year-old male with moderate dementia exhibited signs of distress, though he was unable to communicate the source of his pain. Nursing staff employed observational pain assessment techniques, noting changes in behaviour and facial expressions. Recognising the emotional impact of his condition, nurses utilised distractions—such as music therapy and reminiscence therapy—to alleviate anxiety and potential pain (Reis da Silva, 2024c). This approach not only calmed the patient but also fostered a better environment for assessing and managing his pain effectively. This case underscores the profound effect that emotional intelligence and understanding can have on pain management in patients with cognitive impairments (Chatchumni et al., 2020; (Yamanaka, 2018).

Case Study 3: Post-operative Pain Management in an Older Patient

A 74 years old male who underwent hip replacement surgery exhibited inadequate pain management post-operatively, as indicated by self-reports and behavioural observations. The nursing team integrated a multimodal analgesic approach, using non-opioid analgesics alongside non-pharmacological interventions such as guided imagery and ice application. Regular assessments led to adjustments in his pain management plan, significantly reducing his reliance on opioids and enhancing his recovery trajectory (Chatchumni et al., 2020; Yin et al., 2015). This case illustrates the importance of continual evaluation and adjustment of pain management strategies based on comprehensive assessments of both physiological and emotional aspects of pain.

Case Study 4: Addressing Cancer-Related Pain in a Seventy-Year-Old Female

A 69-year-old female receiving palliative care for metastatic breast cancer experienced debilitating pain despite opioid therapy. The nursing team collaborated with the specialist pain team to explore alternative and complementary strategies, including the incorporation of mindfulness meditation and acupuncture sessions. Education was provided to the patient regarding self-management of pain, which empowered her to take an active role in her treatment. This integrative approach led to reduced pain levels, improved emotional well-being, and enhanced quality of life, demonstrating the benefits of a multidisciplinary strategy in pain management (Yamanaka, 2018).

Case Study 5: Physiotherapy and Emotional Intelligence (EI) in Dementia

This case study focuses on an 80-year-old male patient diagnosed with dementia who participated in a physiotherapist-led program incorporating sensory-motor exercises, affective music, and reminiscence-based movement therapy. Research highlights that engaging patients with dementia in activities that stimulate sensory processing, and emotional connections can significantly improve their overall well-being. Observational scales such as the Pain Assessment in Advanced Dementia (PAINAD) were employed, indicating a noticeable reduction in patient agitation and an improvement in sleep quality (Kozlowski et al., 2017). The employed interventions focused on enhancing emotional communication, which is particularly important in dementia care, as evidence suggests that emotionally intelligent approaches can significantly contribute to the efficacy of therapeutic interventions (Kozlowski et al., 2017). Moreover, the incorporation of music and movement not only serves as a form of physical exercise but also facilitates emotional expression and connection, highlighting the role of EI in therapeutic contexts.

Integrating EI into physiotherapy can lead to enhanced therapeutic alliances and improved patient engagement. The physiotherapist's ability to assess and respond to the emotional needs of the patient is paramount, underscoring the rationale for training healthcare providers in EI competencies (Kozlowski et al., 2017). The benefits observed in this case study align with findings that well-structured emotional intelligence training can augment the clinical effectiveness of health professionals, thereby fostering environments that promote patient-centred care (Sela et al., 2020).

Case Study 6: Multimodal Pain Plan for Isolated Older Woman

This case study centres on a 74-year-old woman suffering from osteoarthritis, who faced challenges exacerbated by digital exclusion and social isolation. A community nurse-led home visit program was initiated, which developed a multimodal pain management plan encompassing physical therapy, emotional support, and digital literacy classes. Research indicates that older adults experience significant barriers in accessing pain management and healthcare services due to technological challenges, which can result in elevated levels of distress and inadequate pain management (Jung & Matthews, 2021). In tailoring the pain plan to the patient's needs, the program aimed to enhance her physical mobility through targeted physical therapy interventions while also addressing her emotional and psychological wellbeing.

The incorporation of emotional support proved crucial as studies highlight the significant role of emotional factors in pain perception and coping strategies among older adults (Lewis et al., 2017). Furthermore, connecting this individual with digital literacy classes not only supported her ability to access healthcare resources but also facilitated social integration, thereby mitigating feelings of isolation. Such holistic approaches align with evidence-based practices that stress the importance of addressing both physical and psychological needs in geriatric care (Athanasakis, 2019). By fostering emotional resilience through supportive interactions, healthcare providers can significantly enhance the quality of life for patients like her, emphasising the importance of interdisciplinary collaboration in effective pain management (Soimah & Utami, 2023; Reis da Silva, 2025h).

Case Study 7: Interdisciplinary Pain Clinic

This case study discusses a rural outreach program that integrates various health professionals, including speech therapists, social workers, and psychologists, into a home-based palliative care model for older adults suffering from cancer-related pain. The collaborative framework employed within this plan underscores the value of interdisciplinary approaches in managing complex pain, particularly in rural settings where access to specialized care may be limited (Joo & Liu, 2021). Research demonstrates that interdisciplinary teams can effectively enhance patient experiences through enhanced communication, emotional support, and tailored interventions that meet the multifaceted needs of patients (Joo & Liu, 2021).

In this setting, emotional expression and nutritional support formed the core of the pain management strategy. The involvement of psychologists to support emotional expression indicates an awareness of the psychological dimensions of pain, supporting findings that emotional and psychosocial factors are deeply intertwined with pain perception and management (Xu et al., 2021). Providing comprehensive care that integrates emotional support, nutritional guidance, and effective communication strategies has been shown to improve patients' quality of life (QOL) and significantly reduce emergency admissions (Vocci et al., 2021). This holistic care model exemplifies the essential role of interdisciplinary collaboration and emotional intelligence in enhancing the healthcare delivery process, ultimately promoting better patient outcomes in palliative care settings.

6. MULTIDISCIPLINARY AND TECHNOLOGICAL APPROACHES TO PAIN MANAGEMENT

6.1 Multidisciplinary and Technological Approaches to Pain Management

Pain management, particularly in older adults, requires a robust multidisciplinary approach that leverages collaborative practices among healthcare professionals while also incorporating technological advancements (Reis da Silva, 2025f). By utilising artificial intelligence (AI), wearable technologies, telehealth services, and personalised, culturally sensitive interventions, healthcare teams can significantly enhance pain management outcomes (Reis da Silva, 2025f).

6.2 Collaboration Among Healthcare Professionals

Collaboration among various healthcare professionals — including physicians, nurses, physical therapists, pharmacists, and mental health specialists — is essential for providing comprehensive pain management (Reis da Silva, 2024f). This interdisciplinary approach allows for a multifaceted assessment of pain, wherein diverse perspectives inform treatment plans tailored to individual patient needs (Xu et al., 2018; Burton & Shaw, 2015). Effective communication and teamwork among professionals can lead to improved pain relief, increased patient satisfaction, and a decrease in opioid use, as noted in systematic reviews (Burton & Shaw, 2015; Zahari et al., 2020).

Research highlights that the integration of diverse disciplines can enhance the effectiveness of pain management programs. For instance, coordinated care models, where pain management specialists work alongside primary care providers, have shown promise in optimising treatment plans by ensuring that all health aspects, including psychological and social factors related to pain, are addressed (Zahari et al., 2020; Chatchumni et al., 2020). Moreover, this collaboration can leverage shared decision-making strategies, empowering patients and their families to participate actively in pain management decisions, which is especially important in culturally diverse populations (Xu et al., 2018).

6.3 Home Adaptation and Community Support for Older Adults with Chronic Pain

Older adults with chronic pain often require tailored home adaptations to maintain their independence and ensure safety (Reis da Silva, 2023b; Reis da Silva, 2023c). Occupational therapists and nurses play a vital role in assessing the needs of these individuals, implementing changes that may include adaptive seating, grab bars, modified kitchen tools, and ergonomic furniture (Reis da Silva, 2023c). Such modifications not only support physical functionality but also contribute to enhancing the quality of life of older adults, allowing them to remain in their preferred living environments rather than transition to assisted living facilities (Leeuwen et al., 2019; Reis da Silva, 2023b). The desire among many older adults to adapt their home environments rather than move reflects a profound preference for maintaining autonomy, emphasising the significance of community support systems and familial involvement in sustaining adherence to home modifications (Reis da Silva, 2023b).

Involving caregivers and community services amplifies the effectiveness of these adaptations, as these additional resources can further reduce hospitalisations. A systematic review reiterates that engagement in community-dwelling programs, while incorporating social support, has a reciprocal impact on both the effective management of chronic conditions and the overall health outcomes for older adults (Tang et al., 2019). These structures not only support physical health but also instil emotional resilience and connectivity, critical factors in managing the multifaceted experience of chronic pain in ageing populations (Campbell et al., 2015; Reis da Silva, 2025h).

Additionally, adapting certain aspects of the home environment can substantially influence an older individual's capacity to perform daily activities and manage their pain effectively. Evidence suggests that when older adults are equipped with the right tools and modifications, their self-efficacy regarding pain management increases, leading to improved adherence to prescribed therapies and potentially better overall health outcomes (Campbell et al., 2015).

6.4 Role of AI, Wearable Technologies, and Telehealth

The application of artificial intelligence in pain management is being explored as a means to enhance decision-making and predictive analytics for treatment outcomes (Reis da Silva, 2025a; Reis da Silva, 2025g). AI algorithms can process large datasets, identifying patterns and trends that inform personalized pain management strategies (Reis da Silva, 2025b). For instance, AI can assist in predicting which patients may experience certain types of pain based on their medical histories and associated conditions. Moreover, wearable technologies have emerged as a crucial tool for continuous pain monitoring (Reis da Silva, 2025f). Devices equipped with sensors can track physiological parameters such as heart rate variability and movement patterns, providing real-time data that can indicate pain levels (Reis da Silva, 2025a). This technology offers patients the ability to self-monitor their conditions, leading to more accurate assessments of their pain experiences and allowing healthcare providers to tailor interventions responsively (Reis da Silva, 2025f).

Telehealth also plays a transformative role in pain management, particularly highlighted during the COVID-19 pandemic (Reis da Silva, 2025a). Remote consultations have made it possible for patients to access pain management services without the barriers of travel, which can be particularly challenging for older adults. Telehealth platforms promote continuous patient engagement and follow-up care, allowing for timely adjustments in pain management strategies (Crawford et al., 2016). In an era increasingly dependent on technology, telehealth is proving indispensable for managing chronic pain in patients who may have limited physical mobility (Reis da Silva, 2025f).

6.5 Digital Literacy and Technological Barriers in Pain Management

While modern technology offers significant advantages for managing chronic pain, such as through wearables, telehealth, and mobile health (mHealth) applications, digital illiteracy poses a considerable barrier for many older adults (Reis da Silva, 2025a; Reis da Silva, 2025f). Research indicates that the difficulties associated with accessing technology, combined with a lack of digital skills and trust in digital health tools, can severely limit the potential benefits these technologies might provide (Dermody et al., 2020; Reis da Silva, 2025f). Interventions aimed at enhancing digital literacy—such as training programs that simplify interfaces and culturally adapt tools—are essential for enabling older populations to take full advantage of these innovations (Zwakhalen et al., 2018).

Considerable efforts are underway across platforms to address these gaps. For instance, programs established by Age UK and the NHS Digital Participation initiative are recognised as useful models for fostering digital literacy among older adults. These programs emphasise the importance of providing older adults with the skills necessary to utilize modern technology effectively, thereby improving their capacity to engage in self-monitoring and self-management for pain relief (Dermody et al., 2020). By improving access to technology, healthcare providers can foster a more inclusive environment for pain management and increase older adults' confidence in their ability to access necessary healthcare services remotely (Reis da Silva, 2025a).

Furthermore, it is imperative for healthcare professionals to be aware of and actively address the technological barriers faced by older patients (Reis da Silva, 2025a). Studies have shown that older adults who successfully navigate these digital challenges can experience enhanced pain management outcomes through telehealth consultations and access to personalised health data, ultimately contributing to an improved quality of life (Bowen et al., 2019). Bridging the digital divide is thus integral not just for enhancing pain management, but for fostering a sense of agency and autonomy among older adults living with chronic pain (Reis da Silva, 2025f).

6.6 Personalised and Culturally Sensitive Interventions

The move toward personalised medicine in pain management is crucial, particularly when addressing the needs of older adults from diverse cultural backgrounds (Burton & Shaw, 2015; Henschke et al., 2016). Individualised treatment plans that consider cultural perceptions of pain, health beliefs, and community practices can significantly enhance patient engagement and treatment adherence (Torres-Cueco & Nohales-Alfonso, 2021; Henschke et al., 2016).

Cultural sensitivity is particularly important in pain assessment and management; healthcare providers must be trained to recognise and respond to culturally informed coping strategies that patients may employ (Torres-Cueco & Nohales-Alfonso, 2021). For example, studies have suggested employing culturally relevant pain assessment tools and methodologies that reflect the unique experiences and values of diverse communities (Burton & Shaw, 2015; Henschke et al., 2016). This can facilitate more effective interventions and improve patient outcomes by fostering trust and understanding in the patient-provider relationship. One illustrative example is the integration of family involvement in decision-making regarding pain management, which is particularly valued in many cultures. Strategies that empower patients and their families to engage actively in discussions about pain management can yield improved satisfaction and outcomes in pain management (Xu et al., 2018).

6.7 Assessment Instruments and Communication Aids

Effective pain assessment in older adults necessitates accommodating communication limitations that often accompany ageing. Instruments such as the Doloplus-2, PAINAD (Pain Assessment in Advanced Dementia), the Abbey Pain Scale, and the McGill Pain Questionnaire are critical in capturing the nuances of pain experiences across diverse populations (Burton et al., 2019). These tools are designed to be sensitive to the specific needs of older adults, ensuring that pain is adequately assessed, even in individuals with cognitive impairments or communication challenges (Burton et al., 2019).

The employment of culturally responsive communication strategies is also essential in enhancing the effectiveness of pain assessment instruments (Burton & Shaw, 2015). Research has shown that training healthcare professionals in culturally competent practices leads to improved patient engagement and more accurate assessments of pain (Henschke et al., 2016). Training initiatives should encompass awareness of linguistic nuances, non-verbal expressions of pain, and the psychosocial contexts that influence how pain is perceived and reported by older adults. Such comprehensive training can greatly enhance the efficacy of pain management strategies and contribute to informed, patient-centered care (Burton & Shaw, 2015; Henschke et al., 2016).

Furthermore, the integration of technology in pain assessment should not overlook these critical factors. Audio-visual aids, mobile applications, and telehealth systems have the potential to streamline communication processes and introduce more adaptive and responsive pain assessment strategies. However, these technologies must be implemented with careful consideration of the specific communication needs and sensory-motor capabilities of older adults to enhance their pain management experiences (Burton & Shaw, 2015; Henschke et al., 2016).

In summary, the intersection of home adaptation, community support, digital literacy, and effective assessment instruments represents a comprehensive approach to managing chronic pain in older adults. These elements underscore the necessity for an integrated care model that emphasises not only physical adaptations but also emotional and psychological support through community engagement and technology. By fostering environments that prioritise independence, enhance digital competencies, and employ culturally sensitive communication strategies, healthcare systems can significantly improve the quality of life for older adults navigating chronic pain. The collective focus on these areas offers a pathway toward optimizing support for one of society's most vulnerable populations.

7. INTEGRATIVE AND NON-PHARMACOLOGICAL INTERVENTIONS FOR PAIN MANAGEMENT IN OLDER ADULTS

Effective pain management, particularly in older adults, often requires a multi-faceted approach that integrates non-pharmacological therapies alongside conventional treatments. These interventions address physical sensations of pain, as well as incorporate emotional and psychosocial support. The following discussion delves into several effective strategies, including mind-body approaches, acupuncture, physical therapy, and emotional and spiritual support, while providing insights into their potential benefits and limitations.

7.1 Mind-Body Approaches

Mind-body interventions, such as mindfulness meditation, Qigong, Yoga, and cognitive behavioural therapy (CBT), have gained attention for their effectiveness in managing chronic pain conditions (Zeidan & Vago, 2016). Mindfulness-based stress reduction (MBSR) is one of the most well-documented approaches, effectively reducing pain perception and improving the overall quality of life. Research has shown that mindfulness meditation can lead to significant reductions in pain intensity and improve psychological health by fostering a greater sense of self-regulation and coping strategies (Zeidan & Vago, 2016; Adler-Neal & Zeidan, 2017).

The benefits of these interventions are manifold. They effectively reduce chronic pain and related symptoms such as anxiety and depression (Garland et al., 2020) and empower individuals by promoting self-management of their condition (Meehan & Carter, 2021). However, not all older adults may find these practices accessible. Advanced cognitive impairments or mobility limitations can hinder participation (Vitoula et al., 2018; Chen & Michalsen, 2017). Furthermore, while the existing evidence base is promising, some studies vary in quality, underscoring the need for more rigorous trials to confirm long-term efficacy (Feng et al., 2021).

7.2 Acupuncture

Acupuncture, a practice rooted in traditional Chinese medicine, is another valuable non-pharmacological option for pain relief (Reis da Silva, 2025g). It involves the insertion of fine needles at specific points on the body to promote healing and alleviate discomfort. Acupuncture has shown particular efficacy in managing conditions common in older adults, such as osteoarthritis and chronic low back pain (Chen & Michalsen, 2017). Its holistic approach is appealing to many, especially because it avoids the side effects commonly associated with pharmacological treatments (Lin et al., 2021; Chen & Michalsen, 2017). Evidence supports its ability to improve quality of life and reduce pain severity (Goh et al., 2019). Still, patient responses can vary significantly. While some experience substantial relief, others report minimal to no benefit (Ardestani et al., 2021). Additionally, fear or anxiety related to needles may dissuade some individuals from pursuing this therapy.

7.3 Physical Therapy

Physical therapy remains a cornerstone of multidisciplinary pain management. It includes a variety of techniques—such as therapeutic exercises, manual manipulation, and mobility-enhancing modalities—aimed at improving function and alleviating pain (Vitoula et al., 2018). In older adults, physical therapy is particularly valuable due to its capacity for customisation, allowing tailored plans that respect individual capabilities and limitations (Vitoula et al., 2018; Yeh & Horwitz, 2017). Consistent participation can enhance mobility, reduce disability, and support overall recovery (Brosseau et al., 2017). Nonetheless, practical challenges exist. Transportation difficulties or physical limitations may affect attendance and adherence (Lumley & Schubiner, 2019). Moreover, some individuals may experience temporary pain exacerbation if therapy is not administered appropriately (Lumley & Schubiner, 2019).

7.4 Emotional and Spiritual Support

Incorporating emotional and spiritual support into pain management strategies is essential for addressing the holistic needs of older patients (Reis da Silva, 2024g). Emotional distress often accompanies chronic pain, and unaddressed psychological or spiritual concerns can intensify the experience of suffering (Yeh & Horwitz, 2017). Interventions such as counselling, guided reflection, or spiritual care contribute to more comprehensive, compassionate care and can lead to greater patient satisfaction (Yeh & Horwitz, 2017). Supporting patients emotionally fosters resilience and helps them develop coping mechanisms for both physical pain and its emotional ramifications (Reis da Silva, 2025h). However, acceptance of these interventions varies widely depending on individual values, beliefs, and cultural backgrounds (Garland et al., 2020). Moreover, the effective delivery of such support requires specialised training, which may not always be available in healthcare settings (Wei et al., 2020).

Taken together, these approaches—mind-body practices, acupuncture, physical therapy, and emotional and spiritual support—highlight the importance of a multidisciplinary, person-centred strategy in managing pain among older adults. Tailoring interventions to the individual's preferences, abilities, and values ensures a more ethical, effective, and dignified model of care.

8. ETHICAL AND PERSON-CENTRED CARE CONSIDERATIONS IN PAIN MANAGEMENT

Pain management, especially for older adults, necessitates a focus on ethical considerations and person-centred approaches that respect the dignity, autonomy, and specific needs of each individual. This entails ensuring informed consent within the context of pain relief and striving for equity in access to pain relief technologies.

8.1 Autonomy, Consent, and Dignity in Pain Care

Autonomy in pain management refers to the respect for the patient's right to make informed decisions about their treatment options (Corey & McQueen, 2017). This is particularly crucial in geriatric care, where older individuals may be experiencing cognitive decline, potentially impacting their decision-making abilities (Reis da Silva, 2024f). Providing clear and concise information about treatment options is essential for obtaining informed consent, especially when discussing pain relief options that may involve complex medications or interventions.

In practice, healthcare providers should adopt an approach that enhances the patient's autonomy (Reis da Silva, 2024h). This includes asking open-ended questions to gauge the patient's understanding and values regarding pain management choices. Shared decision-making models can also be beneficial, where patients are actively involved in discussions about their pain relief options, thus fostering a sense of control over their care (Corey & McQueen, 2017). Furthermore, acknowledging the inherent dignity of patients ensures they are treated with respect and that their experiences of pain are validated, which is crucial for effective care (Corey & McQueen, 2017).

8.2 Challenges to Autonomy

Barriers to achieving patient autonomy in pain management often stem from cognitive impairments, cultural factors, and systemic healthcare issues. For instance, patients with advanced dementia may struggle to articulate their pain, limiting their ability to provide informed consent (Nahin et al., 2016). Culturally informed care is also essential, as different cultural backgrounds may influence how pain is perceived and reported, impacting the autonomy individuals experience in decision-making (Nahin et al., 2016).

8.3 Equity in Access to Pain Relief Technologies

Access to effective pain management technologies is another critical ethical consideration. There exists significant disparity in access to pain relief technologies across different geographic regions and socioeconomic groups (Corey & McQueen, 2017). For example, older adults living in rural areas may lack access to advanced pain relief modalities, such as integrative therapies or newer pharmacological treatments, exacerbating existing health inequities (Aldamluji et al., 2020).

8.4 Addressing Disparities

To address these disparities, there needs to be a focus on policy changes that promote equitable access to pain management technologies. Telehealth services have become a vital tool in bridging this gap, allowing patients from underserved areas to receive consultation and advice from pain specialists without the need to travel long distances (Madsen et al., 2017; Reis da Silva, 2025a). Additionally, advocacy for broader insurance coverage for alternative and integrative pain management modalities, such as acupuncture and physical therapy, can facilitate improved access for low-income patients facing chronic pain (Eccleston et al., 2017).

Furthermore, providing education and resources about available pain management options in multiple languages and formats can empower patients from diverse backgrounds to seek appropriate care. Establishing community-based pain management programs may also help ensure that vulnerable populations receive both educational support and access to needed interventions (Menezes et al., 2024).

9. CONCLUSION AND FUTURE DIRECTIONS IN PAIN MANAGEMENT

Pain management, particularly in older adults, commands significant attention in healthcare policy and practice, given the unique complexities associated with ageing populations. This concluding section discusses policy implications, identifies existing research gaps, and emphasises the areas where innovation potential lies.

9.1 Policy Implications

Effective pain management is subject to a myriad of policies that influence access to treatment, guidelines for practitioners, and funding for research initiatives (Sakamoto et al., 2018). Individuals with chronic pain, especially older adults, face barriers to obtaining adequate pain relief, underscoring the critical need for policies that promote access to multidisciplinary pain management resources (Reis da Silva, 2024f). Such policies should emphasise the integration of pharmacological and non-pharmacological treatments, recognising that effective pain management often requires a comprehensive approach that addresses both the physiological and psychosocial aspects of pain (Yin et al., 2015; Sakamoto et al., 2018).

Furthermore, pain management protocols should include clear pathways for the use of integrative therapies, such as acupuncture and mind-body interventions, which have been shown to be beneficial yet are often underutilised in conventional settings (Leis & Morrison, 2021). Policymakers should advocate for the funding of integrative care models and educational programs to train healthcare providers in these approaches. Such initiatives could reduce reliance on opioids and mitigate the associated risks of misuse and dependency among older adults (Elbers et al., 2018). Additionally, ensuring that pain relief technologies, such as telehealth platforms and mobile health applications, are included in public health initiatives is vital (Reis da Silva, 2025a). Equity in access to these technologies can significantly enhance pain management outcomes for underrepresented and underserved populations, especially those in rural or low-income areas (Dunham et al., 2021).

9.2 Research Gaps and Innovation Potential

Despite the growing body of literature on pain management, significant gaps remain that necessitate further investigation and innovation. One primary gap is the limited understanding of pain mechanisms in older adults and the need for personalised pain management strategies tailored to individual experiences and medical histories (Sakamoto et al., 2018; Devan et al., 2019). Research should focus on the biopsychosocial model of pain, which considers biological, psychological, and social factors influencing the pain experience (Farzad et al., 2021). More studies exploring how to effectively integrate these dimensions into comprehensive care plans may yield valuable insights (Hurley-Wallace et al., 2021).

Additionally, there is a pressing need for longitudinal research assessing the effectiveness of non-pharmacological interventions over time, particularly concerning their long-term impacts on pain management and quality of life in diverse older populations (Amponsah et al., 2019). Innovations in wearable health technologies that monitor physiological responses can enhance existing models of pain management by facilitating real-time assessments and timely interventions (Tsai et al., 2020). Furthermore, extensive research is required to evaluate the efficacy of digital health interventions, including mHealth applications, in supporting self-management of pain among older adults (Tsai et al., 2020). Understanding patient engagement with such technologies will help refine them to meet user needs more effectively and increase the likelihood of adherence to pain management protocols (Buck et al., 2021).

Lastly, there is a critical need for more research exploring the cultural perceptions of pain and the acceptability of various pain management strategies across different populations. Ensuring culturally sensitive interventions can help tailor pain management approaches to fit the unique needs of diverse communities, thus promoting equity in healthcare provision (Probyn et al., 2017).

9.3 Limitations and Future Implications

The assessment and management of pain presents notable limitations and future implications across various populations. One significant challenge is the inconsistency of pain assessment tools, which can lead to ineffective pain management strategies. For instance, studies indicate that healthcare professionals often rely on subjective interpretations or invalidated tools rather than adhering to standardised assessments, particularly in vulnerable groups such as those with cognitive impairments or advanced dementia (Tsai et al., 2020; Burns & McIlfatrick, 2015). This inconsistency is exacerbated by cultural attitudes towards pain and barriers in communication, which complicate accurate assessments in older populations and nursing homes (Vaismoradi et al., 2016; Mataqi & Aslanpour, 2019).

Moreover, there remains a significant gap in the education and training of healthcare providers regarding effective pain management practices, highlighting a need for incorporating comprehensive Analgesia pharmacology and pharmacodynamics curricula in healthcare education – for example, Nursing, Medicine, Pharmacy (Shipton et al., 2018). Future efforts should focus on developing and validating more objective assessment tools that cater specifically to these populations and enhance the communication skills of healthcare providers to better understand and manage patients' pain experiences effectively (Hanson et al., 2016; Martin et al., 2020). Integration of advanced technology and psycho-social considerations in pain assessment models could facilitate a more holistic approach to pain management, which remains crucial moving forward (Wideman et al., 2019; Eccleston et al., 2021).

9.4 Recommendations

Chronic pain in older adults is a multidimensional phenomenon requiring nuanced, evidence-based, and person-centred approaches. Only through integration of psychological, emotional, physical, social, and technological domains can healthcare professionals adequately support this growing population. Future directions should include an inclusion of EI training in all healthcare curricula; further research on kinesiophobia in older adults, funding for digital literacy interventions and policies promoting equity in access to multidisciplinary pain care.

9.5 Conclusion

The future directions in pain management for older adults highlight the need for a robust ethical framework and innovative solutions that prioritize person-centred care. Policies must address accessibility, while research should focus on the evolving landscape of pain management strategies, fostering a holistic understanding of pain that incorporates diverse treatments and patient experiences. Emphasising these directions will lead to improved health outcomes and enhanced quality of life for older adults living with chronic pain.

REFERENCES

Adler-Neal, A., & Zeidan, F. (2017). Mindfulness meditation for fibromyalgia: Mechanistic and clinical considerations. *Current Rheumatology Reports*, *19*(9), 59. Advance online publication. DOI: 10.1007/s11926-017-0686-0 PMID: 28752493

Aldamluji, N., Burgess, A., Pogatzki-Zahn, E., Ræder, J., & Beloeil, H. (2020). Prospect guideline for tonsillectomy: Systematic review and procedure-specific postoperative pain management recommendations. *Anaesthesia*, *76*(7), 947–961. DOI: 10.1111/anae.15299 PMID: 33201518

Amponsah, A., Björn, A., Bam, V., & Axelin, A. (2019). The effect of educational strategies targeted for nurses on pain assessment and management in children: An integrative review. *Pain Management Nursing*, *20*(6), 604–613. DOI: 10.1016/j.pmn.2019.03.005 PMID: 31103495

Anderson, A., Deng, J., Anthony, R., Atalla, S., & Monroe, T. (2017). Using complementary and alternative medicine to treat pain and agitation in dementia. *Critical Care Nursing Clinics of North America*, *29*(4), 519–537. DOI: 10.1016/j.cnc.2017.08.010 PMID: 29107312

Ardestani, S., Karkhaneh, M., Stein, E., Punja, S., Junqueira, D., Kuzmyn, T., & Vohra, S. (2021). Systematic review of mind-body interventions to treat myalgic encephalomyelitis/chronic fatigue syndrome. *Medicina*, *57*(7), 652. DOI: 10.3390/medicina57070652 PMID: 34202826

Athanasakis, E. (2019). A meta-synthesis of how registered nurses make sense of their lived experiences of medication errors. *Journal of Clinical Nursing*, *28*(17-18), 3077–3095. DOI: 10.1111/jocn.14917 PMID: 31099064

Berger, A., Liu, Y., Mosel, L., Champagne, K., Ruoff, M., Cornett, E., Kaye, A. D., Imani, F., Shakeri, A., Varrassi, G., Viswanath, O., & Urits, I. (2021). Efficacy of dry needling and acupuncture in the treatment of neck pain. *Anesthesiology and Pain Medicine*, *11*(2). Advance online publication. DOI: 10.5812/aapm.113627 PMID: 34336626

Beswick, E., Park, E., Wong, C., Mehta, A., Dakin, R., Chandran, S., Newton, J., Carson, A., Abrahams, S., & Pal, S. (2020). A systematic review of neuropsychiatric and cognitive assessments used in clinical trials for amyotrophic lateral sclerosis. *Journal of Neurology*, *268*(12), 4510–4521. DOI: 10.1007/s00415-020-10203-z PMID: 32910255

Booker, S., & Herr, K. (2015). The state-of-“cultural validity” of self-report pain assessment tools in diverse older adults: Table 1. *Pain Medicine*, *16*(2), 232–239. DOI: 10.1111/pme.12496 PMID: 25219949

Booker, S., & Herr, K. (2016). Assessment and measurement of pain in adults in later life. *Clinics in Geriatric Medicine*, *32*(4), 677–692. DOI: 10.1016/j.cger.2016.06.012 PMID: 27741963

Booker, S., Herr, K., & Horgas, A. (2021). A paradigm shift for movement-based pain assessment in older adults: Practice, policy and regulatory drivers. *Pain Management Nursing*, *22*(1), 21–27. DOI: 10.1016/j.pmn.2020.08.003 PMID: 32948452

Bowen, E., Nayfe, R., Milburn, N., Mayo, H., Reid, M., Fraenkel, L., Weiner, D., Halm, E. A., & Makris, U. (2019). Do decision aids benefit patients with chronic musculoskeletal pain? a systematic review. *Pain Medicine*, *21*(5), 951–969. DOI: 10.1093/pm/pnz280 PMID: 31880805

Brant, J. (2018). Assessment and management of cancer pain in older adults: Strategies for success. *Asia-Pacific Journal of Oncology Nursing*, *5*(3), 248–253. DOI: 10.4103/apjon.apjon_11_18 PMID: 29963586

Brosseau, L., Taki, J., Desjardins, B., Thevenot, O., Fransen, M., Wells, G., Imoto, A. M., Toupin-April, K., Westby, M., Gallardo, I. C. Á., Gifford, W., Laferrière, L., Rahman, P., Loew, L., Angelis, G. D., Cavallo, S., Shallwani, S. M., Aburub, A., Bennell, K. L., & McLean, L. (2017). The Ottawa panel clinical practice guidelines for the management of knee osteoarthritis. part one: Introduction, and mind-body exercise programs. *Clinical Rehabilitation*, *31*(5), 582–595. DOI: 10.1177/0269215517691083 PMID: 28183188

Bruckenthal, P., Marino, M., & Snelling, L. (2016). Complementary and integrative therapies for persistent pain management in older adults: A review. *Journal of Gerontological Nursing*, *42*(12), 40–48. DOI: 10.3928/00989134-20161110-08 PMID: 27898135

Buck, C., Keweloh, C., Bouras, A., & Simões, E. (2021). Efficacy of short message service text messaging interventions for postoperative pain management: Systematic review. *JMIR mHealth and uHealth*, *9*(6), e20199. DOI: 10.2196/20199 PMID: 34132646

Burton, A., & Shaw, R. (2015). Pain management programmes for non-English-speaking black and minority ethnic groups with long-term or chronic pain. *Musculoskeletal Care*, *13*(4), 187–203. DOI: 10.1002/msc.1099 PMID: 25784618

Burton, E., Farrier, K., Galvin, R., Johnson, S., Horgan, F., Warters, A., & Hill, K. (2019). <p>physical activity programs for older people in the community receiving home care services: Systematic review and meta-analysis</p>. *Clinical Interventions in Aging*, *14*, 1045–1064. DOI: 10.2147/CIA.S205019 PMID: 31239654

Campbell, A., Godfryd, A., Buys, D., & Locher, J. (2015). Does participation in home-delivered meals programs improve outcomes for older adults? results of a systematic review. *Journal of Nutrition in Gerontology and Geriatrics*, *34*(2), 124–167. DOI: 10.1080/21551197.2015.1038463 PMID: 26106985

Cao, S., Fisher, D., Yu, T., & Dong, H. (2019). The link between chronic pain and Alzheimer's disease. *Journal of Neuroinflammation*, *16*(1), 204. Advance online publication. DOI: 10.1186/s12974-019-1608-z PMID: 31694670

Carley, J., Karp, J., Gentili, A., Marcum, Z., Reid, M., Rodríguez, E., Rossi, M. I., Shega, J., Thielke, S., & Weiner, D. (2015). Deconstructing chronic low back pain in the older adult: step by step evidence and expert-based recommendations for evaluation and treatment: part iv: depression. *Pain Medicine*, *16*(11), 2098–2108. DOI: 10.1111/pme.12935 PMID: 26539754

Carragher, J., & Gormley, K. (2016). Leadership and emotional intelligence in nursing and midwifery education and practice: A discussion paper. *Journal of Advanced Nursing*, *73*(1), 85–96. DOI: 10.1111/jan.13141 PMID: 27607451

Chary, S. (2021). What do we need to consider for pain management?.. https://doi.org/DOI: 10.5772/intechopen.93640

Chatchumni, M., Eriksson, H., & Mazaheri, M. (2020). A scoping review of pain management education programs (PMEPS): Do they prepare nurses to deal with patients' postoperative pain? *Pain Research & Management*, *2020*, 1–7. DOI: 10.1155/2020/4062493 PMID: 33123303

Chen, L., & Michalsen, A. (2017). Management of chronic pain using complementary and integrative medicine. *BMJ (Clinical Research Ed.)*, *j1284*, j1284. DOI: 10.1136/bmj.j1284 PMID: 28438745

Cirillo, A., Collins, J., Sawatzky, B., Hamdy, R., & Dahan-Oliel, N. (2019). Pain among children and adults living with arthrogryposis multiplex congenita: A scoping review. *American Journal of Medical Genetics. Part C, Seminars in Medical Genetics*, *181*(3), 436–453. DOI: 10.1002/ajmg.c.31725 PMID: 31347265

Corey, J. and McQueen, K. (2017). Pain relief in areas of deprivation and conflict.. https://doi.org/DOI: 10.1093/med/9780190217518.003.0028

Cravello, L., Santo, S., Varrassi, G., Benincasa, D., Marchettini, P., Tommaso, M., & Caltagirone, C. (2019). Chronic pain in the elderly with cognitive decline: A narrative review. *Pain and Therapy*, *8*(1), 53–65. DOI: 10.1007/s40122-019-0111-7 PMID: 30666612

Crawford, C., Boller, J., Jadalla, A., & Cuenca, E. (2016). An integrative review of pain resource nurse programs. *Critical Care Nursing Quarterly*, *39*(1), 64–82. DOI: 10.1097/CNQ.0000000000000101 PMID: 26633161

D'Cruz, K., Meikle, L., White, M., Herrmann, A., McCallum, C., & Romero, L. (2020). Tailoring education of adults with cognitive impairment in the inpatient hospital setting: A scoping review. *Australian Occupational Therapy Journal*, *68*(1), 90–102. DOI: 10.1111/1440-1630.12698 PMID: 33029784

da Silva, T. H. R. (2022). Emotional awareness and emotional intelligence. *British Journal of Community Nursing*, *27*(12), 573–574. DOI: 10.12968/bjcn.2022.27.12.573 PMID: 36519463

Dermody, G., Whitehead, L., Wilson, G., & Glass, C. (2020). The role of virtual reality in improving health outcomes for community-dwelling older adults: Systematic review. *Journal of Medical Internet Research*, *22*(6), e17331. DOI: 10.2196/17331 PMID: 32478662

Devan, H., Farmery, D., Peebles, L., & Grainger, R. (2019). Evaluation of self-management support functions in apps for people with persistent pain: Systematic review. *JMIR mHealth and uHealth*, *7*(2), e13080. DOI: 10.2196/13080 PMID: 30747715

Dillane, I., & Doody, O. (2019). Nursing people with intellectual disability and dementia experiencing pain: An integrative review. *Journal of Clinical Nursing*, *28*(13-14), 2472–2485. DOI: 10.1111/jocn.14834 PMID: 30786087

Dunham, M., Bonacaro, A., Schofield, P., Bacon, L., Spyridonis, F., & Mehrpouya, H. (2021). Smartphone applications designed to improve older people's chronic pain management: An integrated systematic review. *Geriatrics (Basel, Switzerland)*, *6*(2), 40. DOI: 10.3390/geriatrics6020040 PMID: 33917697

Eccleston, C., Fisher, E., Howard, R., Slater, R., Forgeron, P., Palermo, T., Birnie, K. A., Anderson, B. J., Chambers, C. T., Crombez, G., Ljungman, G., Jordan, I., Jordan, Z., Roberts, C., Schechter, N., Sieberg, C. B., Tibboel, D., Walker, S. M., Wilkinson, D., & Wood, C. (2021). Delivering transformative action in paediatric pain: A lancet child & adolescent health commission. *The Lancet. Child & Adolescent Health*, *5*(1), 47–87. DOI: 10.1016/S2352-4642(20)30277-7 PMID: 33064998

Eccleston, C., Fisher, E., Thomas, K., Hearn, L., Derry, S., Stannard, C., Knaggs, R., & Moore, A. (2017). Interventions for the reduction of prescribed opioid use in chronic non-cancer pain. *Cochrane Database of Systematic Reviews, 2021*(5). Advance online publication. DOI: 10.1002/14651858.CD010323.pub3 PMID: 29130474

Elbers, S., Wittink, H., Pool, J., & Smeets, R. (2018). The effectiveness of generic self-management interventions for patients with chronic musculoskeletal pain on physical function, self-efficacy, pain intensity and physical activity: A systematic review and meta-analysis. *European Journal of Pain (London, England), 22*(9), 1577–1596. DOI: 10.1002/ejp.1253 PMID: 29845678

Eldufani, J., & Blaise, G. (2019). The role of acetylcholinesterase inhibitors such as neostigmine and rivastigmine on chronic pain and cognitive function in aging: A review of recent clinical applications. *Alzheimer's & Dementia: Translational Research & Clinical Interventions, 5*(1), 175–183. DOI: 10.1016/j.trci.2019.03.004 PMID: 31194017

Farzad, M., MacDermid, J., Ring, D., & Shafiee, E. (2021). A scoping review of the evidence regarding assessment and management of psychological features of shoulder pain. *Rehabilitation Research and Practice, 2021*, 1–15. DOI: 10.1155/2021/7211201 PMID: 34631168

Feng, B., Hu, X., Lu, W., Wang, Y., & Ip, W. (2021). Are mindfulness treatments effective for pain in cancer patients? a systematic review and meta-analysis. *European Journal of Pain (London, England), 26*(1), 61–76. DOI: 10.1002/ejp.1849 PMID: 34369040

Fredriksen-Goldsen, K., Jen, S., Bryan, A., & Goldsen, J. (2016). Cognitive impairment, Alzheimer's disease, and other dementias in the lives of lesbian, gay, bisexual and transgender (LGBT) older adults and their caregivers: Needs and competencies. *Journal of Applied Gerontology, 37*(5), 545–569. DOI: 10.1177/0733464816672047 PMID: 27729400

Garland, E., Brintz, C., Hanley, A., Roseen, E., Atchley, R., Gaylord, S., Faurot, K. R., Yaffe, J., Fiander, M., & Keefe, F. (2020). Mind-body therapies for opioid-treated pain. *JAMA Internal Medicine, 180*(1), 91. DOI: 10.1001/jamainternmed.2019.4917 PMID: 31682676

Goh, S., Persson, M., Stocks, J., Hou, Y., Welton, N., Lin, J., Hall, M. C., Doherty, M., & Zhang, W. (2019). Relative efficacy of different exercises for pain, function, performance and quality of life in knee and hip osteoarthritis: Systematic review and network meta-analysis. *Sports Medicine (Auckland, N.Z.), 49*(5), 743–761. DOI: 10.1007/s40279-019-01082-0 PMID: 30830561

Golden, R., Emery-Tiburcio, E., Post, S., Ewald, B., & Newman, M. (2019). Connecting social, clinical, and home care services for persons with serious illness in the community. *Journal of the American Geriatrics Society, 67*(S2). Advance online publication. DOI: 10.1111/jgs.15900 PMID: 31074858

Hanson, E., Hellström, A., Sandvide, Å., Jackson, G., MacRae, R., Jack-Waugh, A., & Tolson, D. (2016). The extended palliative phase of dementia – an integrative literature review. *Dementia (London), 18*(1), 108–134. DOI: 10.1177/1471301216659797 PMID: 27460046

Henschke, N., Lorenz, E., Pokora, R., Michaleff, Z., Quartey, J., & Oliveira, V. (2016). Understanding cultural influences on back pain and back pain research. *Best Practice & Research. Clinical Rheumatology, 30*(6), 1037–1049. DOI: 10.1016/j.berh.2017.08.004 PMID: 29103548

Hurley-Wallace, A., Nowotny, E., Schoth, D., & Liossi, C. (2021). Online multidisciplinary interventions for paediatric chronic pain: A content analysis. *European Journal of Pain (London, England), 25*(10), 2140–2154. DOI: 10.1002/ejp.1827 PMID: 34155745

Jiménez-Picón, N., Romero-Martín, M., Ponce-Blandón, J., Ramírez-Baena, L., Palomo-Lara, J., & Gómez-Salgado, J. (2021). The relationship between mindfulness and emotional intelligence as a protective factor for healthcare professionals: Systematic review. *International Journal of Environmental Research and Public Health, 18*(10), 5491. DOI: 10.3390/ijerph18105491 PMID: 34065519

Johnson, M. (2019). The landscape of chronic pain: Broader perspectives. *Medicina, 55*(5), 182. DOI: 10.3390/medicina55050182 PMID: 31117297

Joo, J., & Liu, M. (2021). Nurses' barriers to caring for patients with covid-19: A qualitative systematic review. *International Nursing Review, 68*(2), 202–213. DOI: 10.1111/inr.12648 PMID: 33420749

Jung, M., & Matthews, A. (2021). Understanding nurses' experiences and perceptions of end-of-life care for cancer patients in Korea: A scoping review. *Journal of Palliative Care, 36*(4), 255–264. DOI: 10.1177/08258597211027021 PMID: 34182840

Jurček, A. and Urek, M. (2021). Integrating the needs of LGBT+ older adults into health and social care education., 81-88. https://doi.org/DOI: 10.26493/978-961-293-129-2.81-88

Kang, Y., & Demiris, G. (2017). Self-report pain assessment tools for cognitively intact older adults: Integrative review. *International Journal of Older People Nursing, 13*(2), e12170. Advance online publication. DOI: 10.1111/opn.12170 PMID: 28980440

Kemp, H., Laycock, H., Costello, A., & Brett, S. (2019). Chronic pain in critical care survivors: A narrative review. *British Journal of Anaesthesia, 123*(2), e372–e384. DOI: 10.1016/j.bja.2019.03.025 PMID: 31126622

Khammissa, R., Ballyram, R., Fourie, J., Bouckaert, M., Lemmer, J., & Feller, L. (2020). Selected pathobiological features and principles of pharmacological pain management. *The Journal of International Medical Research, 48*(5), 0300060520903653. Advance online publication. DOI: 10.1177/0300060520903653 PMID: 32408839

Kim, H., Jung, S., Kim, H., & Abraham, I. (2020). Systematic review of longitudinal studies on chemotherapy-associated subjective cognitive impairment in cancer patients. *Psycho-Oncology, 29*(4), 617–631. DOI: 10.1002/pon.5339 PMID: 32017297

Kozlowski, D., Hutchinson, M., Hurley, J., Rowley, J., & Sutherland, J. (2017). The role of emotion in clinical decision making: An integrative literature review. *BMC Medical Education, 17*(1), 255. Advance online publication. DOI: 10.1186/s12909-017-1089-7 PMID: 29246213

Kwon, C., Lee, B., Suh, H., Chung, S., & Kim, J. (2018). Efficacy and safety of auricular acupuncture for cognitive impairment and dementia: a systematic review. *Evidence-Based Complementary and Alternative Medicine*, 2018(1). https://doi.org/ DOI: 10.1155/2018/3426078

Lauder, G. (2017). A review of intravenous lidocaine infusion therapy for paediatric acute and chronic pain management.. DOI: 10.5772/66771

Leeuwen, K., Loon, M., Nes, F., Bosmans, J., Vet, H., Ket, J., & Ostelo, R. (2019). What does quality of life mean to older adults? a thematic synthesis. *PLoS One, 14*(3), e0213263. DOI: 10.1371/journal.pone.0213263 PMID: 30849098

Leis, J., & Morrison, C. (2021). An integrative review of arts-based strategies for addressing pain and substance use disorder during the opioid crisis. *Health Promotion Practice, 22*(1, suppl), 44S–52S. DOI: 10.1177/1524839921996065 PMID: 33942641

Lewis, P., Gaffney, R., & Wilson, N. (2017). A narrative review of acute care nurses' experiences nursing patients with intellectual disability: Underprepared, communication barriers and ambiguity about the role of caregivers. *Journal of Clinical Nursing, 26*(11-12), 1473–1484. DOI: 10.1111/jocn.13512 PMID: 27533751

Lin, L., Li, H., Yang, J., Hao, X., Yan, S., Wang, Y., Yu, F.-T., Shi, G.-X., & Liu, C. (2021). Acupuncture for psychological disorders caused by chronic pain: A review and future directions. *Frontiers in Neuroscience*, *14*, 626497. Advance online publication. DOI: 10.3389/fnins.2020.626497 PMID: 33584181

Lumley, M., & Schubiner, H. (2019). Psychological therapy for centralized pain: An integrative assessment and treatment model. *Psychosomatic Medicine*, *81*(2), 114–124. DOI: 10.1097/PSY.0000000000000654 PMID: 30461545

Mallari, B., Spaeth, E., Goh, H., & Boyd, B. (2019). Virtual reality as an analgesic for acute and chronic pain in adults: A systematic review and meta-analysis. *Journal of Pain Research*, *12*, 2053–2085. DOI: 10.2147/JPR.S200498 PMID: 31308733

Martin, C., Bakker, C., Breth, M., Gao, G., Lee, K., Lee, M., Tiase, V. L., Tunby, L. J., Wyatt, T. H., & Janeway, L. (2020). The efficacy of mobile health interventions used to manage acute or chronic pain: A systematic review. *Research in Nursing & Health*, *44*(1), 111–128. DOI: 10.1002/nur.22097 PMID: 33341989

Mataqi, M., & Aslanpour, Z. (2019). Factors influencing palliative care in advanced dementia: A systematic review. *BMJ Supportive & Palliative Care*, *10*(2), 145–156. DOI: 10.1136/bmjspcare-2018-001692 PMID: 30944119

McGuire, D., Kaiser, K., Haisfield-Wolfe, M., & Iyamu, F. (2016). Pain assessment in noncommunicative adult palliative care patients. *The Nursing Clinics of North America*, *51*(3), 397–431. DOI: 10.1016/j.cnur.2016.05.009 PMID: 27497016

McMaughan, D., Oloruntoba, O., & Smith, M. (2020). Socioeconomic status and access to healthcare: Interrelated drivers for healthy aging. *Frontiers in Public Health*, *8*, 231. Advance online publication. DOI: 10.3389/fpubh.2020.00231 PMID: 32626678

Meehan, E., & Carter, B. (2021). Moving with pain: What principles from somatic practices can offer to people living with chronic pain. *Frontiers in Psychology*, *11*, 620381. Advance online publication. DOI: 10.3389/fpsyg.2020.620381 PMID: 33569028

Menezes, C., Silva, A., Santos, A., Gonçalves, D., Teles, E., Silva, E., … & Maciel, K. (2024). Colágeno como agente de mudança na osteoartrite: perspectivas de uma revisão integrativa.. https://doi.org/DOI: 10.58871/CONSAMU24.C43

Morone, N. (2019). Not just mind over matter: Reviewing with patients how mindfulness relieves chronic low back pain. *Journal of Evidence-based Integrative Medicine*, *24*, 2515690X19838490. Advance online publication. DOI: 10.1177/2515690X19838490 PMID: 30942087

Nahin, R., Boineau, R., Khalsa, P., Stussman, B., & Weber, W. (2016). Evidence-based evaluation of complementary health approaches for pain management in the United States. *Mayo Clinic Proceedings*, *91*(9), 1292–1306. DOI: 10.1016/j.mayocp.2016.06.007 PMID: 27594189

Niknejad, B., Bolier, R., Henderson, C.Jr, Delgado, D., Kozlov, E., Löckenhoff, C., & Reid, M. (2018). Association between psychological interventions and chronic pain outcomes in older adults. *JAMA Internal Medicine*, *178*(6), 830. DOI: 10.1001/jamainternmed.2018.0756 PMID: 29801109

Pask, S., Dell'Olio, M., Murtagh, F., & Boland, J. (2020). The effects of opioids on cognition in older adults with cancer and chronic noncancer pain: A systematic review. *Journal of Pain and Symptom Management*, *59*(4), 871–893.e1. DOI: 10.1016/j.jpainsymman.2019.10.022 PMID: 31678462

Prezerakos, P. (2018). Nurse managers' emotional intelligence and effective leadership: A review of the current evidence. *The Open Nursing Journal*, *12*(1), 86–92. DOI: 10.2174/1874434601812010086 PMID: 29997711

Probyn, K., Bowers, H., Mistry, D., Caldwell, F., Underwood, M., Patel, S., Sandhu, H. K., Matharu, M., & Pincus, T. (2017). Non-pharmacological self-management for people living with migraine or tension-type headache: A systematic review including analysis of intervention components. *BMJ Open*, *7*(8), e016670. DOI: 10.1136/bmjopen-2017-016670 PMID: 28801425

Reis da Silva, T. H. (2023a). Falls assessment and prevention in the nursing home and community. *British Journal of Community Nursing*, *28*(2), 68–72. DOI: 10.12968/bjcn.2023.28.2.68 PMID: 36735363

Reis da Silva, T. H. (2023b). Ageing in place: Ageing at home and in the community. *British Journal of Community Nursing*, *28*(5), 213–214. DOI: 10.12968/bjcn.2023.28.5.213 PMID: 37130715

Reis da Silva, T. H. (2023c). Moving and Handling in the Community. *British Journal of Community Nursing*, *28*(8), 369. DOI: 10.12968/bjcn.2023.28.8.369 PMID: 37527217

Reis da Silva, T. H (2024a). Oncology and Cancer Medicine: Understanding the complexities in Older Patients. *Biomed J Sci & Tech Res* 55(3)-2024. DOI: https://doi.org/DOI: 10.26717/BJSTR.2024.55.008720

Reis da Silva, T. H. (2024b). Falls prevention in older people and the role of nursing. *British Journal of Community Nursing*, *29*(7), 335–339. DOI: 10.12968/bjcn.2024.0005 PMID: 38963269

Reis da Silva, T. H. (2024c). Enhancing the mental health of refugees and asylum seekers through music interventions. *Mental Health Practice*. Advance online publication. DOI: 10.7748/mhp.2024.e1717

Reis da Silva, T. H. (2024d). Chapter 8 – Emotional Intelligence in Teaching Geriatric Nursing: Humanising Technology for Compassionate Care in Higher Education. In Tikadar, S.; Liu, H.; Bhattacharya, P.; Bhattacharya, S. *Humanizing Technology With Emotional Intelligence*. Pp. 141-160. IGI Global Scientific Publishing. https://doi.org/DOI: 10.4018/979-8-3693-7011-7.ch008

Reis da Silva, T. H. (2024e). Chapter 12 – Emotional Intelligence in Integrative Medicine: Enhancing Patient-Centred Care Through Humanised Technology. In Tikadar, S.; Liu, H.; Bhattacharya, P.; Bhattacharya, S. *Humanizing Technology With Emotional Intelligence*. Pp. 263-280. IGI Global Scientific Publishing. https://doi.org/DOI: 10.4018/979-8-3693-7011-7.ch012

Reis da Silva, T. H. (2024f). Chapter 11 - Integrating business essentials into Gerontological Nursing: Enhancing Care for Older Adults in Diverse Settings. In Sedky, A. *Resiliency Strategies for Long-Term Business Success*. Pp. 283-316. IGI Global. DOI: https://doi.org/DOI: 10.4018/979-8-3693-9168-6.ch011

Reis da Silva, T. (2024g). The Evolution of Nursing for Older Adult: A Historical Perspective. *Associative J Health Sci*. 3(3). AJHS. 000561. 2024. DOI: . Link: https://crimsonpublishers.com/ajhs/pdf/AJHS.000561.pdfDOI: 10.31031/AJHS.2024.03.000561

Reis da Silva, T. H. (2024h). Chapter 6 – Navigating Healthcare Complexity: Integrating Business Fundamentals into Nursing Leadership. In Sedky, A. *Resiliency Strategies for Long-Term Business Success*. Pp. 145-168. IGI Global. https://doi.org/DOI: 10.4018/979-8-3693-9168-6.ch006

Reis da Silva, T. M. (2025a). Integrative Approaches to Geriatric Care: Enhancing Physical and Mental Health Through AI-Driven Insights. In Jermsittiparsert, K., & Marzo, R. (Eds.), *Physical Health, Mental Health, and Human Well-Being in the Age of AI* (pp. 113–136). IGI Global Scientific Publishing., DOI: 10.4018/979-8-3693-6190-0.ch007

Reis da Silva, T. H. (2025b). AI-Powered Emotional Intelligence in Nursing: Bridging the Gap in Older People Care. In Jermsittiparsert, K., & Marzo, R. R. (Eds.), *Physical Health, Mental Health, and Human Well-Being in the Age of AI*. IGI Global Scientific Publishing., DOI: 10.4018/979-8-3693-6190-0.ch9

Reis da Silva, T. M. H. (2025c). The Role of Emotional Intelligence in Promoting Mental Peace, Healthy Work Environments, and Emotional Well-Being Among Entrepreneurs. In Tunio, M. N. (Ed.), *Supporting Psychological and Emotional Well-being Among Entrepreneurs*. IGI Global Scientific Publishing., DOI: 10.4018/979-8-3693-3673-1.ch21

Reis da Silva, T. H. (2025d). Emotional Intelligence and AI in Geriatric Nursing: Bridging Technology and Compassionate Care. In Jermsittiparsert, K., & Marzo, R. R. (Eds.), *Physical Health, Mental Health, and Human Well-Being in the Age of AI*. IGI Global Scientific Publishing., DOI: 10.4018/979-8-3693-6190-0.ch10

Reis da Silva, T. M. (2025e). Fostering Emotional Intelligence for Competency Development in Nursing Education. In Aldosemani, T., Lytras, M., & Ordóñez de Pablos, P. (Eds.), *Innovative Educational Frameworks for Future Skills and Competencies* (pp. 39–62). IGI Global Scientific Publishing., DOI: 10.4018/979-8-3693-7555-6.ch002

Reis da Silva, T. H. (2025f). Integrating Artificial Intelligence in Geriatric Care: Enhancing Physical and Mental Health Outcomes. In Jermsittiparsert, K., & Marzo, R. R. (Eds.), *Physical Health, Mental Health, and Human Well-Being in the Age of AI*. IGI Global Scientific Publishing., DOI: 10.4018/979-8-3693-6190-0.ch11

Reis da Silva, T. H. (2025g). Promoting Emotional Well-Being in Older Adults: The Role of AI in Supporting Emotional Intelligence and Mental Health. In Jermsittiparsert, K., & Marzo, R. R. (Eds.), *Physical Health, Mental Health, and Human Well-Being in the Age of AI* (pp. 137–167). IGI Global Scientific Publishing., DOI: 10.4018/979-8-3693-6190-0.ch8

Reis da Silva, T. M. (2025h). Fostering Emotional Resilience and Mindful Leadership in Gerontology Nursing: A Model for Change and Innovation. In Baez, M. (Ed.), *Strategic Approaches to Mindful Leadership and Change Management* (pp. 259–280). IGI Global Scientific Publishing., DOI: 10.4018/979-8-3693-7066-7.ch009

Reis da Silva, T. M., Hammett, R., & Low, G. (2025). Emotional Intelligence in Business: Enhancing Leadership, Collaboration, and Performance. In Sedky, A. (Ed.), *Building Business Knowledge for Complex Modern Business Environments* (pp. 149–178). IGI Global Scientific Publishing., DOI: 10.4018/979-8-3693-6447-5.ch006

Rostad, H., Utne, I., Grov, E., Puts, M., & Halvorsrud, L. (2017). Measurement properties, feasibility and clinical utility of the doloplus-2 pain scale in older adults with cognitive impairment: A systematic review. *BMC Geriatrics*, *17*(1), 257. Advance online publication. DOI: 10.1186/s12877-017-0643-9 PMID: 29096611

Sakamoto, J., Ward, H., Vissoci, J., & Eucker, S. (2018). Are nonpharmacologic pain interventions effective at reducing pain in adult patients visiting the emergency department? a systematic review and meta-analysis. *Academic Emergency Medicine*, *25*(8), 940–957. DOI: 10.1111/acem.13411 PMID: 29543359

Scher, C., Petti, E., Meador, L., Cleave, J., Liang, E., & Reid, M. (2020). Multidimensional pain assessment tools for ambulatory and inpatient nursing practice. *Pain Management Nursing*, *21*(5), 416–422. DOI: 10.1016/j.pmn.2020.03.007 PMID: 32448737

Scurrah, A., Shiner, C., Stevens, J., & Faux, S. (2017). Regional nerve blockade for early analgesic management of elderly patients with hip fracture – a narrative review. *Anaesthesia*, *73*(6), 769–783. DOI: 10.1111/anae.14178 PMID: 29278266

Sela, Y., Grinberg, K., & Nissanholtz-Gannot, R. (2020). Attracting Israeli nursing students to community nursing. *Israel Journal of Health Policy Research*, *9*(1), 44. Advance online publication. DOI: 10.1186/s13584-020-00400-6 PMID: 33059759

Shipton, E., Bate, F., Garrick, R., Steketee, C., Shipton, E., & Visser, E. (2018). Systematic review of pain medicine content, teaching, and assessment in medical school curricula internationally. *Pain and Therapy*, *7*(2), 139–161. DOI: 10.1007/s40122-018-0103-z PMID: 30058045

Soimah, S. and Utami, S. (2023). The emotional intelligent and social support as predictor of stress at work among nurses during post pandemic., 145-152. https://doi.org/DOI: 10.2991/978-94-6463-186-9_18

Strand, L., Gundrosen, K., Lein, T., Laekeman, M., Lobbezoo, F., Defrin, R., & Husebø, B. (2018). Body movements as pain indicators in older people with cognitive impairment: A systematic review. *European Journal of Pain (London, England)*, *23*(4), 669–685. DOI: 10.1002/ejp.1344 PMID: 30450680

Suntai, Z., Won, C., & Noh, H. (2020). Access barrier in rural older adults' use of pain management and palliative care services: A systematic review. *The American Journal of Hospice & Palliative Care*, *38*(5), 494–502. DOI: 10.1177/1049909120959634 PMID: 32959683

Tang, S., Tse, M., Leung, S., & Fotis, T. (2019). The effectiveness, suitability, and sustainability of non-pharmacological methods of managing pain in community-dwelling older adults: A systematic review. *BMC Public Health*, *19*(1), 1488. Advance online publication. DOI: 10.1186/s12889-019-7831-9 PMID: 31703654

Torres-Cueco, R., & Nohales-Alfonso, F. (2021). Vulvodynia—It is time to accept a new understanding from a neurobiological perspective. *International Journal of Environmental Research and Public Health, 18*(12), 6639. DOI: 10.3390/ijerph18126639 PMID: 34205495

Tsai, Y., Browne, G., & Inder, K. (2020). The effectiveness of interventions to improve pain assessment and management in people living with dementia: A systematic review and meta-analyses. *Journal of Advanced Nursing, 77*(3), 1127–1140. DOI: 10.1111/jan.14660 PMID: 33222273

Turton, B., Williams, S., Burton, C., & Williams, L. (2017). Arts-based palliative care training, education and staff development: A scoping review. *Palliative Medicine, 32*(2), 559–570. DOI: 10.1177/0269216317712189 PMID: 28604224

Vachon-Presseau, É., Centeno, M., Ren, W., Berger, S., Tétreault, P., Ghantous, M., Baria, A., Farmer, M., Baliki, M. N., Schnitzer, T. J., & Apkarian, A. (2016). The emotional brain as a predictor and amplifier of chronic pain. *Journal of Dental Research, 95*(6), 605–612. DOI: 10.1177/0022034516638027 PMID: 26965423

Vaismoradi, M., Skär, L., Söderberg, S., & Bondas, T. (2016). Normalizing suffering: A meta-synthesis of experiences of and perspectives on pain and pain management in nursing homes. *International Journal of Qualitative Studies on Health and Well-being, 11*(1), 31203. DOI: 10.3402/qhw.v11.31203 PMID: 27173102

Vitoula, K., Venneri, A., Varrassi, G., Paladini, A., Sykioti, P., Adewusi, J., & Zis, P. (2018). Behavioral therapy approaches for the management of low back pain: An up-to-date systematic review. *Pain and Therapy, 7*(1), 1–12. DOI: 10.1007/s40122-018-0099-4 PMID: 29767395

Vocci, M., Gallo, I., Spiri, W., Borgato, M., & Fontes, C. (2021). Vulnerabilities of nurses in an intensive care unit: An integrative review. *Revista Brasileira de Enfermagem, 74*(3), e20200724. Advance online publication. DOI: 10.1590/0034-7167-2020-0724 PMID: 34161500

Wei, G., Farooq, J., & Kumar, A. (2020). Impact of mind-body treatment interventions on quality of life in neurofibromatosis patients: A systematic review and meta-analysis. *Dermatologic Therapy, 34*(1). Advance online publication. DOI: 10.1111/dth.14613 PMID: 33258517

Wideman, T., Edwards, R., Walton, D., Martel, M., Hudon, A., & Seminowicz, D. (2019). The multimodal assessment model of pain. *The Clinical Journal of Pain, 35*(3), 212–221. DOI: 10.1097/AJP.0000000000000670 PMID: 30444733

Xu, H., Stjernswärd, S., & Glasdam, S. (2021). Psychosocial experiences of front-line nurses working in hospital-based settings during the covid-19 pandemic - a qualitative systematic review. *International Journal of Nursing Studies Advances*, *3*, 100037. DOI: 10.1016/j.ijnsa.2021.100037 PMID: 34308373

Xu, X., Luckett, T., Wang, A., Lovell, M., & Phillips, J. (2018). Cancer pain management needs and perspectives of patients from Chinese backgrounds: A systematic review of the Chinese and English literature. *Palliative & Supportive Care*, *16*(6), 785–799. DOI: 10.1017/S1478951517001171 PMID: 29338806

Yamanaka, M. (2018). A concept analysis of self-management of cancer pain. *Asia-Pacific Journal of Oncology Nursing*, *5*(3), 254–261. DOI: 10.4103/apjon.apjon_17_18 PMID: 29963587

Yang, S., & Chang, M. (2019). Chronic pain: Structural and functional changes in brain structures and associated negative affective states. *International Journal of Molecular Sciences*, *20*(13), 3130. DOI: 10.3390/ijms20133130 PMID: 31248061

Yeh, G., & Horwitz, R. (2017). Integrative medicine for respiratory conditions. *The Medical Clinics of North America*, *101*(5), 925–941. DOI: 10.1016/j.mcna.2017.04.008 PMID: 28802471

Yin, H., Tse, M., & Wong, F. (2015). Systematic review of the predisposing, enabling, and reinforcing factors which influence nursing administration of opioids in the postoperative period. *Japan Journal of Nursing Science*, *12*(4), 259–275. DOI: 10.1111/jjns.12075 PMID: 25781037

Zahari, Z., Ishak, A., & Justine, M. (2020). The effectiveness of patient education in improving pain, disability and quality of life among older people with low back pain: A systematic review. *Journal of Back and Musculoskeletal Rehabilitation*, *33*(2), 245–254. DOI: 10.3233/BMR-181305 PMID: 31356191

Zeidan, F., & Vago, D. (2016). Mindfulness meditation–based pain relief: A mechanistic account. *Annals of the New York Academy of Sciences*, *1373*(1), 114–127. DOI: 10.1111/nyas.13153 PMID: 27398643

Zwakhalen, S., Docking, R., Gnass, I., Sirsch, E., Stewart, C., Allcock, N., & Schofield, P. (2018). Pain in older adults with dementia. *Schmerz (Berlin, Germany)*, *32*(5), 364–373. DOI: 10.1007/s00482-018-0290-x PMID: 29931391

ADDITIONAL READING

Booker, S., & Herr, K. (2016). Assessment and measurement of pain in adults in later life. *Clinics in Geriatric Medicine*, *32*(4), 677–692. DOI: 10.1016/j.cger.2016.06.012 PMID: 27741963

Booker, S. and Herr, K. (2019). Pain in older patients., 319-338. DOI: 10.1093/med/9780199768912.003.0020

Booker, S., Herr, K., & Horgas, A. (2021). A paradigm shift for movement-based pain assessment in older adults: Practice, policy and regulatory drivers. *Pain Management Nursing*, *22*(1), 21–27. DOI: 10.1016/j.pmn.2020.08.003 PMID: 32948452

Bruckenthal, P., Marino, M., & Snelling, L. (2016). Complementary and integrative therapies for persistent pain management in older adults: A review. *Journal of Gerontological Nursing*, *42*(12), 40–48. DOI: 10.3928/00989134-20161110-08 PMID: 27898135

Burns, M., & McIlfatrick, S. (2015). Palliative care in dementia: Literature review of nurses' knowledge and attitudes towards pain assessment. *International Journal of Palliative Nursing*, *21*(8), 400–407. DOI: 10.12968/ijpn.2015.21.8.400 PMID: 26312536

Dunham, M., Bonacaro, A., Schofield, P., Bacon, L., Spyridonis, F., & Mehrpouya, H. (2021). Smartphone applications designed to improve older people's chronic pain management: An integrated systematic review. *Geriatrics (Basel, Switzerland)*, *6*(2), 40. DOI: 10.3390/geriatrics6020040 PMID: 33917697

Reis da Silva, T. H. (2024). Chapter 11 - Integrating business essentials into Gerontological Nursing: Enhancing Care for Older Adults in Diverse Settings. In Sedky, A. Resiliency Strategies for Long-Term Business Success. Pp. 283-316. IGI Global. DOI: https://doi.org/DOI: 10.4018/979-8-3693-9168-6.ch011

Reis da Silva, T. H. (2025). AI-Powered Emotional Intelligence in Nursing: Bridging the Gap in Older People Care. In Jermsittiparsert, K., & Marzo, R. R. (Eds.), *Physical Health, Mental Health, and Human Well-Being in the Age of AI*. IGI Global Scientific Publishing., DOI: 10.4018/979-8-3693-6190-0.ch9

Reis da Silva, T. M., Hammett, R., & Low, G. (2025). Emotional Intelligence in Business: Enhancing Leadership, Collaboration, and Performance. In Sedky, A. (Ed.), *Building Business Knowledge for Complex Modern Business Environments* (pp. 149–178). IGI Global Scientific Publishing., DOI: 10.4018/979-8-3693-6447-5.ch006

Tang, S., Tse, M., Leung, S., & Fotis, T. (2019). The effectiveness, suitability, and sustainability of non-pharmacological methods of managing pain in community-dwelling older adults: A systematic review. *BMC Public Health*, *19*(1), 1488. Advance online publication. DOI: 10.1186/s12889-019-7831-9 PMID: 31703654

KEY TERMS AND DEFINITIONS

Pain: An unpleasant sensory and emotional experience associated with actual or potential tissue damage, categorised into acute and chronic forms.

Older Adults: Defined as individuals aged 65 and above, often experience unique pain management challenges due to physiological changes and comorbidities.

Acute Pain: Arising suddenly and typically short-lived, contrasts with chronic pain, characterised by persistent pain lasting over three months.

Nociceptive Pain: Results from actual or potential tissue damage, while neuropathic pain arises from nerve injuries or dysfunctions. Psychogenic pain, conversely, is influenced by psychological factors rather than direct tissue damage.

Integrative Therapy: Encompasses holistic approaches that combine conventional practices with alternative and complementary methods to enhance treatment outcomes.

Dignity: Healthcare refers to the inherent worth and respect afforded to individuals, particularly within pain management contexts.

Functionality: Describes a person's ability to perform daily activities, often impacted by pain.

Quality of Life: Encompasses overall well-being, including emotional, social, and physical health, significantly affected by pain conditions.

Chapter 9

Empowering Patients Through Knowledge: Educational Strategies in Rehabilitation

R. Vettriselvan
https://orcid.org/0009-0000-8016-212X
Academy of Maritime Education and Training, India

R. Ramya
https://orcid.org/0000-0002-1324-136X
Saraswathi Institute of Medical Sciences, India

V. Selvalakshmi
https://orcid.org/0000-0002-6684-1609
Saveetha Institute of Medical and Technical Sciences, India

P. Jyothi
Saveetha Engineering College, India

Palanivel Rathinasabapathi Velmurugan
https://orcid.org/0000-0002-0395-9060
Berlin School of Business and Innovation, Germany

ABSTRACT

Educational strategies play a crucial role in the rehabilitation process, offering patients the tools and knowledge necessary to actively participate in their recovery journey. By providing a comprehensive understanding of their conditions, treatment options, and the importance of lifestyle changes, patients are empowered to make informed decisions. This active involvement fosters greater motivation, self-efficacy,

DOI: 10.4018/979-8-3693-6432-1.ch009

and adherence to rehabilitation programs. Moreover, educational interventions tailored to individual needs can enhance emotional well-being, reduce anxiety, and promote long-term health management. This approach focuses not only on the physical aspects of recovery but also on the psychological and social dimensions, leading to holistic health outcomes. Ultimately, empowering patients with knowledge helps them take control of their healing process, making them more resilient and capable of achieving lasting improvements in their health and quality of life.

INTRODUCTION

Over the past few decades rehabilitation has undergone major progress by shifting from traditional biomedical approaches towards patient-oriented whole-person healthcare models. The modern healthcare approach looks beyond physical therapy because sustainable recovery demands full assessment of psychological together with emotional and cognitive and social health needs. Manmade rehabilitation methods now demonstrate expanded perspectives on patient requirements while promoting care programs that span across entire health durations (Nader et al., 2000). During previous years rehabilitation programs focused almost exclusively on physical wellness but failed to recognize how emotional along with cognitive elements influence recovery equally significantly. Current research demonstrates that healthcare professionals must use holistic approaches when treating patients because symptoms tend to exist within a whole person framework. Current healthcare developments have made patient education the essential foundation of rehabilitation to share information while enabling patients to gain autonomy and modify their behaviors (Stepanian et al., 2023). Through educational procedures patients gain the abilities they need to understand their medical situations and learn about their treatment processes and acquire self-care competencies. When patients acquire additional knowledge from their caregivers their treatment compliance improves as does their motivation and their rehabilitation results become more positive. Patients who receive complete information about their condition actively collaborate in medical care while building effective communication with healthcare providers and dedicating themselves to their rehabilitation targets (François et al., 2024). The research evidence indicates that educated patients make superior healthcare decisions and perform health activities as recommended and practice wellness choices (Nicolau et al., 2023). Digital technology advancements have bettered both outreach and performance of rehabilitative educational methods. Users now benefit from mobile health applications and tele-rehabilitation platforms and interactive e-learning modules because these digital tools provide them with steady access to instructional materials and assessment tools and rehabilitation program guidance.

The modern innovations serve especially well for people who live in remote or underserved areas since they do not have much contact with medical professionals (Xin et al., 2022). The digital learning environment provides enhanced adaptability together with tailored programs that enable convenience for patients which leads to superior participation and independence. Through education-based rehabilitation methods healthcare organizations create a healthcare system which delivers inclusive accessible patient-focused care. Educational programs perform two functions by providing information while simultaneously awakening patient capabilities which results in better patient autonomy during recovery periods. Such empowered patients exhibit better health results and keep better functional status alongside demonstrating active behaviors. As such, patient education is not merely an ancillary feature of modern rehabilitation it is an essential pillar of a truly patient-centered healthcare model (Ricci et al., 2022).

Research Aim and Objectives

This chapter performs a comprehensive assessment of educational strategies in rehabilitation and their positive effects on patient results due to empowerment. This research examines structured patient education interventions because they enhance motivation together with autonomy and foster prolonged self-care practices among rehabilitation patients in our behavioral healthcare system. The chapter evaluates the placement of these strategies through theoretical and empirical evidence to create links between information transmission and enduring behavioral transformations in rehabilitation contexts.

This chapter pursues two specific objectives which support the main objective.

- The analysis reviews rehabilitation-oriented educational approaches and assessments their theoretical bases and practical outcomes for recovery enhancement.
- The research investigates education as a means to empower patients through examination of teaching approaches which build autonomy while boosting motivation and enabling self-managed care.
- This study explores the gaps in rehabilitation procedures regarding educational method adoption and establishes practical solutions that eliminate institutional along with patient-related barriers.
- This review examines digital technology systems that utilize mobile applications combined with e-learning platforms together with tele-rehabilitation tools to deliver patient education for different community demographics (Giovannoni et al., 2024).

The chapter achieves a complete understanding of educational and rehabilitation relationships through its outlined goals. The text provides guidelines for healthcare experts and educators and policymakers about creating and conducting evaluations of educational recovery solutions which put patient autonomy at their center.

Structure of the Chapter

To achieve a coherent and systematic exploration of the topic, the chapter is organized into the following key sections:

Conceptual Framework: This section establishes the foundational concepts relevant to rehabilitation, empowerment, and holistic health. It outlines the progression from health literacy to empowerment and behavioral change, offering a visual and narrative model to contextualize the role of education in rehabilitation.

Theoretical Framework: Here, major behavioral and psychological theories are discussed to understand how education drives patient engagement. These include Social Cognitive Theory (Bandura, 2001), the Health Belief Model (Rosenstock, 1974), the Theory of Planned Behavior (Ajzen, 1991), and the Self-Determination Theory. The section will also incorporate the Integrated Care model to demonstrate how coordinated educational approaches support holistic recovery.

Research Methodology: This section outlines the systematic approach used to conduct the literature review, guided by the PRISMA 2020 checklist. It includes details on search strategies, inclusion and exclusion criteria, data sources, and thematic synthesis of the selected studies.

Solutions and Recommendations: Based on the findings, this section presents evidence-based recommendations for improving the design and implementation of educational strategies in rehabilitation. It highlights the need for personalization, digital integration, interdisciplinary collaboration, and culturally sensitive approaches.

Future Research Directions: Anticipating the evolving nature of healthcare delivery and patient engagement, this section outlines future research avenues. These include investigating long-term outcomes of educational interventions, exploring innovations in health technology, and tailoring strategies to diverse populations and institutional contexts.

Conclusion: The final section synthesizes the key insights of the chapter, emphasizing the transformative potential of education in rehabilitation and providing guidance for future policy and practice development in patient-centered care.

CONCEPTUAL FRAMEWORK

Rehabilitation represents a complex method which helps patients regain functional abilities as well as enhances their life quality while building their independence during their recovery from sicknesses and injuries or persistent medical issues. The treatment approach extends to physical therapy as well as occupational therapy and psychological counseling and social support services (Nicolau et al., 2022). Patient healthcare needs have become increasingly intricate so rehabilitation now needs to support physical restoration together with working through emotional challenges and cognitive as well as social difficulties that affect recovery. The rehabilitation process remains dependent on fundamental educational strategies because these methods enable patients to understand their medical conditions and make well-informed care decisions and take active control of their healthcare (Stepanian et al., 2023). Conventionally rehabilitation services limited their focus to treating patients' physical dysfunction although they dismissed important psychosocial aspects of recovery. More research shows that education serves as the cornerstone for providing necessary knowledge and abilities required by patients for successful self-management. When patients enter rehabilitation programs with knowledge of their conditions they demonstrate better compliance and enhanced interaction with medical staff while developing long-lasting healthy practices after their release from hospital care (Clark & Roberts, 2023). Educational programs integrated within the therapeutic process help patients grasp their medical condition and rehabilitation assignments and the effect their work will have on their lasting health outcomes (Giovannoni et al., 2024). Understanding these facts leads patients to both gain competence and develop stronger motivation to stay involved throughout the recovery process.

Empowerment Through Education in Rehabilitation

The core concept of patient-centered rehabilitation bases its approach on empowerment as the process to boost a person's independence for healthcare choices regarding their health situation. Healthcare empowerment requires healthcare providers to develop patient autonomy while boosting self-confidence and actively involving individuals in their treatments (Sagen et al., 2024). Empowerment in patients creates enhanced adherence to medical prescriptions along with improved behavior maintenance toward better care satisfaction. Empowered patients experience better rehabilitation results since they achieve superior functional outcomes, show decreased hospital admissions rates and demonstrate better mental health status according to Hiragami (2023). The power of education serves as a fundamental mechanism for developing empowerment in people. The provision of suitable information that is accessible to patients enables them to make smart medical decisions while establishing doable goals that foster control of their health progression. The combination of condition understanding and knowing therapeutic purpose together with active participation benefits leads patients to develop self-guided activities which strengthen their recovery (Fancourt & Steptoe, 2019). Successful patient ownership contributes to reduced nervousness and helplessness and simultaneously generates increased motivation and confidence (Gaalema et al., 2022). Current conceptual frameworks show that health literacy operates as an intellectual foundation for empowerment as an emotional response that enables patient engagement until it leads to behavioral modifications (Hickmann et al. 2022). The educational process activates multiple positive outcomes because it serves as the central piece that leads to improved understanding and freedom and maintained behavioral changes. The insufficient delivery of education to patients will prevent their full participation in healthcare which can decrease the success rates of rehabilitation procedures.

Holistic Health Recovery as a Foundation

The incorporation of holistic health principles within rehabilitation practices enhances the reasons for making education a priority. Holistic rehabilitation understands that complete recovery needs physical restoration together with emotional equilibrium and mental well-being and social readjustment and spiritual achievement respectively (Fancourt & Steptoe, 2019). This model accepts the multiple connected systems and develops combined patient-centered treatment approaches which focus on addressing all domains at once. The method shows specific importance for people with ongoing medical conditions or patients who require recovery from sophisticated surgical procedures. Patients who struggle with cardiovascular disease and diabetes experience extended medical issues which include anxiety together with depression and social isolation effects. Holistic rehabilitation programs featuring counseling alongside peer support and stress reduction training with lifestyle education demonstrate powerful effects in resilience improvement and emotional coping abilities and general health condition (Grant et al., 2021; Xin et al., 2023). The key function of education for healing involves teaching patients about how their behaviors together with their emotional state and social activity patterns affect their health outcomes. Patients who understand stress-induced enhancement of chronic pain and recovery motivation importance through social support become better able at taking comprehensive proactive steps for healing (Giovannoni et al., 2024). According to Sagen et al. (2024), patients gain hope and emotional strength while recovering through spiritual care agendas which present meaning for their needs based on their cultural and religious perspectives. Therapeutic environments which include physical and virtual spaces make up one aspect of holistic rehabilitation approaches. The feeling of control together with engagement improves when physical infrastructures encourage emotion-based safety and provide comfort along with accessibility. Patients become more likely to participate in their recovery journey because the environment combines rehabilitation centers that offer relaxation along with user-friendly digital platforms (Gaalema et al., 2022).

THEORETICAL FRAMEWORK

Theoretical grounding provides essential knowledge about how education strategies inside rehabilitation settings influence patient behaviors as well as engagement and end results. The behaviors and care models presented in this section describe how educational methods empower patients to achieve lasting recovery. Behavioral and care theories used to study educational strategies include Social Cognitive Theory as well as the Health Belief Model, the Theory of Planned Behavior, the Patient-Centered Care Model, Self-Determination Theory, and the Integrated Care Model. The combination of this selected set of frameworks gives a complete perspective for both designing and evaluating educational rehabilitation programs.

Social Cognitive Theory (Bandura, 2001)

Alleged by Albert Bandura Social Cognitive Theory (SCT) declares self-efficacy as the essential aspect because it represents an individual's confidence to conduct activities which result in favorable outcomes. The concept of self-efficacy stands central in rehabilitation since it determines patient participation in physical therapy activities and medication adherence and sustained health behavior adoption (Ghazi et al., 2018). Every study dedicated to rehabilitation evaluates how patients with higher self-efficacy maintain better rehabilitation protocol adherence and succeed in their functional recovery (Giovannoni et al., 2024). SCT also highlights observational learning, reinforcement, and cognitive processes as pivotal influences on behavior. Healthcare professionals play the role of behavioral models to display proper techniques and provide support which boosts patient drive and confidence (Gaalema et al., 2022). SCT-based educational methods construct self-efficacy by allowing patients to develop skills gradually while receiving positive feedback and defining clear recovery objectives to acquire active recovery control.

Health Belief Model (Rosenstock, 1974)

The Health Belief Model (HBM) offers a suitable model to understand how people evaluate risks against benefits and barriers which determines their health behaviors. HBM explains that people engage in beneficial health behaviors when they understand their condition risks alongside its seriousness and find action benefits greater than costs and receive proper prompts to develop actions (Rosenstock, 1974). Patients tend to follow prescribed therapy and life changes during rehabilitation according to the beliefs they hold (Gaalema et al., 2022). Educational methods that employ the HBM model modify the way patients perceive their situation. Through discussions about rehabilitation advantages and long-term consequences of non-compliance clinicians help patients view health behavior changes in new positive light that drives treatment engagement. When interventions address expected obstacles including pain and inconvenience together with a lack of knowledge patients re-think their ability to engage in treatment (Fancourt & Steptoe, 2019). Patient adherence to treatment schedules becomes more consistent through the combination of reminder alerts along with motivational supports and professional follow-up services which enhance both patient commitment and medical responsibility (Paul et al., 2023; Xin et al., 2022).

Theory of Planned Behavior (Ajzen, 1991)

TPB constructs behavior through three fundamental linkages including attitudes toward giving nurses feedback to team leaders (Ajzen, 1991). The rehabilitation outcomes depend on these three elements because they affect patient commitment and retention in therapy programs. TPB-based educational interventions aim to transform attitudes by delivering solid evidence which explains the importance of recommended activities to increase perceived importance and relevance. People in rehabilitation programs need especially strong perceived behavioral control following their recovery efforts because they often face feelings of distress and discouragement. The combination of small achievements and customized resources enables patients to understand their personal capacity to succeed according to Rich et al. (2023). Subjective norms within patient rehabilitation receive influence through family member and peer support group involvement which demonstrates to patients that their caring network expects them to become actively engaged (Paul et al., 2023).

Patient-Centered Care Model (Epstein et al., 2010)

The Patient-Centered Care (PCC) Model supports healthcare systems to create person-centered care by honoring patients' personal preferences along with their values and their individual requirements (Epstein et al., 2010). The model proves highly effective for rehabilitation purposes due to its ability to boost patient engagement and their commitment to treatment. The Patient-Centered Care approach promotes shared practice between patients and clinicians for goal creation and therapy decisions and performance assessments allowing for learning to evolve beyond traditional information dissemination. The educational approaches linked to PCC implement personalized communication methods alongside cultural and contextual awareness and emotional patient support. Rehabilitation programs designed to adjust their content based on patients' abilities and life needs and specific goals demonstrate superior long-term patient engagement potential according to Lo et al. (2022). The implementation of telemedicine along with digital tools brings greater access to educational content which patients can access through flexible familiar environments (Hwang & Lee, 2023). Educational programs maintain their relevance without losing efficacy because of their adjustable nature which works among patients from numerous backgrounds.

Self-Determination Theory (Deci & Ryan, 1985)

SDT introduces motivational aspects to educational research within the field of patient education. According to SDT optimal behavioral engagement develops from feeling autonumous and experiencing competence along with sensing relatedness to others two intrinsic psychological needs (Deci & Ryan, 1985). Medical rehabilitation programs which address these needs tend to generate sustained motivation from within patients together with increased adherence to care regimens. SDT-based educational approaches enable patients to select their learning methods while validating their ideas and developing mastery through incremental education. Patients who can choose educational material timing and format receive autonomy support as a result. Exercise programs which simultaneously advance physical abilities and mental skills help patients become more competent. Healthcare education delivered with emotional support produces connectedness between patients and caregivers (François et al. 2024). These elements function together to build a motivational setting which keeps patients engaged independently from external pressures or rewards.

Integrated Care Model

The Integrated Care Model delivers coordinated healthcare through interdisciplinary teams following personalized patient-centered approaches that handle entire patient care requirements across medicine, psychology and social aspects (Epstein et al., 2010). This rehabilitation model recommends that physicians and therapists and nurses and social workers and educators should work together to synchronize their care plans. The educational methods deployed through integrated care models function independently from other aspects of service provision. These educational messages exist within each touch point starting from physical therapy appointments until psychological counseling and receive ongoing reinforcement through present messaging. Patients receive cohesive guidance as a result of this integration which reduces their confusion while building trust (Lo et al., 2022). Shared database systems enable educational content modification based on patient achievements through real-time assessment and continuous learning functionality.

Synthesis of Theoretical Insights

Educational theories show that interventions in rehabilitation produce complex dynamics in educational approaches. These theories shape belief systems along with motivational factors and inclusive care design (HBM, TPB, SCT, SDT) which support evidence-based patient-centered educational strategies. Educational methods which follow these established frameworks have better success rates in patient engagement together with empowerment enhancement and behavioral change outcomes which results in improved clinical outcomes and prolonged health improvement.

RESEARCH METHODOLOGY

A systematic literature review served as the research method to evaluate educational strategies in rehabilitation. The review followed the methodological standards of Preferred Reporting Items for Systematic Reviews and Meta-Analyses (PRISMA) 2020 that enabled transparent and reproducible research throughout the study process. The main goal of this study was to gather current research that evaluates educational approaches affecting patient empowerment levels and engagement rates and health outcome success across different rehabilitation environments.

Search Strategy and Data Sources

TA comprehensive literature search accessed at least five major scholarly databases which included PubMed and Scopus together with Web of Science CINAHL in addition to Google Scholar in order to retrieve a wide range of interdisciplinary studies. Domain experts formed a list of keywords and Medical Subject Headings (MeSH) terms through collaboration which contained the following search parameters: "patient education" with "rehabilitation" and "self-management" and "patient empowerment" and "digital health education" combined with "rehabilitation outcomes." Boolean operators enabled the refinement of information through the usage of AND/OR combination rules. The research focused on peer-reviewed publications from January 2020 to March 2025 to maintain a modern and applicable collection of materials. Research publications in English language that investigated adult rehabilitation participants from physical, neurological and chronic care fields were acceptable for evaluation.

Inclusion and Exclusion Criteria

- Studies were included based on the following criteria:
- Focused on educational interventions aimed at patients undergoing rehabilitation.
- Reported measurable outcomes related to empowerment, adherence, functional recovery, or psychological well-being.
- Employed either qualitative, quantitative, or mixed-methods research designs.
- Published in peer-reviewed journals between 2020 and 2025.

Studies were excluded if they:

- Focused exclusively on provider education without patient involvement.
- Lacked empirical data (e.g., opinion pieces, editorials).
- Were duplicates or conference abstracts without full texts.

Screening and Selection Process

PRISMA flow diagram served as the method for disclosing the article selection procedure. The start of the research resulted in 734 initial findings but duplicate removal reduced this number to 612. Each article went through title-screening followed by abstract-screening conducted independently by two reviewers. Detailed review involved 176 articles that researchers retrieved for analysis. Forty-two studies passed the inclusion and exclusion criteria which resulted in their selection for final synthesis. The reviewers checked their inclusion decisions by having discussions to reach consensus and brought in a third person for consultation when needed.

Data Extraction and Synthesis

Researchers applied a unified data extraction template that organized details about study plans along with demographic information of participants and their education programs and measurement tools and final study results. Among the analyzed research studies there was an equal distribution of quantitative results (n=25) and qualitative results (n=10) and mixed-methods findings (n=7). The intervention effectiveness on mobility improvement and pain reduction and adherence rates as well as psychosocial functioning received statistical evidence from quantitative studies (Al Kuwaiti et al., 2023). In-depth qualitative studies revealed patient perspectives about education and examined the factors which help or hinder their involvement in the program (Silver et al., 2024). The integration of multiple research methods in mixed-methods studies generated comprehensive knowledge through the connection of statistical outcome data to patient self-reported feedback and preferences about the intervention treatment. The researchers used thematic analysis to bring together all research findings. Research data revealed four main themes: self-efficacy importance as well as student engagement combined with digital technology integration and customized educational approaches and collaborative interprofessional partnerships for educational success.

Ethical Considerations

As this was a review of publicly available data, no ethical approval was required. However, all included studies were published in peer-reviewed journals and adhered to institutional or national ethical standards.

PRACTICAL REAL CASE STUDIES ON EDUCATIONAL STRATEGIES IN REHABILITATION

Case Study 1: Rehabilitation of a Stroke Patient Using Patient-Centered Education

Background: Mr. A, a 63-year-old male, suffered a stroke that impaired his right arm and leg, leading to partial paralysis. He also experienced aphasia, which affected his ability to communicate effectively. He was admitted to a rehabilitation center where a patient-centered approach was implemented as part of his rehabilitation plan.

Educational Strategy: In his rehabilitation process, a patient-centered educational approach was used to ensure that Mr. A fully understood his condition and recovery plan. The rehabilitation team, including physiotherapists, speech therapists, and occupational therapists, worked together to educate him about his stroke, its effects, and the importance of active participation in his rehabilitation. The team used visual aids and simplified language to explain complex medical terms related to his condition. Given Mr. A's aphasia, the communication was tailored to his specific needs, and alternative communication methods, such as picture cards and simple gestures, were incorporated. In addition, the team encouraged Mr. A to take an active role in setting his rehabilitation goals. This helped him feel more in control and motivated, which increased his adherence to the prescribed exercises. The team also provided him with educational materials that explained stroke recovery and the importance of continued exercise for improving mobility and speech.

Outcome: The patient demonstrated a significant improvement in both physical and communication abilities after six months. His mobility improved with the help of regular physiotherapy exercises, and his communication abilities gradually returned as speech therapy helped him regain some of his language skills. Mr. A reported feeling more confident and empowered, largely due to the patient-centered educational interventions. He was also able to manage his daily activities more independently, contributing to a better quality of life.

Case Study 2: Use of Digital Tools in the Rehabilitation of an Elderly Patient with Osteoarthritis

Background: Mrs. B, a 75-year-old woman, was diagnosed with osteoarthritis, which affected her knees and hands. She had difficulty performing basic tasks like walking, climbing stairs, and grasping objects. Due to her age, Mrs. B had limited access to rehabilitation services and faced difficulties attending in-person therapy sessions due to mobility issues.

Educational Strategy: Mrs. B's rehabilitation team introduced digital tools, including a mobile app specifically designed for elderly patients with osteoarthritis. The app included instructional videos on joint exercises, educational content about osteoarthritis, reminders for daily exercises, and the ability to track her progress. The app allowed Mrs. B to complete exercises at home, significantly reducing her need to travel for therapy sessions. The app was also paired with a wearable device that tracked her physical activity and sent real-time feedback to both her and her rehabilitation team. This continuous feedback helped adjust the difficulty of her exercises based on her progress. Additionally, the app provided educational modules that explained the importance of managing osteoarthritis and the impact of exercise on joint health.

Outcome: Mrs. B adhered to her exercise regimen, which she found easy to integrate into her daily routine due to the convenience of the mobile app. Over the course of three months, her pain decreased, and her mobility improved. She regained the ability to walk longer distances, manage household chores, and use her hands more effectively. The digital tools not only improved her rehabilitation outcomes but also empowered her to take control of her health and engage in self-management.

Case Study 3: Empowerment through Education in the Rehabilitation of a Young Athlete with a Knee Injury

Background: Mr. C, a 22-year-old collegiate athlete, tore his anterior cruciate ligament (ACL) during a football match. The injury required surgery, followed by an extensive rehabilitation program. As a young, competitive athlete, Mr. C was highly motivated but had limited knowledge about the rehabilitation process and the steps needed for recovery.

Educational Strategy: Mr. C's rehabilitation team provided detailed education on the ACL injury, the surgery he had undergone, and the rehabilitation milestones he needed to reach to safely return to sport. The rehabilitation process was broken down into phases, and Mr. C was educated about each phase's objectives, such as regaining strength, flexibility, and coordination. The team also used motivational interviewing techniques to assess his readiness for change and to establish goals that were realistic but challenging. One of the main focuses of the education was on self-efficacy building Mr. C's belief in his ability to follow through with the rehabilitation program. He was given access to educational materials, including video tutorials and written guidelines, which explained the exercises and their role in strengthening his knee and preventing re-injury.

Outcome: By actively participating in his rehabilitation process and understanding the rationale behind each exercise, Mr. C showed remarkable progress. He adhered to his rehabilitation schedule, and after six months, he was able to return to full athletic participation. His recovery was not only physical but also psychological, as he felt more confident in his ability to prevent future injuries and manage his rehabilitation independently.

Case Study 4: Community-Based Educational Program for Post-Surgical Recovery

Background: Mrs. D, a 55-year-old woman, underwent hip replacement surgery due to severe osteoarthritis. After the surgery, she struggled to regain strength and mobility. Mrs. D was not familiar with the rehabilitation process and was unsure about how to manage her recovery at home.

Educational Strategy: Mrs. D participated in a community-based rehabilitation program that provided group education sessions to post-surgical patients. The program combined group learning, peer support, and expert-led educational sessions. During the sessions, Mrs. D learned about the importance of post-surgical exercises, pain management strategies, and lifestyle adjustments to ensure a smooth recovery. In addition, the program incorporated hands-on workshops where patients practiced mobility exercises with assistance from physical therapists. A critical element of this program was the support network of other patients who had undergone similar surgeries, offering Mrs. D emotional encouragement and motivation.

Outcome: Mrs. D made significant progress in her recovery due to the combination of structured education and peer support. Her range of motion and strength improved, and she regained the ability to walk with minimal assistance. The group setting provided her with a sense of community and belonging, which improved her motivation and adherence to the rehabilitation plan. She felt less isolated and more empowered to take control of her recovery.

Case Study 5: The Impact of Interdisciplinary Education on a Patient with Chronic Pain

Background: Mr. E, a 45-year-old male, was suffering from chronic lower back pain. His condition had been ongoing for several years, and despite several treatments, including physical therapy and medication, his pain persisted. Mr. E had a limited understanding of the nature of chronic pain and the role of lifestyle changes in its management.

Educational Strategy: An interdisciplinary team, including a pain specialist, physiotherapist, psychologist, and nutritionist, worked together to provide Mr. E with a comprehensive education program. The team educated him about chronic pain mechanisms, the importance of posture and ergonomics, and the impact of psychological factors such as stress on pain perception. The team also used cognitive-behavioral therapy (CBT) techniques to help Mr. E develop coping strategies for managing pain. He was educated on pacing his activities to avoid flare-ups and was introduced to mindfulness practices to reduce stress and muscle tension. Additionally, the nutritionist provided information on the role of diet in managing inflammation and supporting musculoskeletal health.

Outcome: Mr. E experienced a significant reduction in pain and improved overall well-being after completing the education program. His understanding of pain management strategies allowed him to make more informed decisions about his lifestyle and treatment, leading to better pain control. The interdisciplinary approach ensured that all aspects of his health were addressed, contributing to a more holistic and sustainable recovery process.

SOLUTIONS AND RECOMMENDATIONS

The achievement of optimal rehabilitation program results depends on personalized evidence-driven educational methods which form part of comprehensive health care delivery models. This part proposes functional recommendations to enhance educational rehabilitation practices by adopting evidence-based and best practice strategies alongside theoretical approaches from previous sections. Each proposed method concentrates on two main aspects: patient engagement along with accessibility to programs and motivation and long-term adherence enhancement.

1. Tailored Educational Programs

The fundamental value within successful rehabilitation programs consists of personalized education. Individualized adaptations in healthcare interventions that match each patient's learning type and cultural base and cognitive strength and health initiative goals produce superior comprehension and engagement according to Ricci et al. (2022). The educational content needs presentation methods which match individual preferences between visual (infographics and videos) and auditory (voice recordings) along with kinesthetic (interactive tasks). Information delivery strategies that match individual needs help patients understand better while strengthening their ability to remember along with improving their emotional engagement in education (Gaalema et al., 2022). The implementation of personalized treatment methods must resolve issues related to language diversity and health literacy and neurological disability. Healthcare providers can achieve this goal through simplified language and translation services combined with cognitive support tools which include pictorial guides. The early implementation of assessments helps healthcare providers create patient-specific learning paths which match patients' ability levels and drive their dedication and result improvement (Xin et al., 2022).

2. Integration of Digital Tools and E-Learning Platforms

Healthcare institutions can provide accessible patient-focused rehabilitation interventions through digital educational platforms. Digital applications together with virtual reality solutions and teaching systems through the internet deliver convenient educational resources that include video-based exercises and evaluation dashboards and patient self-assessment features (Arntz et al., 2023). The technology supports independent learning through guided access to educational resources which patients can review any time they need reinforcement of their understanding. The programming of mobile apps includes automatic reminder features together with milestone alerting and teleconsultation interface tools which create perpetual patient involvement. E-learning platforms together with tele-rehabilitation services enable flexibility because patients with mobility restrictions can receive care without needing in-person clinic visits thus improving their accessibility (Devi et al., 2025). Through interactive quizzes and feedback loops patients gain the ability to self-monitor their behavior while recovering through an improved participation process (Fancourt & Steptoe, 2019). Digital intervention platforms need designed accessibility features to accommodate elderly patients along with those who have limited technological literacy. Voice navigation and adjustable font sizes together with culturally appropriate content enable better user engagement by minimizing digital exclusion according to Soltani et al. (2022).

3. Interdisciplinary Collaboration in Education Delivery

The delivery of thorough patient education in rehabilitation requires an integrated approach between different healthcare professionals. SD-mouth rehabilitation education strategies succeed by uniting physical therapists with occupational therapists as well as psychologists and speech therapists alongside social workers and nurses for supporting patients with all recovery needs (Vettriselvan et al., 2025). Interdisciplinary education models create a single support system which combines clear patient messages through the elimination of information duplication. Patients who receive educational therapy from physical therapists learn exercise mechanics and pacing principles but simultaneously receive psychological guidance for coping strategies as well as emotional resilience training and stress management techniques from psychologists according to Lo et al. (2022). Joint educational efforts between these professionals create both superior educational value and increased trust from patients in their healthcare providers. Patients tend to view their care experiences as whole and customized when health education comes from an integrated team of healthcare providers. Clinical collaboration enables internal health team members to communicate through unified care plans and electronic health records which delivers precise consistent information to patients throughout their recovery process according to Grant et al. (2021).

4. Community-Based Educational Programs and Peer Support

Community-based education programs have proven themselves as crucial additions to standard rehabilitation services. Such educational programs use peer and group sessions combined with experiential learning opportunities to help patients provide mutual reinforcement and support (Grant et al., 2021). Đây represents one of the vital aspects of care for patients with chronic conditions because peer support matches the importance of clinical guidance. The group education format enables members of the program to discuss methods and at the same time strengthen their collective achievements. The environment based on collective responsibility and belonging creates benefits for those who might be experiencing social isolation and stigma and motivation loss (Xin et al., 2022). The delivery of educational programs in community settings eliminates institutional obstacles and offers programming that better meets cultural needs especially for diverse minority groups who lack proper healthcare services. Formal rehabilitation frameworks that adopt community-based programs increase educational outreach coverage and enable healthcare providers to sustain their support networks after discharge. Successful recoveries from peer mentors show others the way to stay committed while acting as models for recovery success (Soltani et al., 2022).

5. Continuous Feedback and Progress Monitoring

Effectual learning together with behavior modification depends on ongoing feedback as its vital component. Real-time progress tracking becomes possible through continuous feedback systems in educational techniques which also strengthens beneficial patient behavioral changes. Modern technologies which include wearable devices together with smart home sensors and digital diaries produce strong evidence about activity levels while showing adherence patterns and physiological changes (Rodgers et al., 2019). Real-time assessment of patient performance and preferences by healthcare providers leads to immediate rehabilitation plan modifications that include goal or intervention adjustments. Tangible progress records distributed to patients help increase their motivation and strengthen their confidence while lowering their recovery-related doubts (Giovannoni et al., 2024). The customized feedback systems notify providers about patient difficulties which enables them to step in promptly. Through both patient-clinician dialogues and app-generated reports patients obtain useful feedback that maintains their dedication to rehabilitation therapy and sustains their therapeutic support. Research indicates that routine feedback delivery enhances patient adherence as well as boosts their care satisfaction ratings (Grant et al., 2021). The solutions support rehabilitation patient education through three key areas which combine customized treatment with technological integration and community engagement across specialized reorder. Strategies brought into practice enable patient empowerment and enhance both patient engagement and recovery results thus transforming rehabilitation education from a required aspect to an essential success factor.

FUTURE RESEARCH DIRECTIONS

Educational interventions in rehabilitation show short-term benefits according to existing studies but research lacks clarity about their long-term effects and their usefulness with different patient groups and technological integration. The establishment of future-ready rehabilitation education frameworks depends on filling the existing knowledge gaps. Further investigation should concentrate on the following critical areas to advance knowledge.

1. Long-Term Impact of Educational Interventions

Existing studies about rehabilitation education mainly evaluate its effects on immediate functional outcomes and student engagement as well as learning acquisition. The long-term aspects of rehabilitation education effects require more comprehensive study for patients with chronic diseases and those moving to independent post-treatment homes. New research needs to use extensive time frameworks to evaluate how educational training programs lead to lasting modifications of behaviors and better self-care abilities and health quality improvement (Rich et al., 2024). Research should examine if patients continue health-promoting habits after rehabilitation termination and understand how these practices affect their reduced hospital admissions and decreased complications instead of hospital readmissions and their emotional strength following rehabilitation. Research into patient responses during extended tracking periods enables the assessment of how they handle educational development changes brought on by altering cognitive and physical capabilities. Research using diverse population groups and settings including home-based care and community health centers and rural territories will expand knowledge about lasting impact of educational programs in healthcare (Fu et al., 2024).

2. Cultural and Socioeconomic Influences on Educational Outcomes

Different educational approaches succeed only when the culture and socioeconomic status of the audience creates a match with their learning environment. Future examinations need to study cultural elements that impact patient health views and rehabilitation understanding together with the ways these understandings affect educational material reception (Fancourt & Steptoe, 2019). Patients from collective-oriented cultures allow family members to make healthcare choices about their health while patients from certain cultures choose to follow traditional medical practices instead of contemporary biomedical medicine. The participation and benefits derived from education-based rehabilitation programs experience substantial effects due to factors including level of income as well as digital literacy capabilities and healthcare infrastructure access (Khokale et al., 2023). Investigative studies should determine how culturally appropriate educational materials should be structured and delivered to support low-literate and multilingual and disadvantaged population groups. The identification of health inequalities alongside their remedies will help create inclusive rehabilitation training systems which suit diverse patient populations (Soltani et al., 2022).

3. Leveraging Technological Innovation in Education Delivery

The recent advances in technology create new possibilities to restructure rehabilitation education. Healthcare education benefits from the application of artificial intelligence (AI) together with machine learning as well as data-driven personalization tools that customize educational materials according to patient illness and individual learning requirements and speed of progress while matching motivational characteristics (Silver et al., 2024). The AI-powered platforms generate adjustable learning curriculum structures and realize individual patient needs which enable instantaneous feedback for therapeutic decision-making. Immersive technology tools namely virtual reality and augmented reality show potential to enhance experiential learning opportunities in education and healthcare. Patients gain confidence and skill development through virtual environments which reproduce real-life activities with the help of these tools (Khokale et al., 2023). VR-based rehabilitation education strengthening patient attention and decreasing their anxiety marks an efficient method to develop muscle memory needed for functional activities. Research into these technologies should focus specifically on their ability to retain knowledge and patient adherence rates together with accessibility and cost-effectiveness measures and ability to serve various age groups and disability levels (Johnson et al., 2023).

4. Development of Interdisciplinary Educational Models

The current practice of multidisciplinary rehabilitation requires the adoption of new interdisciplinary educational approaches which enable medical professionals to create unified patient-focused educational methods. Traditional multidisciplinary work methods where professionals work independently differ from interdisciplinary models which incorporate shared educational goals among professionals and joint curriculum development and unified messages across fields (Ghazi et al., 2018). Future scientific investigations must examine how medical teams combining physiotherapists along with psychologists and speech therapists and social workers and nutritionists should collaborate to develop recovery education programs which represent the full recovery experience (Lo et al., 2022). Such models deliver better continuous patient care while reducing conflicting recommendations while generating trust between patients and their healthcare providers. The analysis needs research to study ways digital platforms enhance collaboration between professionals through jointly maintained digital data and discussion tools and educative content creation systems (Bendowska & Baum, 2023). Professional development evaluation for educational design teams with communication skills will be vital to establish optimal collaboration among healthcare providers. Endorsing standardized best practice protocols in this field will produce enhanced interactions for patients and providers which drives optimized results in rehabilitation treatments. Medical rehabilitation education is set for progress through its capacity for adaptation to diverse patient groups and advancing technological elements and changing treatment settings. Research stakeholders who focus on long-term evaluation alongside cultural competency education combined with digital innovation and interdisciplinary collaboration will drive the field toward improved education models which focus on inclusivity and personalization and effective results. This strategic direction maintains alignment with present worldwide healthcare patterns to provide critical support which enables every patient group to reclaim their independence and achieve long-term recovery.

CONCLUSION

The chapter emphasizes educational strategies in present-day rehabilitation because they empower patients and maintain long-term involvement leading to advanced recovery results. Literature reviews show rehab models evolving from physical-focused approaches to holistic care that treats health through mental, emotional, psychological and social aspects (Stepanian et al., 2023). Within this strategic framework education operates as a core system that enables patients to acquire needed knowledge while building confidence and autonomy which helps them successfully deal with their rehabilitation process. The tools patients learn in educational programs enable them to grasp their medical diagnoses and decide intelligently about their health which leads to their active involvement in their recovery path. By understanding their condition patients improve their treatment compliance and therapeutic activities participation when they combine this knowledge with self-efficacy and goal-oriented behavior (Ghazi et al., 2018). Heathcare providers improve clinical outputs and patient satisfaction through delivering patient-specific educational material which aligns with individual learning methods together with cognitive capacity and cultural backgrounds (Gaalema et al., 2022).

The research shows that assessment of cultural elements along with socioeconomic conditions together with psychological aspects produces essential value during intervention program development. Rehabilitation programs require adaptable educational approaches which include all patients to succeed in their objectives. Throughout the entire recovery process patients need the support and respect that comes from healthcare delivery and content which incorporates understanding of social determinants of health (Fancourt & Steptoe, 2019). The acquisition of patient empowerment through education creates permanent alterations to individual behaviors. Health outcomes in rehabilitation improve when patients gain self-confidence because they can effectively manage their conditions, sustain lifestyle changes and keep appointments effectively (Giovannoni et al., 2024). More self-directed control and mental well-being with increased resilience and better control power are key recovery elements that education enables through its enhancement of autonomy. The implementation of emerging technologies including virtual reality (VR) and mobile applications and artificial intelligence (AI) and wearable devices creates an effective way to transform education delivery in rehabilitation programs. The innovations introduce dynamic patient-driven and accessible learning spaces which adapt their content for better engagement and interaction (Khokale et al., 2023). Digital tools enhance knowledge acquisition and simultaneously improve rehabilitation technique learning when used effectively according to Arntz et al. (2023). The implementation of technology needs to be supported by thorough investigations of user-friendly practices and equal access to guarantee universal patient benefits irrespective of background characteristics or technological capabilities. Future studies need to focus on thorough investigations of sustained educational effects on patient behavior as well as life quality and healthcare service usage. Design and delivery of every program must focus on meeting the needs of marginalized populations by evaluating cultural needs and financial obstacles (Rich et al., 2024). Research should focus on AI-based adaptive teaching methods as well as virtual reality and augmented reality systems to develop patient motor skills and maintain their active involvement during safe and controlled therapeutic sessions.

Educational approaches in rehabilitation achieve success because they heavily depend on the quality of interdisciplinary teamwork. Additional studies need to analyze how integrated healthcare teams should approach joint educational intervention development and delivery with a unified approach that targets multiple patient needs (Ghazi et al., 2018). Future approaches to education and team-based training must become essential because they will develop needed competencies for sustaining collaborative work efforts. Modern rehabilitation depends fundamentally on education rather than considering it optional. Healthcare systems become more efficient when patients receive individualized educational instruction that uses evidence-based practices and welcomes everyone. This strategy delivers superior health outcomes for patients. The evolution of rehabilitation science requires adaptive innovative and human-centered educational practices to lead the way. The continuing development of research and policy and practice innovation requires investment to establish rehabilitation education as an equitable system that supports lifelong recovery for all patients (Soltani et al., 2022).

REFERENCES

Ajzen, I. (1991). The theory of planned behavior. *Organizational Behavior and Human Decision Processes*, *50*(2), 179–211. DOI: 10.1016/0749-5978(91)90020-T

Al Kuwaiti, A., Nazer, K., Al-Reedy, A., Al-Shehri, S., Al-Muhanna, A., Subbarayalu, A. V., Al Muhanna, D., & Al-Muhanna, F. A. (2023). A Review of the Role of Artificial Intelligence in Healthcare. *Journal of Personalized Medicine*, *13*(6), 951. DOI: 10.3390/jpm13060951 PMID: 37373940

Arntz, A., Weber, F., Handgraaf, M., Lällä, K., Korniloff, K., Murtonen, K. P., Chichaeva, J., Kidritsch, A., Heller, M., Sakellari, E., Athanasopoulou, C., Lagiou, A., Tzonichaki, I., Salinas-Bueno, I., Martínez-Bueso, P., Velasco-Roldán, O., Schulz, R. J., & Grüneberg, C. (2023). Technologies in Home-Based Digital Rehabilitation: Scoping Review. *JMIR Rehabilitation and Assistive Technologies*, *10*, e43615. DOI: 10.2196/43615 PMID: 37253381

Bendowska, A., & Baum, E. (2023). The Significance of Cooperation in Interdisciplinary Health Care Teams as Perceived by Polish Medical Students. *International Journal of Environmental Research and Public Health*, *20*(2), 954. DOI: 10.3390/ijerph20020954 PMID: 36673710

Devi, M., Manokaran, D., Sehgal, R. K., Shariff, S. A., & Vettriselvan, R. (2025). Precision Medicine, Personalized Treatment, and Network-Driven Innovations: Transforming Healthcare With AI. In Kanthavel, R., & Dhaya, R. (Eds.), *AI for Large Scale Communication Networks* (pp. 303–322). IGI Global Scientific Publishing., DOI: 10.4018/979-8-3693-6552-6.ch014

Epstein, R. M., Fiscella, K., Lesser, C. S., & Stange, K. C. (2010). Why the nation needs a policy push on patient-centered health care. *Health Affairs (Project Hope)*, *29*(8), 1489–1495. DOI: 10.1377/hlthaff.2009.0888 PMID: 20679652

Fancourt, D., & Steptoe, A. (2019). Cultural engagement and mental health: Does socio-economic status explain the association?. Social science & medicine (1982), 236, 112425. https://doi.org/DOI: 10.1016/j.socscimed.2019.112425

François, J., Audrain-Pontevia, A., Boudhraâ, S., & Vial, S. (2024). Assessing the Influence of Patient Empowerment Gained Through Mental Health Apps on Patient Trust in the Health Care Provider and Patient Compliance With the Recommended Treatment: Cross-sectional Study. *Journal of Medical Internet Research*, *26*, e48182. DOI: 10.2196/48182 PMID: 38345851

Fu, W., Baldwin, T. F., Brechter, J. H., Erickson, M. R., Kobal, K., LaFay, V., Miller, T. M., & Morales, J. (2024). Effects of Educational Interventions Designed to Develop Physical Therapist Learners' Clinical Reasoning: A Systematic Review. *Physical Therapy*, *105*(3), pzae182. Advance online publication. DOI: 10.1093/ptj/pzae182 PMID: 39718199

Gaalema, D. E., Savage, P. D., O'Neill, S., Bolívar, H. A., Denkmann, D., Priest, J. S., Khadanga, S., & Ades, P. A. (2022). The Association of Patient Educational Attainment With Cardiac Rehabilitation Adherence and Health Outcomes. *Journal of Cardiopulmonary Rehabilitation and Prevention*, *42*(4), 227–234. DOI: 10.1097/HCR.0000000000000646 PMID: 34840247

Ghazi, C., Nyland, J., Whaley, R., Rogers, T., Wera, J., & Henzman, C. (2018). Social cognitive or learning theory use to improve self-efficacy in musculoskeletal rehabilitation: A systematic review and meta-analysis. *Physiotherapy Theory and Practice*, *34*(7), 495–504. DOI: 10.1080/09593985.2017.1422204 PMID: 29308969

Giovannoni, G., Ford, H. L., Schmierer, K., Middleton, R., Stennett, A. M., Pomeroy, I., Fisniku, L., Scalfari, A., Bannon, C., Stross, R., Hughes, S., Williams, A., Josephs, S., Peel, C., & Straukiene, A. (2024). MS care: Integrating advanced therapies and holistic management. *Frontiers in Neurology*, *14*, 1286122. DOI: 10.3389/fneur.2023.1286122 PMID: 38351950

Grant, E., Johnson, L., Prodromidis, A., & Giannoudis, P. V. (2021). The Impact of Peer Support on Patient Outcomes in Adults With Physical Health Conditions: A Scoping Review. *Cureus*, *13*(8), e17442. DOI: 10.7759/cureus.17442 PMID: 34589348

Hiragami, F. (2023). Developing Skills in Intra-Workplace Rehabilitation Education: II. *Open Journal of Therapy and Rehabilitation*, *11*(3), 98–121. DOI: 10.4236/ojtr.2023.113009

Khokale, R. S., Mathew, G., Ahmed, S., Maheen, S., Fawad, M., Bandaru, P., Zerin, A., Nazir, Z., Khawaja, I., Sharif, I., Abdin, Z. U., & Akbar, A. (2023). Virtual and Augmented Reality in Post-stroke Rehabilitation: A Narrative Review. *Cureus*, *15*(4), e37559. DOI: 10.7759/cureus.37559 PMID: 37193429

Nader, T., Rothenberg, S., Averbach, R., Charles, B., Fields, J. Z., & Schneider, R. H. (2000). Improvements in chronic diseases with a comprehensive natural medicine approach: A review and case series. *Behavioral Medicine (Washington, D.C.)*, *26*(1), 34–46. DOI: 10.1080/08964280009595751 PMID: 10971882

Nicolau, C., Mendes, L., Ciríaco, M., Ferreira, B., Baixinho, C. L., Fonseca, C., Ferreira, R., & Sousa, L. (2022). Educational Intervention in Rehabilitation to Improve Functional Capacity after Hip Arthroplasty: A Scoping Review. *Journal of Personalized Medicine*, *12*(5), 656. DOI: 10.3390/jpm12050656 PMID: 35629079

Paul, B., Kirubakaran, R., Isaac, R., Dozier, M., Grant, L., & Weller, D.RESPIRE Collaboration. (2023). A systematic review of the theory of planned behaviour interventions for chronic diseases in low health-literacy settings. *Journal of Global Health*, *13*, 04079. DOI: 10.7189/jogh.13.04079 PMID: 37681679

Ricci, L., Villegente, J., Loyal, D., Ayav, C., Kivits, J., & Rat, A. C. (2022). Tailored patient therapeutic educational interventions: A patient-centred communication model. *Health Expectations*, *25*(1), 276–289. DOI: 10.1111/hex.13377 PMID: 34816546

Rodgers, M. M., Alon, G., Pai, V. M., & Conroy, R. S. (2019). Wearable technologies for active living and rehabilitation: Current research challenges and future opportunities. *Journal of Rehabilitation and Assistive Technologies Engineering*, *6*, 2055668319839607. DOI: 10.1177/2055668319839607 PMID: 31245033

Sagen, J. S., Kjeken, I., Habberstad, A., Linge, A. D., Simonsen, A. E., Lyken, A. D., Irgens, E. L., Framstad, H., Lyby, P. S., Klokkerud, M., Dagfinrud, H., & Moe, R. H. (2024). Patient Involvement in the Rehabilitation Process Is Associated with Improvement in Function and Goal Attainment: Results from an Explorative Longitudinal Study. *Journal of Clinical Medicine*, *13*(2), 320. DOI: 10.3390/jcm13020320 PMID: 38256454

Silver, J. K., Dodurgali, M. R., & Gavini, N. (2024). Artificial Intelligence in Medical Education and Mentoring in Rehabilitation Medicine. *American Journal of Physical Medicine & Rehabilitation*, *103*(11), 1039–1044. DOI: 10.1097/PHM.0000000000002604 PMID: 39016292

Soltani, S., Moghadam, M. M., Amani, S., Akbari, S., Shiani, A., & Soofi, M. (2022). Socioeconomic disparities in using rehabilitation services among Iranian adults with disabilities: A decomposition analysis. *BMC Health Services Research*, *22*(1), 1449. DOI: 10.1186/s12913-022-08811-8 PMID: 36447232

Stepanian, N., Larsen, M. H., Mendelsohn, J. B., Mariussen, K. L., & Heggdal, K. (2023). Empowerment interventions designed for persons living with chronic disease - a systematic review and meta-analysis of the components and efficacy of format on patient-reported outcomes. *BMC Health Services Research*, *23*(1), 911. DOI: 10.1186/s12913-023-09895-6 PMID: 37626346

Vettriselvan, R., Deepan, A., Jaiswani, G., Balakrishnan, A., & Sakthivel, R. (2025). Health Consequences of Early Marriage: Examining Morbidity and Long-Term Wellbeing. In Uddin, E. (Ed.), *Social, Political, and Health Implications of Early Marriage* (pp. 189–212). IGI Global Scientific Publishing., DOI: 10.4018/979-8-3693-3394-5.ch008

Xin, W., Xu, D., Dou, Z., Jacques, A., Umbella, J., & Hill, A. M. (2024). Effectiveness of Community-Based Rehabilitation (CBR) Centers for Improving Physical Fitness for Community-Dwelling Older Adults: A Systematic Review and Meta-Analysis. *Annals of Rehabilitation Medicine*, *48*(1), 5–21. DOI: 10.5535/arm.23148 PMID: 38433005

ADDITIONAL READING

Reber, P. A., DiPietro, E. A., Paraway, Y., Obst, B. P., Smith, R. A., & Koller, C. L. (2011). Communication: the key to effective interdisciplinary collaboration in the care of a child with complex rehabilitation needs. Rehabilitation nursing: the official journal of the Association of Rehabilitation Nurses, 36(5), 181–213. https://doi.org/DOI: 10.1002/j.2048-7940.2011.tb00192.x

Vainauskienė, V., & Vaitkienė, R. (2021). Enablers of Patient Knowledge Empowerment for Self-Management of Chronic Disease: An Integrative Review. *International Journal of Environmental Research and Public Health*, *18*(5), 2247. DOI: 10.3390/ijerph18052247 PMID: 33668329

KEY TERMS AND DEFINITIONS

Rehabilitation: Rehabilitation is a process that helps individuals regain their functional abilities after experiencing illness, injury, or disability. It aims to restore physical, mental, and social function, supporting patients in leading an independent and fulfilling life through various therapeutic interventions and support systems.

Patient Empowerment: Patient empowerment refers to the process by which individuals gain control over their health and treatment decisions. It involves providing patients with the knowledge, skills, and confidence necessary to actively participate in their healthcare, fostering autonomy and improving overall rehabilitation outcomes.

Self-Efficacy: Self-efficacy is the belief in one's ability to perform actions required to achieve a desired outcome. In rehabilitation, it is crucial as individuals with high self-efficacy are more likely to engage in rehabilitation activities and persist in their recovery process, improving long-term health outcomes.

Holistic Health: Holistic health is an approach to healthcare that recognizes the interconnectedness of the body, mind, and spirit. It involves treating the whole person by considering all aspects of their well-being physical, emotional, social, and spiritual—in order to promote overall healing and recovery.

Health Literacy: Health literacy is the ability to understand and apply health-related information in making informed decisions about one's care. This includes the ability to interpret medical instructions, understand health risks, and navigate healthcare systems, all of which are vital for effective rehabilitation and long-term health management.

Patient-Centered Care: Patient-centered care focuses on the individual needs, preferences, and values of the patient. It involves collaborating with patients in decision-making processes and ensuring that care plans are tailored to meet their unique circumstances, thus improving their experience and outcomes in rehabilitation.

Behavioral Change: Behavioral change refers to the process by which individuals modify their actions or habits in response to interventions. In rehabilitation, this can involve adopting healthier lifestyles, engaging in prescribed exercises, or following treatment plans, all of which are key to successful recovery.

Motivational Interviewing: Motivational interviewing is a counseling approach designed to enhance an individual's motivation to change behavior. It focuses on fostering a supportive environment that encourages patients to explore their feelings and develop intrinsic motivation to engage in rehabilitation and self-care practices.

Assistive Technology: Assistive technology refers to tools or devices that aid individuals in performing tasks they are unable to do independently due to physical or cognitive limitations. In rehabilitation, these technologies support mobility, communication, and daily activities, facilitating greater independence for patients.

Interdisciplinary Collaboration: Interdisciplinary collaboration involves the teamwork of healthcare professionals from different disciplines, such as physicians, nurses, therapists, and psychologists, working together to deliver comprehensive care. In rehabilitation, this collaborative approach ensures that all aspects of the patient's health and recovery are addressed, leading to improved patient outcomes and holistic care.

Chapter 10
Patient and Healthcare Professional Perceptions:
Qualitative Study

Daniela Vieira
https://orcid.org/0000-0001-8263-0927
Escola Superior de Saúde Fernando Pessoa, Portugal

Eduarda C. T. Sousa
https://orcid.org/0009-0003-6820-0519
Portuguese Oncology Institute of Porto, Portugal

André Laranja
Portuguese Oncology Institute of Porto, Portugal

André Soares
Radiation Department, Portuguese Oncology Institute of Porto, Portugal

Mário Dinis-Ribeiro
Portuguese Oncology Institute of Porto, Portugal

Eurico Monteiro
Portuguese Oncology Institute of Porto, Portugal

ABSTRACT

The perception of patients, ENT doctors and speech therapists about the experience of living with dysphagia and dysphonia after chemoradiotherapy (CRT) for oropharyngeal cancer is little studied. This perception is essential for improving care and influencing health policies. A descriptive qualitative study was carried out using semi-structured interviews. The interviews were recorded, transcribed and analysed thematically using NVivo®. The themes 'swallowing and dysphagia' and 'voice and dysphonia' emerged, with sub-themes related to quality of life, eating, socialising and communication. The most frequently reported difficulties were hoarseness, choking, thick saliva and coughing when drinking liquids. The need for a holistic approach and continuous monitoring from the start of treatment, involving patients and families, is emphasised.

DOI: 10.4018/979-8-3693-6432-1.ch010

INTRODUCTION

The subjective experience of individuals living with oropharyngeal cancer remains significantly under-explored, despite its critical importance for informing person-centered care and effectively supporting patients throughout the continuum of treatment and recovery. Over recent decades, researcher has increasingly focused on the effects of chemoradiotherapy (CRT) for head and neck cancers, identifying common complications such as dysphagia (swallowing difficulties) and dysphonia (voice impairment) (Checklin et al., 2020; Lazarus, 2009; Nund et al., 2015). While there has been a shift towards comprehending the functional outcomes and, to some extent, the patient's lived experience during rehabilitation, a comprehensive appreciation of the individual's journey is often still lacking (Nund et al., 2014; Nund et al., 2015; Soldatova & Mirza, 2019).

A significant lacuna in the extant literature pertains to the subjective experience of oropharyngeal cancer survivors specifically. Much of the existing research has focused on laryngeal cancers, thereby creating a knowledge deficit concerning non-laryngeal head and neck cancers, including oropharyngeal carcinoma (Soldatova & Mirza, 2019). The detrimental impact of dysphagia and dysphonia on quality of life (QoL) – manisfestating before, during, and after CRT, and persisting over extended periods – is well decumented (de Oliveira Faria et al., 2021; Nund et al., 2015). Consequently, a deeper understanding of how these functional impairments shape patients' daily lives, personal identities, and overall well-being is imperative (Nund et al., 2014).

Common voice chalenges reported by survivors include reduce vocal loudness, difficulties being heard in noisy environments, variability in vocal quality, and reduced speech intelligibility. Swallowing difficulties frequently entail the necessity for liquids to facilitate bolus passage, the perception of food becoming impeded, and persistent xerostomia (dry mouth) (Soldatova & Mirza, 2019). Although validated QoL questionnaires have been used to assess these issues (Hunter et al., 2013), such instruments may not adequately reflect the nuanced, context-specific, and personally meaningful aspects of an individual's lived experience (Sandelowski, 2000).

These instruments, while providing standardized and quantifiable data, are limited by their reliance on predefined categories and response options, potentially overlooking emergent and individualized themes that arise from personal narratives (Patton, 2002). This limitation is further underscored by studies identifying discrepancies between patients' self perceptions and the assessments of formal caregivers, such as speech-language pathologists (SLPs) and other health professionals (Constantinescu et al., 2017). Such discrepancy highlight the the critical need for research that prioritizes the voices of survivors, providing them with a platform to articulate their lived reality.

Consequently, it is imperative to explore voice and swallowing changes directly from the perspective of individuals living with oropharyngeal cancer, as clinical measurements of dysphagia and dysphonia alone may not fully capture the real-life impact of these conditions. A more profound and exhaustive comprehension will not only be benefit for the individuals affected but also inform healthcare professionals and caregivers, thereby facilitating more empathetic, tailored, and effective support across all stages of care trajectory (Nund et al., 2015).

The present chapter endeavors to contribute to this understanding by exploring the perspectives of both oropharyngeal cancer survivors and health professionals, specifically ear, nose, and throat (ENT) doctors and speech-language pathologists (SLPs). The ultimate aim is to inform the scientific community and promote improvements in the organization and delivery of healthcare services, fostering a more person-centered approach to oropharyngeal cancer care.

BACKGROUND

To better explore the experience of living with dysphagia and dysphonia in oropharyngeal cancer patients treated by non-surgical methods, survivors, and healthcare professionals (ENT doctors and SLPs) were enrolled using a person-centered approach in which the person is the focus based on Standards for Reporting Qualitative Research (SRQR) guidelines (O'Brien et al., 2014). Considering the individual, exploratory and subjective nature of the study, a phenomenological approach was chosen to access the everyday experience from an individual perspective (Patton, 2002). In the context of scientific inquiry, phenomenology aims to explore and describe the lived experiences of individuals to uncover the essence and meaning of a phenomenon as perceived by those who directly experience it.

This approach is particularly well-suited to studies seeking to understand subjective experiences, perceptions, and meanings as they are constructed within the participants' everyday lifeworld. Prioritising depth, context, and individual perspective over the generalizability of findings, phenomenology allows researchers to capture the richness and complexity of human experience (Creswell & Poth, 2018). Through "bracketing", the deliberate suspension of preconceived notions and theoretical assumptions, researchers endeavor to approach the phenomenon with an open perspective, focusing intently on participants' descriptions and narratives (Finlay, 2011). Data are typically gathered via in-depth interviews, and subsequent analysis involves identifying significant statements, clustering these into emergent themes, and ultimately developing a composite description that illuminates the essence of the experience (Moustakas, 1994). A phenomenological approach was therefore selected for the present study, given its inherent alignment with the exploratory, individual, and subjective nature of the research question. This methodology facilitates an in-depth understanding of the phenomenon as lived by the participants, fundamentally prioritizing their voices and experiences in the interpretation of meaning (van Manen, 2016).

The study was approved by the Ethics Committee of the Portuguese Oncology Institute (IPO), Porto (CES.265R/020), and participants were recruited in the ENT Department of this hospital after giving signed informed-consent. At the beginning of the study, the interview script was reviewed by a panel of experts and then administered to a member of each group (patients, SLPs and ENT doctors). All interviews were conducted and recorded by the first author on a face-to-face basis. The first author has academic and professional training to conduct an interview. Interviews were conducted in a medical office in the outpatient ENT clinic on a follow-up appointment. Only interviewees and the first author were present in the room. The interview script was based on a literature review as well as on the clinical practice of the researchers and consisted of open questions about a set of topics related to swallowing and voice disorders in cancer patients undergoing non-surgical treatment, along with a closed question related to symptoms.

Sample

To cover the diversity in oropharyngeal cancer patients, we followed maximum variation sampling - saturation - in which all data collected are considered relevant because they capture the core and central shared experiences of a population (Patton, 2002). The sociodemographic data collected were gender (male/female), age (in years), geographical location (district), education (level), number of months since treatment and TNM cancer staging. For the formal caregivers (ENT doctors and SLPs), data regarding gender (male/female), age (in years), geographical location (district) and years of professional experience were collected.

Participants

Patients with Oropharyngeal Cancer

All patients who underwent CRT with curative intent for oropharyngeal tumors in the IPO, Porto, were included. Exclusion criteria were previous surgical treatment; a pre-treatment condition with impact on voice or swallowing (e.g. neurological disease); palliative care; not giving informed consent; and cognitive deficit or difficulty understanding the Portuguese language.

Formal Caregivers

Formal caregivers recruited for this study included five ENT doctors and five SLPs with more than five years of experience in treating patients with oropharyngeal cancer who had undergone curative treatment with CRT. Exclusion criteria were not performing clinical functions in the study area and not consenting to participate. Details of maximum variation sampling are described in Table 1. Four men and one female participated in the patient group (aged 49-64 years; treatment duration = 3-6 years), the SLPs were all female (n = 5) and the ENT group comprised three men and two females.

Table 1. Socio-demographic data of the participants.

Socio-demographic data	Category	Patient	SLP	ENT
Sex	Male	4	0	3
	Female	1	5	2
Age	<50 years	2	4	3
	>50 years	3	1	2
Geographic location - district	Porto	1	2	3
	Braga	3	----	---
	Vila Real	1	----	----
	Faro	----	1	----
	Coimbra	-----	1	1
	Lisboa	-----	1	----
	Viana do Castelo	----	---	1
Time since complete treatment	<4 years old	3	-----	----
	>4 years old	2	-----	----
Years of work experience	<5 years old	-----	1	0
	>5 years old	----	4	5

Procedures

The patients participated through an individual semi-structured in-depth interview with the principal investigator; formal caregivers responded to the interview via email. A few topics were listed at the beginning of the interview to stimulate personal reflection (Patton, 2002). A script interview was used to ensure standardization and that all topics were covered, striving to maintain a fluid style in face-to-face interviews (Patton, 2002). Participants were encouraged to speak freely and comment on voice and swallowing changes and their caregivers experienced in their clinical practice. Face-to-face interviews lasted 15-40 minutes, were audio-recorded and transcribed for analysis by the first author and checked by the second author (Braun & Clarke, 2006). In the case of formal caregivers, they freely answered the interview script. The Ethics Committee of the IPO, Porto, authorized this study and each participant gave his/her consent.

Data Analysis

The literal transcripts of the patients' interviews and the formal caregivers' responses were analyzed using thematic analysis (Braun & Clarke, 2006). An inductive approach was followed to identify patterns in the data collected and directly extracted from the interviews (Braun & Clarke, 2006; Patton, 2002). Coding was performed with the support of NVivo® software. A list of categories emerged, which were refined by the co-investigator until consensus was reached. All interview transcripts were recoded using the category listing and themes were developed based on the relationships between the categories(Braun & Clarke, 2006). Using NVivo®, the number of references of a node was determined for each group, according to the coding of the user, and the coverage percentage, which indicates how much of the source content is coded at this node.

MAIN FOCUS OF THE CHAPTER

The aim of this study was to investigate the viewpoints and experience of living with swallowing and voice disturbances secondary to CRT treatment by SLPs and ENT doctors. Data resulting from the semi-structured interviews were used to answer this question. No repeat interviews were conducted. All stakeholders invited to participate accepted the invitation. Data were rich in reporting the experiences of living with swallowing and voice disorders. All patients were treated with CRT for oropharyngeal cancer, and most of the professionals had more than five years of professional experience in the care and follow-up of these patients.

Regarding the symptoms associated with CRT treatment experienced/selected by our participants, the results are shown in Graph 1. Hoarseness, getting food stuck in the throat, having thick saliva or sputum, choking while drinking liquids and coughing were the most frequently reported difficulties by all groups (patients, SLPs and ENT doctors). All symptoms except vomiting were listed by the present study cohort.

Table 2. Symptoms experienced/selected by participants.

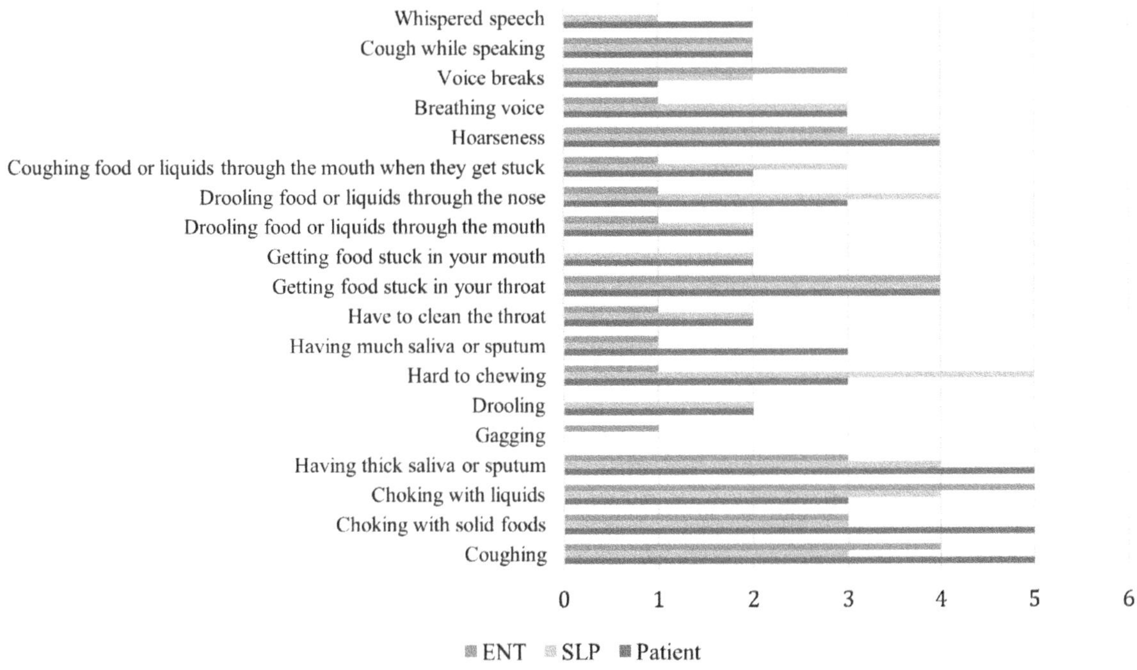

Thematic analysis revealed data regarding swallowing and voice disorders and the experience of living with them after non-surgical treatment for oropharyngeal tumors. Two overarching themes emerged from the interviews, detected by the two researchers, which captured the experiences of patients and caregivers. The first theme was "swallowing and dysphagia" and the second was "voice and dysphonia", which cut across all three groups (patients, SLPs and ENT doctors) and underpinned several sub-themes (Figure 1).

Figure 1. Themes and sub-themes merged.

Voice and dysphonia

- Communication
- Voice quality
- Social life
- Family life

Deglutition and dysphagia

- Burden
- Eating desire
- Fear
- Food selection
- Dysphagia symptoms
- Eating duration
- Social life
- Family life

According to the word frequency analysis a word cloud was formed with the main ideas addressed by the participants being used in the coding, such as deglutition disorders/swallowing, voice/vocal, difficulty(s) and life (Figure 2).

Figure 2. Word cloud from the qualitative analysis.

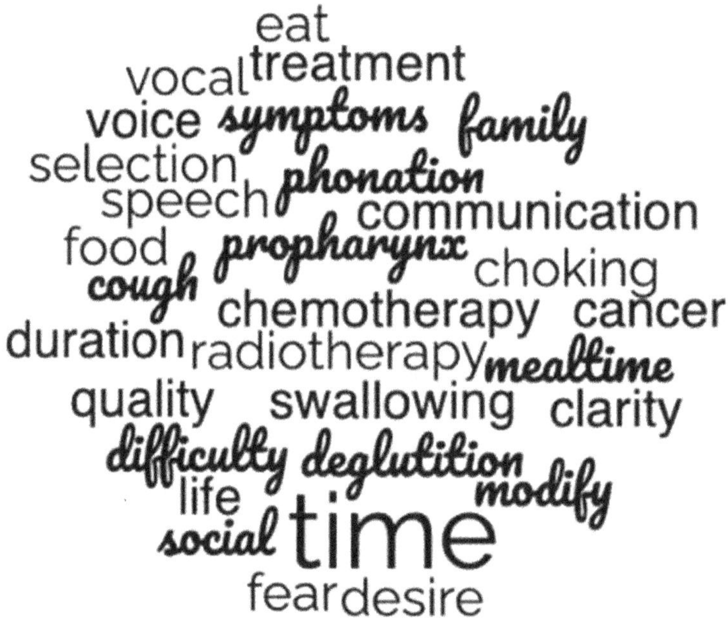

By analyzing the interviews, 273 coding's were performed, and some topics most frequently referenced by the participants (highest coverage) stand out, namely: "swallowing and dysphagia" and "burden" for both the SLP and patient groups;

"dysphagia symptoms", "communication" and "vocal quality" for all three groups; and "mealtime" for the ENT group (Table 2).

Table 3. Number of references and percentage of coverage for each of the codes assigned.

Codes	Nr. of references				% Coverage			
	ENT	SLP	Patient	Total	ENT	SLP	Patient	Total
Swallowing and dysphagia	5	6	6	17	5,43	6,67	6,67	18,77
Burden	5	5	5	15	5,43	5,56	5,56	16,55
Food selection	5	6	9	20	5,43	6,67	10	22,1
Desire to eat	5	5	5	15	5,43	5,56	5,55	16,54
Fears	5	5	5	15	5,43	5,56	5,56	16,55
Dysphagia symptoms	15	12	12	39	16,3	13,33	13,33	42,96
Mealtimes	6	5	5	16	6,52	5,56	5,56	17,64
Family life swallowing	5	5	5	15	5,43	5,56	5,56	16,55
Social life swallowing	4	5	5	14	4,35	5,56	5,56	15,47
Voice and dysphagia	5	5	5	15	5,43	5,56	5,56	16,55
Communication	10	10	10	30	10,87	11,11	11,11	33,09
Voice quality	12	12	9	33	13,04	13,33	10	36,37
Family life voice	5	4	5	14	5,43	4,44	5,56	15,43
Social life voice	5	5	5	15	5,43	5,56	5,56	16,55
Total	92	90	91	273	100	100	100	-----

P- Patient; SLP - Speech and Language Pathologist; ENT – otorhinolaryngologists; Nr. Of reference - number of references of a node for each group, according to the coding done by the user; % coverage - indicate how much of the source content is coded at this node.

The themes and sub-themes are described below, with examples of the participants' responses.

Theme 1: Swallowing and Dysphagia

The participants described changes in swallowing after treatment with CRT for oropharyngeal cancer, which were present over time, representing one of the themes of this thematic analysis. In this first theme, eight sub-themes emerged, all related to swallowing, whether with the swallowing action itsclf (symptoms), with eating (food selection, mealtimes, desire to eat) or with the impact (fears and burden) on their daily lives, both at the family and social levels. Tables 3-10 present the results in more detail. The presence of swallowing disorders reported in the three groups of participants is illustrated below:

... after the treatment with radio and chemotherapy I had difficulty swallowing ... [P1]
... after treatment with radio and chemotherapy the patient with oropharyngeal cancer presents difficulties in swallowing ... [ENT1]
... in general, after treatment with radio and chemotherapy the patient with oropharyngeal cancer presents difficulties in swallowing ... [SLP1]

Symptoms of Dysphagia

The sub-theme "dysphagia symptoms" stems from the symptoms that the participants mentioned throughout the interviews, related to difficulty in progression of the bolus, the quantity and quality of saliva, changes in taste and smell, the need to use strategies to facilitate swallowing, oral health, and the presence of signs of altered safety in swallowing and in the formation of the bolus (Table 3).

Table 4. Descriptions about the sub-theme dysphagia symptoms.

Patient	... the food would get stuck, I couldn't swallow, I choked very easily...I had no saliva, but then little by little it came back, I still get a dry mouth and I must hydrate a lot... [P1] ...at the beginning I could not smell or taste food... [P2] ...I don't get the whole flavor... [P3] ...cracked mouth, lost taste... [P4] ...apart from taste, my saliva also fails a lot, I must help swallow with water, until today... [P5]
SLP	...difficulty in the oral phase of swallowing due to xerostomia, loss of dental parts, difficulty in propelling the bolus, sensation of "food stuck in the throat", coughing and hawking when swallowing liquids (most of the time devalued by the patient) ... ... choking with liquids ... poor oral containment ... sensory alteration ... dry saliva and sputum ... mastication may be impaired ... tongue motility alteration ... pharyngeal motility alteration ... nasal regurgitation... [SLP1] ...difficulty in projecting food, feeling it gets stuck somewhere in the throat...everything tastes the same, metal... [SLP2] ...opening the mouth, pain when swallowing, taking a long time to eat, previous escape of food, difficulty in eating solid food, not being able to do oral feeding... complaints in swallowing dense solids and pasty... need to intersperse with liquid... staying with food in the mouth at the end of all meals that they cannot swallow and need to rinse the mouth at the end to clean... [SLP3] ...food uptake... trismus and in chewing and propelling food... radiomucositis... candidiasis... [SLP4]
ENT	...xerostomia ... difficulty in forming a bolus ... odynophagia very frequent ... mucositis ... [ENT1] ...pain, xerostomia, choking ... coughing, choking and sensation of food in the hypopharynx (especially small dry foods) ... [ENT2] ...xerostomia, difficulty swallowing dry food, food stuck in throat, choking episodes ... presence of thick/cloudy sputum and getting food stuck in throat because of xerostomia (most frequent sequelae of radiotherapy) [ENT3] ...coughing, choking when eating food and drinking liquid, has thicker saliva and sputum, problems chewing, must clear throat and gets food stuck in throat and coughs food or liquids out of mouth when they get stuck...anorexia [ENT4] ...odynophagia, dysphagia, aspiration pneumonia...dysgeusia...pain [ENT5]

P- Patient; SLP - Speech and Language Pathologist; ENT doctors

Food Selection

This sub-theme arises from the reported difficulty in preparing and selecting foods that they can swallow safely and without pain. The foods that most condition the diet of this cohort of participants are solid, dry, hard, and fibrous foods (Table 4).

Table 5. Descriptions of the sub-theme food selection.

Patient	... mainly more solid things, everything that is not creamy, food must be accompanied with sauces, for example [P1]. ... dry ... [P3] ... it's always soup, I miss eating nuts, lupins ... [P4]
SLP	...difficulty in selecting foods rich in protein, as there is difficulty in cooking more fibrous foods, such as meat... [SLP1] ...understanding which are the easiest to pass, so that they do not get lumpy... [SLP2] ... Difficulty in adapting the foods they like into the consistency they can eat... [SLP3] ... as to consistency, the amount of administration, eating certain foods at colder temperatures... [SLP4]
ENT	...balance between solid food versus xerostomia... avoidance of liquids (choking episodes... [ENT2] ...eliminating the drier, more solid foods from the diet, making a pasty/creamy diet... [ENT3] ...difficulty in food selection, e.g., in choice of textures... ... [ENT4] ...look for foods that I can swallow, usually those that cause less pain... ... [ENT5]

P- Patient; SLP - Speech and Language Pathologist; ENT doctors

Desire to Eat

When questioned, participants mentioned that their desire to eat was altered, either by issues related to the lack of food variability and consistency, to ensure safety at the time of swallowing, or by changes in taste and smell (Table 5).

Table 6. Descriptions about the sun-theme desire to eat.

Patient	...my desire to eat changed, but it gradually improved... ... [P3]
SLP	...the desire to eat changes, everything tastes the same, the metal... [SLP2] ...they often cannot eat what they want and do not like because the food is presented in another consistency... [SLP3]
ENT	...the urge to eat is diminished... [ENT2] ... sometimes there is even anorexia, but mostly it has to do with the associated dysgeusia and xerostomia, making meals sometimes a sacrifice... [ENT3] ...the will to eat changes and some patients present with anorexia... [ENT4] ...due to dysgeusia they lose their appetite, as well as the will to eat due to the complications that arise along the meal (pain, discomfort) ... [ENT5]

P- Patient; SLP - Speech and Language Pathologist; ENT doctors

Mealtimes

Another aspect considered to be impacted was "mealtimes", which was frequently mentioned by the participants, usually due to the difficulties inherent in the process of chewing and swallowing, which proved to be time consuming (Table 6).

Table 7. Descriptions about the sub-theme mealtime.

Patient	...at the beginning it took longer at meals... [P1] ...it takes longer during meals... [P2] ...it takes me much longer now... [P4] ...I think I even eat faster now; I changed it was quantity because I eat less... [P45]
SLP	...increased meal duration, with associated fatigue... [SLP1] ...meals are longer in the initial phase; with the continuity of RT, they sometimes end up giving up VO (oral route) feeding ... [SLP2] ...very long time/duration of meals due to all swallowing mechanics being altered and use of strategies to be able to swallow... [TF3]
ENT	...takes longer due to dysphagia caused by mucositis ... [ENT1] ...the mealtime is increased ... [ENT2] ...meals take longer... ... [ENT3] ...time/duration of meals is changed. If switched to alternative route, meals take less time. If he keeps the oral route, sometimes the mealtime takes longer due to the added difficulties... [ENT5]

P- Patient; SLP - Speech and Language Pathologist; ENT doctors

Fear

After CRT treatment, many participants mention fear of relapse and fear related to comorbidities associated with dysphagia, namely pneumonia, asphyxia or choking (Table 7).

Table 8. Descriptions about the sub-theme fears.

Patient	...at that time yes, I was afraid, I was afraid of not getting it right, but I believed, an optimistic way of thinking, I did not consider myself to be ill without a solution, that it was temporary... ... [P3] ...I had fears of not recovering, initially I was always hoping to get my taste buds back, but I don't think about it so much anymore... [P5]
SLP	...fear of food getting stuck in the throat and choking... [SLP1] ...they are afraid of dying from losing so much weight and not getting it back... [SLP2] ...they are afraid of choking, but a large proportion of the users think it goes well and take a big risk... [SLP3] ...they are afraid for the fight against the oncological disease; the having to use NG... [SLP4]
ENT	...they have fears, of choking... the fact that they are hungry and are afraid to eat, because they fear the risk of choking... [ENT1]

P- Patient; SLP - Speech and Language Pathologist; ENT doctors

Burden

Participants were unanimous about the burden of dysphagia on persons' lives after CRT treatment (Table 8).

Table 9. Descriptions about the sub-theme burden.

Patient	...difficulties in swallowing were a burden for me... [P1] ...have been a burden to me... [P4]
SLP	...swallowing difficulties are a burden for the patient... [SLP5]
ENT	...swallowing difficulties are a burden ... [ENT1]

P- Patient; SLP - Speech and Language Pathologist; ENT doctors

Social Life: Swallowing

When asked about eating in public and their social participation, the answers point to a decrease in most situations, with avoidance associated with food selection and signs of dysphagia (coughing, choking) (Table 9).

Table 10. Descriptions about the sub-theme social life - swallowing.

Patient	...at the beginning ...it didn't come out, I don't know if it was because of the difficulty in swallowing, but I travelled regularly and had to deal with the problem, I went with NG for congresses... [P1] ...I can't control it because I don't know when I'm going to choke, if it's more solid or tastes bad it can usually happen...[P2] ...in that period of treatment, I did not leave the house, I had no strength or willpower... I was driving, it was only at the end of the last 15 that my daughter and son kept me company... [P3] ... I don't feel like going out to eat so often because the food doesn't mean anything to me... [P5]
SLP	...decreased participation in family and friend gatherings, and going to restaurants due to eating difficulties, bearing in mind that the texture of the food sometimes has to be changed, and users do not always feel comfortable with the exposure of eating difficulties... [SLP1] ...they do not leave the house for home, and often do not like to eat at the same time as the rest of the family... [SLP2] ...they stop having the meal with the family at the table and go out to eat... [SLP3] ...if they use NG or have difficulties many have reservations at meals in front of others. Therefore, they sometimes do not go to social gatherings that also include the meal... [SLP4] ...they inhibit themselves from social relationships and deprive themselves of family gatherings... [SLP5]
ENT	...the patient feels ashamed... [ENT1] ...avoid dining out and ashamed of dining in a group - social boundary... [ENT2] ...greatly affects social life, in the sense that the patient feels ashamed of the way he eats, with associated coughing, regurgitation, by the very selection of food and the time it takes to eat... [ENT3]

P- Patient; SLP - Speech and Language Pathologist; ENT doctors

Family Life: Swallowing

When asked about the family dynamics associated with swallowing disorders, the answers, as in a wider context, point to changes related to the need to adapt food preparation and to avoidance, with a tendency to decrease participation in family events and in routines related to meals. However, the family emerged as an important element of support (Table 10).

Table 11. Descriptions about the sub-theme family life - swallowing.

Patient	...at the beginning having no previous history who is with us must learn how to produce food for a cancer patient... [P2] ...the woman had to change the cooking and adapt the food to my difficulties... [P5]
SLP	...decreased participation in family events... [SLP1] ...do not share meals with family... [SLP2] ...family life is affected by the need to make several different dishes, different consistencies, concern about how to prepare meals and what foods the wearer can eat... [SLP3]
ENT	...change in the family's eating routines... [ENT1] ...takes longer to eat, the feeling of upset/challenge due to needing different food/meal... [ENT2] ... eats separately and requires appropriate diet just for you... [ENT4] ...often do not have their meals in common with the rest of the family members... ... [ENT5]

P- Patient; SLP - Speech and Language Pathologist; ENT doctors

Theme 2: Voice and Dysphonia

Participants also described changes in "voice and dysphonia" after treatments with CRT for oropharyngeal cancer, which represents the second theme of this thematic analysis. In this second theme, four sub-themes emerged, all related to voice, whether with communication in general (ability to make themselves heard and understood), changes in voice quality (dysphonia symptoms) or with impact on their daily lives, both at family and social levels. Tables 11-14 present the results in more detail. Below, we illustrate the presence of voice disorders reported in the three groups of participants:

... My voice sounded different after the radio and chemotherapy, it's different ... [P1]

... my voice became hoarse, thicker, slower ... [P2]

... the patient's voice changes after being treated with radio and chemotherapy ... [ENT2]

... the patient after treatment with radio and chemotherapy loses vocal projection ... [ENT4]

... After treatment with radio and chemotherapy the voice of the users is diminished in volume, with gaps in the voice ... [SLP2]

Communication

This sub-theme stems from the participants' statements mentioning factors that hindered their ability to communicate, namely in noisy environments, changes related to saliva characteristics, which limited articulatory ability, and phone communication, where they felt difficulties in expression (Table 11).

Table 12. Descriptions about the sub-theme communication.

Patient	...people had difficulty understanding what I was saying, when I am tired it is worse, especially at home at the end of the day they notice... [P1] ...if I am in noisy places people find it more difficult to hear me... [P2] ...difficulty when I speak for a long time with lack of saliva, it even atrophies me, I can't find the words, I always must drink... [P3] ...people had difficulty understanding me... [P4] ...in noisy environments it becomes more difficult for them to hear me... [P4]
SLP	...when there is more background noise, hospital corridors always have a lot of background noise, patients find it difficult to make themselves heard... [SLP2] ...they have difficulties in making themselves heard on the phone, in noisy environments or if the person listening is not paying attention... [SLP3] ...patients have difficulties in making themselves heard in noisy places, if the interlocutor is not looking at them/ wearing a mask does not facilitate... [SLP4] ...Sometimes people find it difficult to understand the patient... [SLP5]
ENT	...the patient has difficulty making himself heard, especially on the telephone... [ENT1] ...in noisy environment, patients have difficulty making themselves heard... ... [ENT2] ...sometimes people have difficulty understanding the patient... [ENT3]

P- Patient; SLP - Speech and Language Pathologist; ENT doctors

Voice Quality

During the interviews, several vocal characteristics associated with CRT treatment in patients with oropharyngeal cancer were listed by the three groups of participants, namely: hoarseness, breathiness, harshness, changes in vocal frequency and intensity, resonance, and vocal projection (Table 12).

Table 13. Descriptions about the sub-theme vocal quality.

Patient	...I find it hoarser, there are words that are difficult to say more, less clear... [P1] ...hoarse, thicker, slower... [P2] ...I felt it scratching... [P4] ...stayed hoarse to this day... [P5] ...I feel the voice inside sounds lower... [P3]
SLP	...hoarser, rougher, and blown out voice, with reduction of the frequency amplitude and vocal intensity... increase of the roughness associated to soprosity... compromising the phonation in the acute phase, by inflammation not only of the vocal folds, but also of the oropharynx, as well as in the medium and long term by alteration of the myoelastic characteristics of the vocal folds, and edema of the vocal folds that sometimes does not revert, translating into hoarseness. The blowing voice and speech with air can occur due to alteration of the myoelastic characteristics of the vocal folds, which provokes a reduction in the vibration frequency of the mucous wave, and from there the blowing. It can also occur due to vocal fold paralysis caused by recurrent laryngeal nerve damage caused by radiation. Whispering speech can often arise in the acute phase of radiotherapy, and when there is laryngeal nerve involvement... [SLP1] ...diminished volume with voice failure... voice becomes more "dirty" sometimes due to saliva quality... [SLP2] ...voice quality/clarity changes, becomes more nasalized depending on the location of RT... [SLP3] ...unless they must use SNG there may be slight symptoms due to oedema of the retrocricoid region... discreet hoarseness and murmuring, there may be a wet voice if there are alterations in swallowing/ accumulation of food at the laryngeal level (vallecula and piriform sinuses) and because of alterations in the pharyngeal and esophageal phase due to radiomucositis... Because of excessive muscular tension/ anxiety, because of previous habits which may not favor the voice during the RT period, such as speaking fast, with strong intensity and being very talkative. [SLP4]
ENT	...the clarity of the voice is altered; the voice is more muffled... rougher and there are breaks in the voice... [ORL1] ...the voice besides being rougher and more muffled, more severe presents breaks by the associated mucositis and the frank decrease of salivary secretion in the oral cavity and oropharynx, as well as the accumulation of thicker secretions in the oro and hypopharynx and larynx... [ENT1] ...presents hoarseness, roughness, decreased vocal projection... becomes rougher... [ENT2] ...gets a lower timbre, roughness, and less intensity/difficulty in vocal projection... voice quality decreases ... patients notice voice alteration, but rarely value these symptoms, when they present concomitant problems in swallowing... [ENT3] ...voice quality worsens, loses sonority... [ENT4] ...wet voice and dysphonia (+ harshness) ... [ENT5]

P- Patient; SLP - Speech and Language Pathologist; ENT doctors

Social Life: Voice

When asked about the implications of voice alterations on their daily life, we came across decreased communicative intention, isolation, and work impact (Table 13).

Table 14. Descriptions about the sub-theme social life - voice.

Patient	...I take some care when I go out and when I am with other people, but I try to be prepared for this difficulty, and it has already become normal... [P1] ...the changes in the voice have always affected, although now not as much as in the beginning, because at the time it was a catastrophic scenario... [P2]
SLP	...can interfere at work level if there is increased vocal use or in noisier environments... [SLP1] ...does not want to speak in public... [SLP2] ...patients become embarrassed and isolate themselves... [SLP3] ...may not be able to speak for the same number of hours due to vocal fatigue or excess muscle tension... avoiding conversation either face-to-face or on the telephone... [SLP4]
ENT	...less desire to socialize... shame and vocal fatigue... [ENT2] ...can lead to isolation... [ENT4] ...the patient with vocal alteration sometimes inhibits himself from social relationships because he cannot be heard and is unnoticeable to others... ... [ENT5]

P- Patient; SLP - Speech and Language Pathologist; ENT doctors

Family Life: Voice

In terms of the impact of voice alterations on the family dynamics, our findings indicate the presence of social avoidance and reduced vocal endurance. These observations highlight the significant role of the family as a crucial source of support during such circumstances (Table 14).

Table 15. Descriptions about the sub-theme family life - voice.

Patient	...in convivial situations I can't talk for a long time... [D2]
SLP	...can affect day-to-day life, depending on the characteristics of the household (communication with the elderly, education of younger children, larger house) ... [SLP1] ... when the family does not understand it ... ... [SLP3]
ENT	...most of the time has little impact the voice per se ... [ENT1] ...less willingness to socialize ... shame and vocal fatigue ... [ENT2] ...isolation, but less than at the social level... [ENT4]

P- Patient; SLP - Speech and Language Pathologist; ENT doctors

The results are discussed according to the literature, clinical implications, and recommended future research. The aim of this study was to investigate the perception of patients, SLPs and ENT doctors about the effects of non-surgical treatments in patients with oropharyngeal cancer. Five patients treated with CRT for oropharyngeal cancer, as well as five SLPs and five ENT doctors with experience in caring for these patients, participated in the study by responding to interviews. From the interviews, two main themes were identified, related to swallowing and voice changes. This study provided a patient, SLP and ENT focused description of the effects of non-surgical treatments for oropharyngeal tumors as an opportunity to improve service delivery, as well as highlighting positive aspects and limitations

(Messing et al., 2019). Despite this, and some studies on the patient's perspective and a biopsychosocial approach (Dornan et al., 2021; Fitchett et al., 2018; Jacobson, 2018; Lang et al., 2013), this research sought to understand and compare the data from three groups (patient, SLP and ENT).

Analysis of patient's data revealed that sociodemographic factors, including age, gender, and family support, saliently influenced their perception and experience of swallowing and voice changes. Older participants in this study reported a tendency to socialize less during mealtimes, often describing these occasions as periods of discomfort or isolation. This tendency was often attributed to diminished adaptability and apprehensions of choking or coughing. Male participants frequently highlighted the loss of autonomy and the frustration of relying on others for meal preparation or effective communication. In contrast, the sole female participant in this cohort placed greater emphasis on the emotional burden experienced and the perceived invisibility of her voice difficulties to others. Furthermore, despite having transitioned beyond the acute phase of treatment, participants consistently reported significant ongoing impacts on their quality of life, particularly in the domains of social interaction and food enjoyment. This observation suggests that the duration since treatment completion does not invariable equate to full functional or emotional recovery. Notably, patients with reported robust family support tended to exhibit more positive coping strategies and a more pronounced desire to re-engage socially. These latter findings underscore the potentially protective role of strong social and familial networks in facilitating long-term rehabilitation and adjustment.

Analysis of the answers of the participants in this study allowed us to verify the presence of changes in swallowing and voice (Lazarus et al., 2007; Nund et al., 2015; Nund et al., 2014), which may be prolonged over time, affecting daily activities and interactions, thus impacting QoL (Kraaijenga et al., 2016).

One of the difficulties listed by the participants is related to food selection: after the treatments, they must choose foods with a certain consistency or taste, either due to swallowing safety limitations or dysgeusia; solid and dry foods are often rejected (Ottosson et al., 2013); and swallowing difficulties in turn interfere with the meal duration, which becomes longer (Nund et al., 2014; Ottosson et al., 2013). The limitations in food selection and taste affect the ability to enjoy the action of eating and drinking (Ottosson et al., 2013) and therefore the pleasure that eating can bring, impacting on socialization, with implications in terms of QoL and decreased social interactions at mealtimes. Another influenced aspect is related to the desire to eat - the desire and pleasure that is removed from eating - with food providing merely a nourishing and hydrating action, as previous studies have shown (Nund et al., 2014; Ottosson et al., 2013). Reported in previous studies, mealtimes and their preparation may be altered, with the patient avoiding family events or even not having meals at the table with the family. Participants describe feeling a loss of family mealtimes, isolating themselves, with an impact on family dynamics and their relationships (Baijens et al., 2021; Dornan et al., 2021; Nund et al., 2014).

The fear of disease relapse and course is a factor that is present in these patients, as well as uncertainty about the effects of the toxicity of long-term treatments (Nund et al., 2014; Ottosson et al., 2013). Social and even family avoidance occurs due to the difficulties related to the textures and flavors that they can ingest, as most restaurants do not have adapted options. The presence of feelings of shame, coughing and choking during meals also contributes to the social and family impact, as reported by some participants and in previous studies (Baijens et al., 2021; Nund et al., 2014; Ottosson et al., 2013).

Patients decrease the time and number of interactions, both due to swallowing and communication disorders (Baijens et al., 2021). All these changes have a negative impact on the perception of living with swallowing disorders, which are felt as a burden in their lives, as other research has shown (Nund et al., 2014; Ottosson et al., 2013).

Consistent with previous research, participants in this study described several frequent and common vocal quality changes after treatment, such as hoarseness, poor pitch, vocal fatigue, and xerostomia (Nund et al., 2015). The participants in these studies addressed a few challenges in daily life arising from the vocal changes, which in turn have implications for communication effectiveness, decreasing social participation and interaction, and thus affecting both social and family life due also to not being understood by the message receiver. Patients become frustrated because people do not ask for clarification, but rather ignore it, and so the patient feels left out of the conversation. In this context also, noisy environments were frequently mentioned as having an impact on keeping the conversation going. These communicative difficulties occur not only in a social context, namely at social gatherings and at work level, but also among family, with shared emphasis on familiar relationships and their roles and responsibilities in the family dynamic. At the social level, communication difficulties decrease participation in social gatherings or talking on the phone, leading to the avoidance of communication, as if life were on hold (Constantinescu et al., 2017; Nund et al., 2015).

About the analysis of symptoms, according to Graph 1 these were similar between the groups, showing that even when CRT does not directly affect the larynx, vocal changes such as hoarseness occur (Kraaijenga et al., 2016). The same is true of swallowing, with symptoms such as getting food stuck in the throat, having thick saliva or sputum, choking when drinking liquids and coughing (Zebralla et al., 2021). Thus, clinicians should attend to the symptoms reported by patients and make the respective referrals to other specialties. It is possible that by using a larger cohort of participants, with similar characteristics, different data could be produced. In this study, quantitative assessment was not able to verify a reduction of QoL. One of the limitations was related to the length of the answers in the interviews, because some participants were quite concise. Another limitation relates to the small number of participants in each group; furthermore, in the case of the group of patients, there was only one woman. This may reflect the prevalence of the disease in the male population (Mehanna et al., 2010) and the eventual differences in perception between men and women. Another aspect was the participation of patients with palliative intent, which is suggested for study in future research. In addition, no distinction was made between acute and long-term post-treatment experience.

The participants in this study consistently reported that both swallowing and voice disorders significantly impacted their professional identities and their capacity to return to work. The described communication challenges, including vocal fatigue, hoarseness, and reduced intelligibility which consequently limited their ability to engage effectively in work-related conversations, lead meetings, or perform customer-facing tasks. For instance, one participant described a deliberate avoidance of telephone calls due to embarrassment associated with voice changes, while in another noted that frequent coughing episodes during meals induced anxiety in social work settings. Swallowing issues also contributed to a sense of vulnerability in professional environments, particularly when eating with colleagues or managing prolonged speaking demands. Cumulatively, these limitations prompted some individuals to curtail their working hours, transition to different roles, or, in some cases, exit the workforce entirely. To address these barriers, occupational rehabilitation strategies should include interdisciplinary care involving speech-language pathologists, occupational therapists, and vocational counselors. A comprehensive treatment approach is imperative, encompassing voice therapy tailored to specific work-related demands training in alternative communication strategies, fatigue management and techeniques, and structured, gradual return-to-work programs developed in collaboration with employers. Furthermore, the provision of psychological support and the implementation of peer mentoring programs have demonstrated a pivotal role in the restoration of confidence among this patient population. Crucially, enhancing employer awareness of the often subtle yet pervasive consequences of head and neck cancer treatment is fundamental to cultivating inclusive and supportive work environments that accommodate the needs of survivors.

Comparative Analysis Between the Groups

This comparative. analysis of perspectives from patients, SLPs, and ENT specialists reveals critical areas of convergence and divergence, collectively underscoring the importance of coordinated interdisciplinary care in oropharyngeal cancer survivorship.

A central theme emerging from the data was the profound disruption caused by dysphagia. Patients consistently reported significant distress, encompassing dietary restrictions, a diminished enjoyment of eating, and persistent fears, particularly of choking or aspiration. These experiences were strong echoed by SLPs who emphasized the frequency and severity of post-treatment dysphagia symptoms, including xerostomia, pain, and delayed swallow reflexes. Both patients and SLPs identified mealtimes as emotionally and socially charged moments, often characterized by anxiety or social withdrawal. In contrast, ENTs, while acknowledging dysphagia, tended to focus on primary oncologic treatment outcomes, sometimes underestimating the long-term functional and psychosocial impacrt or the persistent nature of dysphagia, especially when objective laryngoscopic findings did not fully align with patients' subjective reports of suffering.

Further elaborating on dysphagia, both patients and SLPs agreed emphasized its "invisible" nature - a distressing symptom that, dispite often lacking overt external signs, profoundly affects family life and social participation, particularly in contexts involving shared meals or public eating. In contrast, ENTs were less likely to describe the social and emotional dimensions of dysphagia in such depth. This discrepancy highlights a potential gap in holistic patient assessment and care, reinforcing the need for structured, empathetic communication across disciplines to fully appreciate the patient's lived experience (Govender et al., 2017; Nund et al., 2014).

A related subtheme concerned the challenging process of relearning to eat and swallow following treatment. Patients described extensive efforts to adapt, such as modifying food texture, adopting lower eating paces, and avoiding social dining situations, all reflecting the significant burden and meticulous mealtime management dysphagia imposes. SLPs reported patients through these compensatory strategies while also noting significant variability in individual motivation and emotional resilience. This potential divergence between clinical rehabilitation goals and patient's readiness or capacity for intervention suggests the need for highly personalized care plans, developed through shared decision-making processes that respect patient autonomy and psychosocial status(Patterson & Lawton, 2023; Manduchi et al., 2024).

Regarding voice and dysphonia, communication challenges were reported less commonly by patients than swallowing problems; however, when present, they deeply affected social roles, family dynamics, and self-perception. Issues, such as hoarseness or reduced vocal strength, led to difficulty being understood, participating in conversations, or returning to occupational duties. SLPs typically identified these challenges early, especially in patients with laryngeal involvement or extensive mucosal damage from treatment. ENTs, on the other hand, addressed these issues primarily through laryngoscopic evaluation and, where indicated, surgical or pharmacological interventions. This difference in approach highlights the importance of systematically integrating functional voice rehabilitation, led bt SLPs, into standard post-treatment care pathways to address the functional impact of dysphonia.

Importantly, while all participants groups identified interdisciplinary collaboration as essential for optimal care, each group also described significant fragmentation in its pratical application. Patients reported receiving conflicting advice or feeling "lost among specialists". SLPs noted challenges such as delayed referrals or linsuficient follow-up from ENTs. Meanwhile, some ENTs expressed uncertainty regarding the precise scope and optimal timing of SLP interventions. These findings suggest a persistent disconnect in interdisciplinary care, despite shared recognition of its importance. Optimizing patient outcomes in oropharyngeal cancer survivorship requires a more robustly coordinated, interdisciplinary model. Such a model should promote early and systematic involvement of SLPs, establish clear protocols for structured handovers between professionals, and integrate patient-reported outcome measures (PROMs) into routine follow-up assessments. While this study offers a rich insights into lived experiences and clinical perceptions surrounding oropharyngeal cancer susvivoiship, its exploratory nature and limited sample size constrains the generalizability of its findings. The convergence across groups regarding the significant burden and often "invisible" nature of dysphagia, alongside the divergence in perceived priorities and timelines for intervention, strongly underscores the pressing need for interdisciplinary, patient-centered approaches. These approaches must holistically address both physiological and psychosocial dimensions of recovery to truly support individuals navigating life after oropharyngeal cancer.

A series of **clinical actions** could been proposed on the basis of patient experiences with the aim of enhancing the quality of care and QoL for persons undergoing CRT for oropharyngeal cancer. First, patients emphasized the need for earlier and clearer information about potential long-term swallowing and voice consequences, highlighting the importance of pre-treatment counseling and expectation management. The integration of SLPs at the point of diagnosis has the potential to facilitate early assessment, personalized education, and baseline functional documentation. Furthermore, patients reported feelings of isolation and a lack of preparation for managing symptoms with the domestic environment underscore the necessity for structured post-treatment follow-up and the strategic utilization of remote support tools, such as mobile applications or telehealth check-ins. A comprehensive approach to dysphagia therapy should incorporate specific exercises alongside counseling on dietary adaptation, emotional coping mechanisms, and strategies for social reintegration. Similarly, voice rehabilitation must address both technical and psychosocial aspects, implementing strategies to rebuild communication confidence. Finally, interdisciplinary collaboration - particularly between oncologists, SLPs, and ENTs – is essential to ensure a more holistic and continuous care experience that aligns with patients' lived realities beyond the completion of acute treatment.

This study underscores the pivotal role of patient narratives in fostering more empathetic and responsive clinical care, emphasizing the necessity to incorporate patient-centered listening into the training of health professionals. The insights shared by patients reveal gaps in communication, emotional support, and continuity of care. These issues can only be addressed by professionals who are attuned not just to clinical outcomes but also to lived experiences. Consequently, it is recommended that health education curricula - particularly in SLP, ENT, oncology, and nursing - include structured training on patient-centered communication, interdisciplinary collaboration, and rehabilitation planning based on functional and psychosocial needs. The integration of case-based learning, reflective practice, and direct exposure to patient testimonies has the potential to facilitate the development of the sensitivity and skills required to promote holistic recovery in individuals undergoing complex treatments such as CRT. Such curricular emphasis would cultivate a new generation of health professionals better equipped to deliver care that aligns clinical objectives with patient well-being and individualized needs.

We tried to follow a maximum variation sample to capture the central themes across a range of patients, SLPs and ENT doctors, and all patient participants were recruited from the same service so that their experiences and perceptions were representative compared with those obtained from professionals at different institutions (Patton, 2002).

The findings of this study align with current healthcare paradigms that emphasize patient-centered care, the integratiom of Patient-Reported Outcome Measures (PROMs), and interdisciplinary collaboration as foundations pillars for improving quality of care. Patient narratives, as captured in this research, disclosed functional and emotional dimensions that are not always captured through clinical observation alone. In this context, PROMs have the potential to be systematically integrated into follow-up protocols, thereby facilitating more effective tracking of long-term functional and psychosocial outcomes after CRT. This, in turn, could lead to the development of a more responsive and adaptive care model.

However, the study underscores critical deficiencies in the healthcare system, particularly the absence of structured protocols for long-term rehabilitation and inadequate support for patients post-discharge. The reports of patients feeling unprepared to manage symptoms at home, in conjunction with the inconsistent interdisciplinary coordination, highlight systemic weaknesses in continuity of care. These challenges are further compounded by the fragmented communication between ENTs and SLPs, which includes delays in referrals and uncertainty about roles. This, in turn, compromises the efficiency and effectiveness of interventions. The European White Paper on Oropharyngeal Dysphagia offers pertinent suggestinons for intervention in this domain (Baijens et al., 2021). In light of the themes identified in the present study, the following practical recommendations are proposed:

- The integration of SLPs at the time of diagnosis is of paramount importance, as it facilitates the provision of anticipatory guidance and baseline assessments.
- The development and implementation of clesr, interdisciplinary care pathways are imperative. These pathways must encompass standardized referral timelines and structured handover procedures between healthcare professionals.
- The expansion of training programs is imperative to include modules on patient-centered communication, interdisciplinary teamwork, and the functional impact of dysphagia and dysphonia.
- The implementation of remote monitoring strategies, such as telehealth follow-ups and digital symptom diaries, is crucial to extend support beyond the hospital setting.
- The promotion of awareness campaigns and continuing education for health professionals and employers is essential for fostering a greater understanding of the hidden impacts of oropharyngeal cancer treatment.
- These recommendations reflect an opportunity to align clinical practices with the real-world needs and priorities of patients, ultimately supporting holistic and sustained recovery.

LIMITATIONS OF THE STUDY AND FUTURE RESEARCH DIRECTIONS

It is imperative to acknowledge the limitations of this study when interpreting the findings and assessing their applicability to broader populations. A salient limitation pertains to the modest and imbalanced sample size, comprising five oropharyngeal cancer patients, five SLPs, and five ENTs. The preponderance of male participants and the absence of diversity in variables such as treatment duration and family support serve to limit the generalizability of the results and restrict the representativeness of different patient and professional experiences. The methodological decision to employ a small, qualitative sample was deliberate, aiming to facilitate an exhaustive thematic analysis. However, future research endeavors should consider incorporating larger and more heterogeneous samples to enhance the generalizability of the findings. This would facilitate a more comprehensive understanding of the variability of lived experiences across different clinical and social contexts.

Another methodological limitation pertains to the mode of data collection. Patient interviews were conducted in person, while the interviews with SLPs and ENTs specialists were completed asynchronously via email. While this approach enabled the involvement of professionals with limited availability and facilitated thoughtful responses, it introduced inconsistency in data collection methods. The disparities in format might have exerted an influence on the depth, spontaneity, and richness of the data. In the interest of enhancing the comparability and overall quality of the data, it is recommended that the method of data collection be standardized across participant groups in future studies. Synchronous virtual interviews are a viable solution that would facilitate this standardization.

Furthermore, the cross-sectional nature of this study provides only a limited perspective on the experiences of participants after treatment. Future research endeavors would benefit from a prospective design, entailing the conduction of interviews at regular intervals throughout the treatment and recovery process. This approach would facilitate a more dynamic and reliable analysis of how experiences with dysphagia and dysphonia evolve over time, offering a deeper understanding of their trajectory and impact on QoL.

Incorporating nutritional status as a variable is also recommended in future studies, particularly to examine differences between patients who rely solely on oral feeding and those who do not. A comprehensive understanding of the interplay between feeding modality and overall well-being may offer valuable insights into patients' physical, psychological, and social experiences.

Moreover, the findings of this study underscore the necessity for modifications in clinical practice. Patients should undergo systematic monitoring from the commencement of their oncological treatment, encompassing not only physical symptoms but also their personal perceptions and lived experiences with dysphagia and/or dysphonia. These conditions have the potential to exert a substantial influence on various aspects of psychosocial functioning, including socialization, personal relationships, and self-concept. Consequently, they can exert a notable impact on QoL. The implementation of validated QoL assessment tools in routine clinical care would facilitate healthcare providers' identification of patients in need of support, education, or rehabilitation to better adapt to post-treatment changes (Kraaijenga et al., 2016; Zebralla et al., 2021).

Finally, it is imperative to consider the role of families and support networks. It has been demonstrated that alterations in mealtime routines and communication can profoundly affect patients and their families (Dornan et al., 2021; Zebralla et al., 2021). Future studies should explore the experiences and needs of these networks, as they often represent crucial sources of emotional and practical support (Lang et al., 2013). The provision of structured education and information, such as through support groups, has been demonstrated to facilitate a more realistic adjustment of expectations and assist both patients and their families in navigating the challenges associated with treatment and recovery.

CONCLUSION

The patient's perspective is of inestimable value in expanding our understanding of how individuals experience swallowing and voice challenges across various domains of life, including family, social, and professional. Recovery from CRT for oropharyngeal cancer is often protracted and unpredictable, engendering doubt and emotional strain for both patients and caregivers. This study underscores the need for extended, personalized follow-up care that prioritizes swallowing and voice rehabilitation - not just during acute phases, but throughout the survivorship trajectory. Furthermore, it underscores the extensive deleterious effects that these conditions can exert, a phenomenon that has been repeatedly corroborated by patients, SLPs, and ENTs. The alignment observed across participant groups lends further credence to the validity of these findings and underscores the pressing need to develop interdisciplinary, person-centered responses.

These insights are in alignment with contemporary clinical and educational trends that emphasize holistic, integrated, and patient-driven care. Within the thematic framework of Holistic Approaches to Health Recovery, this chapter makes a significant contribution by illustrating how the subjective experience of dysphagia and dysphonia -often overlooked - can inform not only clinical practices but also the structure of healthcare systems. This knowledge should inform training curricula, with the objective of cultivating professionals who are better prepared to listen to and advocate for patients' individual trajectories. Moreover, the findings reveal systemic challenges in oncology care networks, including fragmented service delivery and inadequate rehabilitation pathways. These findings underscore the necessity for more coordinated and empathetic models of care. The management of care based solely on observable disorders is insufficient; meaningful recovery and support can only be offered through holistic engagement with the lived experience of illness.

ACKNOWLEDGMENT

This research received no specific grant from any funding agency in the public, commercial, or not-for-profit sectors.

REFERENCES

Baijens, L. W. J., Walshe, M., Aaltonen, L. M., Arens, C., Cordier, R., Cras, P., Crevier-Buchman, L., Curtis, C., Golusinski, W., Govender, R., Eriksen, J. G., Hansen, K., Heathcote, K., Hess, M. M., Hosal, S., Klussmann, J. P., Leemans, C. R., MacCarthy, D., Manduchi, B., & Clavé, P. (2021). European white paper: Oropharyngeal dysphagia in head and neck cancer. *European Archives of Oto-Rhino-Laryngology*, *278*(2), 577–616. DOI: 10.1007/s00405-020-06507-5 PMID: 33341909

Braun, V., & Clarke, V. (2006). Using thematic analysis in psychology. *Qualitative Research in Psychology*, *3*(2), 77–101. DOI: 10.1191/1478088706qp063oa

Checklin, M., Bain, J., Bath, L., & Lethbridge, K. (2020). Patients' Perspectives on What Makes a Better Care Experience While Undergoing Treatment for Oropharyngeal Dysphagia Secondary to Head and Neck Cancer. *Dysphagia*, *35*(4), 702–716. DOI: 10.1007/s00455-019-10077-y PMID: 31748827

Constantinescu, G., Rieger, J., Winget, M., Paulsen, C., & Seikaly, H. (2017). Patient Perception of Speech Outcomes: The Relationship Between Clinical Measures and Self-Perception of Speech Function Following Surgical Treatment for Oral Cancer. *American Journal of Speech-Language Pathology*, *26*(2), 241–247. DOI: 10.1044/2016_AJSLP-15-0170 PMID: 28359083

Creswell, J. W., & Poth, C. N. (2018). *Qualitative inquiry and research design: Choosing among five approaches* (4th ed.). SAGE Publications.

de Oliveira Faria, S., Hurwitz, G., Kim, J., Liberty, J., Orchard, K., Liu, G., Barbera, L., & Howell, D. (2021). Identifying Patient-Reported Outcome Measures (PROMs) for Routine Surveillance of Physical and Emotional Symptoms in Head and Neck Cancer Populations: A Systematic Review. *Journal of Clinical Medicine*, *10*(18), 4162. Advance online publication. DOI: 10.3390/jcm10184162 PMID: 34575271

Dornan, M., Semple, C., Moorhead, A., & McCaughan, E. (2021). A qualitative systematic review of the social eating and drinking experiences of patients following treatment for head and neck cancer. *Supportive Care in Cancer*, *29*(9), 4899–4909. DOI: 10.1007/s00520-021-06062-7 PMID: 33646367

Finlay, L. (2011). *Phenomenology for therapists: Researching the lived world.* Wiley-Blackwell. DOI: 10.1002/9781119975144

Fitchett, R. C., Aldus, E. J., Fitchett, L. R., & Cross, J. (2018). The lived experience of head and neck cancer patients receiving curative radiotherapy: A systematic review and meta-ethnography. *Psycho-Oncology, 27*(9), 2077–2086. DOI: 10.1002/pon.4790 PMID: 29883989

Govender, R., Wood, C. E., Taylor, S. A., Smith, C. H., Barratt, H., & Gardner, B. (2017). Patient Experiences of Swallowing Exercises After Head and Neck Cancer: A Qualitative Study Examining Barriers and Facilitators Using Behaviour Change Theory. *Dysphagia, 32*(4), 559–569. DOI: 10.1007/s00455-017-9799-x PMID: 28424898

Hunter, K. U., Schipper, M., Feng, F. Y., Lyden, T., Haxer, M., Murdoch-Kinch, C.-A., Cornwall, B., Lee, C. S. Y., Chepeha, D. B., & Eisbruch, A. (2013). Toxicities Affecting Quality Of Life After Chemo-Imrt Of Oropharyngeal Cancer: Prospective Study Of Patient-Reported, Observer-Rated, And Objective Outcomes. International Journal Of Radiation Oncology*Biology*Physics 85, 935–940. Https://Doi.Org/10.1016/J.Ijrobp.2012.08.030

Jacobson, M. C. (2018). The experience of head and neck cancer survivorship (including laryngectomy): An integrated biopsychosocial model. *Current Opinion in Supportive and Palliative Care, 12*(1), 65–73. DOI: 10.1097/SPC.0000000000000322 PMID: 29232259

Kraaijenga, S. A., Lapid, O., van der Molen, L., Hilgers, F. J., Smeele, L. E., & van den Brekel, M. W. (2016). Feasibility and potential value of lipofilling in post-treatment oropharyngeal dysfunction. *The Laryngoscope, 126*(12), 2672–2678. DOI: 10.1002/lary.26003 PMID: 27076387

Lang, H., France, E., Williams, B., Humphris, G., & Wells, M. (2013). The psychological experience of living with head and neck cancer: A systematic review and meta-synthesis. *Psycho-Oncology, 22*(12), 2648–2663. DOI: 10.1002/pon.3343 PMID: 23840037

Lazarus, C. L. (2009). Effects of chemoradiotherapy on voice and swallowing. *Current Opinion in Otolaryngology & Head & Neck Surgery, 17*(3), 172–178. DOI: 10.1097/MOO.0b013e32832af12f PMID: 19337126

Lazarus, C. L., Ward, E. C., & Yiu, E. M. (2007). Speech and swallowing following oral, oropharyngeal, and nasopharyngeal cancers. In *Head and Necl Cancer - treatment, rehabilitation, and outcomes* (pp. 103–122). Plural Publishing.

Manduchi, B., Che, Z., Ringash, J. G., Fitch, M. I., Howell, D., & Martino, R. (2024). Patient-reported outcome measures for dysphagia in head and neck cancer: A systematic review and appraisal of content validity and internal structure. *Head & Neck*, *46*(4), 951–972. DOI: 10.1002/hed.27693 PMID: 38356437

Mehanna, H., West, C. M., Nutting, C., & Paleri, V. (2010). Head and neck cancer—Part 2: Treatment and prognostic factors. *BMJ (Clinical Research Ed.)*, *341*(sep28 2), c4690. DOI: 10.1136/bmj.c4690 PMID: 20876637

Messing, B. P., Ward, E. C., Lazarus, C., Ryniak, K., Kim, M., Silinonte, J., Gold, D., Thompson, C. B., Pitman, K. T., Blanco, R., Sobel, R., Harrer, K., Ulmer, K., Neuner, G., Patel, K., Tang, M., & Lee, G. (2019). Establishing a Multidisciplinary Head and Neck Clinical Pathway: An Implementation Evaluation and Audit of Dysphagia-Related Services and Outcomes. *Dysphagia*, *34*(1), 89–104. DOI: 10.1007/s00455-018-9917-4 PMID: 29922848

Moustakas, C. (1994). *Phenomenological research methods*. SAGE Publications. DOI: 10.4135/9781412995658

Nund, R. L., Rumbach, A. F., Debattista, B. C., Goodrow, M. N., Johnson, K. A., Tupling, L. N., Scarinci, N. A., Cartmill, B., Ward, E. C., & Porceddu, S. V. (2015). Communication changes following non-glottic head and neck cancer management: The perspectives of survivors and carers. *International Journal of Speech-Language Pathology*, *17*(3), 263–272. DOI: 10.3109/17549507.2015.1010581 PMID: 25764915

Nund, R. L., Ward, E. C., Scarinci, N. A., Cartmill, B., Kuipers, P., & Porceddu, S. V. (2014). The lived experience of dysphagia following non-surgical treatment for head and neck cancer. *International Journal of Speech-Language Pathology*, *16*(3), 282–289. DOI: 10.3109/17549507.2013.861869 PMID: 24345002

O'Brien, B. C., Harris, I. B., Beckman, T. J., Reed, D. A., & Cook, D. A. (2014). Standards for reporting qualitative research: A synthesis of recommendations. *Academic Medicine*, *89*(9), 1245–1251. DOI: 10.1097/ACM.0000000000000388 PMID: 24979285

Ottosson, S., Laurell, G., & Olsson, C. (2013). The experience of food, eating and meals following radiotherapy for head and neck cancer: A qualitative study. *Journal of Clinical Nursing*, *22*(7-8), 1034–1043. DOI: 10.1111/jocn.12151 PMID: 23480499

Patterson JM, Lawton M. (2023). Dysphagia Advances in Head and Neck Cancer. Curr Otorhinolaryngol Rep. Feb 15:1-8. . Epub ahead of print. PMID: 36816911; PMCID: PMC9930077.DOI: 10.1007/s40136-023-00445-6

Patton, M. Q. (2002). *Qualitative research and evaluation methods* (3rd ed. ed.). Thousand Oaks, CA: Sage Publications.

Soldatova, L., & Mirza, N. (2019). Long-Term Voice And Swallowing Outcomes For Oral And Oropharyngeal Cancer Following Primary Or Adjuvant Chemoradiation. *The Annals of Otology, Rhinology, and Laryngology, 128*(9), 802–810. Https://Doi.Org/10.1177/0003489419842256. DOI: 10.1177/0003489419842256 PMID: 31007044

van Manen, M. (2016). *Researching lived experience: Human science for an action sensitive pedagogy* (2nd ed.). Routledge.

Zebralla, V., Wichmann, G., Pirlich, M., Hammermüller, C., Berger, T., Zimmermann, K., Neumuth, T., Mehnert-Theuerkauf, A., Dietz, A., Hinz, A., & Wiegand, S. (2021). Dysphagia, voice problems, and pain in head and neck cancer patients. *European Archives of Oto-Rhino-Laryngology, 278*(10), 3985–3994. DOI: 10.1007/s00405-020-06584-6 PMID: 33452920

KEY TERMS AND DEFINITIONS

Head and Neck Cancer: Soft tissue tumors or cancer arising from the mucosal surfaces of the lip; oral cavity; pharynx; larynx; and cervical esophagus. other sites included are the nose and paranasal sinuses; salivary glands; thyroid gland and parathyroid glands; and melanoma and non-melanoma skin cancers of the head and neck.

Speech Language Pathology: The study of speech or language disorders and their diagnosis and correction.

Patient Reported Outcome Measures: Assessment of the quality and effectiveness of health care as measured and directly reported by the patient.

Oropharyngeal Dysphagia: Difficulty in swallowing which may result from neuromuscular disorder or mechanical obstruction. dysphagia is classified into two distinct types: oropharyngeal dysphagia due to malfunction of the pharynx and upper esophageal sphincter; and esophageal dysphagia due to malfunction of the esophagus.

Quality of Life: A generic concept reflecting concern with the modification and enhancement of life attributes, e.g., physical, political, moral, social environment as well as health and disease.

Chapter 11

The Concept of Vulnerability and the Importance of the Sensitivity Index for Public Health Decision-Making

Fabrício Pimenta da Cunha
Universidade do Estado do Rio de Janeiro, Brazil

Maria Conceição Manso
https://orcid.org/0000-0002-1774-1337
Universidade Fernando Pessoa, RISE-Health, Portugal

Alfredo Akira Ohnuma
https://orcid.org/0000-0002-0772-9334
Universidade do Estado do Rio de Janeiro, Brazil

ABSTRACT

The concept of vulnerability is commonly used to refer to people's susceptibility to environmental problems, health damage and the degree of risk to which a population tends to suffer damage from natural disasters. Urban areas are vulnerable to climate change. The propensity of a given population/location can be adversely affected by climate change, based on three fundamental elements: sensitivity, adaptive capacity and exposure. The degree of vulnerability of a area, depends on indicators of exposure, sensitivity and adaptive capacity in a stepwise manner. Vulnerability is thus

DOI: 10.4018/979-8-3693-6432-1.ch011

presented as the degree of susceptibility or risk to which a population is exposed to suffering damage from natural disasters. This vulnerability concept is explained through the application of a case study carried out in the city of Rio de Janeiro, Brazil, to produce maps that have made it possible to identify the most vulnerable areas in the territory, thus facilitating decision-making by public authorities, intervention and the adoption of measures to minimise the vulnerability of these areas.

INTRODUCTION

In its AR6 report, the Intergovernmental Panel on Climate Change (IPCC, 2022) presents data indicating that extreme events are becoming more frequent and intense, thereby increasing the likelihood of natural disasters resulting in loss of human life (Virissini et al., 2023). As observed by Vicent et al. (2005), the rise in economic losses and loss of human life resulting from extreme events has prompted the scientific community at large to engage in the systematic aggregation of data, research, and work, intending to elucidate these phenomena and formulate resilience strategies for populations residing in urban settings.

The climate change emergency presents novel and significant challenges for urban areas, which must formulate strategic policies to mitigate the effects of climate change and enhance resilience to these occurrences (World Bank, 2011; Tyler and Moench, 2012; EEA, 2016; Cunha et al., 2024). The consequences of these climatic events are acknowledged as one of the most pressing challenges currently facing humanity. The impact of climate change is not limited to rural or urban areas; it also influences scenarios and contexts in these settings. There is a clear and established relationship between climate change and urbanisation (Hoornweg et al., 2011).

Urban areas are particularly susceptible to the effects of climate change and extreme weather events (Leal Filho et al., 2019), given that over 50% of the global population resides in these environments. By 2050, this proportion could reach 75% (UNDRR, 2019). As a consequence of this urban expansion and the prevailing global trend of urbanisation, the various risks associated with these spaces impact populations and impede cities' capacity to adapt to and mitigate climate change (Landauer et al., 2015; Li and Bouzeid, 2013).

The consequences of these climatic events are widely acknowledged as one of the most pressing challenges currently facing humanity. Climate change exerts a profound influence on a multitude of scenarios and contexts, both in rural and urban settings. There is a growing body of evidence that a direct link exists between climate change and urbanisation (Hoornweg et al., 2011).

It is of paramount importance to gain an understanding of the areas of vulnerability in cities in the current scenario, as this will inform both mitigation and adaptation actions. As defined by Tobin and Montz (1997), vulnerability can be understood as the probability that a community, structure, service, or geographical area will be damaged or disturbed by the impact of a given hazard.

The concept of vulnerability can be defined as the propensity of a given population or location to be adversely affected by climate change. This is a function of three fundamental elements: sensitivity index, adaptive capacity and exposure index (IPCC, 2022). The intrinsic relationship between these three elements can be expressed as follows:

$$V = f(E,S,AC)$$

where:

E = Exposure Index

S = Sensitivity Index

AC = Adaptive Capacity

The IPCC (2022) defines the exposure index as comprising all climate changes related to the components that cause meteorological drought. These include changes in average rainfall (either an increase or a decrease), variability (which makes it more difficult to maintain the hydrological balance, especially in relation to soil moisture levels) and the occurrence of climatic extremes.The sensitivity index is defined as the biophysical effect of climate change, taking into account the socioeconomic context, demographic structure, health conditions and the occurrence of climate-related diseases such as dengue and leptospirosis, among others, in a given population (IPCC, 2022). The adaptive capacity index is defined as the ability of human systems to respond and reorganise in the face of potential climate extremes, natural disasters and climate change (IPCC, 2022). However, Moser (1998) proposes that in order to determine the degree of vulnerability of a given area, it is essential to cross-reference the indicators of exposure, sensitivity and adaptive capacity. However, the cross-referencing of indicators should not be conducted in a linear manner, but rather in a staggered fashion. It is first necessary to correlate the exposure and sensitivity data in order to generate the potential impacts. Subsequently, the cross-referencing with the adaptive capacity of the territory and populations must be undertaken in order to arrive at the degree of vulnerability of the area. This process is illustrated in the flowchart shown in Figure 1.

Figure 1. Socio-environmental vulnerability

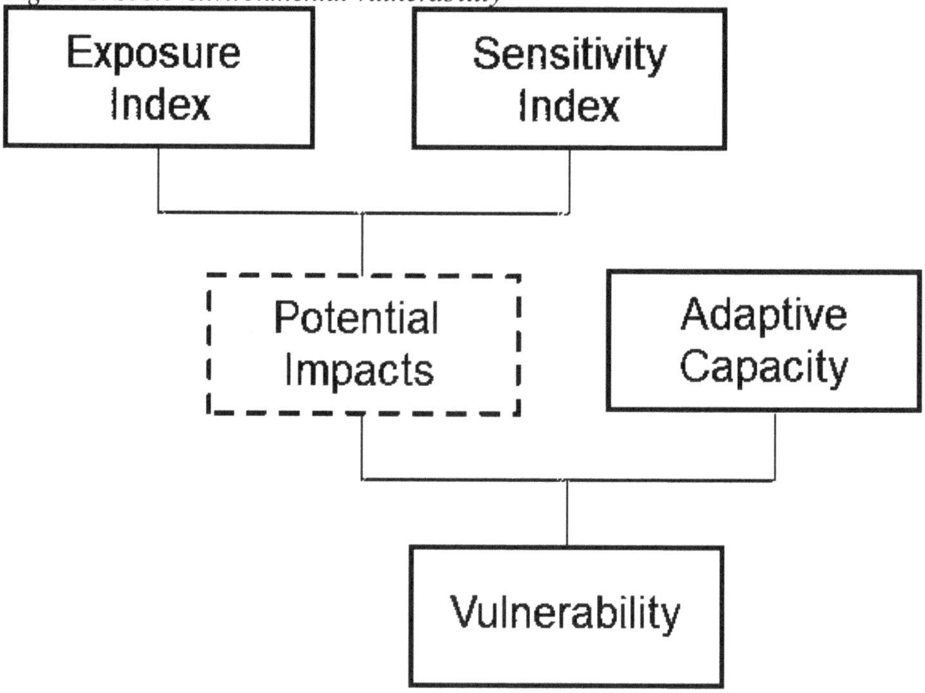

Source: MOSER (1998)

Vulnerability is defined as the degree of susceptibility or risk to which a population is exposed to damage from natural disasters. Furthermore, it encompasses the correlation between the severity of the damage and the magnitude of the threat, adverse event, or accident (Bertolazzi, 2009).

The authors conducted a study to identify and map the sensitivity index of a Brazilian metropolis (Rio de Janeiro) and its links with the concept of vulnerability. This enabled the most sensitive areas to be prioritised, thus facilitating the implementation of more effective interventions and action by the public authorities.

BACKGROUND

The study of vulnerability is of the utmost importance for understanding the weaknesses of the territory where we live, but in the area of public health, the sensitivity index to which populations are exposed is of great importance. It is important to note that the sensitivity index is a component of vulnerability that can assist public officials in making informed decisions.

This prompts the question of which techniques are employed to identify and map the sensitivity index for the purposes of public health planning.

The indicators that comprise sensitivity indices are associated with a number of factors, including health conditions, the population's exposure to climate-related diseases, poverty, and socio-demographic circumstances. It is therefore evident that the indicators which comprise this index are of paramount importance in order to identify the areas in which action is required in order to minimise risk and vulnerability.

In the case of Freitas et al. (2012) and also explained by Mytko (2024), the influence of sensitivity, as a component of vulnerability, on the physical and structural characteristics of the occupation of a given region is profound. The interaction between the physical environment and social dynamics is of fundamental importance in determining the susceptibility of a location to adverse events.

The spatialisation (mapping) of the indicators that make up the sensitivity index allows us to understand the dynamics of population occupation correlated with the geographical and logistical characteristics of the territory, which is extremely necessary in the area of public health, allowing, for example, in the area of epidemiology, the identification of people and characteristics that place them at greater or lesser risk of exposure to health events in certain territories (Bertolozzi, 2009).

The mapping of indicators is conducted using Geographic Information Systems (GIS), which facilitate the utilisation of a substantial volume of data from disparate formats and sources in a coherent and georeferenced manner. This enables the confrontation and connection of numerous factors and deterministic variables pertaining to physical conditions (Weiss and Pippi, 2018), which are indispensable planning tools for the management and planning of cities in the present era (Mileu and Queirós, 2018).

For GIS, as with any data analysis tool, the reliability of the information uploaded and the appropriateness of the proposed analyses are of paramount importance. Cross-referencing data in this environment often fails to reflect the reality of urban areas. Therefore, to ensure the validity of the results obtained from the analyses of this system, it is essential to define a methodology based on reviews of scientific work and its subsequent validation in the urban space (Schmidt and Barbosa, 2016).

The use of public data on an appropriate scale is extremely important for this analysis. The data referring to the sensitivity index is normally collected by the public administration in order to monitor and understand the population dynamics of its territory, but the analysis of this data in the light of spatialisation in GIS and multi-criteria cross-referencing of the indicators that make up the sensitivity index has the potential to guide the intervention of the public authorities in the territory in an assertive and effective manner (Duarte et al., 2021; Cocco et al., 2023).

The objective of multicriteria analysis (MCA) is to deconstruct intricate urban issues (indices) into more manageable components (indicators) and their underlying elements. Subsequently, it enables experts and decision-makers to ascertain the relative significance of each element within the constructed hierarchy (Schmidt and Barbosa, 2016). These judgments are translated into numerical values, which are subsequently referred to as "weights." The fundamental premise of this technique is to assess the weightings of experts on a given topic by comparing all the factors or elements in a paired manner. The resulting vector of values represents the relative importance of each factor in relation to the others, following the normalisation and combination of the paired data set (Schmidt and Barbosa, 2016).

Ultimately, the utilisation of a GIS environment and multi-criteria analysis, which defines the weights of each indicator and cross-references them, enables the sensitivity index to be spatially mapped. This is a crucial step in understanding the territory and the most pertinent mitigation, adaptation and public health actions.

MAPPING THE SENSITIVITY INDEX: A CASE STUDY IN THE CITY OF RIO DE JANEIRO – BRAZIL

The sensitivity index, as demonstrated in the case study conducted in Rio de Janeiro, Brazil, indicates the locations of the highest incidence of tropical diseases (Dengue), areas with the highest levels of poverty and the greatest socio-demographic vulnerability. The constituent indicators of each index are presented in Table 1.

Table 1. Sensitivity index indicators for Rio de Janeiro

	Indexes	Indicator
Sensitivity Index	Climate-related Diseases Index (Dengue)	Number of cases
	Poverty Index	Rate of population likely to die before the age of 40 years
		Rate of population over 25 illiterate
		Proportion of sectors with poor sanitation
		Infant mortality rate
		Income below the poverty line
	Sociodemographic Vulnerability Index	Female head of household rate
		Head of household rate Young people (10 to 29 years)
		(Present) Elderly population rate
		Population rate of children under 5
		Disabled population rate

Source: the authors

METHODOLOGY

The study used the following methodological approach:

1. spatialisation of the indicators for each index,
2. assigning a weight to each indicator, which was obtained through questionnaires submitted to a panel of experts, using Delphi methodology to process the data,
3. map algebra in a GIS (Geographic Information System) environment
4. map construction.

In the initial phase, public databases were employed for the spatialisation/mapping of the indicators, which ranged in scale from 1:25,000 to 1:50,000. These data sets were made available by the Brazilian Institute of Geography and Statistics (IBGE) and the Rio de Janeiro City Hall, and were subsequently processed in a GIS environment.

Figures 2 to 12 depict the mapping of the eleven indicators in the city of Rio de Janeiro, using gradients in shades of gray, with the darker color (black) representing Very High vulnerability and the lighter gray representing Very Low vulnerability.

Figure 2. Number of cases of Dengue

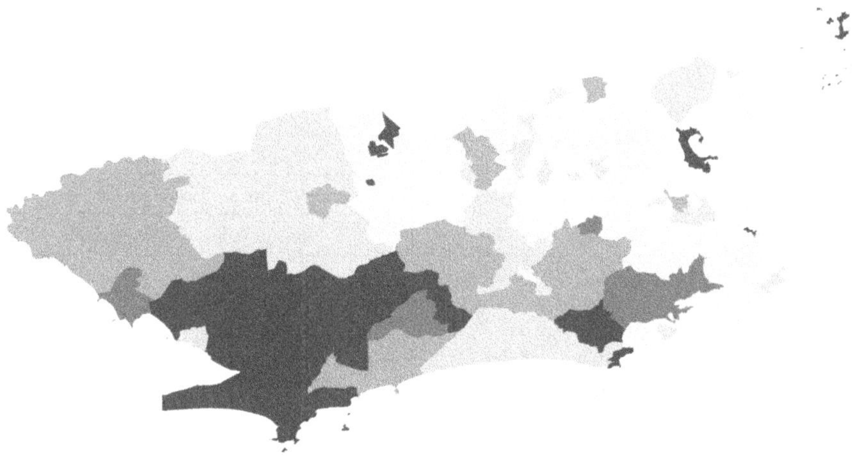

Figure 3. Rate of population likely to die before the age of 40 years old

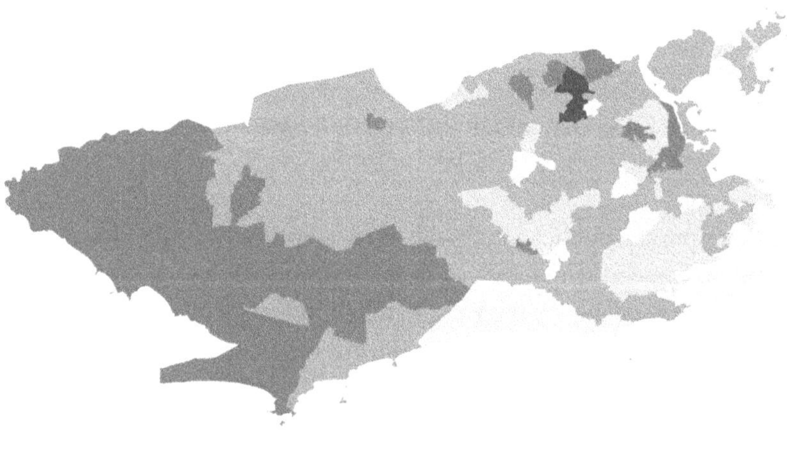

Figure 4. Rate of illiterate population over 25 years old

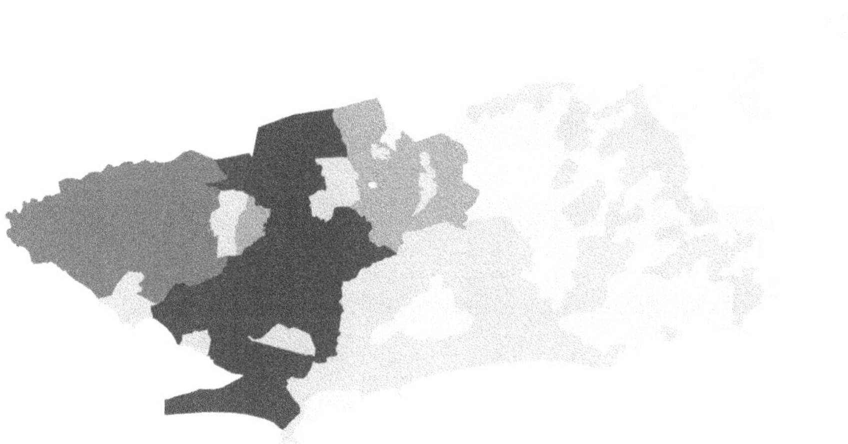

Figure 5. Proportion of sectors with poor sanitation

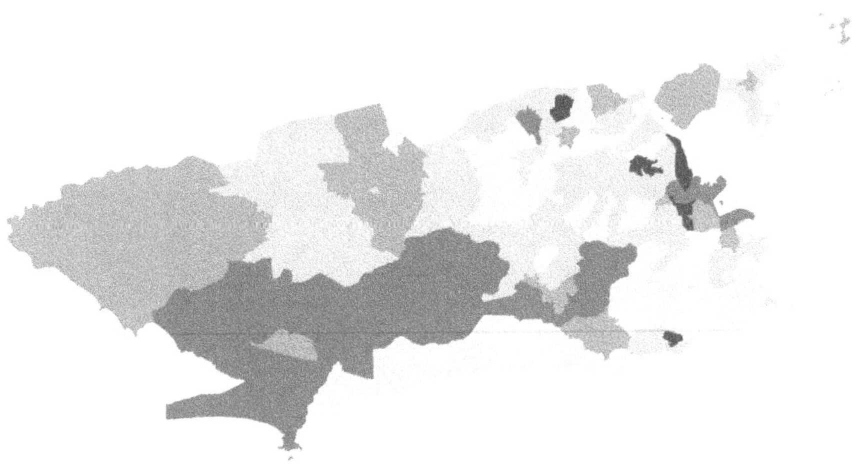

Figure 6. Infant mortality rate

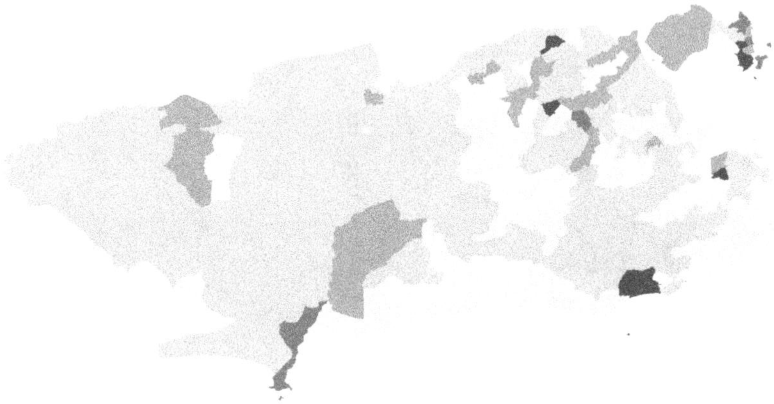

Figure 7. Income below the poverty line

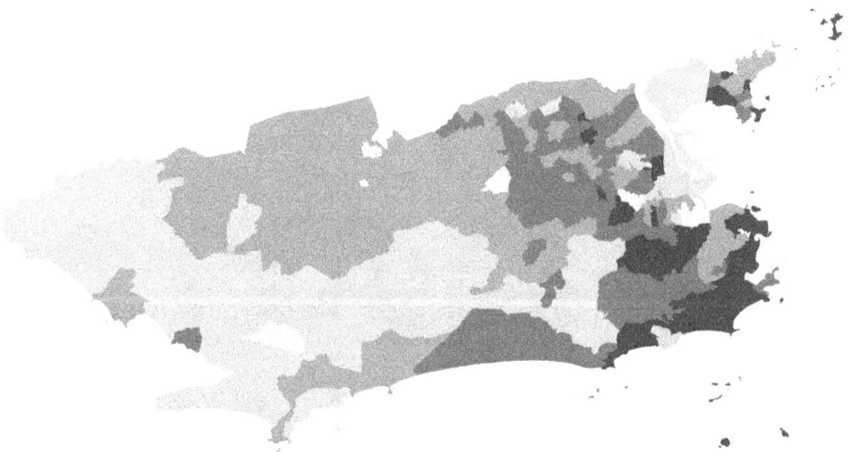

Figure 8. Rate of female heads of household

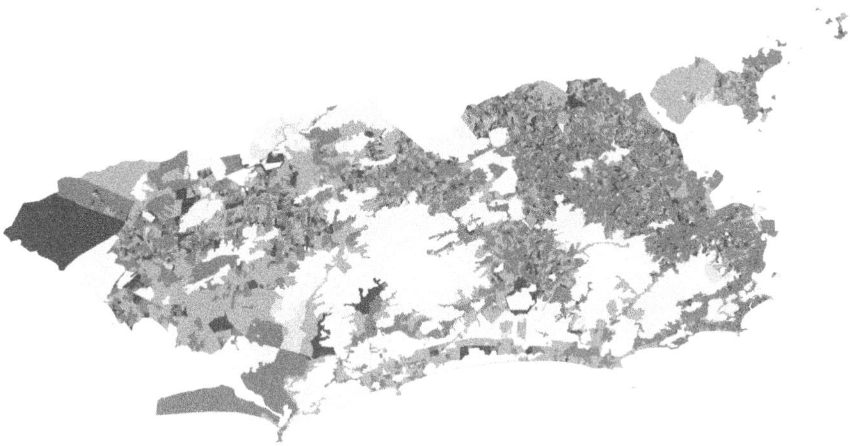

Figure 9. Head of household rate Young people (10 to 29 years old)

Figure 10. Elderly population rate

Figure 11. Population rate of children under 5 years old

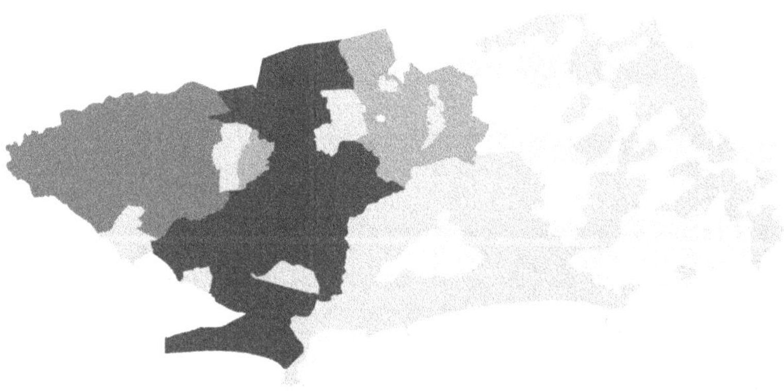

Figure 12. Disabled population rate

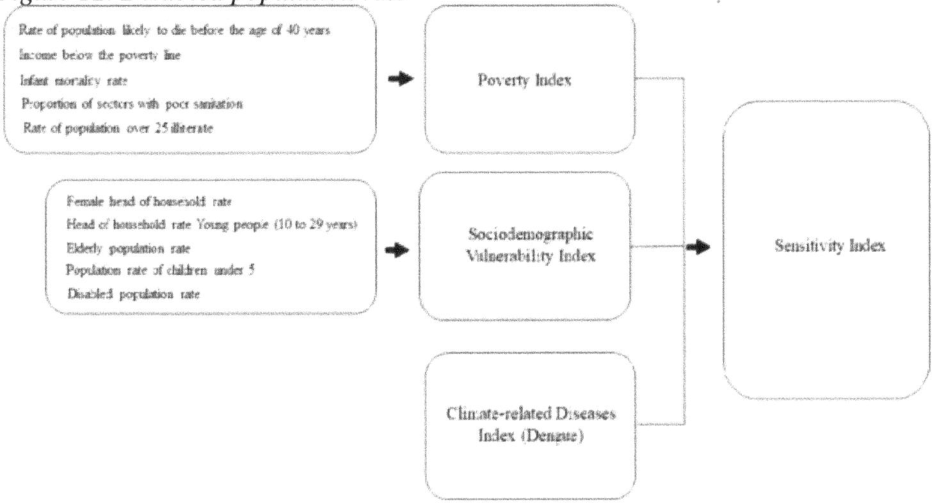

Once the mapping of the indicators had been completed, the second stage consisted of consulting a panel of experts.

The panel of experts was made up of university professors and professionals in the field of environmental planning, who assigned degrees of importance to the indicators and listed them all in a paired analysis. Gupta & Clarke (1996) emphasise the crucial role of a panel of experts in ensuring impartiality in research. They highlight the potential for personal communication barriers and problems, such as the persuasiveness and psychological dominance of some panel members, the natural reluctance to express unpopular opinions or modify views, and the influence of convincing minorities, whose opinions and arguments are pivotal to the process.

This analysis was carried out by means of questionnaires distributed to the panel, using the Delphi method of data collection and processing. After consolidating the data, the results in terms of importance obtained in the paired analysis, the scale used has 5 (five) vulnerability classifications: (i) 1/5 - very low, (ii) 1/3 - low, (iii) 1 - equal, (iv) 3 - high and (v) 5 - very high.

RESULTS

Figure 13 shows the construction of the Vulnerability Index and the Table 2, 3 and 4 show the matrix data on the level of importance of the indicators resulting from the consultation with the expert panel.

Figure 13. Formation of the Sensitivity Index

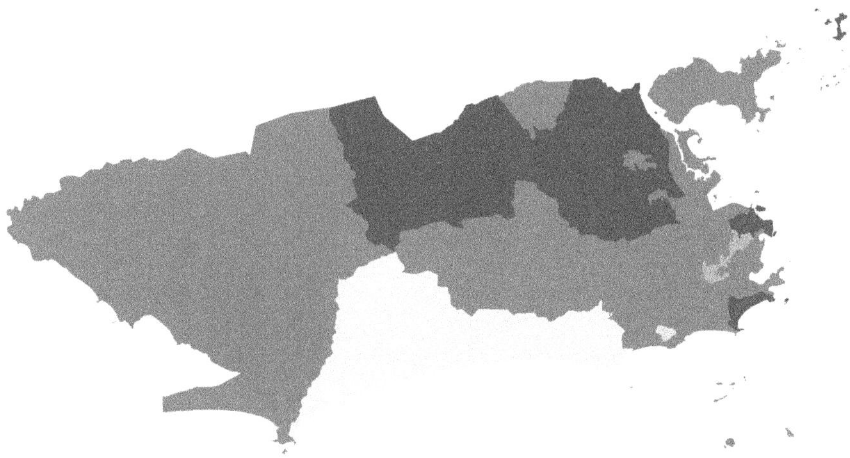

Table 2. Matrix of the indicators of the Poverty Index

	Rate of population likely to die before the age of 40 years	**Rate of population over 25 illiterate**	**Proportion of sectors with poor sanitation**	**Infant mortality rate**	**Income below the poverty line**
Rate of population likely to die before the age of 40 years	1				
Rate of population over 25 illiterate	1/3	1			
Proportion of sectors with poor sanitation	1	3	1		
Infant mortality rate	3	5	5	1	
Income below the poverty line	3	3	5	5	1

Table 3. Matrix of the indicators of the Sociodemographic Vulnerability Index.

	Female head of household rate	**Head of household rate Young people (10 to 29 years old)**	**Elderly population rate**	**Population rate of children under 5**	**Disabled population rate**
Female head of household rate	1				
Head of household rate Young people (10 to 29 years)	1	1			
Elderly population rate	3	5	1		
Population rate of children under 5	5	3	1	1	
Disabled population rate	3	3	1	1	1

Table 4. Sensitivity Index Pairwise Comparison Matrix

	Climate-related Diseases Index (Dengue)	**Poverty Index**	**Sociodemographic Vulnerability Index**
Climate-related Diseases Index (Dengue)	1		
Poverty Index	3	1	
Sociodemographic Vulnerability Index	3	1	1

In the third stage, the specialised indicators were cross-referenced using multi-criteria analysis (MCA) in a GIS environment, utilising the weights derived from the panel of experts. This enabled the visual representation of the areas of the territory most vulnerable to the sensitivity index (Figure 14).

Figure 14. Building the Sensitivity Index

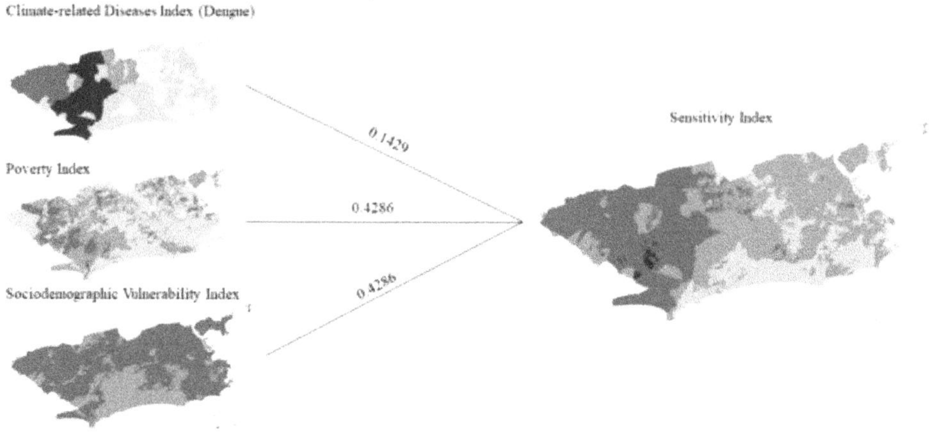

Finally, in stage four, the result was the spatialisation of the sensitivity index, demonstrating the areas of the territory most sensitive to this index (Figure 15). Again, the darker color (black) represents Very High sensitivity and the lighter gray representing Very Low sensitivity.

Figure 15. Map of the Sensitivity Index for Rio de Janeiro (the darker color (black) represents Very High sensitivity and the lighter gray representing Very Low sensitivity)

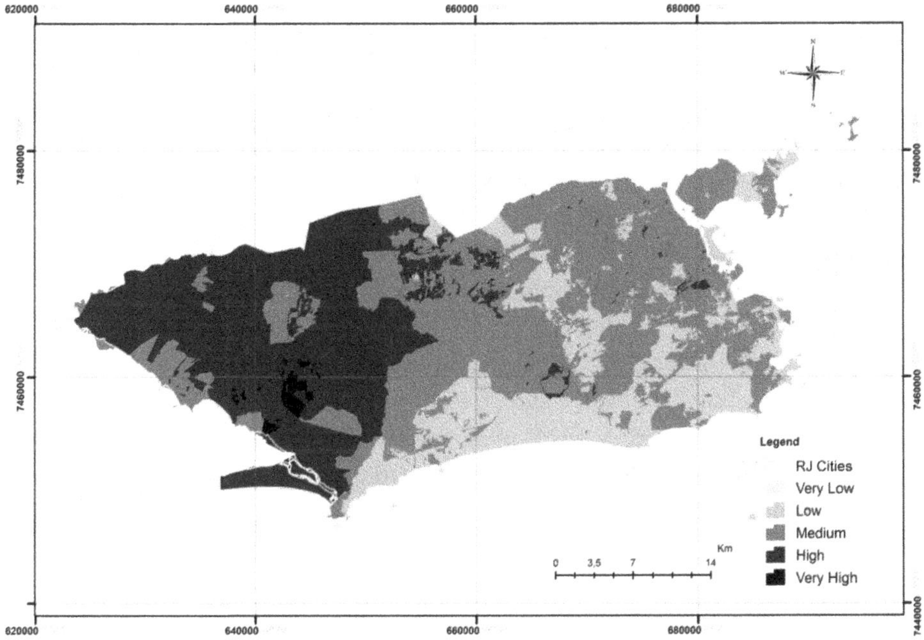

The results obtained through map algebra enabled the identification of areas within the territory that are most vulnerable. This facilitated decision-making by public authorities, intervention and the adoption of measures to minimise the fragility of these spaces.

The sensitivity index is inherently associated with public health concerns, including the identification of regions with inadequate sanitation, susceptibility to tropical diseases, and socio-environmental vulnerability. The combination of this information with strategic public health planning facilitates the decision-making process for the allocation of public facilities, health care infrastructure and public health campaigns.

The identification of the most sensitive areas in the territory enables more assertive and timely decision-making by public authorities, which in turn facilitates the minimisation of the vulnerability of these spaces. Furthermore, it allows for the identification of short-, medium- and long-term actions that can be taken to reduce the degree of the sensitivity index of these urban spaces.

DISCUSSION

Analysis of the sensitivity index reveals how specific indicators contribute to vulnerability patterns across Rio de Janeiro, providing crucial insights for targeted interventions.

In this case, in relation to the climate-related diseases index (Dengue), the spatial distribution of dengue cases correlates strongly with infrastructure deficiencies and environmental conditions. These disease hotspots serve as both indicators of current vulnerability and predictors of susceptibility to other climate-sensitive vector-borne diseases. This relationship demonstrates how disease transmission vulnerability is embedded in urban planning and environmental management contexts.

As well, the poverty indicators reveal significant interrelationships between socioeconomic factors and health outcomes. Poor sanitation shows a strong spatial correlation with infant mortality and poverty rates, illustrating how these factors create reinforcing cycles of vulnerability. Adult illiteracy notably correlates with higher rates of climate-related diseases, highlighting how educational disadvantage can compromise health literacy and preventive behaviors. Areas with the highest composite poverty scores represent priority zones where integrated interventions would yield maximum impact.

Regarding sociodemographic vulnerability index components, age-related vulnerability indicators (children under 5 and elderly populations) frequently overlap with areas of elevated disease risk and poverty. The female-headed household indicator reveals vulnerability patterns not always captured by traditional poverty measures, suggesting the need for specialized support services. The disabled population indicator identifies communities requiring accessible healthcare facilities and specialized emergency response planning.

And, the synergistic relationships, e.g., the multi-criteria analysis demonstrates how interactions between indicators create vulnerability hotspots greater than the sum of individual factors. The expert-assigned weights highlight how certain indicators—particularly infant mortality and extreme poverty—exert disproportionate influence on overall sensitivity. This nuanced understanding enables authorities to develop location-specific intervention strategies addressing the most significant vulnerability drivers in each area, optimizing the impact of public health resources and infrastructure investments

This study's integrated methodology combining Geographic Information Systems (GIS), multi-criteria analysis (MCA), and expert consultation via the Delphi method demonstrates both strengths and limitations for public health vulnerability assessment (Cocco et al, 2024).

GIS effectively visualized complex vulnerability patterns across Rio de Janeiro by integrating multi-source data, revealing spatial relationships between indicators not apparent in tabular analyses. This visual representation facilitates intuitive understanding for decision-makers. However, GIS approaches depend heavily on data currency and may mask fine-scale vulnerability variations within administrative units.

Multi-criteria analysis enabled the systematic integration of diverse indicators into composite indices, acknowledging vulnerability's multidimensional nature through transparent weighting. Nevertheless, MCA introduces subjectivity in weight determination, and linear aggregation methods may not fully capture complex interactions between vulnerability factors (Duarte et al, 2021; Cocco et al, 2024).

The Delphi methodology brought valuable interdisciplinary insights to the weighting process while mitigating individual bias through structured consensus-building. However, panel composition inevitably influences outcomes, potentially reflecting particular disciplinary orientations despite diversity efforts (Linstone & Turoff, 2002).

The integration of these complementary approaches creates a more robust methodology than any single approach alone, particularly valuable for public health applications in identifying priority intervention areas. Therefore, based on the previous, the authors acknowledge that future iterations could benefit from incorporating community-based participatory research to validate expert-derived assessments with residents' lived experiences in high-sensitivity areas (Farias et al, 2020; Bolina et al, 2021; Malta & Marques, 2021).

The sensitivity index mapping supports evidence-based policymaking by identifying highly vulnerable areas, enabling strategic governance. Public health can use it to focus interventions like vaccinations and education, maximizing impact. Infrastructure planning benefits by directing resources to communities most in need, addressing broader health determinants. For emergencies, it guides prioritized responses in high-risk zones. Over time, it supports policy evaluation and refinement. It also fosters cross-sectoral collaboration by providing a shared understanding of vulnerability, and offers a replicable model for cities to integrate resilience into planning (Visserini et al, 2023; Mytko, 2024)

FUTURE RESEARCH DIRECTIONS

A decision support system is currently being developed in APP format. The objective is to facilitate the accessibility of vulnerability data and the sensitivity, adaptive capacity and exposure indices in georeferenced map format, thereby enabling decision-makers and the general population to identify the risks and vulnerabilities associated with their respective areas of residence or travel.

CONCLUSION

The study provided a comprehensive approach to the concept of vulnerability, highlighting the importance of the sensitivity index as a strategic tool for public health planning and decision-making. Using the case of Rio de Janeiro, it was demonstrated how the spatialization of sensitivity indicators, through geographic information systems and multi-criteria analysis, can facilitate the identification of the most vulnerable areas, thereby enabling more targeted public interventions.

The findings underscore that integrating socioeconomic, demographic, and environmental data is essential to understanding territorial dynamics and implementing actions that minimize risks associated with natural disasters and extreme climate events. Furthermore, by identifying priority regions for investment in infrastructure and healthcare services, the sensitivity index proves its relevance in reducing inequalities and promoting health equity.

Finally, this study emphasizes the need for continuous methodological improvement and the expanded use of technologies such as GIS to support public management. Future research may explore new variables and methods to refine vulnerability indices, contributing to the formulation of increasingly effective and resilient public policies in the face of challenges posed by climate change and rapid urbanization.

ACKNOWLEDGMENT

This research received no specific grant from any funding agency in the public, commercial, or not-for-profit sectors.

REFERENCES

Bertolozzi, M.R, Nichiata, L.Y., Takahashi, R.F., Ciosak, S.I., Hino, P., Ferreira do Val, F. & Guanillo, M.C.v(2009). The vulnerability and the compliance in Collective Health. *Revista da Escola de Enfermagem da USP, 43*(spe2),1320-1324.

Bolina, A. F., Rpdrigues, R. A. P., Tavares, D. M., & Haas, V.J. (2021). Índices de vulnerabilidade social e programático para idosos que vivem no domicilio. Enfermería Global. Nº 65 Enero 2022 P153.

Cocco, R. M., Weiss, R., & Pippi, L. G. A. (2024). Análise Multicritério e Geoprocessamento no Planejamento do Sistema de Espaços Livres Urbano. *Engenharia Urbana Em Debate*, *4*(2), 58–68. DOI: 10.14244/engurbdebate.v4i2.116

Cunha, F. P., Manso, M. C., & Ohnuma Júnior, A. A. (2024). Analysis of The Occurrence of Extreme Events in The City of Rio de Janeiro/RJ. *Revista de Gestão Social e Ambiental*, *18*(4), e04730. DOI: 10.24857/rgsa.v18n4-066

Duarte, D. C. de O., Oliveira, J. C., & de, ., Lani, J. L., Uberti, M. S., Marques, Éder T. & Abreu, M. V. S. (2021). Multi-Criteria Evaluation Applied to the Determination of Areas of Suitability for Real Estate Appreciation. Brazilian. *Journal of Cardiography*, *73*(2), 516–529.

Duarte, L., Sanchez, J.G., Fonte, J., & Teodoro, A.C. (2021). A GIS pen-source application to enhance the identification of archaeological crop marks using remote sensing data. *SPIE*, v11863.

European Environment Agency. (2016). *Urban adaptation to climate change in Europe 2016*. EEA.

Farias, H. S., Vargas, K. B., Marino, T. B., Souza, G. M., & Lucena, A. J. (2020). *Vulnerabilidade socioambiental no Oeste Metropolitano do Rio de Janeiro: estratégias de prevenção a riscos* (19th ed.). Espaço e Economia.

Freitas, C. M., Lopes de Carvalho, M., Ximenes, E. F., Arraes, E. F., & Gomes, J. O. (2012). Vulnerabilidade socioambiental, redução de riscos de desastres e construção da resiliência: Lições do terremoto no Haiti e das chuvas fortes na Região Serrana, Brasil. *Ciencia & Saude Coletiva*, *17*(6), 1577–1586. DOI: 10.1590/S1413-81232012000600021 PMID: 22699648

Gupta, U. G., & Clarke, R. E. (1996). Theory and Applications of the Delphi Technique: A Bibliography (1975–1994). *Technological Forecasting and Social Change*, *53*(2), 185–211. DOI: 10.1016/S0040-1625(96)00094-7

Hoornweg, D., Sugar, L., & Gomez, C. L. T. (2011). Cities and greenhouse gas emissions: Moving forward. *Environment and Urbanization*, *23*(1), 207–227. DOI: 10.1177/0956247810392270

IPCC. (2022). *Climate Change 2022: Impacts, Adaptation, and Vulnerability. Contribution of Working Group II to the Sixth Assessment Report of the Intergovernmental Panel on Climate Change*. Cambridge University Press.

Landauer, M., Juhola, S., & Söderholm, M. (2015). Inter-Relationships Between Adaptation and Mitigation: A Systematic Literature Review. *Climatic Change*, *131*(4), 505–517. DOI: 10.1007/s10584-015-1395-1

Leal Filho, W., Mifsud, M., Molthan-Hill, P., & Nagy, J, G., Ávila, L.V. & Salvia, A.L. (. (2019). O ceticismo das mudanças climáticas nas universidades: Um estudo global. *Sustainability*, *11*, 2981. DOI: 10.3390/su11102981

Li, D., & BouZeid, E. (2013). Synergistic interactions between urban heat islands and heat waves: The impact in cities is larger than the sum of its parts. *Journal of Applied Meteorology and Climatology*, *52*(9), 2051–2064. DOI: 10.1175/JAMC-D-13-02.1

Linstone, H. A., & Turoff, M. (2002). *The Delphi Method: techniques and applications*. Listone and Turof.

Malta, F. S., & Marques, C. (2021). E. Socio-Environmental Vulnerability Index: An Application to Rio de Janeiro-Brazil. *International Journal of Public Health*, *66*, 1–11. DOI: 10.3389/ijph.2021.584308 PMID: 34744556

Mileu, N., & Queirós, M. (2018). Integrating risk assessment into spatial planning: Risk The decision support system. *ISPRS International Journal of Geo-Information*, *7*(5), 184–202. DOI: 10.3390/ijgi7050184

Moser, C. O. N. (1998). The asset vulnerability framework: Reassessing urban poverty reduction strategies. *World Development*, *26*(1), 1–19. DOI: 10.1016/S0305-750X(97)10015-8

Mytko, A. (2024). *Vulnerabilidade do sistema urbano costeiro frente a ameaças relacionadas à mudança climática*. PUC-Rio. DOI: 10.17771/PUCRio.acad.68292

Schmidt, M. A. R., & Barbosa, G. R. (2016). Use of artificial neural networks in initial ponderation of AHP techniques applied to analysis of watershed vulnerability. *Boletim de Ciências Geodésicas*, *22*(3), 511–525. DOI: 10.1590/S1982-21702016000300029

Tobin, G., & Montz, B. (1997). *Natural hazards*. Guilford.

Tyler, S., & Moench, M. (2012). A framework for urban climate resilience. *Climate and Development*, *4*(4), 311–326. DOI: 10.1080/17565529.2012.745389

UNDRR. (2019). *United Nations Office for Disaster Risk Reduction*. United Nations.

Vincent, L. A., Peterson, T. C., Barros, V. R., Marino, M. B., Rusticucci, M., Carrasco, G., Ramirez, E., Alves, L. M., Ambrizzi, T., Berlato, M. A., Grimm, A. M., Marengo, J. A., Molion, L., Moncunill, D. F., Rebello, E., Anunciação, Y. M. T., Quintana, J., Santos, J. L., Baez, J., & Karoly, D. (2005). Observed trends in indices of daily temperature extremes in South America 1960-2000. *Journal of Climate*, *18*(23), 5011–5023. DOI: 10.1175/JCLI3589.1

Vissirini, F.S.B., Reis, P.T.B., Cunha, F.P., Gondim, F.R., Ohuma JR.A.A. Formiga, R.M. (2023). Urban Vulnerability and the Tools Required for Hydro-Meteorological Risk Disaster Management. *Journal of Environmental Management and Sustainability, 12*(2), 1-37, e22616.

Weiss, R., & Pippi, L. G. (2019). Análise multicritério na definição de vulnerabilidade ambiental. *TerraPlural*, *13*(3), 272–295. DOI: 10.5212/TerraPlural.v.13i3.0018

World Bank. (2011). *Guide to climate change adaptation in cities*. World Bank.

Chapter 12
Training of Communicative Partners in Early Childhood

Ana Filipa Santos
https://orcid.org/0009-0005-9523-7629
School of Health, Polytechnic of Porto, Portugal & Porto Cerebral Palsy Association, Portugal

Joana Dantas Senra
Porto Cerebral Palsy Association, Portugal

Marta Joana Pinto
https://orcid.org/0000-0003-3900-0481
School of Health, Polytechnic of Porto, Portugal

Eugénia Magina
https://orcid.org/0009-0003-0111-7462
School of Health, Polytechnic of Porto, Portugal

ABSTRACT

Speech-Language Pathologist/Therapist (S-LP/T) is the professional responsible for offering assessment and intervention therapy to children (and adults) with numerous clinical and educational conditions that have an impact on communication competence. Nowadays, S-LP/T can also consider consulting, providing support and empowering people and their families to make informed decisions about communication problems, among other issues. Family members or other caregivers of children with communication disorders are privileged communication partners. It is up to the S-LP/T to train family members as communicative partners so that they can promote the child's communicative and language development and support the

DOI: 10.4018/979-8-3693-6432-1.ch012

family during these critical years. The aim of this chapter is to review the literature on the role of the S-LP/T in empowering parents/caregivers of children with communication and language disorders, knowing the impact of intervention focused on empowering communication partners in early childhood.

INTRODUCTION

The World Health Organization (WHO) identified language as one of the domains of development that is associated not only with development in the first years of life and with learning and academic success, but also with the person's participation in the different domains of their life (health, physical and mental, finances, etc.) (Roberts et al., 2019).

Early childhood is a critical period of rapid brain growth and neuroplasticity (Carvalho et al., 2016; Roberts et al., 2019; Sánchez, 2019) and it is during this period that children most quickly and effectively learn their language (Roberts et al., 2019). However, a part of the population may face some type of difficulty in acquiring language. The literature provides descriptive information about children with neurodevelopmental disorders and the appearance of difficulties in the acquisition and development of specific intellectual, motor or social functions. This will have a negative impact on participation and performance in activities of daily living, interaction with peers, academic performance and self-esteem (Dunst, 2020; Jimenez-Arberas et al., 2024).

The Speech-Language Pathology/Therapy (S-LP/T) plays a fundamental role in the linguistic development of children who have difficulties in language acquisition. These difficulties can manifest themselves in areas such as verbal comprehension and expression, grammar, vocabulary or articulation of the sounds of the language (American Speech-Language-Hearing Association [ASHA], 2016; García-Sánchez et al., 2020; Mora, García & Sánchez, 2023). Therefore, as a specialist, the support of the S-LP/T in early childhood is crucial to minimize the impacts of these difficulties. However, for more effective support, collaborative work with the family and professionals involved should be considered (Coufal & Woods, 2018; Langner & Fukkink, 2022; Yang, Hossain & Sitharthan, 2013).

In early childhood in particular, the S-LP/T role as communication consultant is particularly crucial in promoting language development and supporting families in creating an environment rich in communicative stimuli. This role has evolved beyond direct intervention with the child, currently including training caregivers and consulting professionals (Coufal & Woods, 2018).

The role of the S-LP/T has evolved significantly in recent decades, reflecting changes in society's needs, scientific advances and the recognition of communication as a right. This progress has expanded the S-LP/T field of activity and their work increasingly follows an evidence-based approach and prioritizes collaboration for a more integrated and holistic practice (ASHA, 2016; Mora, García & Sánchez, 2023).

Although there are still marked differences between countries, they all seem to share efforts to improve practice and increase access to speech-language therapy. The United States and Australia appear to be leading in research and innovation, while Spain and Portugal continue to expand the role of the S-LP/T in health and education systems and the consideration of parents/caregivers as fundamental to the success of children's learning and development (APTF, n.d.; Asociación Española de Logopedia, Foniatria y Audiología e Ibero-Amaericana de Fonoaudiología [AELFA-IF], n.d.; ASHA, 2021, 2016.; Mora, García & Sánchez, 2023; Speech Pathology Australia [SPA], 2024.; Sociedade Portuguesa de Terapia da Fala [SPTF], n.d.).

Comparing different countries, it seems to us that the global trend is to promote a preventive, inclusive and accessible approach, recognizing the importance of empowering parents/caregivers and communities as protagonists in the children's communication process.

BACKGROUND

Child development refers to a set of physiological processes that allow the organization, functioning and maturity of the different structures and functions of the human body. Children, through their performance and participation in day-to-day activities, experience and interact with the environment, developing the motor, cognitive and sensory-perceptual skills necessary to face increasingly complex challenges, according to their age, culture and society. This suggests that there is a relationship between the number and type of experiences acquired and the need for support in different aspects of life (Jimenez-Arberas et al., 2024).

A characteristic of human development perspectives is the assertion that participation in everyday activities is important for the child's communicative and linguistic development. Daily activity environments, which constitute the fabric of the lives of children and their families, offer needed experiences and provide children with contexts for learning culturally significant behaviors (Dunst, Trivette, & Hamby, 2007, 2006). Bath time, meals, dressing and undressing, buying food, reading stories, helping with homework, family outings, playing in a park, going to the pool, are some examples of daily activities.

The acquisition of communicative competence is essential for the child's global development (Levey, 2024; Owens, 2016). Specifically, mastering expressive communication will enable the child to express their needs and desires, and interact appropriately in the world around them, with the first three years of life having fundamental importance (Luze et al., 2001).

Communication can be observed from birth through the visual contact established between a baby and its parents. Communication precedes the development of language, and any difficulties are warning signs and serve as indicators for taking preventive actions to involve the baby in communicative exchanges and shared attention. In early childhood, joint attention between the baby and his or her parents is particularly important. It starts with a shared look between the parents and the baby and later starts to involve a third element that can be an object, person or even a pet, in which the caregiver comments the baby's focus of attention. In typical development, the child begins to learn how to get the adult's attention using body movements, vocalizations and their own gaze. Parents, for their part, can use similar means to draw the child's attention to new objects, events, etc. The development of this game of social interaction requires the ability to coordinate attention around an object or activity and share an interest with someone else (Prelock & Nelson, 2012).

The nature of the communicative process thus takes on a bidirectional perspective. All people involved in a communicative interaction are communicative partners and are responsible for communicative success (Klatte et al., 2023; Klatte et al., 2020 Lopez et al., 2021).

The communicative dyad is a rich process of exchanges and joint learning. In the article by Masek et al. (2021) a study is carried out on the diversity of skills learned in this process of parent-child interaction, when exchanges assume a contingent and responsive basis. Communicative contingency is understood as the immediate and significant exchange carried out in the interaction between parents/caregivers and the child, thus promoting the basis for connected and involved communication. Communicative contingency varies throughout development (Mahoney & MacDonald, 2007b; Reed et al., 2016), and initially concerns the synchrony between the affection and behavior of the father/caregiver and baby and, later, concerns attention and rapid response to the child's interests as he begins to explore the environment (Bornstein & Tamis-LeMonda, 1989; Tamis-LeMonda, et al., 2001 cit in Masek et al., 2021). Regardless of the variation in the focus of contingency throughout development, the relationship between contingent exchanges and the impact on communicative and linguistic development is unanimous. Studies in the field of neuroscience demonstrate that the activation of Broca's area is related to conversational exchanges and not to the amount of linguistic input from the caregiver (Masek et al., 2021).

It should be noted that joint attention plays a fundamental role in establishing the relationship between communicative contingency and linguistic development. Masek et al. (2021) propose a reciprocal model, in which contingency and joint attention are related and affect each other, thus constituting the basis for learning.

The nature of communication between parents/caregivers and children during interactions, namely the adult's contingent and responsive interactions, are highlighted in several studies as the basis for children's linguistic acquisition and development (Cologon et al., 2016; Masek et al., 2021; Muhinyi & Rowe, 2019; Contingency and responsiveness contribute to improving language and literacy development, as well as the generalization of skills across multiple contexts (Cologon et al., 2016; Mahoney & MacDonald, 2007b).

For children, the privileged communicative partners, in their daily lives, are above all their parents/caregivers, and constitute their main support, and the communicative process can be a real challenge for both, adult and child (Simões, 2011). It is therefore essential that parents have the skills and confidence to interact and communicate with their children, in order to stimulate linguistic development. Evidence indicates that the quantity and quality of interaction between parents and children influences the child's language skills (Espe-Sherwindt & Serrano, 2016; Klatter et al, 2023; Leivickis et al., 2023; Madigan et al., 2019).

MAIN FOCUS OF THE CHAPTER

Communicative Partners

A child's maximum development potential is determined by the quality of experiences that parents provide for their children. Regardless of how stimulating the toys a child has at home, or how exceptional the learning activities a child receives in school, therapy or other formal learning contexts, it is in the interaction with parents that the greatest learning potential develops (Carvalho et al., 2016; Mahoney & MacDonald, 2007a).

Development programs attached to nursery, pre-school and therapies can only play an important role in promoting the development and well-being of children, when they consider the involvement of parents in the entire process, both in situations of children in risk or with some developmental disorder, such as for children with typical development (Mahoney & MacDonald, 2007a).

Mahoney and MacDonald (2007a) mention three main reasons for the fundamental role that parents play in their children's learning potential: (1) Parents establish a relationship of affection and bonding with the child that no one else can or should try to replace. This connection places parents in a privileged position, being the most powerful influencers in their children's lives. (2) Children's learning and development is an ongoing process that can occur in any everyday situation in which the child is actively involved. Learning new skills is very little related to the adult's intention to create learning experiences, but rather when there are elements such as attention, interest and motivation on the part of the child. Therefore, every moment of the day is a potential moment for learning and parents are the people most likely to be present. (3) Even if parents have limited time to spend with the child, due to professional or other responsibilities, parents have many more opportunities to interact with and promote the child's development than any other adult or professional. Considering that parents are the privileged caregivers, in daily and permanent contact with their children, they are therefore in a favourable position to promote the child's development and learning.

Considering, furthermore, that it is in activities of daily living, in the family and in the community, where significant experiences that provide opportunities for language acquisition occur, interventions, particularly at the level of linguistic skills, must include active involvement between children and parents/caregivers (Dunst, 2020; Dunst et al., 2016; Espe-Sherwindt & Serrano, 2016; Gail et al., 2022; Heidlage et al., 2020; Weisberg et al., 2016).

Thus, although there is no indication that professionals' clinical practices should be interrupted or eliminated, it is essential that the S-LP/T daily practice considers families and establishes an intervention process based on collaborative practices, highlighting the need for professionals to add time to these practices to spend with parents and help them support their child's development in responsive interactions during their daily routines (Langner & Fukkink, 2023; Mahoney and MacDonald, 2007a).

In the first years of life, most children progress in acquiring communication skills with the use of gestures (e.g. pointing, gesturing) to linguistic skills, such as the appearance of the first word, following instructions, constructing complex sentences, sharing of ideas, expressing feelings, engaging in dialogue with others and high-quality interactions with their parents and caregivers. However, although most children acquire language relatively quickly and sequentially, some children may have difficulty for a variety of reasons, including genetic, neurological or environmental (American Psychiatric Association, 2013; Law et al., 2019; Roberts et al., 2019).

The family-centered approach considers parents/caregivers as fundamental elements in the intervention process and is a fundamental principle of early childhood intervention (An et al., 2017; Carvalho et al., 2016; Division for Early Childhood [DEC], 2014; Dunst & Espe-Sherwindt, 2016; Individuals with Disabilities Education Improvement Act, 2004). This approach focuses on empowering parents/caregivers, aiming for parents to achieve responsive patterns of interaction and communication with their children in natural environments that enhance the child's language development (Akemoglu et al., 2019; Carvalho et al., 2026; DEC, 2014; Espe-Sherwindt & Serrano, 2016). The social-interactionist approach to language development also reinforces the role of the environment and social engagement and emphasizes the role of caregivers (and significant others) in children's language learning (Cologon et al., 2016).

Greater communicative responsiveness on the part of parents/caregivers, and consequently less directive or controlling approaches, have also been associated with increased initiative and communication, as well as growth in the child's vocabulary (Cologon et al., 2016; MacGuillion et al., 2017).

Cologon et al. (2016), reinforces that caregivers need information and support to facilitate this responsiveness, and it is necessary to implement an intervention focusing on caregivers, improving their communicative skills, through the establishment of interaction patterns that support communication opportunities in natural contexts and reduce directive approaches (An et al., 2017; Cologon et al., 2016).

Intervention programs focused on parents/caregivers have demonstrated an impact on reducing directness and increasing reciprocity in communicative interaction, such as turn-taking (Cologon et al., 2016; Te Kaat-van den Os et al., 2016). In the systematic review carried out by Te Kaat-van den Os et al. 016) evidence of the positive impact of caregiver training on the child's communicative skills is mentioned. All programs included in the study are focused on parent-child interaction, parent/caregiver responsiveness, linguistic input used in interaction, and training and strategies that support linguistic development. The study carried out by Akemoglu et al. (2019) also states that the use of a naturalistic approach in implementing strategies resulted in an improvement in the child's communicative and social skills. Namely, the positive impact on the child's ability to initiate interaction (verbally or non-verbally) (Vismara et al., 2013; Akemoglu et al., 2019) and imitation skills (Ingersoll et al. 2016; Vismara et al. 2012, 2013; Wainer and Ingersoll 2013, 2015). Furthermore, in the meta-analysis by Roberts and Kaiser (2011), which involved different intervention programs focused on the skills of parents/caregivers - Hanen Program®, Parent-Based Intervention, Child Talk, Social Pragmatic Joint Attention, Heidelberg Parent-Based Language Intervention, Focused Stimulation, Parent Sensitivity and Responsiveness, Enhanced Milieu Teaching and Parent Video Home Training - found a significant and positive impact on the child's language skills.

Also, the results of the systematic review and meta-analysis carried out by Roberts et al. (2019), in which caregiver training was associated with children's language development, revealed a positive association between the variables studied.

Cologon et al. (2016) add to the extensive research that has been carried out on the effectiveness of the Hanen Program®, on the caregiver's linguistic input and the development of vocabulary and language with different groups of children with results in increased responsiveness and decreased directness of the caregiver after the intervention. The implementation of the Hanen Program® supported the caregiver's communicative approach that facilitated the child's communication, resulting in an increase in the child's communicative initiatives and interactions and leading to greater joint activity around the child's interests, compared to children in control groups. Furthermore, children used more combinations of initial words and morphemes compared to control groups, increasing the structural complexity of the language. Improvements were also reported in other areas of development such as behavior and, therefore, a reduction in caregiver stress. Therapists' reports also indicated an increase in self-confidence and self-esteem of parents/caregivers and the strengthening of the adult-child relationship after the intervention, as well as parent/caregiver-therapist relationships, allowing for more effective and positive collaboration during planning the intervention. intervention (Cologon et al., 2016). Akemoglu et al. (2019) adds that this effectiveness is transversal to different socio-economic contexts, ages (0-8), diagnoses and communicative levels.

In order to obtain more positive intervention results, it is essential that early childhood intervention programs consider all components of family-centred practices (Akhbari Ziegler and Hadders-Algra, 2020; DEC, 2014).

Role of Speech and Language Pathologists/ Therapists With Communicative Partners

Parents/caregivers, as adult learners, need a teaching approach that is participatory, flexible and respectful of their autonomy and experience, which highlights the extreme relevance of andragogy in training caregivers. Adult learning must be contextual and oriented towards solving practical problems, and professionals must adapt their approaches according to the needs and capabilities of caregivers (García-Sánchez et al., 2020).

Knowles et al., (2005 cit. in García-Sánchez et al., 2020) propose six basic principles of adult learning to consider: (1) The adult's need to know: the child's main caregivers feel the need to understand what, why and how the child has these behaviours; (2) The learner's self-concept: feeling autonomous, maintaining self-direction of learning. Adults need to be responsible for their educational decisions and to be involved in planning and evaluating their instruction; (3) The learner's previous experience: giving them resources and mental models. This previous experience, including error, provides the basis for future learning actions; (4) Readiness to learn: the adult is especially prepared to learn what relates to their life, to their own development as a person; (5) Learning orientation: problem-centred, being contextual. Adult learning is problem-centred rather than content-centred; (6) Motivation to learn: especially that which has intrinsic value, which is a personal pay-off. Adults respond better to internal motivators than to external motivators.

They are more interested in learning topics that have immediate relevance to their jobs or personal lives (García-Sánchez et al., 2020).

Over the years, a number of studies have been carried out trying to understand not only the factors that can influence collaborative practices, but also the needs and expectations, the perception of difficulties of both families and professionals, and also the type of practices that are important in the intervention (Davies et al., 2017; Klatte et al., 2023; Klatte et al., 2020; Kwok et al., 2021; Kookorelias et al., 2019). As a result, there are proposals in the literature for collaborative strategies and models to support the practices of professionals, particularly S-LP/T (An et al., 2017; An & Palisano, 2014; García-Sánchez et al., 2020; (Harniess, 2021; Rush & Shelden, 2011).

The S-LP/T is described as a facilitator of learning for parents/caregivers. They use empowering strategies that allow caregivers to develop their own skills to deal with the child's needs (García-Sánchez et al., 2020). In addition, the S-LP/T plays a key role in accompanying the family, helping parents to feel safe and able to promote the child's development (García-Sánchez et al., 2020).

Collaborative practices are a key element of family-centred intervention and are essential for the family's concerns and the child's development needs to be reflected in the assessment and intervention (An & Palisano, 2014; García-Sánchez et al., 2020; Klatte et al., 2023; Klatte et al., 2023; Kokorelias et al., 2019).

Definitely, the importance of collaborative practices in clinical practice has been increasingly recognised. However, its implementation is challenging for both professionals and parents/caregivers (Klatte, 2023). Although S-LP/T recognise the importance of family involvement throughout the therapeutic process, studies to date have shown that the professional still takes the lead, particularly during assessment and when drawing up a therapeutic plan (Ferreira, 2021; Singer et al., 2022).

Collaboration between professionals and family members requires an individual and flexible approach to the individual specificities of each family and the professionals themselves. From this point of view, there are also possible conflicts in the expectations of both regarding their roles in the intervention (Davies et al., 2017; Klatte et al., 2023).

S-LP/T can use effective helpgiving practices to boost family empowerment: relational practices, participatory practices and technical quality (An et al., 2016; Dunst & Trivette, 2009; García-Sánchez et al., 2020; Klatte et al., 2023; Mas et al., 2022; Pinto, 2018; Pinto & Serrano, 2022).

Relational practices refer to the professional's interpersonal behaviours, as well as positive convictions and beliefs about the family's skills and abilities. Active and reflective listening, empathy, understanding, authenticity and showing warmth and interest are behaviours associated with good communication skills and describes relational practices (Carvalho et al., 2016; García-Sánchez et al., 2020; Pinto, 2018;

Pinto & Serrano, 2022). These practices also respect beliefs about the family's abilities to deal with their concerns and needs on a day-to-day basis. The professional recognises and validates existing strengths and uses the family's abilities to improve their functioning (Dunst et al., 2002).

In turn, participatory practices add the possibility of the family's active participation in the intervention process, promoting new capacities and positively influencing the control that the family experiences in their family functioning. They are, therefore, professional behaviours aimed at involving the family in the decision-making and informed choice process and at using existing strengths and developing skills to achieve the resources, support and services desired by the family. Professionals should work in collaboration with the family to identify their needs and collaborate in obtaining the desired resources, leaving the family to make informed decisions about identifying the most appropriate resources and supports to meet those needs. These practices also include the professional's responsiveness and flexibility in the face of changing circumstances in the family's life (Carvalho et al., 2016; Pinto, 2018; Pinto & Serrano, 2022). They provide the family with opportunities to discuss intervention options, there is collaboration and sharing in decision-making, there is family participation in the implementation of decisions (An et al., 2016; Carvalho et al., 2016; García-Sánchez et al., 2020; Pinto, 2018).

With regard to the technical quality of the professional, this refers to theoretical and practical knowledge about the area in which they work, and they should always value and act in accordance with the latest evidence that indicates the importance of an authentic assessment of the child's functional competences, in a natural environment and with their privileged interlocutors, and the construction of a therapeutic plan that aims to improve the child's participation in daily activities and consequently the inclusion and quality of life of the whole family (García-Sánchez et al, 2020; Pinto, 2018; Pinto & Serrano, 2022).

The simultaneous use of all three components is essential for the intervention to be effective, if we want to achieve results in terms of empowering family members (Dunst & Espe-Sherwindt, 2016).

The importance of professionals, including S-LP/T using effective helpgiving practices to support families in early childhood intervention has resulted in a variety of studies that show that professionals use relational practices and that participatory practices have been increasingly considered and used (Dunst & Espe-Sherwindt, 2016; Ferreira, 2021; Mas et al., 2018; Pinto, 2018). Other research has added to the benefits of professionals adopting family-centred practices to support children and their parents/carers (Dunst et al., 2014, 2007; Dunst & Espe-Sherwindt, 2016; Leite, 2018; Serrano et al., 2017).

Lee et al. (2022) add that there are several core components of family-centred intervention programmes: (a) the therapist must implement relational practices in which they establish relationships of trust and respect with the carers; (b) the intervention must be based on participation, taking place in natural contexts and addressing goals to increase the child's participation in their daily routines; (c) caregivers and the therapist should collaborate together to determine intervention goals and contexts; (d) sessions should build on carers' strengths and increase their capacity to support their children; (e) the therapist should use coaching strategies, including guided practice, to support carers' learning (Dunst, 2007; Schertz et al., 2011; Tomeny et al., 2020).

In this sense, in the intervention process, which is intended to be collaborative in a family-centred approach, the planning, implementation and evaluation of interventions are highlighted as key strategies for professionals (Espe-Sherwindt & Serrano, 2016; Escorcia et al., 2016a; García-Sánchez et al., 2020; Rush & Shelden, 2011):

- Active listening. Open and honest communication with parents/caregivers should be encouraged, promoting a two-way exchange of information;
- Direct observation. During visits, professionals should observe interactions between the child and the parents/carers in order to adjust interventions effectively;
- Analysing strategies. Throughout the intervention, at a time when it is deemed appropriate, it will be useful to reflect on the strategies. An analysis of existing strategies to determine whether they are consistent with evidence-based practices, whether they are being effective, and whether they may need to be altered or modified to achieve the desired result;
- Feedback. Understood as information provided by the professional based on direct observation of the parent/cargiver. It is often useful, by helping to strengthen the caregiver's capacity, if the observation is followed by reflective advice or feedback on the observed behaviour. These comments from the professional on the adult communicative partner's behaviour should take place after the family member has reflected on the situation and can include further information or ideas for future actions/behaviours;
- Reflection and problem-solving strategy. The parents/carers, with indirect guidance from the professional (again, for example, through guided questions), evaluate specific alternatives to the concern or goal to be achieved. These strategies, common in coaching, encourage parents/caregivers to generate ideas on how to improve the use of the intervention strategy they are using and how to generalise the strategy to new routines. Each idea is valued and contributes to the discussion;

- Communicative style. As we can easily deduce from the strategies discussed so far, communication is the cornerstone of all work with families. The success or failure of the intervention process depends to a large extent on the fluidity and authenticity of this communication.

The communicative style that the S-LP/T assumes with the parents/caregivers will also determine the type of relationship that will be established with them. Therefore, it is necessary to take into account some basic aspects in our interaction with caregivers: (1) simplicity in the use of language, deliberately devoid of unnecessary technical details; (2) brevity, using short sentences and objective speech; (3) the use of order. If possible, treat objectives or needs differently, opening up new topics when previous ones have been adequately and/or sufficiently addressed; (4) balanced use of speaking time. As a general idea, in collaborative work there should be a proportionality between speaking time and listening time, almost in equal parts, between the family and the S-LP/T; (5) informing, not being right. The S-LP/T working under the paradigm of family-centred practices must understand the importance and profound significance of accepting that the family, and they alone, should have the final say in the decisions they consider most appropriate for themselves and their child. This is the essence of promoting informed decisions. The S-LP/T provides information and, based on this, the family freely chooses the course of action to follow; the aim is not to convince the family; (6) non-judgement. Derived from the previous point, which emphasises respect for the family's decisions, even if the professional, based on their own beliefs, values or experience, may disagree. Not judging the family is one of the fundamental principles on which the therapeutic relationship is built and sustained. The error of judgement can be made in many different ways, whether verbal or non-verbal, such as a sudden change in body position or intonation. To avoid this, the S-LP/T must be aware of their own non-verbal communication; (7) empathetic listening. This is more than just attentive listening. When practising empathic listening, you don't just listen to words or observe behaviour, you speculate on the emotions and needs behind those words and behaviours, even if you can't understand exactly what the other person's experience is. The focus is on offering the other person a safe space so that they can express themselves and gain clarity about their situation, without imposing our own opinions, judgements, experiences and immediate solutions; (8) flowing at the family's pace. Each family is unique and has its own rhythm, and there are aspects of the intervention that the S-LP/T may need to adjust, such as: the length of the session, the amount of information to be shared, the number of objectives to be addressed, the time dedicated to each objective, the degree of formality or even the possible use of a certain sense of humour (García-Sánchez et al., 2020).

In addition to optimising learning, coaching strategies that support parents/caregivers in problem-solving and reflecting on intervention procedures can support the independence and competence of the parent/caregiver in their child's development and also facilitate relationships between the parent/caregiver and the S-LP/T (Lorio et al., 2020; Salisbury et al., 2017). However, Akhbari Ziegler and Hadders-Algra (2020) point out that only a limited range of available strategies are usually used.

In other studies, professionals have reported that they rarely use strategies such as guided practice to teach parents/caregivers, although they value collaborative practices. However, when strategies are applied incompletely, they can put at risk the achievement of positive results in the child's communication. Collaboration and problem-solving between S-LP/T and parents/caregivers, without effective instruction to the latter, can limit their ability to support their child's developmental needs (Meadan et al., 2018; Sawyer & Campbell, 2012).

Tomeny et al. (2020) report that although professionals use strategies to develop the capacities of parents/caregivers through guided practice, they do not include them in planning or decision-making, which can minimise the effect of the intervention on the child's participation in their daily routines or result in practices that are misaligned with the family's values and beliefs.

Synthesising research on adult learning principles and early childhood intervention has revealed benefits in using specific coaching strategies to achieve planned goals. Coaching strategies that allow opportunities for practice and provide feedback on parent/caregiver performance optimise learning (Brown & Woods, 2016; Sone et al., 2021). However, S-LP/T rarely report using these strategies (Meadan et al., 2018; Sawyer & Campbell, 2012). The study by Lee et al. (2022) finds that professionals tend to lead the intervention to the detriment of the use of coaching strategies and a family-centred approach, this being pointed out by the therapists as a consequence of the characteristics of the parents/caregivers themselves and their preference for traditional models of intervention.

Strategies such as joint interaction, in which parents/caregivers and therapists interact with the child, and the exchange of information, in which topics related to the child's development and evolution are discussed, suggest the incomplete use of coaching strategies. The moments of joint attention could be accompanied by strategies such as guided practice and observation (Brown & Woods, 2016; Sone et al., 2021) and the discussion of topics without the use of problem-solving, planning and reflection strategies may not indicate the involvement of parents/caregivers in decision-making to address intervention needs (Lee et al., 2022).

Analysing clinicians' beliefs about family-centred practices reveals potential explanations for the infrequent use of coaching strategies. Parent/caregiver characteristics (e.g. expectations, comfort and availability) are cited as the most frequent barriers to optimal parent/caregiver empowerment by professionals in several studies

(Douglas et al., 2019; Fleming et al., 2011; Lee et al., 2022; Meadan et al., 2018). In contrast, other studies report caregivers' interest in learning strategies, high satisfaction and lower levels of stress among parents/caregivers when taught how to use intervention strategies with their children (Abouzeid et al., 2020; Cycyk & Huerta, 2020; Sawyer and Campbell, 2012).

Some beliefs of S-LP/T suggest that they may believe that there is an ideal 'norm' of session structure for which the intervention should be designed for all families. For example, the need for appropriate materials and, by contrast, the lack of these in families' contexts, limits the use of participation-based sessions (Lee et al, 2022).

In fact, instead of encouraging the child to perform 'ideal' behaviours to facilitate learning according to normative developmental milestones, S-LP/T using family-centred practices should focus on strengthening the skills of parents/caregivers and improving communication between them and the child in natural activities in their environment.

FUTURE RESEARCH DIRECTION

Future research could focus on examining the factors that hinder or support collaboration between professionals and parents/caregivers in fostering children's learning and development. Such studies might include a diverse, global participant pool to compare practices and analyze both individual and organizational aspects. Potentially key areas of exploration sould encompass professional training, communication and information-sharing processes, workload and time limitations, attitudes towards teamwork, as well as policies and administrative frameworks. Additionally, it is essential to incorporate the perspectives and experiences of parents and caregivers in these investigations.

CONCLUSION

Family-centred practices are intended to be a model that emphasizes the collaboration and involvement of the family in the therapeutic process and have shown evidence of effectiveness in the development of children's communication and language when professionals and parents/caregivers collaborate in this process. We now know that intervention centred on parents/caregivers, while including daily routines, activities, places and people in the child's life, has more effective results in terms of the child's development, quality of family life and inclusion.

However, there is still a long way to go for professionals to use these practices, as research still indicates a leadership role for S-LP/T throughout the therapeutic process, which seems to be related to professionals' beliefs and the difficulty in breaking free from the norms of traditional models. Specialized and reflective training could be a possible solution for adopting a more family-centred model. Training that not only includes content on assessment models and intervention planning in natural living contexts according to the child's developmental needs, but also allows professionals to pay attention to the parents' concerns. Only when professionals recognize that their beliefs and values are not the same as those of the families they support, will they be able to be empathetic and create more meaningful relationships and consequently more effective results throughout the therapeutic process.

ACKNOWLEDGMENT

This research received no specific grant from any funding agency in the public, commercial, or not-for-profit sectors.

REFERENCES

Akemoglu, Y., Muharib, R., & Meadan, H. (2019). A Systematic and Quality Review of Parent-Implemented Language and Communication Interventions Conducted via Telepractice. *Journal of Behavioral Education*, *28*(2), 282–316. DOI: 10.1007/s10864-019-09356-3

American Speech and Hearing Association. (2021). SLP Health Care Survey Report: Workforce Trends 2005–2021. https://www.asha.org/siteassets/surveys/2021-slp-health-care-survey-workforce-trends-2005-2021.pdf

American Speech-Language-Hearing Association. (2016). *Scope of practice in speech-language pathology* [Scope of Practice]. https://www.asha.org/policy/

An, M., & Palisano, J. R. (2014). Family–professional collaboration in pediatric rehabilitation: A practice model. *Disability and Rehabilitation*, *36*(5), 434–440. DOI: 10.3109/09638288.2013.797510 PMID: 23713990

An, M., Palisano, R. J., Yi, C., Chiarello, L. A., Dunst, C. J., & Gracely, E. J. (2017). Effects of a Collaborative Intervention Process on Parent Empowerment and Child Performance: A Randomized Controlled Trial. *Physical & Occupational Therapy in Pediatrics*, *0*(0), 1–15. 101080/01942638.2017.1365324 PMID: 28929830

Associação Portuguesa de Terapeutas da Fala. (n.d.). https://www.oterapeutadafalapodefazeradiferenca.org/home

Carvalho, L., Almeida, I. Ch., Felgueiras, I., Leitão, S., Boavida, J., Santos, P. C., Serrano, A., Brito, A. T., Lança, C., Pimentel, J. S., Pinto, A. I., Grande, C., Brandão, T., & Franco, V. (2016). *Práticas recomendadas em intervenção precoce na infância: Um guia para profissionais*. Associação Nacional de Intervenção Precoce.

Cologon, K., Wicks, L., & Salvador, A. (2017). Supporting caregivers in developing responsive communication partnerships with their children: Extending a caregiver-led interactive language program. *Child Language Teaching and Therapy*, *33*(2), 157–169. DOI: 10.1177/0265659016650978

Coufal, K. L., & Woods, J. J. (2018). Interprofessional collaborative practice in early intervention. *Pediatric Clinics of North America, 65*(1), 143–155. DOI: 10.1016/j.pcl.2017.08.027 PMID: 29173715

Crawford, M. F. (2013). *Individuals with disabilities education improvement act of 2004 noncompliance determination complaints in commonwealth states* [Doctoral thesis Capella University. https://www.proquest.com/docview/1348696289

Davies, K. E., Marshall, J., Brown, L. J. E., & Goldbart, J. (2017). Co-working: Parents' conception of roles in supporting their children's speech and language development. *Child Language Teaching and Therapy, 33*(2), 171–185. DOI: 10.1177/0265659016671169

Division for Early Childhood Intervention. (2014). *DEC Recommended Practices.* https://www.dec-sped.org/dec-recommended-practices

Dunst, C. J. (2020). Everyday learning opportunities of young children with and without developmental disabilities or delays. *International Journal of Early Childhood Environmental Education, 7*(3), 23–41.

Dunst, C. J., Boyd, K., Trivette, C. M., & Hamby, D. W. (2002). Family-oriented program models and professional helpgiving practices. *Family Relations, 51*(3), 221–229. DOI: 10.1111/j.1741-3729.2002.00221.x

Dunst, C. J., & Espe-Sherwindt, M. (2016). Family-centered practices in early childhood intervention. In Reichow, B., Boyd, B. A., Barton, E. E., & Odom, S. L. (Eds.), *Handbook of early childhood special education* (pp. 37–55). Springer. DOI: 10.1007/978-3-319-28492-7_3

Dunst, C. J., & Trivette, C. M. (2009). Capacity-Building Family-Systems Intervention Practices. *Journal of Family Social Work, 12*(789296667), 119–143. DOI: 10.1080/10522150802713322

Dunst, C. J., Trivette, C. M., & Hamby, D. W. (2006). Technical manual for measuring and evaluating family support program quality and benefits. Winterberry Monograph Series. Winterberry Press. https://library.bsl.org.au/jspui/bitstream/1/4994/1/DunstC_Technical-manual-for-measuring-and-evaulating_Winterberry-2006.pdf

Dunst, C. J., Trivette, C. M., & Hamby, D. W. (2007). Meta-Analysis of family-centered helpgiving practices research. *Mental Retardation and Developmental Disabilities Research Reviews, 13*(4), 370–378. DOI: 10.1002/mrdd.20176 PMID: 17979208

Española de Logopedia, A. Foniatria y Audiología e Ibero-Americana de Fonoaudiología. (n.d.). https://www.aelfa.org/

Espe-Sherwindt, M., & Serrano, A. M. (2016). It takes two: The role of family-centered practices in communication intervention. *Revista de Logopedia, Foniatría y Audiología, 36*(4), 162–169. DOI: 10.1016/j.rlfa.2016.07.006

Ferreira, L. P. (2021). Terapeutas da Fala em contexto clínico: *Práticas Centradas na Família* [Master's dissertation, Instituto Politécnico do Porto]. Repositório Científico do Instituto Politécnico do Porto. https://recipp.ipp.pt/bitstream/10400.22/17254/1/DM_Liliana%20Ferrreira.pdf

Gail, J., Soderberg, J., Abbott, R., Garzon, R., & Scott, C. (2022). Improving language support for infants and toddlers. Results of FIND coaching in childcare. *Infants and Young Children, 35*(2), 91–105. https://doi.org/https://doi.org/10.1097/IYC.0000000000000214. DOI: 10.1097/IYC.0000000000000214

García-Sánchez, F. A., Mora, C. T. E., & Castellano, I. F. (2020). Reflexiones y estrategias de acompañamiento familiar en Atención Temprana. *Revista de Logopedia, Foniatría y Audiología, 40*(3), 118–127. DOI: 10.1016/j.rlfa.2020.02.004

Heidlage, J. K., Cunningham, J. E., Kaiser, A. P., Trivette, C. M., Barton, E. E., Frey, J. R., & Roberts, M. Y. (2020). The effects of parent-implemented language interventions on child linguistic outcomes: A meta-analysis. *Early Childhood Research Quarterly, 50*, 6–23. DOI: 10.1016/j.ecresq.2018.12.006

Jimenez-Arberas, E., Casais-Suarez, Y., Fernandez-Mendez, A., Menendez-Espina, S., Rodriguez-Menendez, S., Llosa, J. A., & Prieto-Saborit, J. A. (2024). Evidence-based implementation of the family-centered model and the use of tele-intervention in early childhood services: A systematic review. *Health Care, 12*(1), 112. DOI: 10.3390/healthcare12010112 PMID: 38201017

Klatte, S. I., Bloemen, M., Groot, A., Mantel, T. M., Ketelaar, M., & Gerrits, E. (2024). Collaborative working in speech and language therapy for children with DLD—What are parents' needs? *International Journal of Language & Communication Disorders, 59*(1), 340–353. DOI: 10.1111/1460-6984.12951 PMID: 37715545

Klatte, S. I., Ketelaar, M., Groot, A., Bloemen, M., & Gerrits, E. (2023). Collaboration: How does it work according to therapists and parents of young children? A systematic review. *Child: Care, Health and Development, 50*(1), 1–20. DOI: 10.1111/cch.13167 PMID: 37724049

Klatte, S. I., Lyons, R., Davies, K., Harding, S., Marshall, J., McKean, C., & Roulstone, S. (2020). Collaboration between parents and SLTs produces optimal outcomes for children attending speech and language therapy: Gathering the evidence. *International Journal of Language & Communication Disorders, 00*(0), 1–11. DOI: 10.1111/1460-6984.12538 PMID: 32383829

Kokorelias, K., Gignac, M. A. M., Naglie, G., & Cameron, J. I. (2019). Towards a universal model of family centered care: A scoping review. *BMC Health Services Research, 19*(1), 564. DOI: 10.1186/s12913-019-4394-5 PMID: 31409347

Kwok, E., Bootsma, J., Cahill, P., & Rosenbaum, P. (2021). A scoping review of qualitative studies on parents' perspectives on speech, language, and communication interventions. *Disability and Rehabilitation, 44*(25), 8084–8093. DOI: 10.1080/09638288.2021.1989061 PMID: 34669539

Langner, J., & Fukkink, R. G. (2022). A realist synthesis of interprofessional collaborative practices in early intervention for children with speech, language and communication needs. *International Journal of Language & Communication Disorders, 58*(2), 516–541. DOI: 10.1111/1460-6984.12789 PMID: 36217271

Law, J., McKean, C., Murphy, C., & Thordardottir, E. (Eds.). (2019). *Managing children with developmental language disorder: Theory and practice across europe and beyond*. Routledge. DOI: 10.4324/9780429455308

Lee, J., Kaat, A. J., & Roberts, M. Y. (2022). Involving caregivers of autistic toddlers in early intervention: Common practice or exception to the norm? *American Journal of Speech-Language Pathology, 31*(4), 1755–1770. DOI: 10.1044/2022_AJSLP-21-00246 PMID: 35749738

Leite, C. S. C. (2018). *Benefícios da intervenção precoce: Perspetiva de famílias portuguesas* [Doctoral thesis, Universidade do Minho]. Repositório da Universidade do Minho. https://hdl.handle.net/1822/56328

Levey, S. (2024). *Introdution to Language Development* (3rd ed.). Plural Publishing Inc.

Lopez, K. M. J., Lyons, R., Novogrodsky, R., Baena, S., Feilberg, J., Harding, S., Kelić, M., Klatte, I. S., Mantel, T. C., Tomazin, M. O., Ulfsdottir, T. S., Zajdó, K., & Rodriguez-Ortiz, I. R. (2021). Exploring parental perspectives of childhood speech and language disorders across 10 countries: A pilot qualitative study. *Journal of Speech, Language, and Hearing Research: JSLHR, 64*(5), 1739–1747. DOI: 10.1044/2020_JSLHR-20-00415 PMID: 33823117

Luze, G. J., Linebarger, D. L., Greenwood, C. R., Carta, J. J., Walker, D., Leitschuh, C., & Atwater, J. B. (2001). Developing a general outcome measure of growth in expressive communication of infants and toddlers. *School Psychology Review, 30*(3), 383–406. DOI: 10.1080/02796015.2001.12086122

MacGuillion, M., Pine, J., Herbert, J., & Matthews, D. (2017). A randomised controlled trial to test the effect of promoting caregiver contingent talk on language development in infants from diverse socioeconomic status backgrounds. *Journal of Child Psychology and Psychiatry, and Allied Disciplines*, *58*(10), 1122–1131. DOI: 10.1111/jcpp.12725 PMID: 28429816

Madigan, S., Prime, H., Graham, S. A., Rodrigues, M., Anderson, N., Khoury, J., & Jenkins, J. M. (2019). Parenting behavior and child language: A meta-analysis. *Pediatrics*, *144*(4), e20183556. DOI: 10.1542/peds.2018-3556 PMID: 31551396

Mahoney, G., & MacDonald, J. D. (2007a). *Autism and developmental delays in young children: The responsive teaching curriculum for parents and professionals, Curriculum guide*. Pro-ed.

Mahoney, G., & MacDonald, J. D. (2007b). Autism and developmental delays in young children. [file:///C:/Users/Utilizador/Downloads/Autism_and_Developmental_Delays_in_Young_Children.pdf]. *International Journal of Early Childhood Special Education*, *1*, 1.

Mas, J. M., Canadas, M., Balcells-Balcells, A., Gine, C., Serrano, A. M., & Dunst, C. J. (2018). Psychometric properties of the Spanish version of the family-centred practices scale for use with families of young children receiving early childhood intervention. *Journal of Applied Research in Intellectual Disabilities*, *31*(5), 851–861. DOI: 10.1111/jar.12442 PMID: 29532976

Masek, L. R., McMillan, B. T. M., Paterson, S. J., Tamis-LeMonda, C. S., Golinkoff, R. M., Hirsh-Pasek, K. (2021) Where language meets attention: How contingent interactions promote learning. *Developmental Review*, 60, 0273-2297. DOI: 10.1016/j.dr.2021.100961

Mora, C. T. E., García, L. R., & Sánchez, F. A. G. (2023). *Guía de intervención logopédica en atención temprana centrada en la familia*. Editorial Síntesis.

Muhinyi, A., & Rowe, M. L. (2019). Shared reading with preverbal infants and later language development. *Journal of Applied Developmental Psychology*, *64*, 101053. Advance online publication. DOI: 10.1016/j.appdev.2019.101053

Owens, R. E. (2016). *Language Development: An Introduction* (9th ed.). Pearson.

Pinto M. & Serrano, A.M. (2022). Perceção dos profissionais acerca da participação das famílias no apoio pelas equipas de intervenção precoce. *Zero-a-Seis*, 24 (n. Especial), 740-768. DOI: 10.5007/1518-2924.2022.e83100

Pinto, M. J. S. (2018). *Participação das famílias no apoio prestado pelo Sistema Nacional de Intervenção Precoce na Infância* [Doctoral thesis, Universidade do Minho]. Repositório da Universidade do Minho. https://hdl.handle.net/1822/65351

Prelock, P. J., & Nelson, N. W. (2012). Language and Communication in Autism: An Integrated View. *Pediatric Clinics of North America, 59*(1), 129–145. DOI: 10.1016/j.pcl.2011.10.008 PMID: 22284798

Reed, J., Hirsh-Pasek, K., & Golinkoff, R. M. (2016). Meeting Children Where They Are: Adaptive Contingency Builds Early Communication Skills. In Witt, P. (Ed.), *Communication and Learning - Handbooks of Communication Science* (pp. 601–627). Gruyter Mouton. DOI: 10.1515/9781501502446-025

Roberts, M. Y., Curtis, P. R., Sone, B. J., & Hampton, L. H. (2019). Association of parent training with child language development: A systematic review and meta-analysis. *JAMA Pediatrics, 173*(7), 671–680. DOI: 10.1001/jamapediatrics.2019.1197 PMID: 31107508

Roberts, M. Y., & Kaiser, A. P. (2011). The Effectiveness of Parent-Implemented Language Interventions: A Meta-Analysis. *American Journal of Speech-Language Pathology, 20*(3), 180–199. DOI: 10.1044/1058-0360(2011/10-0055) PMID: 21478280

Rush, D. D. & Shelden, M'L. L. (2011). *The Early Childhood Coaching Handbook*. Paul H Brookes Publishing Co.

Sánchez, F. A. G. (2019). Neurociencias y atención temprana. In Mora, C. T. E., & García, L. R. (Eds.), *Prácticas de atención temprana centradas en la familia y en entornos naturales* (pp. 33–50). UNED.

Sawyer, S., & Tapia, A. (2005). The sociotechnical nature of mobile computing work: Evidence from a study of policing in the United States. *International Journal of Technology and Human Interaction, 1*(3), 1–14. DOI: 10.4018/jthi.2005070101

Simões, M. C. B. (2011). *Rotinas familiares privilegiadas na comunicação de crianças com perturbação do espectro do autismo. Uma perspectiva parental* [Monografia, Universidade Atlântida]. Repositório Científico Universidade Atlântida.

Singer, I., Klatte, I. S., Vries, R., Lugt, R., & Gerrits, E. (2022). Using co-design to develop a tool for shared goal-setting with parents in speech and language therapy. *International Journal of Language & Communication Disorders, 57*(6), 1281–1303. DOI: 10.1111/1460-6984.12753 PMID: 35859264

Sociedade Portuguesa de Terapia da Fala. (n.d.). *Linguagem na criança*. https://sptf.org.pt/departamento-linguagem-na-crianca/

Sosa, A. V. (2016). Association of the Type of Toy Used During Play With the Quantity and Quality of Parent-Infant Communication. *JAMA Pediatrics*, *170*(2), 132–137. DOI: 10.1001/jamapediatrics.2015.3753 PMID: 26720437

Speech Pathology Australia. (2024). *Let's talk about speech pathology*. https://www.speechpathologyaustralia.org.au/

Tamis-LeMonda, C. S., Kuchirko, Y., & Song, L. (2014). Why Is Infant Language Learning Facilitated by Parental Responsiveness? *Current Directions in Psychological Science*, *23*(2), 121–126. DOI: 10.1177/0963721414522813

Te Kaat-van den Os, D., Jongmans, M., Volman, M. C. J. M., & Lauteslager, P. E. M. (2017). Parent-implemented language interventions for children with developmental delay: A systematic review. *Journal of Policy and Practice in Intellectual Disabilities*, *14*(2), 129–137. DOI: 10.1111/jppi.12181

Weisberg, D. S., Hirsh-Pasek, K., Golinkoff, R. M., Kittredge, A. K., & Klahr, D. (2016). Guided play: Principles and practices. *Current Directions in Psychological Science*, *25*(3), 177–182. DOI: 10.1177/0963721416645512

Yang, C.-H., Hossain, S. Z., & Sitharthan, G. (2013). Collaborative practice in early childhood intervention from the perspectives of service providers. *Infants and Young Children*, *26*(1), 57–73. DOI: 10.1097/IYC.0b013e3182736cbf

Ziegler, S. A., & Hadders-Algra, M. (2020). Coaching approaches in early intervention and pediatric rehabilitation. *Developmental Medicine and Child Neurology*, *62*(5), 569–574. DOI: 10.1111/dmcn.14493 PMID: 32065385

ADDITIONAL READING

Levickis, P., Eadie, P., Mensah, F., McKean, C., Bavin, E. L., & Reilly, S. (2023). Associations between responsive parental behaviors in infancy and toddlerhood, and language outcomes at age 7 years in a population-based sample. *International Journal of Language & Communication Disorders*, *58*(4), 1098–1112. DOI: 10.1111/1460-6984.12846 PMID: 36726027

Chapter 13
Women's Health Across the Lifespan:
An Integrative Role of Physiotherapy in Pelvic Health and Other Health Conditions

Fátima Santos
https://orcid.org/0000-0001-6816-2071
Escola Superior Saúde Fernando Pessoa, Portugal

Mário Esteves
https://orcid.org/0000-0001-9138-3972
Escola Superior de Saúde Fernando Pessoa, Portugal

Clarinda S. D. S. F. Festas
https://orcid.org/0000-0001-5244-1914
Escola Superior de Saúde Fernando Pessoa, Portugal

Sara Viana
Unidade Local de Saúde São João, Portugal & Escola Superior de Saúde Fernando Pessoa, Portugal

Diana Bernardo
https://orcid.org/0000-0002-3832-7581
Escola Superior de Saúde, Instituto Politécnico de Bragança, Portugal

Telma Pires
Escola Superior de Saúde, Instituto Politécnico de Bragança, Portugal

Rui Viana
https://orcid.org/0000-0002-2542-8068
Unidade Local de Saúde São João, Escola Superior de Saúde Fernando Pessoa, Portugal

ABSTRACT

Physiotherapists can contribute significantly to women's pelvic health and other health conditions throughout the life stages, including adolescence, adulthood, pregnancy, childbirth, postpartum, menopause, and post-menopause. Their roles

DOI: 10.4018/979-8-3693-6432-1.ch013

encompass education, rehabilitation, counselling, and empowerment, promoting health and facilitating recovery in various women's health conditions. The chapter underscores physiotherapy interventions during pregnancy and postpartum recovery, along with rehabilitation for pelvic floor and oncological conditions, emphasising the importance of tailored physical activity and exercise prescriptions. Additionally, it addresses physiotherapy's role in managing often underrepresented conditions, such as dysmenorrhoea and endometriosis. Emphasising a holistic approach, the chapter highlights physiotherapy's important role in supporting lifelong wellness and addressing the unique health needs of women within a collaborative, multidisciplinary healthcare team.

INTRODUCTION

Throughout the female life cycle, women undergo continuous physical, physiological, psychological, and emotional transformations that significantly impact their well-being. From the rapid development experienced during adolescence and youth, through the changes associated with pregnancy and postpartum, to the transition of menopause these processes profoundly affect both the body and mind (Thiyagarajan et al., 2024). Regardless of whether a woman experiences pregnancy, the transformations across all life stages influence not only physical and mental health but also her evolving role in society, shaping her self-perception and place in the world.

Given the diverse challenges women face throughout their life cycle, the inclusion of a specialized physiotherapist in pelvic and women's health is important within multidisciplinary healthcare teams. Physiotherapists, drawing on their comprehensive understanding of the complex interactions between bodily systems, particularly in relation to movement and function, can delivered tailored interventions that positively impact women's health and well-being (Boissonnault et al., 2020, International Organization of Physiotherapists in Pelvic and Women's Health [IOPPWH], 2013, 2023).

The objective of this review is to underscore the role of specialist physiotherapists in women's and pelvic floor health, highlighting their contributions within a multidisciplinary team. The subsequent section will detail physiotherapy interventions across a range of conditions throughout the female lifespan, illustrating their role in addressing and preventing health issues, as well as promoting long-term health outcomes, all underpinned by current evidence. Thus, the following topics are covered: Physiotherapy in pregnancy, childbirth and postpartum; Physiotherapy in menopause and elderly Women; Physiotherapy in pelvic floor disorders; Physiotherapy in oncological rehabilitation; Physiotherapy in aesthetic and reconstructive health and Physiotherapy in other Conditions.

MAIN FOCUS OF THE CHAPTER

Physiotherapy in Pregnancy, Childbirth and Postpartum

Pregnancy, childbirth and postpartum period presents distinct physical, psychological, and emotional challenges for women. Physiotherapists, working as part of a multidisciplinary team, can help optimise the function and quality of life for the woman, the newborn and the family.

It is well known that health literacy plays a crucial role during pregnancy, as the mother's health behaviours impact both her own health and that of her child. A systematic review reveals that high-quality studies or interventions in this area are rare or do not exist, so the healthcare providers are in a privilege position to play a key role in promote greater literacy (Nawabi et al., 2021). As defined by some authors, maternal health literacy is a multifaceted and comprehensive concept, encompassing skills that enable women to access, understand, evaluate, and apply health information related to pregnancy, which is essential for making decisions to improve and maintain both maternal and fetal health (Putri & Lu, 2024). Alongside other healthcare professionals, physiotherapists contribute by providing specialised knowledge in movement and function, particularly regarding the physiological and physical changes in the musculoskeletal system, including the pelvic floor, as well as offering expertise in breathing adaptions, relaxation techniques, non-pharmacological pain management strategies and physical activity and exercise (Boissonnault et al., 2020). By fostering a deep understanding of how women's bodies change and the implications of these changes during pregnancy, labour, childbirth, and the postnatal period, physiotherapists contribute to promoting informed decision-making and empowering women to take an active role in managing their health (IOPPWH, 2013, 2023).

During pregnancy, the body undergoes a wide range of physical changes, including postural adaptations, joint laxity, and shifts in the centre of gravity, which can lead to discomfort and potential dysfunctions. Physiotherapists provide instruction on adopting ergonomic postures, adapting movements to avoid strain and enhance energy conservation, and incorporating exercises that strengthen key muscle groups and proper activate specific muscles like pelvic floor muscles. This intervention can contribute to prevent common pregnancy-related issues such low back pain, pelvic girdle pain and pelvic floor conditions (incontinence, pelvic organ prolapse and sexual dysfunctions), while also promoting optimal physical health for labour and postpartum recovery (IOPPWH, 2013).

Even during pregnancy, the physiotherapist's role also involves raising awareness about the benefits of movement and postures for labour and childbirth. Following the World Health Organization recommendations for positive birth experience, low risk pregnant women should be encouraged to adopt mobility and upright position during labour (World Health Organization, 2018), since there is strong evidence that is a reduction of second stage duration in cases of a flexible sacrum birthing position (Berta et al., 2019). Therefore, deeper body awareness trough movement and postures should be encouraged by the educational physiotherapy´s sessions during pregnancy. By understanding how the body responds to stress and pain during labour and how movement and postures ca help, women are empowered to make informed choices that can contribute to a more positive birth experience.

This increased awareness of the importance of movement in pregnancy and childbirth aligns with recent shifts in how physical activity during pregnancy is understood. In recent years, the perspective on physical activity (PA) during pregnancy has undergone significant changes (Newton & May, 2017). In the past, pregnant women were often advised to reduce or even stop PA, based on the justification that it could lead to complications for both the mother and the fetus.

Currently, scientific evidence confirms that regular PA during pregnancy is safe for both the mother and the fetus and significantly improves important pregnancy outcomes. PA is closely associated with a reduced risk of obesity and excessive gestational weight gain (Ruchat et al., 2018), hypertension, diabetes (American College of Obstetricians and Gynecologists [ACOG], 2015), cardiovascular diseases (Nascimento et al., 2012), and preeclampsia (ACOG, 2015a). It also enhances emotional well-being, lowers the risk of postpartum depression (ACOG, 2015a), reduces the likelihood of caesarean delivery (ACOG, 2020), and can induce beneficial physiological changes in the fetus that positively impact its future health trajectory (Halfon et al., 2014).

The principles of exercise prescription for pregnant women do not differ significantly from those for the general population. In the absence of obstetric or medical complications, it is recommended that pregnant women accumulate at least 150 minutes of moderate-intensity aerobic exercise per week, or 75 minutes of vigorous-intensity aerobic exercise per week, spread over most days of the week (American College of Sports Medicine [ACSM], 2018). Pregnant women who were previously inactive should be encouraged to start with low-intensity exercises and gradually increase the duration or intensity based on their tolerance (ACOG, 2020).

Given the well-documented benefits of exercise (Brown et al, 2022; Yang et al., 2022), especially in preventing significant disorders such as gestational diabetes mellitus, preeclampsia, and gestational hypertension, as well as in improving outcomes for conditions that negatively impact maternal quality of life - including anxiety, prenatal depression, lumbopelvic pain, and urinary incontinence (Ribeiro et al., 2021), physiotherapists can also develop tailored exercise programmes that promote safe physical activity while accommodating pre-existing conditions, thereby mitigating associated risk.

Physiotherapists play also an important role on educate pregnant women on the normal and abnormal musculoskeletal consequences of pregnancy and childbirth in and individual context or offer educational sessions at prenatal classes (Critchley, 2022).

During postpartum period, physiotherapists can support women in their recovery by focusing on restoring pelvic floor and core function, regardless of whether the birth was vaginal or via caesarean section.

Research highlights the benefits of pelvic floor muscle training in managing postpartum urinary incontinence (Diz-Teixeira et al., 2023) as well as improving sexual function and quality of life (Hadizadeh-Talasaz et al., 2019). Additionally, abdominal and pelvic floor muscle training may improve body image, physical function, and abdominal strength in women with diastasis recti, although there remains no consensus on the most effective exercise approach (Gluppe et al., 2021). Furthermore, in cases of caesarean delivery, manual therapy has been shown to be beneficial in the treatment of scar tissue (Deflorin et al., 2020; Olszewska et al., 2020).

Physiotherapists can also manage a range of musculoskeletal conditions in the postpartum period, including pelvic and back pain (Choo et al., 2020). Regarding other conditions, the results of a systematic review and meta-analysis concluded that myofascial therapy can effectively reduce rectus abdominis separation, alleviate pelvic floor muscle dysfunction, enhance lumbar function, relieve pain, and improve the ability to perform daily living activities (Wang et al., 2023).

Their role extends beyond treatment to include education, providing guidance on ergonomics for daily activities such as optimal postures for feeding the baby (whether breastfeeding or not), as well as carrying the baby.

Educating women may also help reduce the stigma and embarrassment surrounding pelvic and abdominal health, enabling women to recognise these sensitive issues as legitimate conditions (Critchley, 2022).

During the postpartum period, physiotherapists can also offer specialised care, focusing on safely supporting women in their return to physical exercise (Dipietro et al., 2019). The practice of physical exercise in the postpartum period has shown considerable benefits. PA contributes to improved cardiorespiratory condition, reduces fatigue, reduce weight retention enhances sleep quality, and decreases the risk of depression (Dipietro et al., 2019). Moreover, specific exercises for the pelvic floor are effective in preventing and reducing genitourinary dysfunctions (Sobhgol et al., 2019).

Physiotherapy plays an important role within the multidisciplinary team, supporting not only the mother and her baby but also healthcare professionals and improving the efficiency of health services. By preventing or treating common pregnancy-related musculoskeletal conditions (IOPPWH, 2013), expert physiotherapists help reduce musculoskeletal complaints that could otherwise require medical intervention.

Even during labour, promoting body awareness and encouraging optimal birthing positions and movements in low-risk pregnant women can facilitate delivery (Berta et al., 2019), potentially reducing reliance on medical pain relief or interventions. In the postpartum period, physiotherapists accelerate maternal recovery through personalised rehabilitation, addressing musculoskeletal conditions such as pelvic dysfunction, back pain, and complications following caesarean delivery (Choo et al., 2020; Critchley, 2022; Deflorin et al., 2020; Diz-Teixeira et al., 2023; Olszewska et al., 2020). This approach helps to alleviate the burden on healthcare professionals and services. Collectively, physiotherapist intervention significantly enhances the collaborative effort of the multidisciplinary team in providing comprehensive maternal healthcare. By reducing the impact of pregnancy and postpartum conditions, improving mobility, and supporting early recovery, physiotherapists may contribute to lowering healthcare costs, shortening hospital stays, and fostering a positive birth experience, all while prioritising woman- and baby-centred care. Further impact studies are needed to demonstrate the effectiveness of specialised women's and pelvic floor health physiotherapy interventions within healthcare services.

Physiotherapy in Menopause and Elderly Women

Menopause is defined as the cessation of menstruation, which can only be confirmed retrospectively. Consequently, women are considered postmenopausal after 12 consecutive months without a menstrual period. The menopausal transition begins with changes in menstrual cycles and culminates one year after the last menstrual period. Although there remains some uncertainty regarding the symptoms associated with menopause, various conditions are commonly reported during the transition to menopause. These include vasomotor symptoms, muscle and joint pain, disturbances in sleep and concentration, fatigue, as well as genitourinary and sexual symptoms, among others, which require a multidisciplinary approach (Hickey et al., 2024).

Many women navigate menopause without requiring medical intervention, however, some do experience symptoms that impact their function and quality of life (Hickey et al., 2024). In a survey conducted across five European countries, the authors concluded that women seeking medical assistance were often primarily motivated by the desire for information rather than by a need for pharmacological treatment, unless their symptoms were particularly severe (Constantine et al., 2016).

Natural menopause is linked to an increased incidence of certain health conditions while reducing the incidence of others (Hickey et al., 2024). It is well established that bone density declines following menopause and there is evidence that strength exercises can be beneficial for improving strength, PA, bone density and hormonal and metabolic levels (Capel-Alcaraz et al., 2023). In this context, specialised physiotherapy programmes play an important role in empowering women during menopause. Among the interventions available, pelvic physiotherapy has been shown to be particularly effective in addressing pelvic floor dysfunctions, which are commonly associated with this stage of life (Mercier et al., 2023). Furthermore, educational programmes offer valuable guidance on managing musculoskeletal disorders, maintaining body composition, and preserving overall functionality (Strand et al., 2024). Manual therapy is also of significance in the alleviation of musculoskeletal symptoms (Espírito Santo et al., 2024). These physiotherapy programmes have been shown to support women in managing the symptoms experienced during the menopausal transition and can further promote active ageing (Strand et al., 2024).

Aging is associated with functional decline, both physical and cognitive, which increases the likelihood of age-related diseases and comorbidities. The reduction in muscle strength, coordination, balance, and gait capacity are consequences of physical deterioration in older adults (Thomas et al., 2019). These factors contribute to a potentially higher risk of falls, especially in women. The higher incidence of falls among women can be attributed to several factors, such as greater longevity, less frequent participation in outdoor activities, more frequent use of medications, including psychotropics, and reduced grip strength (Gai et al., 2009).

PA and exercise programs for older adults have demonstrated significant effectiveness in preventing falls, promoting simultaneous gains in strength and improvements in balance (Sherrington et al., 2008). The ACSM recommend that multicomponent exercises, which combine resistance training, strength, neuromotor components (such as balance, agility, and proprioception), and flexibility, are effective in improving functionality and reducing the risk of falls in older adults (ACSM, 2018).

Some considerations should be considered when prescribing exercise for older adults, particularly: the intensity and duration of PA should be light at the beginning, especially for those who are significantly deconditioned, have functional limitations, or present chronic conditions that affect their ability to perform physical tasks. The progression of PA should be tailored to everyone, considering their tolerance and preferences; a more conservative approach may be necessary for older adults who are severely deconditioned or physically limited (ACSM, 2018).

Physiotherapy in Pelvic Floor Disorders

Currently, the terminology used in the assessment and diagnosis of pelvic floor muscle (PFM) function and dysfunction is still variable. However, the International Continence Society (ICS) has endeavoured to establish important consensus and guidelines on pelvic floor terminology.

PFM-related symptoms can be associated with symptoms of pelvic floor disorders such: (1) urinary incontinence or voiding dysfunction, (2) fecal incontinence or defecatory dysfunction, (3) sexual dysfunction, (4) pelvic organ prolapse, or other disorders of neuromusculoskeletal structures in the pelvis or spine (Frawley et al., 2021).

(1) Urinary Incontinence (UI), have a major impact on society, a public health problem that mostly affects women, especially when they are exposed to certain risk factors, such as pregnancy, vaginal childbirth, menopause and exercise, among other sports. The ICS and the International Urogynecological Association (IUGA), define UI as a symptom, namely the complaint of any involuntary loss of urine (Haylen et al., 2010). UI can have a negative impact on quality of life (QoL), and treatments for this condition are being widely developed to improve symptoms as well as QoL (Viana et al., 2015).

The ICS recommends pelvic physiotherapy as a first line of treatment for UI, including pregnancy and postpartum (Frawley et al., 2021). The program allows significant improvement in the quantity of urinary leakage and an increase in the strength of the PFM (Bø & Hilde, 2013; Pires et al., 2020a).

The effects of exercise have been studied on pelvic floor function in female athletes. Several researchers have established a directly proportional relationship between training intensity/ impact and the prevalence of UI. A systematic review with meta-analysis showed 25.9% prevalence of UI in female athletes in different sports, as well as 20.7% prevalence of stress urinary incontinence (SUI). The most prevalent high impact sport was volleyball, with the value of 75.6%. The prevalence of UI can be high in female athletes, with high-impact sports potentially increasing the risk for SUI (Pires et al., 2020b). So, high-impact sports, such as volleyball, trampolining and basketball, have shown strong associations with increased intra-abdominal pressure and impacts with ground reaction forces, presenting an increased risk of PFM damage compared to low-impact sports (Da Roza et al., 2015; Cardoso et al., 2018). Age, body mass index (BMI) and high-impact sports appear to be the leading factors that promote the onset of SUI, which in turn decrease the QoL in sportswomen (Pires, et al., 2020c). Several studies, including a randomized controlled trial (RCT), show that physiotherapy was effective in treating SUI in elite athletes, as the percentage of urine loss decreased in the experimental group, suggesting that the pelvic floor muscle training (PFMT) protocol can help athletes with SUI (Bø & Hilde, 2013; Pires et al., 2020d).

PFMT alone or associated with multidimensional exercises, bladder training, vaginal cones and sometimes electrostimulation seem to be effective techniques for reducing urinary symptoms and inducing MPP contraction (Bø et al., 2023). Motivation and adherence to pelvic floor physiotherapy intervention is key to maximising treatment results. It should also be noted that the educational component is an important strategy, as it allows women to be informed and able to apply strategies in their daily lives, as well as to modify habits that can minimise UI symptoms (Da Roza et al, 2012; Navarro-Brazález et al., 2021; Reed et al., 2021).

(2) Fecal Incontinence (FI) is a condition that significantly affects the patient's quality of life (QoL). The ICS describes the following symptoms of anorectal incontinence: Anal incontinence as involuntary loss of feces or flatus, which can be classified as: (i) FI as involuntary loss of solid or liquid feces; (ii) Flatus incontinence as involuntary loss of gas; (iii) Double incontinence: complaints of both anal and UI; (iv) Coital fecal (flatal) incontinence: fecal (flatal) incontinence occurring during vaginal sexual intercourse; (v) Passive fecal leakage (unconscious) – soiling (involuntary soiling of liquid or solid stool without sensation or warning or difficulty wiping clean); (vi) Overflow FI: seepage of stool due to fecal impaction (Sultan et al., 2017). Treatments for FI include pharmacological procedures and non- pharmacological interventions. These interventions include dietary adjustments, anal plugs and physiotherapy (PFMT with or without biofeedback, neuromuscular electrical stimulation) (Norton et al., 2010).

Defecation dysfunction includes all defecation disorders, in addition to faecal incontinence. Conservative management strategies—such as establishing an individualised bowel routine, promoting appropriate toileting posture and hygiene habits, and engaging in physiotherapy interventions—should be recommended before surgical options are considered (Crosby & Husk, 2021).

According to the Rome IV criteria, chronic constipation disorders are classified into four subtypes: (a) functional constipation; (b) irritable bowel syndrome with constipation; (c) opioid-induced constipation; and (d) functional defaecation disorders, which include inadequate defaecatory propulsion and dyssynergic defaecation. The initial approach to managing these conditions should focus on non-pharmacological measures, including dietary advice, physical activity, lifestyle modification, and the use of over-the-counter laxatives when appropriate. Pharmacological treatments, with or without biofeedback therapy, may be indicated, although surgical intervention is rarely necessary (Aziz et al., 2020). Health professionals should be encouraged to proactively identify people presenting with symptoms of defaecation dysfunction and ensure that appropriate assessment and treatment are offered (Milsom et al., 2023). Furthermore, anorectal biofeedback is a behavioural training technique that has been shown to be effective in the treatment of dyssynergic defaecation, with reported symptom improvement in approximately 70% of cases. It may also have beneficial effects on slow-transit constipation, which can arise as a secondary manifestation of dyssynergic defaecation (Aziz et al., 2020).

(3) Sexual dysfunction has an increasingly significant dimension and impact on an individual's life. The pelvic floor plays a crucial role in sexual function, with its muscles contributing to vaginal responsiveness, coital satisfaction, and orgasmic responses. Pelvic floor disorders may disrupt sexual arousal, satisfaction, and desire, especially when associated with pain. The professionals can offer emotional support, educate about the physical and emotional changes, their treatments, provide pain

relief techniques and prescribe specific therapies, such as hormone therapy, sex therapy, cognitive-behavioural therapy and pelvic floor exercises (Graziottin, 2023).

In addressing sexuality, we highlight three essential aspects: (i) Encourage open dialogue about the topic, demystify concepts, and create space for questions and concerns, just as we do for any other basic human need; (ii) Promote sexual health education, helping individuals understand how their bodies function so they can comprehend the reasons behind the treatment's implications on their sexuality; (iv) Define intervention strategies to address potential treatment-related toxicity or assist in the redefinition of one's own concept of sexuality (Rogers et al., 2018).

Pelvic rehabilitation will be an asset in reducing or eliminating all these symptoms/disorders: women's sexual interest/desire disorder, sexual aversion disorder, subjective sexual arousal disorder, genital sexual arousal disorder, combined genital and subjective arousal disorder, persistent sexual arousal disorder, women's orgasmic disorder, dyspareunia and vaginismus (Graziottin, 2023).

In his review of the literature, Berghmans (2018) states that physiotherapy, as a holistic approach, can significantly contribute to the management of female sexual dysfunction and pelvic pain. In addition to other physiotherapy techniques, the author highlights that myofascial release and various manual therapy modalities – such as deep-pressure massage, stretching, joint mobilisation, and other trigger point release techniques – can be utilised to address myofascial and pelvic pain.

Regarding chronic pain, there is some evidence that factors related to the autonomic nervous system, such as blood pressure (Bruehl & Chung, 2004) and heart rate variability (Rampazo et al., 2024), can influence pain modulation. A systematic review has proposed that diverse manual therapies can enhance cardiac autonomy in healthy young and middle-aged subjects, as well as in those experiencing discomfort, hypertension, and low back pain associated with myofascial trigger points. The review underscores the necessity for additional randomised controlled studies to further investigate this area (de Sousa et al., 2020). Given the prevalence of myofascial pain in certain pelvic floor conditions, it is imperative to conduct rigorous studies to investigate the impact of manual therapy on autonomic nervous system outcomes that contribute to pelvic pain.

(4) Pelvic Organ Prolapse (POP) is defined, according to the ICS, as an anatomical pelvic alteration, with descent of the anterior and/or posterior vaginal walls, uterus, or vaginal apex, potentially involving the descent of one or more vaginal walls (Haylen et al., 2016). POP can have a multifactorial condition: parity, vaginal delivery, age, and BMI (Vergeldt et al., 2015). Additionally, combinations of anatomical, physiological, genetic, lifestyle, and reproductive factors may contribute to pelvic floor dysfunction (Delancey et al., 2008). It is a health condition that negatively impacts women's QoL. POP treatment can be surgical or conservative. Conservative treatments include the use of pessaries and PFMT (Da Silva et al.,

2024). Several studies have demonstrated the efficacy of PFMT for conservative treatment of POP, including this literature review which concluded: symptom relief, increased strength and support elements of the pelvic organs, better activation of muscle fibers and improvement in patients' QoL, sexual function and body image (da Silva & Livramento, 2023). The treatment of POP should be focused on symptomatic women, while those who are asymptomatic or only mildly symptomatic may be monitored periodically. Therapeutic options include both conservative and surgical approaches, depending on the severity of the prolapse and the associated symptoms. Conservative management, particularly physiotherapy, is recommended for women with mild prolapse (Haylen et al., 2016).

The limited success in treating patients with pelvic floor dysfunction is often attributed to the professional 'compartmentalisation' of the pelvic floor. Consequently, there is a compelling need to adopt a more integrated approach, incorporating PFMT alongside 'core training', lumbopelvic stability exercises, or breathing techniques (Bø et al., 2023).

In addition, new vaginal devices have been developed to help women with their PFM exercises, as well as to monitor their improvement during the rehabilitation period (Antunes et al., 2024; Arantes et al., 2024).

Thus, it is emphasized that pelvic physiotherapy, including lifestyle changes, PFMT and education can be effective in preventing women pelvic floor disorders.

Physiotherapy in Oncological Rehabilitation

Breast and gynaecological cancers are the most frequent malignancies diagnosed in women every year, with a profound impact on several aspects of their lives (Zhu et al., 2024). Thus, holistic approaches involving a multi-professional team are essential to optimize intervention, reduce treatment side effects and improve quality of life (QoL) (Iliescu, 2024). Among those professionals, physiotherapist is a recognized movement specialist, capable of preventing and restoring sensorimotor dysfunctions originated by breast and gynaecological cancers or treatments (Rizzo, 2016). Breast cancer (BC) treatments, particularly surgeries such as mastectomies, significantly impact a woman's body image, affecting her self-esteem, sexuality, and overall QoL. Also, gynaecological problems such as hysterectomy, oophorectomy, and vulvectomy, can lead to significant alterations in a woman's body, affecting her perception of femininity and sexual identity. These changes often result in body image dissatisfaction and lowered self-esteem. Physiotherapy (PT) plays a crucial role in addressing these challenges through targeted interventions that promote physical and emotional rehabilitation (Afshar-Bakshloo et al, 2023). Therefore, physiotherapists implement various strategies to support cancer survivors in improving their body image and overall well-being, by engaging in tailored exercise regimens and other techniques to enhance self-perceived body image, boost self-esteem, and improve physical function in patients (Rizzo, 2016).

Breast Cancer

BC is the most common malignancy, with almost 3 million new cases diagnosed annually, and the leading cause of cancer-related deaths among women worldwide (Wilkinson & Gathani, 2022). Despite the development of new therapeutic techniques, primary treatments continue to lead to significant physical and psychological impairments, including changes in body image, pain, loss of sensation, lymphedema, upper-limb (UL) impairments and fatigue, resulting in decreased physical activity (PA) levels, low self-efficacy and reduced QoL (Senger et al., 2023).

Of these, pain is a common side effect of BC treatment, affecting up to 78% of patients. It can occur acutely after surgery or be prolonged due to chemotherapy and radiation and can limit physical function, while reducing sleep quality (Gallaway et al., 2020). Post-mastectomy pain syndrome (PMPS) is a neuropathic pain, originated by a somatosensory nerve lesion that can be present from the chest to the medial part of UL, affecting 25%-50% of BC survivors (Salati et al., 2023). Chemotherapy-induced peripheral neuropathy (CIPN) is a common dose-limiting toxicity associated with microtubule-targeting agents reported for more than 50% of cancer patients and it is characterized by sensory manifestations in the upper and lower extremities, in a "glove and stocking" fashion (Zhang, 2021). A comprehensive and effective pain management plan including patient education regarding UL positioning, energy conservation strategies and pacing activities is essential to reduce it and to prevent its recurrence (Alhazmi et al., 2021). Transcutaneous electrical nerve stimulation (TENS) and acupuncture can be also useful for pain management, especially in those patients whose medication became ineffective (Püsküllüoğlu et al., 2022). The role of specific exercise therapy and early passive mobilization in pain control was also studied during the perioperative phase with a high-quality RCT showing its positive effect early after surgery (Bruce et al., 2021).

Lymphedema is another deleterious effect of BC treatment, affecting almost 50% of patients, with the vast majority occurring 2 years after anti-cancer therapy (Ren et al., 2022). Complete decongestive therapy (CDT) is the recommended treatment for lymphedema. CDT involves 2 phases: treatment and maintenance. Treatment phase includes skin care, manual lymph drainage, physical exercises and limb bandaging, while maintenance phase involves skin care, physical exercises and bandaging with different elasticity degrees (Yamamoto & Yamamoto, 2007). A more recent meta-analysis showed that low-level laser therapy (LLLT) can also reduce limb swelling and improve QoL of BC survivors and therefore could be a new complementary technique to CDT in patients with established lymphedema of the UL. Indeed, the application of LLLT, directly in regional lymph nodes, can stimulate their function, thus reducing UL swelling (Chiu et al., 2023). UL dysfunctions affect up to 84% in the short term after BC surgery and up to 30% one year after and are characterized by UL pain, reduced shoulder range of motion (ROM), inferior levels of handgrip strength, changes in scapulothoracic kinematics and scapular muscle activation (De Groef et al., 2015). Studies have assessed the effect of PT interventions before and after BC surgery. Prehabilitation consisting of diaphragmatic breathing, postural training and shoulder mobility exercises can attenuate UL dysfunction 1 to 6 months after surgery (Lokapavani et al., 2014). Similarly, PT initiated after surgery involving passive mobilization, stretching, manual therapy, postural and resistance exercises, proprioceptive neuromuscular facilitation and patient´s counselling can improve not only physical function, but also patient's self-perceived body image, self-esteem and self-efficacy (Heimes et al., 2017). More recently, the meta-analysis of Yang and collaborators (2024) also found that the application of kinesiology taping in women with BC-related lymphedema, although it did not reduce UL lymphedema, was an effective technique in improving UL function. Therefore, Kinesiology taping can be an additional emerging technique to be employed by physiotherapists to potentially increase UL function, thus promoting independence and, consequently, improving the QoL of BC survivors (Yang et al., 2024).

Cancer-related fatigue (CRF) is another common, persistent and subjective sense of physical, emotional and/or cognitive tiredness or exhaustion, related to cancer or its treatment, which is not proportional to recent activity pattern (Fabi et al., 2020). A recent meta-analysis assessed the effects of physical exercise on CRF during and after cancer treatment, showing that combining aerobic and resistance exercise is the most effective intervention in reducing CRF during the post-treatment phase (Liu et al., 2022).

Gynaecological Cancers

Gynaecological cancers originate in the female reproductive system and include several heterogeneous types such as ovarian, uterine, cervical, endometrial, fallopian tube and placental (Prat & Mutch, 2018). Patients can develop physical symptoms, including reduced PA levels, physical impairment, functional limitation, pelvic floor (PF) dysfunction and CRF, but also psychological distress, related to the disease and its treatments, low self-esteem, reduced intimacy and changes in sexual life (Gil-Ibanez et al., 2023).The literature reports that PF dysfunction is the main repercussion, which can express incontinence or urinary and fecal retention episodes, vaginal stenosis, genital prolapse, sexual dysfunction and pain (Gil-Ibanez et al., 2023). PT interventions have demonstrated potential to attenuate such symptoms. Specifically, PT for PF improves muscle function in women with urinary incontinence secondary to gynaecological cancers. Accordingly, Yang and collaborators (2012) observed that gynaecologic cancer patients performing a 45-min of PF exercise and a 30-min counselling session per week, for 4 weeks, increased PF strength and improved sexual functioning (Yang et al., 2012). Indeed, when combining PF exercise with other physiotherapy modalities such as manual therapy, tissue mobilization, electrical stimulation and biofeedback, it seems that PF function improved markedly more with higher magnitude in postoperative patients with early-stage gynaecological cancers (Feng et al., 2024). Besides, for women reporting vaginal stenosis and pain affecting their sexual function, manual therapy, information and vaginal dilator therapy may be also useful to recover their intimacy and sexuality, thus optimizing their full recovery (Weare, 2015).

Additionally, it seems that PT intervention after gynaecological cancer surgery, based on early mobilization, as a crucial component of enhanced recovery after surgery (ERAS), reduces the risk of postoperative complications and positively impacts several patient-reported outcomes, such as mobility, balance, locomotion and lower limbs lymphedema (LLL) (Tazreean et al., 2022).

It is estimated that 20-30% of these women will develop LLL. Therefore, the early incorporation of CDT following surgery can also have a preventive effect on LLL installation (Wu et al., 2021). Finally, these patients commonly report CRF, lower extremity muscle weakness and decreased ROM, resulting in locomotion impairment. Generally, aerobic, strengthening and stretching exercises are effective in improving muscle strength, aerobic capacity and mobility (Rose et al., 2023). The physical exercise recommendations for cancer patients include 150 to 300 minutes/week of moderate or an equivalent amount of vigorous intensity aerobic activity (75 to 150 minutes/ week), associated to 2-3 sessions of resistance and flexibility exercises (Patel et al., 2018). In addition to the well-known physical and psychological benefits induced by regular physical exercise, there is increasing evidence emphasizing its role in reducing cancer risk and progression, as well as in improving survival (Spanoudaki et al., 2023). Several mechanisms have been suggested to influence these processes, including the effects of exercise on insulin/glucose metabolism, sex hormones, inflammation, immune function and the tumour microenvironment (Swain et al., 2022). Despite such benefits, PA levels are commonly low in breast and gynaecological cancer patients, which is associated with worst treatment-related side effects, decreased treatment efficacy and reduced QoL (Zainordin et al. 2021). Therefore, flexible approaches are needed for women with breast and gynaecological cancers to achieve the recommended PA levels and, in doing so, increase their QoL and improve survival outcomes.

Physiotherapy in Aesthetic and Reconstructive Health

In many western cultures, ideals of beauty are often characterized by youthfulness, smooth skin, symmetrical features and certain body proportions. These ideals are globalized through media, influencing women worldwide to pursue surgeries like breast augmentation, liposuction, and rhinoplasty to align with these ideals (Swami & Furnham, 2008). Society often pressures women to conform to certain physical standards to be considered "feminine" or attractive. Larger breasts, a narrow waist, and fuller hips are historically tied to notions of femininity and fertility and plays a significant role in shaping perceptions of body image, social norms, media representations, and cultural standards of beauty that often-set unrealistic expectations for physical appearance, particularly for women (Henderson-King & Brooks, 2009).

When individuals feel that they fall short of societal ideals, they may experience dissatisfaction (Grogan, 2021). Body dissatisfaction is a strong predictor of seeking cosmetic surgery. Individuals often compare themselves to others, particularly when exposed to media that presents idealised or edited images, as seen in television, films, fashion magazines, and especially on social media platforms which frequently promote a narrow range of 'ideal' body types and beauty standards. Additionally, influencers and celebrities who openly discuss or undergo cosmetic procedures have contributed to the normalisation of plastic surgery (Perloff, 2014).

Many women feel that their value or success is closely tied to how well they align with societal beauty standards. This association between physical appearance and self-esteem can drive a desire for cosmetic procedures to feel more confident and accepted, or, in some cases, contribute to a distorted perception of one's body, known as body dysmorphic disorder (BDD). This condition results in an obsessive focus on perceived flaws that may be unnoticeable to others. Individuals with BDD are more likely to seek plastic surgery to 'correct' these perceived imperfections, although such procedures rarely address the underlying psychological issues (Jones et al., 2022).

Breast surgeries, including augmentation and reduction, are closely linked to a woman's self-perception and body image. While these procedures can positively impact self-esteem, physiotherapy plays a crucial role in supporting both physical recovery and emotional well-being. By helping women regain confidence in their bodies and restore independence, physiotherapy provides essential emotional support, improves mood, and reduces anxiety, all of which contribute to a more comprehensive and successful recovery (Heimes et al., 2017). This is achieved through tailored exercises, scar management, education, and postural correction, addressing both physical and psychological aspects of recovery (Coelho et al., 2023; Rett et al., 2022).

Aesthetic and reconstructive procedures are closely linked to both physical and psychological such as body image, self-esteem, and emotional well-being (DeVito et al., 2023).

These surgeries are relatively common in breast reconstruction following mastectomies or lumpectomies due to breast cancer; abdominoplasty (tummy tuck) post-pregnancy or following significant weight loss; liposuction, often in combination with other procedures; and reconstructive surgeries for trauma, congenital abnormalities (such as cleft palate), or post-tumour removal (Milazzo et al., 2024).

While cosmetic surgeries are often elective and aimed at enhancing appearance, reconstructive surgeries are typically essential for restoring function and body image, particularly following cancer treatment. These procedures help women regain a sense of normality by restoring both function and mobility (Voineskos et al., 2018). In both cases, physiotherapy is important in postoperative recovery, not only for restoring mobility but also for addressing psychological factors.

In post-breast reconstruction, physiotherapy plays an important role in restoring the range of motion in the shoulders and arms, which is often limited due to surgery and radiation therapy. Techniques such as manual therapy, muscle stretching, and strengthening exercises are used to recovery mobility (Akbas et al., 2021; Bruce et al., 2022). Scar management is also an important aspect of post-operative care, with a focus on improving the flexibility of scar tissue, reducing adhesions, and enhancing the overall appearance of scars. Techniques such as scar massage, specific exercises, and the use of silicone sheets, along with appropriate women counselling, can be effective. Additionally, following surgery or lymph node removal, women are at increased risk of developing lymphedema (a condition characterised by swelling due to the accumulation of lymph fluid). Therefore, the use of manual lymphatic drainage, compression therapy, and specific exercises can be used to both manage and prevent swelling (DiSipio et al., 2013). In pain management, providing relief through various modalities such as electrotherapy, heat or cold therapy, and manual techniques can be employed. Controlled exercises are also used to reduce post-surgical pain by promoting blood flow and facilitating the healing process (De Baets et al. 2022). Improving posture and postural control is also needed in post-chirurgical procedures. Regarding abdominoplasty, strengthening the core is also important to support recovery, prevent complications, and promote functional movement (Devoogdt & De Groef, 2024).

Following surgery, physiotherapists must also promote physical activity and facilitate a gradual and safe return to exercise. Physical activity improves not only physical health but also cardiovascular fitness, which may be compromised by prolonged periods of inactivity. An educational programme that emphasises the importance of posture and works with women to enhance daily living functionality is essential. This programme includes strength and flexibility exercises that facilitate a return to normal activities such as dressing, lifting, and caring for others, significantly improving their independence and overall life satisfaction (Klein et al. 2021).

Physiotherapy in Other Conditions

Menstrual Cycle Symptoms

The female reproductive system undergoes regular cyclic changes known as the menstrual cycle, which prepares the body for ovulation and potential pregnancy. The most noticeable feature of this system is menstruation, or cyclic vaginal bleeding, which occurs alongside a series of coordinated hormonal fluctuations. Menstruation, referred to as menarche when it first begins, typically starts at puberty, with a median onset age of 12.4 years. Normal menstrual frequency is defined as cycles occurring every 24 to 38 days. Menstrual cycles cease at menopause, which, on average, occurs around the age of 51(Thiyagarajan et al., 2024).

The menstrual cycle is a vital indicator of a woman's reproductive health, and any abnormalities require thorough evaluation (Thiyagarajan et al., 2024). Given its significance, the menstrual cycle should be used as an additional vital sign in the assessment of girls and adolescents (ACOG, 2015b). Moreover, understanding the menstrual cycle is essential for guiding women through fertility planning, pregnancy, and the menopausal transition (Thiyagarajan et al., 2024).

Premenstrual syndrome (PMS) is characterised by clinically significant somatic and psychological manifestations during the luteal phase of the menstrual cycle, causing considerable distress and impairment in functional capacity. These symptoms typically disappear within a few days after the onset of menstruation. Globally, the pooled prevalence of PMS among women of reproductive age is 47.8%. Of those affected, approximately 20% experience symptoms severe enough to disrupt daily activities, while the remainder report mild to moderate symptoms. Common symptoms of PMS include changes in appetite, weight gain, abdominal and back pain, headaches, breast tenderness, nausea, constipation, as well as psychological symptoms such as anxiety, irritability, anger, fatigue, restlessness, mood swings, and episodes of crying (Gudipally & Sharma, 2023).

Among these symptoms, dysmenorrhea is a common complaint experienced by menstruating women during their reproductive years. Defined as pain during menstruation, typically located in the lower abdomen and radiating to the inner thighs and back, dysmenorrhea can have a significant negative impact on emotional, psychological, and functional health. In contrast to secondary dysmenorrhea, which is linked to suspected or clinically identifiable pathology, primary dysmenorrhea refers to recurrent lower abdominal pain during the menstrual cycle that is not associated with any underlying disease or pathology (Nagy et al., 2023).

Given that nearly 50 per cent of women of reproductive age experience menstrual-related symptoms that negatively impact their daily lives, it is crucial to provide treatment options that align with their preferences and needs.

In addition to pharmacological treatment, lifestyle modifications—including regular exercise, stress management, healthy sleep habits, and a specific diet, particularly during the premenstrual period— and cognitive-behavioural therapy (CBT) can be use in addressing PMS (Gudipally & Sharma, 2023). For the management of dysmenorrhea, non-pharmacological options such as heat application, exercise, dietary adjustments, acupuncture, transcutaneous electrical nerve stimulation (TENS), and behavioural counselling may also be an option (Nagy et al., 2023). In primary dysmenorrhea, current evidence suggests that conservative treatments, including specific physiotherapy techniques, may lead to a clinically significant reduction in symptoms with the advantage of no side effects (López-Liria et al., 2021).

Physiotherapists can also prescribe and adjust physical exercise to the women needs, teach relaxation techniques and promote healthy lifestyle habits. In an RCT, the authors found that progressive relaxation exercises can effectively reduce primary dysmenorrhea when performed regularly (Çelik & Apay, 2021). On the other hand, in a systematic review, exercise was found to be effective in improving physical menstrual symptoms, such as pain, constipation, and breast tenderness, as well as psychological symptoms, including anxiety and anger (Yesildere et al., 2020). Specifically concerning menstrual pain, current evidence suggests that exercise performed for approximately 45 to 60 minutes per session, three times per week or more, may significantly reduce pain intensity. Therefore, exercise can be considered either alone or in conjunction with other modalities for managing this symptom (Armour et al., 2019).

Endometriosis

Endometriosis is a chronic, inflammatory gynaecological condition characterised by the presence of endometrial-like tissue outside the uterus, affecting approximately 5 to 10% of women during their reproductive years (Horne & Missmer, 2022; Taylor et al., 2021). Traditionally recognised for its pelvic manifestations and frequent association with infertility, growing evidence indicates that this condition has widespread effects throughout the body. As a result, it is becoming increasingly important to understand endometriosis as a systemic condition, requiring a shift in the approach to its management (Taylor et al., 2021).

Endometriosis is often associated to a variety of painful symptoms, including chronic pelvic pain (both cyclical and non-cyclical), painful menstruation (dysmenorrhea), painful sexual intercourse (dyspareunia), and pain during defecation (dyschezia) or urination (dysuria). In addition to experiencing pain within the urogynaecological system, women with endometriosis are also at increased risk of multisite pain (pain in multiple body regions), infertility, fatigue, and the development of other comorbidities (Horne & Missmer, 2022).

The severity of endometriosis ranges from mild to severe, with a significant impact on daily activities and quality of life (Taylor et al., 2018; Horne & Missmer, 2022). Due to its systemic nature, an interdisciplinary approach is required to effectively manage the condition (Horne & Missmer, 2022; Taylor et al., 2021).

Treatment options include pharmacological and hormonal therapies, surgical interventions, dietary intervention and conservative non-pharmacological approaches, such as physiotherapy (Amro et al.,2022; As-Sanie et al., 2019). A systematic review with meta-analysis evaluated the effectiveness of physiotherapy interventions for improving pain intensity and quality of life in women with endometriosis, compared to placebo, sham, or control treatments. The findings showed that non-pharmacologic, conservative therapies were effective in reducing pain and improving quality of life, particularly physical function (Abril-Coello et al., 2023).

In addition to pain, some studies have identified various physical impairments in women with endometriosis. These include decreased flexibility, impaired body balance, reduced muscle thickness and strength in the lumbopelvic and abdominal regions, lower lumbopelvic stability, diminished functional capacity, and higher levels of fatigue compared to healthy women (Álvarez-Salvago et al., 2020; Lara-Ramos et al., 2021).

Despite being underrepresented in the scientific literature, physiotherapy can address the symptoms of endometriosis, particularly musculoskeletal impairments and pelvic floor conditions. The physiotherapy approach focuses on kinesiotherapy, manual therapy, relaxation techniques, exercise prescription, and education to promote a healthier lifestyle, including promoting physical activity and exercise. It can also be used as an intervention in both preoperative and postoperative settings for women undergoing surgery for endometriosis (Wójcik et al.,2022).

Although the beneficial effects of physical exercise on symptoms associated with endometriosis remain ambiguous in the current literature (Tennfjord et al., 2021), a RCT have demonstrated that the quality of life for women with endometriosis can be improved through a supervised therapeutic exercise programme focused on the stabilization of deep abdominal muscles. This study also shown secondary improvements in dyspareunia, local and distal sensitisation, and lumbopelvic impairments (Artacho-Cordón et al., 2023).

SOLUTIONS AND RECOMMENDATIONS

Healthcare professionals should encourage all pregnant women and those in the postpartum period, including those with comorbidities, to seek a physiotherapist specialising in women's and pelvic floor health. In addition to specific physiotherapy interventions during these periods, the physiotherapist can prescribe personalised exercise programmes aimed at promoting health and well-being.

Protocols based on international guidelines for the assessment and treatment of pelvic disorders in pelvic physiotherapy are considered extremely important for the clinical practice of physiotherapists who are experts in this field. Additionally, specific protocols should be developed for pelvic physiotherapy intervention addressing obstetric pelvic floor dysfunctions related to pregnancy and childbirth, as well as conditions like dyssynergic and obstructed defecation.

In elderly woman, individually tailored multicomponent exercise programmes focusing on strength, balance, and flexibility are also recommended to prevent falls and maintain overall health across later life stages.

Regarding oncological rehabilitation, physiotherapy improves breast and gynaecological cancer patient's physical and psychological dimensions and should, therefore, be available from diagnosis, throughout the disease trajectory.

To enhance digital health interventions in physiotherapy, it is recommended to develop telepractice tailored to the diverse health conditions that women may experience throughout their lives. Implementing tele-physiotherapy can provide personalised care, remote monitoring, and real-time feedback. This is particularly valuable for women who prefer or benefit from this complementary approach, as well as those whose health conditions limit their mobility or who live in underserved areas.

Furthermore, physiotherapists should incorporate educational programmes into their approach to empower women regarding their health throughout their lives.

FUTURE RESEARCH DIRECTIONS

Future research should investigate strategies to improve adherence to prenatal exercise programmes, assess personalised postpartum physiotherapy for pelvic floor recovery, and explore safe physical activity to enhance women's mental and physical health. Additionally, studies should examine the effectiveness of personalised exercise plans and technology-based monitoring to support physical activity and prevent falls in older women.

Moreover, further investigation is required into the design of new artificial intelligence technologies and devices, as well as the telemonitoring of muscle function, to optimise the outcomes of PFMT.

Regarding manual therapy intervention, further high-quality RCTs should be conducted to determine the effects of manual therapy modalities, myofascial induction techniques and autonomic nervous system strategies on different health conditions across woman life.

In the realm of oncological rehabilitation, there is a pressing need for research to identify the most suitable physiotherapy interventions. This includes examining the specific techniques used for individual patients and determining the most effective settings for treatment delivery—whether in hospital, home, or community settings—while considering cost-effectiveness and patient safety.

Given the complex symptoms of endometriosis and dysmenorrhoea, future studies should prioritise high-quality RCTs that assess the effectiveness of physiotherapy interventions, including the prescription of tailored physical exercise, on outcomes such as pain relief, musculoskeletal impairments, symptom improvement, quality of life, and patient satisfaction.

CONCLUSION

Physiotherapists can contribute significantly to the health of pregnant and postpartum women, enhancing physical function, mental well-being, and overall quality of life. Their personalised interventions focus on improving function while preventing or treating musculoskeletal conditions. Additionally, they play a key role in prescribing tailored physical activity and exercise programmes suitable for various health conditions across all ages, even in the presence of comorbidities. In particular, pelvic physiotherapy - through comprehensive assessment and treatment - provides significant benefits to women experiencing pelvic disorders at various stages of life.

Moreover, physiotherapy is beneficial for women undergoing cancer treatment, especially in preventing, minimising, and managing adverse effects, thereby improving quality of life and survival outcomes. Its role also extends to supporting recovery after reconstructive and aesthetic surgeries, facilitating physical rehabilitation and promoting psychological well-being.

In conclusion, physiotherapists play an important role in promoting women's health across their lifespan, adopting a holistic approach that addresses not only physical rehabilitation but also psychological well-being. Their contributions within multidisciplinary teams ensure that women receive integrated and effective healthcare solutions, ultimately enhancing their overall quality of life and empowering them to achieve optimal health outcomes.

ACKNOWLEDGMENT

This research received no specific grant from any funding agency in the public, commercial, or not-for-profit sectors.

REFERENCES

Abril-Coello, R., Correyero-León, M., Ceballos-Laita, L., & Jiménez-Barrio, S. (2023). Benefits of physical therapy in improving quality of life and pain associated with endometriosis: A systematic review and meta-analysis. *International Journal of Gynaecology and Obstetrics: the Official Organ of the International Federation of Gynaecology and Obstetrics, 162*(1), 233–243. DOI: 10.1002/ijgo.14645 PMID: 36571475

Afshar-Bakshloo, M., Albers, S., Richter, C., Berninger, O., Blohmer, J. U., Roehle, R., Speiser, D., & Karsten, M. M. (2023). How breast cancer therapies impact body image–real-world data from a prospective cohort study collecting patient-reported outcomes. *BMC Cancer, 23*(1), 705. DOI: 10.1186/s12885-023-11172-y PMID: 37507687

Akbas, A., Dagmura, H., Daldal, E., Dasiran, F. M., Deveci, H., & Okan, I. (2021). Association between Shoulder Range of Motion and Pain Catastrophizing Scale in Breast Cancer Patients after Surgery. *Breast Care (Basel, Switzerland), 16*(1), 66–71. DOI: 10.1159/000506922 PMID: 33716634

Alhazmi, L. S. S., Bawadood, M. A. A., Aljohani, A. M. S., Alzahrani, A. A. R., Moshref, L., Trabulsi, N., & Moshref, R. (2021). Pain Management in Breast Cancer Patients: A Multidisciplinary Approach. *Cureus, 13*(6), e15994. DOI: 10.7759/cureus.15994 PMID: 34336485

Álvarez-Salvago, F., Lara-Ramos, A., Cantarero-Villanueva, I., Mazheika, M., Mundo-López, A., Galiano-Castillo, N., Fernández-Lao, C., Arroyo-Morales, M., Ocón-Hernández, O., & Artacho-Cordón, F. (2020). Chronic fatigue, physical impairments and quality of life in women with endometriosis: A case-control study. *International Journal of Environmental Research and Public Health, 17*(10), 3610. DOI: 10.3390/ijerph17103610 PMID: 32455618

American College of Obstetricians and Gynecologists [ACOG] (2015a). Committee Opinion number 650: Physical Activity an Exercise During Pregnancy and the Postpartum Period. Obstetrics and Gynecology, 126(6), 135–142. https://doi.org/ DOI: 10.1097/AOG.0000000000001214

American College of Obstetricians and Gynecologists [ACOG] (2015b). Committee Opinion No. 651: Menstruation in Girls and Adolescents: Using the Menstrual Cycle as a Vital Sign. *Obstetrics and gynecology, 126*(6), e143–e146. https://doi.org/DOI: 10.1097/AOG.0000000000001215

American College of Obstetricians and Gynecologists [ACOG] (2020). Committee Opinion number 804: Physical activity and exercise during pregnancy and Postpartum Period. Obstetrics and Gynecology, 135(4), 178–188. https://doi.org/DOI: 10.3109/21679169.2013.861509

American College of Sports Medicine [ACSM] (2018). ACSM Guideline for Exercise Testing and Prescription (D. Riebe, M. Nobel, & A. Millholen (eds.); 10h ed.). Wolters Kluwer Health.

Amro, B., Ramirez Aristondo, M. E., Alsuwaidi, S., Almaamari, B., Hakim, Z., Tahlak, M., Wattiez, A., & Koninckx, P. R. (2022). New understanding of diagnosis, treatment and prevention of endometriosis. *International Journal of Environmental Research and Public Health, 19*(11), 6725. DOI: 10.3390/ijerph19116725 PMID: 35682310

Antunes, D., Arantes, R., Seabra, E., Silva, L. F., & Viana, R. (2024). Materials, Functionalities and Processing of a Medical Device to Pelvic Floor Rehabilitation. In Machado, J. (Eds.), *Innovations in Mechatronics Engineering, Lecture Notes in Mechanical Engineering* (pp. 235–241). Springer Nature., DOI: 10.1007/978-3-031-62684-5_21

Arantes, R., Antunes, D., Seabra, E., Viana, R., & Silva, L. F. L. F. (2024). Design of a New Intravaginal Device to Measure and Monitor the Pelvic Floor Muscle Strength, In J. Machado et al. (Eds.), Innovations in Mechatronics Engineering, Lecture Notes in Mechanical Engineering (pp. 288-293). Springer Nature. https://doi.org/DOI: 10.1007/978-3-031-61575-7_26

Armour, M., Ee, C. C., Naidoo, D., Ayati, Z., Chalmers, K. J., Steel, K. A., de Manincor, M. J., & Delshad, E. (2019). Exercise for dysmenorrhoea. *Cochrane Database of Systematic Reviews, 9*(9), CD004142. Advance online publication. DOI: 10.1002/14651858.CD004142.pub4 PMID: 31538328

Artacho-Cordón, F., del Mar Salinas-Asensio, M., Galiano-Castillo, N., Ocón-Hernández, O., Peinado, F. M., Mundo-López, A., & Cantarero-Villanueva, I. (2023). Effect of a multimodal supervised therapeutic exercise program on quality of life, pain, and lumbopelvic impairments in women with endometriosis unresponsive to conventional therapy: A randomized controlled trial. *Archives of Physical Medicine and Rehabilitation*, *104*(11), 1785–1795. DOI: 10.1016/j.apmr.2023.06.020 PMID: 37467936

As-Sanie, S., Black, R., Giudice, L. C., Valbrun, T. G., Gupta, J., Jones, B., & Nebel, R. A. (2019). Assessing research gaps and unmet needs in endometriosis. *American Journal of Obstetrics and Gynecology*, *221*(2), 86–94. DOI: 10.1016/j.ajog.2019.02.033 PMID: 30790565

Aziz, I., Whitehead, W., Palsson, O., Törnblom, H., & Simrén, M. (2020). An approach to the diagnosis and management of Rome IV functional disorders of chronic constipation. *Expert Review of Gastroenterology & Hepatology*, *14*(1), 39–46. DOI: 10.1080/17474124.2020.1708718 PMID: 31893959

Berghmans, B. (2018). Physiotherapy for pelvic pain and female sexual dysfunction: An untapped resource. *International Urogynecology Journal*, *29*(5), 631–638. DOI: 10.1007/s00192-017-3536-8 PMID: 29318334

Berta, M., Lindgren, H., Christensson, K., Mekonnen, S., & Adefris, M. (2019). Effect of maternal birth positions on duration of second stage of labor: Systematic review and meta-analysis. *BMC Pregnancy and Childbirth*, *19*(1), 466. DOI: 10.1186/s12884-019-2620-0 PMID: 31801479

Bø, K., Berghmans, B., Mørkved, S., & Van Kampen, M. (Eds.). (2023). *Evidence-Based Physical Therapy for the Pelvic Floor - Bridging Science and Clinical Practice* (3rd ed.). Elsevier.

Bø, K., & Hilde, G. (2013). Does it work in the long term? — A systematic review on pelvic floor muscle training for female stress urinary incontinence. *Neurourology and Urodynamics*, *32*(3), 215–223. DOI: 10.1002/nau.22292 PMID: 22847318

Boissonnault, J., Kuhn, A., Meeker, M., Strong, S., & Stephenson, R. G. (2020). An international survey of women's and pelvic health physical therapy organizational practice. *Journal of Women's Health Physical Therapy*, *44*(4), 160–175. DOI: 10.1097/JWH.0000000000000174

Brown, W. J., Hayman, M., Haakstad, L. A., Lamerton, T., Mena, G. P., Green, A., Keating, S. E., Gomes, G. A. O., Coombes, J. S., & Mielke, G. I. (2022). Australian guidelines for physical activity in pregnancy and postpartum. *Journal of Science and Medicine in Sport*, *25*(6), 511–519. DOI: 10.1016/j.jsams.2022.03.008 PMID: 35418334

Bruce, J., Mazuquin, B., Canaway, A., Hossain, A., Williamson, E., Mistry, P., Lall, R., Petrou, S., Lamb, S. E., Rees, S., Padfield, E., Vidya, R., & Thompson, A. M. (2021). Exercise versus usual care after non-reconstructive breast cancer surgery (UK PROSPER): Multicentre randomised controlled trial and economic evaluation. *BMJ (Clinical Research Ed.)*, *375*, e066542. DOI: 10.1136/bmj-2021-066542 PMID: 34759002

Bruce, J., Mazuquin, B., Mistry, P., Rees, S., Canaway, A., Hossain, A., Williamson, E., Padfield, E. J., Lall, R., Richmond, H., Chowdhury, L., Lait, C., Petrou, S., Booth, K., Lamb, S. E., Vidya, R., & Thompson, A. M. (2022). Exercise to prevent shoulder problems after breast cancer surgery: The PROSPER RCT. *Health Technology Assessment*, *26*(15), 1–124. DOI: 10.3310/JKNZ2003 PMID: 35220995

Bruehl, S., & Chung, O. Y. (2004). Interactions between the cardiovascular and pain regulatory systems: An updated review of mechanisms and possible alterations in chronic pain. *Neuroscience and Biobehavioral Reviews*, *28*(4), 395–414. DOI: 10.1016/j.neubiorev.2004.06.004 PMID: 15341037

Capel-Alcaraz, A. M., García-López, H., Castro-Sánchez, A. M., Fernández-Sánchez, M., & Lara-Palomo, I. C. (2023). The Efficacy of Strength Exercises for Reducing the Symptoms of Menopause: A Systematic Review. *Journal of Clinical Medicine*, *12*(2), 548. DOI: 10.3390/jcm12020548 PMID: 36675477

Cardoso, A., Lima, C., & Ferreira, C. (2018). Prevalence of urinary incontinence in high-impact sports athletes and their association with knowledge, attitude and practice about this dysfunction. *European Journal of Sport Science*, *18*(10), 1405–1412. DOI: 10.1080/17461391.2018.1496146 PMID: 30025510

Çelik, A. S., & Apay, S. E. (2021). Effect of progressive relaxation exercises on primary dysmenorrhea in Turkish students: A randomized prospective controlled trial. *Complementary Therapies in Clinical Practice*, *42*, 101280. DOI: 10.1016/j.ctcp.2020.101280 PMID: 33310052

Chiu, S. T., Lai, U. H., Huang, Y. C., Leong, C. P., & Chen, P. C. (2023). Effect of various photobiomodulation regimens on breast cancer-related lymphedema: A systematic review and meta-analysis. *Lasers in Medical Science*, *39*(1), 11. DOI: 10.1007/s10103-023-03959-z PMID: 38129368

Choo, H. J., Hwang, S. K., & Hynes, C. K. (2020). Musculoskeletal issues and care for pregnant and postpartum women. *Current Physical Medicine and Rehabilitation Reports*, *8*(4), 493–500. DOI: 10.1007/s40141-020-00286-0

Coelho, F. D., Carvalho, P. H. B., Paes, S. T., & Ferreira, M. E. C. (2023). Esthetic plastic surgery and (in) satisfaction index: A current view. *Revista Brasileira de Cirurgia Plástica*, *32*(1), 135–140. DOI: 10.5935/2177-1235.2017RBCP0019

Constantine, G. D., Graham, S., Clerinx, C., Bernick, B. A., Krassan, M., Mirkin, S., & Currie, H. (2016). Behaviours and attitudes influencing treatment decisions for menopausal symptoms in five European countries. *Post Reproductive Health*, *22*(3), 112–122. DOI: 10.1177/2053369116632439 PMID: 26895640

Critchley, C. J. C. (2022). Physical Therapy Is an Important Component of Postpartum Care in the Fourth Trimester. *Physical Therapy*, *102*(5), pzac021. Advance online publication. DOI: 10.1093/ptj/pzac021 PMID: 35225339

Crosby, E., & Husk, K. (2021). Defecatory Dysfunction. *Obstetrics and Gynecology Clinics of North America*, *48*(3), 653–663. DOI: 10.1016/j.ogc.2021.05.016 PMID: 34416943

Da Roza, T., Brandão, S., Mascarenhas, T., Jorge, R. N., & Duarte, J. A. (2015). Volume of training and the ranking level are associated with the leakage of urine in young female trampolinists. *Clinical Journal of Sport Medicine*, *25*(3), 270–275. DOI: 10.1097/JSM.0000000000000129 PMID: 25010151

Da Roza, T., de Araujo, M., Viana, R., Viana, S., Jorge, R., Bø, K., & Mascarenhas, T. (2012). Pelvic floor muscle training to improve urinary incontinence in young, nulliparous sport students: A pilot study. *International Urogynecology Journal*, *23*(8), 1069–1073. DOI: 10.1007/s00192-012-1759-2 PMID: 22552685

Da Silva, A., & De Moraes Lopes, M. (2024). Treinamento dos músculos do assoalho pélvico associado ao uso do pessário no tratamento do prolapso de órgãos pélvicos: Protocolo de revisão de escopo. *Research. Social Development*, *13*(5), e2813545704–e2813545704.

Da Silva, N. C. S., & Livramento, R. A. (2023). Intervenção Da Fisioterapia Pélvica No Tratamento Do Prolapso Genital: Revisão Integrativa. *Brazilian Journal of Implantology and Health Sciences*, *5*(5), 3402–3414. DOI: 10.36557/2674-8169.2023v5n5p3402-3414

De Baets, L., Vets, N., Emmerzaal, J., Devoogdt, N., & De Groef, A. (2022). Altered upper limb motor behavior in breast cancer survivors and its relation to pain: A narrative review. *The Anatomical Record*, *307*(2), 298–308. DOI: 10.1002/ar.25120 PMID: 36398938

De Groef, A., Van Kampen, M., Dieltjens, E., Christiaens, M. R., Neven, P., Geraerts, I., & Devoogdt, N. (2015). Effectiveness of postoperative physical therapy for upper-limb impairments after breast cancer treatment: A systematic review. *Archives of Physical Medicine and Rehabilitation*, *96*(6), 1140–1153. DOI: 10.1016/j.apmr.2015.01.006 PMID: 25595999

de Sousa, K. A., Cardoso, L. B., Pirola, F. M., Auad, L. G., & de Oliveira, A. S. (2020). Effect of manual therapies on cardiac autonomic control: a systematic review. *Manual Therapy, Posturology & Rehabilitation Journal*, 1-12. https://doi.org/DOI: 10.17784/mtprehabjournal.2021.19.804

Deflorin, C., Hohenauer, E., Stoop, R., Van Daele, U., Clijsen, R., & Taeymans, J. (2020). Physical management of scar tissue: A systematic review and meta-analysis. *Journal of Alternative and Complementary Medicine (New York, N.Y.)*, *26*(10), 854–865. DOI: 10.1089/acm.2020.0109 PMID: 32589450

Delancey, J., Kane Low, L., Miller, J., Patel, D., & Tumbarello, J. (2008). Graphic integration of causal factors of pelvic floor disorders: An integrated life span model. *American Journal of Obstetrics and Gynecology*, *199*(6), 610.e1–610.e5. DOI: 10.1016/j.ajog.2008.04.001 PMID: 18533115

DeVito, R. G., Craft, L., Campbell, C. A., & Stranix, J. T. (2023). Optimizing perioperative outcomes in autologous breast reconstruction. *Gland Surgery*, *12*(4), 508–515. DOI: 10.21037/gs-22-608 PMID: 37200925

Devoogdt, N., & De Groef, A. (2024). Physiotherapy management of breast cancer treatment-related sequelae. *Journal of Physiotherapy*, *70*(2), 90–105. DOI: 10.1016/j.jphys.2024.02.020 PMID: 38519340

Dipietro, L., Evenson, K. R., Bloodgood, B., Sprow, K., Troiano, R. P., Piercy, K. L., Vaux-Bjerke, A., & Powell, K. E. (2019). Benefits of Physical Activity during Pregnancy and Postpartum: An Umbrella Review. *Medicine and Science in Sports and Exercise*, *51*(6), 1292–1302. DOI: 10.1249/MSS.0000000000001941 PMID: 31095086

DiSipio, T., Rye, S., Newman, B., & Hayes, S. (2013). Incidence of unilateral arm lymphoedema after breast cancer: A systematic review and meta-analysis. *The Lancet. Oncology*, *14*(6), 500–515. DOI: 10.1016/S1470-2045(13)70076-7 PMID: 23540561

Diz-Teixeira, P., Alonso-Calvete, A., Justo-Cousiño, L. A., González-González, Y., & Cuña-Carrera, I. D. (2023). Update on Physiotherapy in Postpartum Urinary Incontinence. A Systematic Review. *Archivos Espanoles de Urologia*, *76*(1), 29–39. DOI: 10.56434/j.arch.esp.urol.20237601.2 PMID: 36914417

Espírito Santo, J., Moita, J., & Nunes, A. (2024). The Efficacy of Manual Therapy on Musculoskeletal Pain in Menopause: A Systematic Review. In *Healthcare* (Vol. 12, No. 18, p. 1838). MDPI. https://doi.org/DOI: 10.3390/healthcare12181838

Fabi, A., Bhargava, R., Fatigoni, S., Guglielmo, M., Horneber, M., Roila, F., Weis, J., Jordan, K., & Ripamonti, C. I.ESMO Guidelines Committee. (2020). Cancer-related fatigue: ESMO Clinical Practice Guidelines for diagnosis and treatment. *Annals of Oncology : Official Journal of the European Society for Medical Oncology*, *31*(6), 713–723. DOI: 10.1016/j.annonc.2020.02.016 PMID: 32173483

Feng, L., Hao, Q., Wang, S., Zhao, Y., Wu, H., Cui, Z., Zhang, J., Wang, L., Zhang, D., Zhan, X., & Wei, L. (2024). Effects of Electrical Stimulation, Pelvic Floor Muscle Exercise, and Biofeedback Program on Improving Pelvic Floor Function and Quality of Life in Postoperative Patients with Early-Stage Cervical Cancer. *The Tohoku Journal of Experimental Medicine*, *264*(1), 21–29. DOI: 10.1620/tjem.2024.J044 PMID: 38897964

Frawley, H., Shelly, B., Morin, M., Bernard, S., Bø, K., Digesu, G., Dickinson, T., Goonewardene, S., McClurg, D., Rahnama'i, M. S., Schizas, A., Slieker-ten Hove, M., Takahashi, S., & Voelkl Guevara, J. (2021). An International Continence Society (ICS) report on the terminology for pelvic floor muscle assessment. *Neurourology and Urodynamics*, *40*(5), 1217–1260. DOI: 10.1002/nau.24658 PMID: 33844342

Gai, J., Gomes, L., & Jansen de Càrdenas, C. (2009). Ptofobia - O medo de cair em pessoas idosas. *Acta Medica Portuguesa*, *22*, 83–88. PMID: 19341596

Gallaway, M. S., Townsend, J. S., Shelby, D., & Puckett, M. C. (2020). Pain Among Cancer Survivors. *Preventing Chronic Disease*, *17*, E54. DOI: 10.5888/pcd17.190367 PMID: 32644924

Gil-Ibanez, B., Davies-Oliveira, J., Lopez, G., Díaz-Feijoo, B., Tejerizo-Garcia, A., & Sehouli, J. (2023). Impact of gynecological cancers on health-related quality of life: Historical context, measurement instruments, and current knowledge. *International Journal of Gynecological Cancer : Official Journal of the International Gynecological Cancer Society*, *33*(11), 1800–1806. DOI: 10.1136/ijgc-2023-004804 PMID: 37696648

Gluppe, S., Engh, M. E., & Bø, K. (2021). What is the evidence for abdominal and pelvic floor muscle training to treat diastasis recti abdominis postpartum? A systematic review with meta-analysis. *Brazilian Journal of Physical Therapy*, *25*(6), 664–675. DOI: 10.1016/j.bjpt.2021.06.006 PMID: 34391661

Graziottin, A. (2023). Female sexual dysfunction. In K. Bo, B. Berghmans, S. Mørkved, & M. Van Kampen (Eds.) *(3rd ed.), Evidence-Based Physical Therapy for the Pelvic Floor - Science and Clinical Practice (pp. 266-277). Elsevier.*

Grogan, S. (2021). *Body Image: Understanding Body Dissatisfaction in Men, Women, and Children* (4th ed.). Routledge., DOI: 10.4324/9781003100041

Gudipally, P. R., & Sharma, G. K. (2024 Jan). Premenstrual Syndrome. [Updated 2023 Jul 17] In *StatPearls* [Internet]. StatPearls Publishing., Available from https://www.ncbi.nlm.nih.gov/books/NBK560698/

Hadizadeh-Talasaz, Z., Sadeghi, R., & Khadivzadeh, T. (2019). Effect of pelvic floor muscle training on postpartum sexual function and quality of life: A systematic review and meta-analysis of clinical trials. *Taiwanese Journal of Obstetrics & Gynecology*, *58*(6), 737–747. DOI: 10.1016/j.tjog.2019.09.003 PMID: 31759521

Halfon, N., Larson, K., Lu, M., Tullis, E., & Russ, S. (2014). Lifecourse health development: Past, present and future. *Maternal and Child Health Journal*, *18*(2), 344–365. DOI: 10.1007/s10995-013-1346-2 PMID: 23975451

Haylen, B., De Ridder, D., Freeman, R., Swift, S., Berghmans, B., Lee, J., Monga, A., Petri, E., Rizk, D. E., Sand, P. K., & Schaer, G. (2010). An International Urogynecological Association (IUGA)/International Continence Society (ICS) joint report on the terminology for female pelvic floor dysfunction. *International Urogynecology Journal*, *21*(1), 5–26. DOI: 10.1007/s00192-009-0976-9 PMID: 19937315

Haylen, B., Maher, C., Barber, M., Camargo, S., Dandolu, V., Digesu, A., Goldman, H. B., Huser, M., Milani, A. L., Moran, P. A., Schaer, G. N., & Withagen, M. (2016). An International Urogynecological Association (IUGA)/International Continence Society (ICS) joint report on the terminology for female pelvic organ prolapse (POP). *International Urogynecology Journal*, *27*(2), 165–194. DOI: 10.1007/s00192-015-2932-1 PMID: 26755051

Heimes, A. S., Stewen, K., & Hasenburg, A. (2017). Psychosocial Aspects of Immediate versus Delayed Breast Reconstruction. *Breast Care (Basel, Switzerland)*, *12*(6), 374–377. DOI: 10.1159/000485234 PMID: 29456468

Henderson-King, D., & Brooks, K. D. (2009). Materialism, sociocultural appearance messages, and paternal attitudes predict college women's attitudes about cosmetic surgery. *Psychology of Women Quarterly*, *33*(1), 133–142. DOI: 10.1111/j.1471-6402.2008.01480.x

Hickey, M., LaCroix, A. Z., Doust, J., Mishra, G. D., Sivakami, M., Garlick, D., & Hunter, M. S. (2024). An empowerment model for managing menopause. *Lancet*, *403*(10430), 947–957. DOI: 10.1016/S0140-6736(23)02799-X PMID: 38458214

Horne, A. W., & Missmer, S. A. (2022). Pathophysiology, diagnosis, and management of endometriosis. *BMJ (Clinical Research Ed.)*, *379*, e070750. DOI: 10.1136/bmj-2022-070750 PMID: 36375827

Iliescu, M. G., Stanciu, L. E., Uzun, A. B., Cristea, A. E., Motoască, I., Irsay, L., Iliescu, D. M., Vari, T., Ciubean, A. D., Caraban, B. M., Ciufu, N., Azis, O., & Ciortea, V. M. (2024). Assessment of Integrative Therapeutic Methods for Improving the Quality of Life and Functioning in Cancer Patients—A Systematic Review. *Journal of Clinical Medicine*, *13*(5), 1190. DOI: 10.3390/jcm13051190 PMID: 38592012

International Organization of Physiotherapists in Pelvic & Women's Health [IOP-PWH] (2013). Scope of practice. https://themamasphysio.com/wp-content/uploads/2022/01/womens_health_pt_-_scope_of_practice.pdf

International Organization of Physiotherapists in Pelvic & Women's Health [IOP-PWH], (2023). Recommendations for Education in Pelvic and Women's Health fields. https://ioppwh-website.s3.eu-west-2.amazonaws.com/IOPPWH+Education+Recommendations+June+2023.pdf

Jones, H. E., Faulkner, H. R., & Losken, A. (2022). The Psychological Impact of Aesthetic Surgery: A Mini-Review. *Aesthetic Surgery Journal Open Forum*. Vol. 4 https://doi.org/DOI: 10.1093/asjof/ojac077

Klein, I., Kalichman, L., Chen, N., & Susmallian, S. (2021). A pilot study evaluating the effect of early physical therapy on pain and disabilities after breast cancer surgery: Prospective randomized control trail. *The Breast : Official Journal of the European Society of Mastology*, *59*, 286–293. DOI: 10.1016/j.breast.2021.07.013 PMID: 34340163

Lara-Ramos, A., Álvarez-Salvago, F., Fernández-Lao, C., Galiano-Castillo, N., Ocón-Hernández, O., Mazheika, M., Salinas-Asensio, M. M., Mundo-López, A., Arroyo-Morales, M., Cantarero-Villanueva, I., & Artacho-Cordón, F. (2021). Widespread pain hypersensitivity and lumbopelvic impairments in women diagnosed with endometriosis. *Pain Medicine*, *22*(9), 1970–1981. DOI: 10.1093/pm/pnaa463 PMID: 33675228

Liu, Y. C., Hung, T. T., Konara Mudiyanselage, S. P., Wang, C. J., & Lin, M. F. (2022). Beneficial Exercises for Cancer-Related Fatigue among Women with Breast Cancer: A Systematic Review and Network Meta-Analysis. *Cancers (Basel)*, *15*(1), 151. DOI: 10.3390/cancers15010151 PMID: 36612147

Lokapavani, Y., Krishna, S. R., & Madhavi, K. (2014). Influence of pre operative physical therapy education and exercise on post operative shoulder range of motion and functional activites in subjects with modified radical mastectomy. *International Journal of Physiotherapy*, *1*(4), 170–177. DOI: 10.15621/ijphy/2014/v1i4/54556

López-Liria, R., Torres-Álamo, L., Vega-Ramírez, F. A., García-Luengo, A. V., Aguilar-Parra, J. M., Trigueros-Ramos, R., & Rocamora-Pérez, P. (2021). Efficacy of Physiotherapy Treatment in Primary Dysmenorrhea: A Systematic Review and Meta-Analysis. *International Journal of Environmental Research and Public Health*, *18*(15), 7832. DOI: 10.3390/ijerph18157832 PMID: 34360122

Mercier, J., Dumoulin, C., & Carrier-Noreau, G. (2023). Pelvic floor muscle rehabilitation for genitourinary syndrome of menopause: Why, how and when? *Climacteric*, *26*(4), 302–308. DOI: 10.1080/13697137.2023.2194527 PMID: 37019140

Milazzo, T., Yuan, M., Graham, A., Kim, P., Gallo, L., Uhlman, K., Thoma, A., Coroneos, C., & Voineskos, S. (2024). Reporting of patient-reported outcomes amongst randomized clinical trials in plastic surgery: A systematic review using CONSORT-PRO. *Journal of Plastic, Reconstructive & Aesthetic Surgery; JPRAS*, *99*, 110–121. DOI: 10.1016/j.bjps.2024.09.022 PMID: 39368267

Milsom, I., Altman, D., Cartwright, R., Lapitan, M., Nelson, R., Sjöström, S., & Tikkinen, K. (2023). Epidemiology of urinary incontinence (UI) and other lower urinary tract symptoms (LUTS), pelvic organ prolapse (POP) and anal (AI) incontinence. In: L. Cardozo, E. Rovner, A. Wagg, A. Wein, P. Abrams (Eds.) 7th International Consultation on Incontinence. International Continence Society. https://www.ics.org/ici7/session/7310

Nagy, H., Carlson, K., & Khan, M. A. B. (2024 Jan). Dysmenorrhea. [Updated 2023 Nov 12] In *StatPearls* [Internet]. StatPearls Publishing., Available from https://www.ncbi.nlm.nih.gov/books/NBK560834/

Nascimento, S. L., Surita, F. G., & Cecatti, J. G. (2012). Physical exercise during pregnancy: A systematic review. *Current Opinion in Obstetrics & Gynecology*, *24*(6), 387–394. DOI: 10.1097/GCO.0b013e328359f131 PMID: 23014142

Navarro-Brazález, B., Vergara-Pérez, F., Prieto-Gómez, V., Sánchez-Sánchez, B., Yuste-Sánchez, M. J., & Torres-Lacomba, M. (2021). What influences women to adhere to pelvic floor exercises after physiotherapy treatment? A qualitative study for individualized pelvic health care. *Journal of Personalized Medicine*, *11*(12), 1368. DOI: 10.3390/jpm11121368 PMID: 34945840

Nawabi, F., Krebs, F., Vennedey, V., Shukri, A., Lorenz, L., & Stock, S. (2021). Health Literacy in Pregnant Women: A Systematic Review. *International Journal of Environmental Research and Public Health*, *18*(7), 3847. DOI: 10.3390/ijerph18073847 PMID: 33917631

Newton, E. R., & May, L. (2017). Adaptation of Maternal-Fetal Physiology to Exercise in Pregnancy: The Basis of Guidelines for Physical Activity in Pregnancy. *Clinical medicine insights. Women's health*, *10*, 1179562X17693224. https://doi.org/DOI: 10.1177/1179562X17693224

Norton, C., Whitehead, W., Bliss, D., Harari, D., & Lang, J. (2010). Conservative Management of Fecal Incontinence in Adults Committee of the International Consultation on Incontinence. Management of fecal incontinence in adults. *Neurourology and Urodynamics*, *29*(1), 199–206. DOI: 10.1002/nau.20803 PMID: 20025031

Olszewska, K., Ptak, A., Rusak, A., Dębiec-Bąk, A., & Stefańska, M. (2024). Changes in the scar tissue structure after cesarean section as a result of manual therapy. *Advances in clinical and experimental medicine: Official organ Wroclaw. Medicina Universitaria*, *33*(4), 387–395. DOI: 10.17219/acem/169236 PMID: 37665082

Patel, A. V., Friedenreich, C. M., Moore, S. C., Hayes, S. C., Silver, J. K., Campbell, K. L., Winters-Stone, K., Gerber, L. H., George, S. M., Fulton, J. E., Denlinger, C., Morris, G. S., Hue, T., Schmitz, K. H., & Matthews, C. E. (2019). American College of Sports Medicine Roundtable Report on Physical Activity, Sedentary Behavior, and Cancer Prevention and Control. *Medicine and Science in Sports and Exercise*, *51*(11), 2391–2402. DOI: 10.1249/MSS.0000000000002117 PMID: 31626056

Perloff, R. M. (2014). Social Media Effects on Young Women's Body Image Concerns: Theoretical Perspectives and an Agenda for Research. *Sex Roles*, *71*(11-12), 363–377. DOI: 10.1007/s11199-014-0384-6

Pires, T., Pires, P., Moreira, H., Gabriel, R., Viana, S., & Viana, R. (2020c). Assessment of pelvic floor muscles in sportswomen: Quality of life and related factors. *Physical Therapy in Sport*, *43*, 151–156. DOI: 10.1016/j.ptsp.2020.02.015 PMID: 32200260

Pires, T., Pires, P., Moreira, H., & Viana, R. (2020b). Prevalence of urinary incontinence in high-impact sport athletes: A systematic review and meta-analysis. *Journal of Human Kinetics*, *73*(1), 279–288. DOI: 10.2478/hukin-2020-0008 PMID: 32774559

Pires, T., Pires, P., Moreira, M., Gabriel, R., João, P., Viana, S., & Viana, R. (2020d). Pelvic Floor Muscle Training in Female Athletes: A Randomized Controlled Pilot Study. *International Journal of Sports Medicine*, *41*(4), 264–270. DOI: 10.1055/a-1073-7977 PMID: 31935774

Pires, T. P., Costa, R., & Viana, R. (2020a). Effects of pelvic floor muscle training in pregnant women. *Porto Biomedical Journal*, *5*(5), e077. DOI: 10.1097/j.pbj.0000000000000077 PMID: 33195869

Prat, J., & Mutch, D. G. (2018). Pathology of cancers of the female genital tract including molecular pathology. *International Journal of Gynaecology and Obstetrics: the Official Organ of the International Federation of Gynaecology and Obstetrics*, *143*(S2), 93–108. DOI: 10.1002/ijgo.12617 PMID: 30306579

Püsküllüoğlu, M., Tomaszewski, K. A., Grela-Wojewoda, A., Pacholczak-Madej, R., & Ebner, F. (2022). Effects of Transcutaneous Electrical Nerve Stimulation on Pain and Chemotherapy-Induced Peripheral Neuropathy in Cancer Patients: A Systematic Review. *Medicina (Kaunas, Lithuania)*, *58*(2), 284. DOI: 10.3390/medicina58020284 PMID: 35208610

Putri, A. P., & Lu, Y. Y. (2024). Maternal Health Literacy in Pregnant Women: A Concept Analysis. *Maternal and Child Health Journal*, *28*(8), 1272–1282. DOI: 10.1007/s10995-024-03945-z PMID: 38864987

Rampazo, É. P., Rehder-Santos, P., Catai, A. M., & Liebano, R. E. (2024). Heart rate variability in adults with chronic musculoskeletal pain: A systematic review. *Pain Practice*, *24*(1), 211–230. DOI: 10.1111/papr.13294 PMID: 37661339

Reed, P., Osborne, L. A., Whittall, C. M., & Emery, S. (2021). Impact of patient motivation on compliance and outcomes for incontinence. *Physiotherapy*, *113*, 100–106. DOI: 10.1016/j.physio.2020.10.003 PMID: 34563914

Ren, Y., Kebede, M. A., Ogunleye, A. A., Emerson, M. A., Evenson, K. R., Carey, L. A., Hayes, S. C., & Troester, M. A. (2022). Burden of lymphedema in long-term breast cancer survivors by race and age. *Cancer*, *128*(23), 4119–4128. DOI: 10.1002/cncr.34489 PMID: 36223240

Rett, M. T., Moura, D. P., Oliveira, F. B. D., Domingos, H. Y. B., Oliveira, M. M. F. D., Gallo, R. B. S., & Silva, W. M. D.Junior. (2022). Physical therapy after breast cancer surgery improves range of motion and pain over time. *Fisioterapia e Pesquisa, 29*(1), 46–52. DOI: 10.1590/1809-2950/21001929012022en

Ribeiro, M. M., Andrade, A., & Nunes, I. (2021). Physical exercise in pregnancy: Benefits, risks and prescription. *Journal of Perinatal Medicine, 50*(1), 4–17. DOI: 10.1515/jpm-2021-0315 PMID: 34478617

Rizzo, A. (2016). The Role of Exercise and Rehabilitation in the Cancer Care Plan. *Journal of the Advanced Practitioner in Oncology, 7*(3), 339–342. DOI: 10.6004/jadpro.2016.7.3.20 PMID: 29152403

Rogers, R., Pauls, R., Thakar, R., Morin, M., Kuhn, A., Petri, E., Fatton, B., Whitmore, K., Kingsberg, S. A., & Lee, J. (2018). An International Urogynecological Association (IUGA)/International Continence Society (ICS) joint report on the terminology for the assessment of sexual health of women with pelvic floor dysfunction. *International Urogynecology Journal, 29*(5), 647–666. DOI: 10.1007/s00192-018-3603-9 PMID: 29577166

Rose, G. L., Stewart, E. M., Clifford, B. K., Bailey, T. G., Rush, A. J., Abbott, C. R., Hayes, S. C., Obermair, A., & McCarthy, A. L. (2023). Efficacy of exercise interventions for women during and after gynaecological cancer treatment–a systematic scoping review. *Supportive Care in Cancer, 31*(6), 342. DOI: 10.1007/s00520-023-07790-8 PMID: 37195433

Ruchat, S. M., Mottola, M. F., Skow, R. J., Nagpal, T. S., Meah, V. L., James, M., Riske, L., Sobierajski, F., Kathol, A. J., Marchand, A.-A., Nuspl, M., Weeks, A., Gray, C. E., Poitras, V. J., Jaramillo Garcia, A., Barrowman, N., Slater, L. G., Adamo, K. B., Davies, G. A., & Davenport, M. H. (2018). Effectiveness of exercise interventions in the prevention of excessive gestational weight gain and postpartum weight retention: A systematic review and meta-analysis. *British Journal of Sports Medicine, 52*(21), 1347–1356. DOI: 10.1136/bjsports-2018-099399 PMID: 30337461

Salati, S. A., Alsulaim, L., Alharbi, M. H., Alharbi, N. H., Alsenaid, T. M., Alaodah, S. A., Alsuhaibani, A. S., & Albaqami, K. A. (2023). Postmastectomy Pain Syndrome: A Narrative Review. *Cureus, 15*(10), e47384. DOI: 10.7759/cureus.47384 PMID: 38021812

Senger, J. B., Kadle, R. L., & Skoracki, R. J. (2023). Current Concepts in the Management of Primary Lymphedema. *Medicina (Kaunas, Lithuania), 59*(5), 894. DOI: 10.3390/medicina59050894 PMID: 37241126

Sherrington, C., Whitney, J. C., Lord, S. R., Herbert, R. D., Cumming, R. G., & Close, J. C. (2008). Effective exercise for the prevention of falls: A systematic review and meta-analysis. *Journal of the American Geriatrics Society, 56*(12), 2234–2243. DOI: 10.1111/j.1532-5415.2008.02014.x PMID: 19093923

Sobhgol, S. S., Priddis, H., Smith, C. A., & Dahlen, H. G. (2019). The Effect of Pelvic Floor Muscle Exercise on Female Sexual Function During Pregnancy and Postpartum: A Systematic Review. *Sexual Medicine Reviews, 7*(1), 13–28. DOI: 10.1016/j.sxmr.2018.08.002 PMID: 30301705

Spanoudaki, M., Giaginis, C., Karafyllaki, D., Papadopoulos, K., Solovos, E., Antasouras, G., Sfikas, G., Papadopoulos, A. N., & Papadopoulou, S. K. (2023). Exercise as a promising agent against cancer: Evaluating its anti-cancer molecular mechanisms. *Cancers (Basel), 15*(21), 5135. DOI: 10.3390/cancers15215135 PMID: 37958310

Strand, N. H., D'Souza, R., Gomez, D. A., Whitney, M. A., Attanti, S., Anderson, M. A., & Maloney, J. A. (2024). Pain during menopause. *Maturitas, 108135.* Advance online publication. DOI: 10.1016/j.maturitas.2024.108135 PMID: 39500125

Sultan, A., Monga, A., Lee, J., Emmanuel, A., Norton, C., Santoro, G., Hull, T., Berghmans, B., Brody, S., & Haylen, B. (2017). An International Urogynecological Association (IUGA)/International Continence Society (ICS) joint report on the terminology for female anorectal dysfunction. *International Urogynecology Journal, 28*(1), 5–31. DOI: 10.1007/s00192-016-3140-3 PMID: 27774569

Swain, C. T., Drummond, A. E., Boing, L., Milne, R. L., English, D. R., Brown, K. A., van Roekel, E. H., Dixon-Suen, S. C., Lynch, M. J., Moore, M. M., Gaunt, T. R., Martin, R. M., Lewis, S. J., & Lynch, B. M. (2022). Linking physical activity to breast cancer via sex hormones, part 1: The effect of physical activity on sex steroid hormones. *Cancer Epidemiology, Biomarkers & Prevention, 31*(1), 16–27. DOI: 10.1158/1055-9965.EPI-21-0437 PMID: 34670800

Swami, V., & Furnham, A. (2008). *The Psychology of Physical Attraction* (1st ed.). Routledge.

Taylor, H. S., Adamson, G. D., Diamond, M. P., Goldstein, S. R., Horne, A. W., Missmer, S. A., Snabes, M. C., Surrey, E., & Taylor, R. N. (2018). An evidence-based approach to assessing surgical versus clinical diagnosis of symptomatic endometriosis. *International Journal of Gynaecology and Obstetrics: the Official Organ of the International Federation of Gynaecology and Obstetrics, 142*(2), 131–142. DOI: 10.1002/ijgo.12521 PMID: 29729099

Taylor, H. S., Kotlyar, A. M., & Flores, V. A. (2021). Endometriosis is a chronic systemic disease: Clinical challenges and novel innovations. *Lancet*, *397*(10276), 839–852. DOI: 10.1016/S0140-6736(21)00389-5 PMID: 33640070

Tazreean, R., Nelson, G., & Twomey, R. (2022). Early mobilization in enhanced recovery after surgery pathways: Current evidence and recent advancements. *Journal of Comparative Effectiveness Research*, *11*(2), 121–129. DOI: 10.2217/cer-2021-0258 PMID: 35045757

Tennfjord, M. K., Gabrielsen, R., & Tellum, T. (2021). Effect of physical activity and exercise on endometriosis-associated symptoms: A systematic review. *BMC Women's Health*, *21*(1), 355. DOI: 10.1186/s12905-021-01500-4 PMID: 34627209

Thiyagarajan, D. K., Basit, H., & Jeanmonod, R. (2024 Jan). Physiology, Menstrual Cycle. [Updated 2024 Sep 27] In *StatPearls* [Internet]. StatPearls Publishing., Available from https://www.ncbi.nlm.nih.gov/books/NBK500020/

Thomas, E., Battaglia, G., Patti, A., Brusa, J., Leonardi, V., Palma, A., & Bellafiore, M. (2019). Physical activity programs for balance and fall prevention in elderly: A systematic review. *Medicine*, *98*(27), e16218. DOI: 10.1097/MD.0000000000016218 PMID: 31277132

Vergeldt, T. F., Weemhoff, M., IntHout, J., & Kluivers, K. B. (2015). Risk factors for pelvic organ prolapse and its recurrence: A systematic review. *International Urogynecology Journal*, *26*(11), 1559–1573. DOI: 10.1007/s00192-015-2695-8 PMID: 25966804

Viana, R., Viana, S., Neto, F., & Mascarenhas, T. (2015). Adaptation and validation of the King's Health Questionnaire in Portuguese women with urinary incontinence. *International Urogynecology Journal*, *26*(7), 1027–1033. DOI: 10.1007/s00192-015-2628-6 PMID: 25653033

Voineskos, S. H., Nelson, J. A., Klassen, A. F., & Pusic, A. L. (2018). Measuring Patient-Reported Outcomes: Key Metrics in Reconstructive Surgery. *Annual Review of Medicine*, *69*(1), 467–479. DOI: 10.1146/annurev-med-060116-022831 PMID: 29414263

Wang, Y., Zhang, S., Peng, P., He, W., Zhang, H., Xu, H., & Liu, H. (2023). The effect of myofascial therapy on postpartum rectus abdominis separation, low back and leg pain, pelvic floor dysfunction: A systematic review and meta-analysis. *Medicine*, *102*(44), e35761. DOI: 10.1097/MD.0000000000035761 PMID: 37932976

Weare, K. (2015). Rehabilitation after gynecological cancer treatment. *International Journal of Gynaecology and Obstetrics: the Official Organ of the International Federation of Gynaecology and Obstetrics*, *131*(S2), S164–S166. DOI: 10.1016/j.ijgo.2015.06.015 PMID: 26433675

Wilkinson, L., & Gathani, T. (2022). Understanding breast cancer as a global health concern. *The British Journal of Radiology*, *95*(1130), 20211033. DOI: 10.1259/bjr.20211033 PMID: 34905391

Wójcik, M., Szczepaniak, R., & Placek, K. (2022). Physiotherapy Management in Endometriosis. *International Journal of Environmental Research and Public Health*, *19*(23), 16148. DOI: 10.3390/ijerph192316148 PMID: 36498220

World Health Organization. (2018). *WHO recommendations on intrapartum care for a positive childbirth experience*. World Health Organization.

Wu, X., Liu, Y., Zhu, D., Wang, F., Ji, J., & Yan, H. (2021). Early prevention of complex decongestive therapy and rehabilitation exercise for prevention of lower extremity lymphedema after operation of gynecologic cancer. *Asian Journal of Surgery*, *44*(1), 111–115. DOI: 10.1016/j.asjsur.2020.03.022 PMID: 32402630

Yamamoto, R., & Yamamoto, T. (2007). Effectiveness of the treatment-phase of two-phase complex decongestive physiotherapy for the treatment of extremity lymphedema. *International Journal of Clinical Oncology*, *12*(6), 463–468. DOI: 10.1007/s10147-007-0715-5 PMID: 18071866

Yang, E. J., Lim, J. Y., Rah, U. W., & Kim, Y. B. (2012). Effect of a pelvic floor muscle training program on gynecologic cancer survivors with pelvic floor dysfunction: A randomized controlled trial. *Gynecologic Oncology*, *125*(3), 705–711. DOI: 10.1016/j.ygyno.2012.03.045 PMID: 22472463

Yang, F. A., Wu, P. J., Su, Y. T., Strong, P. C., Chu, Y. C., & Huang, C. C. (2024). Effect of kinesiology taping on breast cancer-related lymphedema: A systematic review and meta-analysis of randomized controlled trials. *Clinical Breast Cancer*, *24*(6), 541–551.e1. Advance online publication. DOI: 10.1016/j.clbc.2024.04.013 PMID: 38834497

Yang, X., Li, H., Zhao, Q., Han, R., Xiang, Z., & Gao, L. (2022). Clinical Practice Guidelines That Address Physical Activity and Exercise During Pregnancy: A Systematic Review. *Journal of Midwifery & Women's Health*, *67*(1), 53–68. DOI: 10.1111/jmwh.13286 PMID: 34841649

Yesildere Saglam, H., & Orsal, O. (2020). Effect of exercise on premenstrual symptoms: A systematic review. *Complementary Therapies in Medicine*, *48*, 102272. DOI: 10.1016/j.ctim.2019.102272 PMID: 31987230

Zainordin, N. H., Karim, N. A., Shahril, M. R., & Abd Talib, R. (2021). Physical Activity, Sitting Time, and Quality of Life among Breast and Gynaecology Cancer Survivors. *Asian Pacific Journal of Cancer Prevention : APJCP*, *22*(8), 2399–2408. DOI: 10.31557/APJCP.2021.22.8.2399 PMID: 34452552

Zhang, S. (2021). Chemotherapy-induced peripheral neuropathy and rehabilitation: A review. *Seminars in Oncology*, *48*(3), 193–207. DOI: 10.1053/j.seminoncol.2021.09.004 PMID: 34607709

Zhu, B., Gu, H., Mao, Z., Beeraka, N. M., Zhao, X., Anand, M. P., Zheng, Y., Zhao, R., Li, S., Manogaran, P., Fan, R., Nikolenko, V. N., Wen, H., Basappa, B., & Liu, J. (2024). Global burden of gynaecological cancers in 2022 and projections to 2050. *Journal of Global Health*, *14*, 04155. DOI: 10.7189/jogh.14.04155 PMID: 39148469

ADDITIONAL READING

Brown, W. J., Hayman, M., Haakstad, L. A., Lamerton, T., Mena, G. P., Green, A., Keating, S. E., Gomes, G. A. O., Coombes, J. S., & Mielke, G. I. (2022). Australian guidelines for physical activity in pregnancy and postpartum. *Journal of Science and Medicine in Sport*, *25*(6), 511–519. DOI: 10.1016/j.jsams.2022.03.008 PMID: 35418334

Pires, T., Pires, P., Moreira, H., Gabriel, R., Reis, A., Viana, S., & Viana, R. (2021). Leg stiffness and muscle power vs manometer in sportswomen with symptoms of stress urinary incontinence. *Clinical Biomechanics (Bristol, Avon)*, *90*, 105471. DOI: 10.1016/j.clinbiomech.2021.105471 PMID: 34610505

Stout, N. L., Santa Mina, D., Lyons, K. D., Robb, K., & Silver, J. K. (2021). A systematic review of rehabilitation and exercise recommendations in oncology guidelines. *CA: a Cancer Journal for Clinicians*, *71*(2), 149–175. DOI: 10.3322/caac.21639 PMID: 33107982

KEY TERMS AND DEFINITIONS

Body Image: Refers to an individual's perceptions, thoughts, and feelings about their physical appearance and body. It encompasses the way one sees themselves in terms of size, shape, and features, as well as the satisfaction or dissatisfaction with these aspects. Body image is influenced by various factors, including societal standards of beauty, personal experiences, and cultural beliefs.

Exercise: A structured and repetitive physical activity aimed at improving or maintaining physical fitness, health, and overall well-being. It encompasses a wide range of activities, including aerobic exercises, strength training, flexibility exercises, and balance training.

Oncological Rehabilitation: Multidimensional healthcare interventions provided throughout the cancer continuum to prevent and mitigate the effects of cancer and cancer treatment, to optimize physical, psychological and social function and to improve patients' survival.

Pelvic Physiotherapy: Specialized intervention with a urogynecological and vesico-sphincteric approach, guided by an expert physiotherapist who values education, manual and instrumental techniques, as well as guidance and supervision of exercises and recommendations.

Women's Health: Refers to the comprehensive well-being of women throughout their lifespan, encompassing the various stages of life, including adolescence, reproductive years, menopause and older life. This holistic approach recognises the interplay of biological, social and cultures factors in women's health, aiming to promote not only the absence of disease but also optimal physical and mental well-being.

Compilation of References

Abou-El-Enein, M., Römhild, A., Kaiser, D., Beier, C., Bauer, G., Volk, H., & Reinke, P. (2013). Good Manufacturing Practices (GMP) manufacturing of advanced therapy medicinal products: A novel tailored model for optimizing performance and estimating costs. *Cytotherapy*, *15*(3), 362–383. DOI: 10.1016/j.jcyt.2012.09.006 PMID: 23579061

Abou-Elsaad, T., Abdel-Hady, H., Baz, H., & ElShabrawi, D. (2017). Language and cognitive outcome for high-risk neonates at the age of 2-3 years - experience from an arab country. *World Journal of Clinical Pediatrics*, *6*(1), 24. DOI: 10.5409/wjcp.v6.i1.24 PMID: 28224092

Abrar-Ul-Hassan, S. (2011). Language Development Hinges on Communication: An Emergentist Perspective. *TESOL Journal*, *2*(4), 510–520. DOI: 10.5054/tj.2011.269749

Abril-Coello, R., Correyero-León, M., Ceballos-Laita, L., & Jiménez-Barrio, S. (2023). Benefits of physical therapy in improving quality of life and pain associated with endometriosis: A systematic review and meta-analysis. *International Journal of Gynaecology and Obstetrics: the Official Organ of the International Federation of Gynaecology and Obstetrics*, *162*(1), 233–243. DOI: 10.1002/ijgo.14645 PMID: 36571475

Adetunji, O., Bishai, D., Pham, C., Taylor, J., Thi, N., Khan, Z., & Bachani, A. (2023). Patient-centered care and geriatric knowledge translation among health-care providers in vietnam: Translation and validation of the patient-centered care measure. *BMC Health Services Research*, *23*(1), 379. Advance online publication. DOI: 10.1186/s12913-023-09311-z PMID: 37076905

Adler-Neal, A., & Zeidan, F. (2017). Mindfulness meditation for fibromyalgia: Mechanistic and clinical considerations. *Current Rheumatology Reports*, *19*(9), 59. Advance online publication. DOI: 10.1007/s11926-017-0686-0 PMID: 28752493

Afshar-Bakshloo, M., Albers, S., Richter, C., Berninger, O., Blohmer, J. U., Roehle, R., Speiser, D., & Karsten, M. M. (2023). How breast cancer therapies impact body image–real-world data from a prospective cohort study collecting patient-reported outcomes. *BMC Cancer, 23*(1), 705. DOI: 10.1186/s12885-023-11172-y PMID: 37507687

Agarwal, A., Durairajanayagam, D., Tatagari, S., Esteves, S. C., Harlev, A., Henkel, R., Roychoudhury, S., Homa, S., Puchalt, N. G., Ramasamy, R., Majzoub, A., Ly, K. D., Tvrda, E., Assidi, M., Kesari, K., Sharma, R., Banihani, S., Ko, E., Abu-Elmagd, M., & Bashiri, A. (2016). Bibliometrics: Tracking research impact by selecting the appropriate metrics. *Asian Journal of Andrology, 18*(2), 296–309. DOI: 10.4103/1008-682X.171582 PMID: 26806079

Agarwal, V. (2018). Complementary and alternative medicine provider knowledge discourse on holistic health. *Frontiers in Communication, 3*, 15. Advance online publication. DOI: 10.3389/fcomm.2018.00015

Agrahari, V., & Hiremath, P. (2017). Challenges associated and approaches for successful translation of nanomedicines into commercial products. *Nanomedicine (London), 12*(8), 819–823. DOI: 10.2217/nnm-2017-0039 PMID: 28338401

Agrawal, G. K., Sarkar, A., Righetti, P. G., Pedreschi, R., Carpentier, S., Wang, T., Barkla, B. J., Kohli, A., Ndimba, B. K., Bykova, N. V., Rampitsch, C., Zolla, L., Rafudeen, M. S., Cramer, R., Bindschedler, L. V., Tsakirpaloglou, N., Ndimba, R. J., Farrant, J. M., Renaut, J., & Rakwal, R. (2013). A decade of plant proteomics and mass spectrometry: Translation of technical advancements to food security and safety issues. *Mass Spectrometry Reviews, 32*(5), 335–365. DOI: 10.1002/mas.21365 PMID: 23315723

Aguiar (2014) *Perturbações da Linguagem e da Fala em crianças dos 4:00A aos 4:11A do Concelho de Oeiras: Fatores de Risco e Necessidades de Encaminhamento para a Terapia da Fala.* Relatório de Investigação. https://repositorio-cientifico.essatla.pt/bitstream/20.500.12253/927/1/Artigo%20Cient%C3%ADfico_Tatiana%20Aguiar_vers%C3%A3o%20final%20corrigida.pdf

Aguiar, J., Kanan, L. A., & Masiero, A. V. (2019). Práticas integrativas e complementares na atenção básica em saúde: Um estudo bibliométrico da produção brasileira. *Saúde em Debate, 43*(123), 1205–1218. DOI: 10.1590/0103-1104201912318

Ahmed, H. M. (2020). Role of verbal and non-verbal communication of health care providers in general satisfaction with birth care: A cross-sectional study in government health settings of Erbil City. *Reproductive Health, 17*(1), 35–44. DOI: 10.1186/s12978-020-0894-3 PMID: 32151284

Ajzen, I. (1991). The theory of planned behavior. *Organizational Behavior and Human Decision Processes, 50*(2), 179–211. DOI: 10.1016/0749-5978(91)90020-T

Akbas, A., Dagmura, H., Daldal, E., Dasiran, F. M., Deveci, H., & Okan, I. (2021). Association between Shoulder Range of Motion and Pain Catastrophizing Scale in Breast Cancer Patients after Surgery. *Breast Care (Basel, Switzerland), 16*(1), 66–71. DOI: 10.1159/000506922 PMID: 33716634

Akemoglu, Y., Muharib, R., & Meadan, H. (2019). A Systematic and Quality Review of Parent-Implemented Language and Communication Interventions Conducted via Telepractice. *Journal of Behavioral Education, 28*(2), 282–316. DOI: 10.1007/s10864-019-09356-3

Al Kuwaiti, A., Nazer, K., Al-Reedy, A., Al-Shehri, S., Al-Muhanna, A., Subbarayalu, A. V., Al Muhanna, D., & Al-Muhanna, F. A. (2023). A Review of the Role of Artificial Intelligence in Healthcare. *Journal of Personalized Medicine, 13*(6), 951. DOI: 10.3390/jpm13060951 PMID: 37373940

Alaniz, M. L., Rosenberg, S. S., Beard, N. R., & Rosario, E. R. (2017). The Effectiveness of Aquatic Group Therapy for Improving Water Safety and Social Interactions in Children with Autism Spectrum Disorder: A Pilot Program. *Journal of Autism and Developmental Disorders, 47*(12), 4006–4017. DOI: 10.1007/s10803-017-3264-4 PMID: 28864911

Alcântara, P., Zonho, A. W., Lobo, M. I. R., Rodrigues, I. N., & Llonch, A. S. (2016). Efeito da interação com palhaços nos sinais vitais e na comunicação não verbal de crianças hospitalizadas. *Revista Paulista de Pediatria : Orgao Oficial da Sociedade de Pediatria de Sao Paulo, 34*, 432–438. DOI: 10.1016/j.rpped.2016.02.001 PMID: 27080219

Alcimed. (2024, April 23). *3 approaches to meet the challenges of food allergy management*. https://www.alcimed.com/en/insights/food-allergy-management/

Aldamluji, N., Burgess, A., Pogatzki-Zahn, E., Ræder, J., & Beloeil, H. (2020). Prospect guideline for tonsillectomy: Systematic review and procedure-specific postoperative pain management recommendations. *Anaesthesia, 76*(7), 947–961. DOI: 10.1111/anae.15299 PMID: 33201518

Alhazmi, L. S. S., Bawadood, M. A. A., Aljohani, A. M. S., Alzahrani, A. A. R., Moshref, L., Trabulsi, N., & Moshref, R. (2021). Pain Management in Breast Cancer Patients: A Multidisciplinary Approach. *Cureus, 13*(6), e15994. DOI: 10.7759/cureus.15994 PMID: 34336485

Allen, K. J., Remington, B. C., Baumert, J. L., Crevel, R. W., Houben, G. F., Brooke-Taylor, S., Kruizinga, A. G., & Taylor, S. L. (2014). Allergen reference doses for precautionary labeling (VITAL 2.0): Clinical implications. ^the %oJournal of Allergy and Clinical Immunology/Journal of Allergy and Clinical Immunology/ the œJournal of Allergy and Clinical Immunology, 133(1), 156–164. DOI: 10.1016/j.jaci.2013.06.042

Allen, K. J., Turner, P. J., Pawankar, R., Taylor, S., Sicherer, S., Lack, G., Rosario, N., Ebisawa, M., Wong, G., Mills, E. N. C., Beyer, K., Fiocchi, A., & Sampson, H. A. (2014). Precautionary labelling of foods for allergen content: are we ready for a global framework? the World Allergy Organization Journal, 7, 10. DOI: 10.1186/1939-4551-7-10

Allen, L., Hatala, A., Ijaz, S., Courchene, E., & Bushie, E. (2020). Indigenous-led health care partnerships in Canada. *Canadian Medical Association Journal*, *192*(9), E208–E216. DOI: 10.1503/cmaj.190728 PMID: 32122977

Alsford, E., Ralephata, A., Bolderson, S., Curtin, M., Parish, E., Klaber, V., Griffin, S., Nash, L., Cullen, R., Musoke, B., Bhalla, S., Walker, L., Duffer, L., O'Sullivan, S., Knowland, V., Cozens, S., McLaren, L., Camilleri, B., Halil, S., & Pring, T. (2017). The wrong side of the tracks: Starting school in a socially disadvantaged London borough. *Child Language Teaching and Therapy*, *33*(2), 145–156. DOI: 10.1177/0265659016654954

Álvarez-Salvago, F., Lara-Ramos, A., Cantarero-Villanueva, I., Mazheika, M., Mundo-López, A., Galiano-Castillo, N., Fernández-Lao, C., Arroyo-Morales, M., Ocón-Hernández, O., & Artacho-Cordón, F. (2020). Chronic fatigue, physical impairments and quality of life in women with endometriosis: A case-control study. *International Journal of Environmental Research and Public Health*, *17*(10), 3610. DOI: 10.3390/ijerph17103610 PMID: 32455618

American College of Obstetricians and Gynecologists [ACOG] (2015a). Committee Opinion number 650: Physical Activity an Exercise During Pregnancy and the Postpartum Period. Obstetrics and Gynecology, 126(6), 135–142. https://doi.org/ DOI: 10.1097/AOG.0000000000001214

American College of Obstetricians and Gynecologists [ACOG] (2015b). Committee Opinion No. 651: Menstruation in Girls and Adolescents: Using the Menstrual Cycle as a Vital Sign. *Obstetrics and gynecology, 126*(6), e143–e146. https://doi.org/DOI: 10.1097/AOG.0000000000001215

American College of Obstetricians and Gynecologists [ACOG] (2020). Committee Opinion number 804: Physical activity and exercise during pregnancy and Postpartum Period. Obstetrics and Gynecology, 135(4), 178–188. https://doi.org/DOI: 10.3109/21679169.2013.861509

American College of Sports Medicine [ACSM] (2018). ACSM Guideline for Exercise Testing and Prescription (D. Riebe, M. Nobel, & A. Millholen (eds.); 10h ed.). Wolters Kluwer Health.

American Music Therapy Association. (2024, July 30th). About music therapy and AMTA. Retrieved from https://www.musictherapy.org/about/

American Psychiatric Association. (2022). *Diagnostic and statistical manual of mental disorders* (5th ed., text rev.)., DOI: 10.1176/appi.books.9780890425787

American Speech and Hearing Association. (2021). SLP Health Care Survey Report: Workforce Trends 2005–2021. https://www.asha.org/siteassets/surveys/2021-slp-health-care-survey-workforce-trends-2005-2021.pdf

American Speech-Language-Hearing Association. (2016). *Scope of practice in speech-language pathology* [Scope of Practice]. https://www.asha.org/policy/

American Speech-Language-Hearing Association. (n.d.). *Augmentative and alternative communication* (Practice portal). Retrieved November, 20, 2024, from www.asha.org/Practice-Portal/Professional-Issues/Augmentative-and-Alternative-Communication/

Amin, M. and Pinilih, S. (2024). Exploring recovery-focused health workers for advancing mental health: literature review., 881-890. https://doi.org/DOI: 10.2991/978-2-38476-273-6_90

Amonkar, N., Su, W. C., Bhat, A. N., & Srinivasan, S. M. (2021). Effects of creative movement therapies on social communication, behavioral-affective, sensorimotor, cognitive, and functional participation skills of individuals with autism spectrum disorder: A systematic review. *Frontiers in Psychiatry*, *12*, 722874. DOI: 10.3389/fpsyt.2021.722874 PMID: 34867515

Amponsah, A., Björn, A., Bam, V., & Axelin, A. (2019). The effect of educational strategies targeted for nurses on pain assessment and management in children: An integrative review. *Pain Management Nursing*, *20*(6), 604–613. DOI: 10.1016/j.pmn.2019.03.005 PMID: 31103495

Amro, B., Ramirez Aristondo, M. E., Alsuwaidi, S., Almaamari, B., Hakim, Z., Tahlak, M., Wattiez, A., & Koninckx, P. R. (2022). New understanding of diagnosis, treatment and prevention of endometriosis. *International Journal of Environmental Research and Public Health, 19*(11), 6725. DOI: 10.3390/ijerph19116725 PMID: 35682310

Anderson, J. A. (1996). Allergic reactions to foods. Critical Reviews in Food Science and Nutrition, 36(sup001), 19–38. DOI: 10.1080/10408399609527757

Anderson, A., Deng, J., Anthony, R., Atalla, S., & Monroe, T. (2017). Using complementary and alternative medicine to treat pain and agitation in dementia. *Critical Care Nursing Clinics of North America, 29*(4), 519–537. DOI: 10.1016/j.cnc.2017.08.010 PMID: 29107312

Andrade, F. B. D., & Ferreira Filho, M. de O., Dias, M. D., Silva, A. O., Costa, I. do C. C., De Lima, É. A. R., & Mendes, C. K. T. (2010). Promoção da saúde mental do idoso na atenção básica: As contribuições da Terapia Comunitária. *Texto & Contexto - Enfermagem, 19*(1), 129–136. https://doi.org/DOI: 10.1590/S0104-07072010000100015

Ang, C., & MacDougall, F. (2022). An evaluation of animal-assisted therapy for autism spectrum disorders: Therapist and parent perspectives. *Psychological Studies, 67*(1), 72–81. DOI: 10.1007/s12646-022-00647-w PMID: 35287312

An, M., & Palisano, J. R. (2014). Family–professional collaboration in pediatric rehabilitation: A practice model. *Disability and Rehabilitation, 36*(5), 434–440. DOI: 10.3109/09638288.2013.797510 PMID: 23713990

An, M., Palisano, R. J., Yi, C., Chiarello, L. A., Dunst, C. J., & Gracely, E. J. (2017). Effects of a Collaborative Intervention Process on Parent Empowerment and Child Performance: A Randomized Controlled Trial. *Physical & Occupational Therapy in Pediatrics, 0*(0), 1–15. 101080/01942638.2017.1365324 PMID: 28929830

An, S., Kanderzhanova, A., Akhmetova, A., Foster, F., & Chan, C. K. (2020). "Chasing hope": Parents' perspectives on complementary and alternative interventions for children with autism in Kazakhstan. *Autism, 24*(7), 1817–1828. DOI: 10.1177/1362361320923494 PMID: 32498539

Antunes, D., Arantes, R., Seabra, E., Silva, L. F., & Viana, R. (2024). Materials, Functionalities and Processing of a Medical Device to Pelvic Floor Rehabilitation. In Machado, J. (Eds.), *Innovations in Mechatronics Engineering, Lecture Notes in Mechanical Engineering* (pp. 235–241). Springer Nature., DOI: 10.1007/978-3-031-62684-5_21

Antunes, M., & Cruz-Santos, A. (2017). Avaliação da comunicação expressiva em crianças dos 6 aos 41 meses de idade na região norte de Portugal: Um estudo exploratório com o Early Communication Indicator. *Revista de Estudios e Investigación en Psicología y Educación*, *79*, 79–84. Advance online publication. DOI: 10.17979/reipe.2017.0.09.2847

Appleby, R., Wright, S., Williams, L., & Stanley, M. (2022). Australian parents' experiences of owning an autism assistance dog. *Health & Social Care in the Community*, *30*(6), e4113–e4121. DOI: 10.1111/hsc.13805 PMID: 35352418

Aranbarri, A., Stahmer, A. C., Talbott, M. R., Miller, M. E., Drahota, A., Pellecchia, M., Barber, A. B., Griffith, E. M., Morgan, E. H., & Rogers, S. J. (2021). Examining US Public Early Intervention for Toddlers With Autism: Characterizing Services and Readiness for Evidence-Based Practice Implementation. *Frontiers in Psychiatry*, *12*, 786138. DOI: 10.3389/fpsyt.2021.786138 PMID: 34975582

Arantes, R., Antunes, D., Seabra, E., Viana, R., & Silva, L. F. L. F. (2024). Design of a New Intravaginal Device to Measure and Monitor the Pelvic Floor Muscle Strength, In J. Machado et al. (Eds.), Innovations in Mechatronics Engineering, Lecture Notes in Mechanical Engineering (pp. 288-293). Springer Nature. https://doi.org/DOI: 10.1007/978-3-031-61575-7_26

Araujo, M. M. T., da Silva, L. F., & Souza, R. C. (2023). Comunicação aumentativa e alternativa na saúde –tecnologia assistiva reduzindo barreiras comunicacionais. *Revista ISAAC, 15*(2), 125–138. https://publicacoes.softaliza.com.br/isaac2023/article/view/7892?utm_source=chatgpt.com

Araújo, M. M. T., Silva, M. J. P., & Puggina, A.C. G. (2007). A comunicação não-verbal enquanto fator iatrogênico. *Revista da Escola de Enfermagem da USP, 41*, 419-425. 07 https://doi.org/DOI: 10.1590/S0080-62342007000300011

Ardestani, S., Karkhaneh, M., Stein, E., Punja, S., Junqueira, D., Kuzmyn, T., & Vohra, S. (2021). Systematic review of mind-body interventions to treat myalgic encephalomyelitis/chronic fatigue syndrome. *Medicina*, *57*(7), 652. DOI: 10.3390/medicina57070652 PMID: 34202826

Armour, M., Ee, C. C., Naidoo, D., Ayati, Z., Chalmers, K. J., Steel, K. A., de Manincor, M. J., & Delshad, E. (2019). Exercise for dysmenorrhoea. *Cochrane Database of Systematic Reviews*, *9*(9), CD004142. Advance online publication. DOI: 10.1002/14651858.CD004142.pub4 PMID: 31538328

Armstrong, R., Scott, J. G., Whitehouse, A. J. O., Copland, D. A., Mcmahon, K. L., & Arnott, W. (2017). Late talkers and later language outcomes: Predicting the different language trajectories. *International Journal of Speech-Language Pathology, 19*(3), 237–250. DOI: 10.1080/17549507.2017.1296191 PMID: 28440674

Arnold, H. S., Conture, E. G., Key, A. P., & Walden, T. (2011). Emotional reactivity, regulation and childhood stuttering: A behavioral and electrophysiological study. *Journal of Communication Disorders, 44*(3), 276–293. DOI: 10.1016/j.jcomdis.2010.12.003 PMID: 21276977

Arntz, A., Weber, F., Handgraaf, M., Lällä, K., Korniloff, K., Murtonen, K. P., Chichaeva, J., Kidritsch, A., Heller, M., Sakellari, E., Athanasopoulou, C., Lagiou, A., Tzonichaki, I., Salinas-Bueno, I., Martínez-Bueso, P., Velasco-Roldán, O., Schulz, R. J., & Grüneberg, C. (2023). Technologies in Home-Based Digital Rehabilitation: Scoping Review. *JMIR Rehabilitation and Assistive Technologies, 10*, e43615. DOI: 10.2196/43615 PMID: 37253381

Arrese, L. C., Carrau, R., & Plowman, E. K. (2017). Relationship Between the Eating Assessment Tool-10 and Objective Clinical Ratings of Swallowing Function in Individuals with Head and Neck Cancer. *Dysphagia, 32*(1), 83–89. DOI: 10.1007/s00455-016-9741-7 PMID: 27538876

Artacho-Cordón, F., del Mar Salinas-Asensio, M., Galiano-Castillo, N., Ocón-Hernández, O., Peinado, F. M., Mundo-López, A., & Cantarero-Villanueva, I. (2023). Effect of a multimodal supervised therapeutic exercise program on quality of life, pain, and lumbopelvic impairments in women with endometriosis unresponsive to conventional therapy: A randomized controlled trial. *Archives of Physical Medicine and Rehabilitation, 104*(11), 1785–1795. DOI: 10.1016/j.apmr.2023.06.020 PMID: 37467936

Asero, R., Ballmer-Weber, B. K., Beyer, K., Conti, A., Dubakiene, R., Fernandez-Rivas, M., Hoffmann-Sommergruber, K., Lidholm, J., Mustakov, T., Elberink, J. N. G. O., Pumphrey, R. S. H., Skov, P. S., Van Ree, R., Vlieg-Boerstra, B. J., Hiller, R., Hourihane, J. O., Kowalski, M., Papadopoulos, N. G., Wal, J., & Vieths, S. (2006). IgE-Mediated food allergy diagnosis: Current status and new perspectives. *Molecular Nutrition & Food Research, 51*(1), 135–147. DOI: 10.1002/mnfr.200600132 PMID: 17195271

ASHA. (1993). *Definitions of communication disorders and variations.* Accessed November 20, 2024. https://www.asha.org/policy/rp1993-00208/

As-Sanie, S., Black, R., Giudice, L. C., Valbrun, T. G., Gupta, J., Jones, B., & Nebel, R. A. (2019). Assessing research gaps and unmet needs in endometriosis. *American Journal of Obstetrics and Gynecology*, *221*(2), 86–94. DOI: 10.1016/j.ajog.2019.02.033 PMID: 30790565

Associação Portuguesa de Terapeutas da Fala. (n.d.). https://www.oterapeutadafalapodefazeradiferenca.org/home

Athanasakis, E. (2019). A meta-synthesis of how registered nurses make sense of their lived experiences of medication errors. *Journal of Clinical Nursing*, *28*(17-18), 3077–3095. DOI: 10.1111/jocn.14917 PMID: 31099064

Auza, B. A., Murata, C., & Peñaloza, C. (2023). Early detection of Spanish-speaking children with developmental language disorders: Concurrent validity of a short questionnaire and a screening test. *Journal of Communication Disorders*, *104*, 106339. DOI: 10.1016/j.jcomdis.2023.106339 PMID: 37247522

Ávila, M., Lucchetti, A., & Lucchetti, G. (2016). Association between depression and resilience in older adults: A systematic review and meta-analysis. *International Journal of Geriatric Psychiatry*, *32*(3), 237–246. DOI: 10.1002/gps.4619 PMID: 27805730

Ayaz, A., Dedebayraktar, D., Inan-Eroglu, E., Besler, H. T., & Buyuktuncer, Z. (2020). How does nutrition education contribute to the consumers' use and attitudes towards food labels? *Nutrition & Food Science*, *51*(3), 517–528. DOI: 10.1108/NFS-05-2020-0174

Azevedo e Silva, G., Giovanella, L., & De Camargo, K. R.Jr. (2020). Brazil's National Health Care System at risk for losing its universal character. *American Journal of Public Health*, *110*(6), 811–812. DOI: 10.2105/AJPH.2020.305649 PMID: 32374681

Aziz, A. A., & Kashinathan, S. (2021). ESL Learners' Challenges in Speaking English in Malaysian Classroom. *International Journal of Academic Research in Progressive Education and Development*, *10*(2), 983–991.

Aziz, I., Whitehead, W., Palsson, O., Törnblom, H., & Simrén, M. (2020). An approach to the diagnosis and management of Rome IV functional disorders of chronic constipation. *Expert Review of Gastroenterology & Hepatology*, *14*(1), 39–46. DOI: 10.1080/17474124.2020.1708718 PMID: 31893959

Bacal, L. R. (2013). The impact of food allergies on quality of life. *Pediatric Annals*, *42*(7). Advance online publication. DOI: 10.3928/00904481-20130619-12 PMID: 23805962

Bahadur, E. (2023). Behavior problems of preschoolers with developmental language disorder. *Turkish Journal of Pediatric Disease*, 1-6. https://doi.org/DOI: 10.12956/tchd.1298463

Baijens, L. W. J., Walshe, M., Aaltonen, L. M., Arens, C., Cordier, R., Cras, P., Crevier-Buchman, L., Curtis, C., Golusinski, W., Govender, R., Eriksen, J. G., Hansen, K., Heathcote, K., Hess, M. M., Hosal, S., Klussmann, J. P., Leemans, C. R., MacCarthy, D., Manduchi, B., & Clavé, P. (2021). European white paper: Oropharyngeal dysphagia in head and neck cancer. *European Archives of Oto-Rhino-Laryngology*, *278*(2), 577–616. DOI: 10.1007/s00405-020-06507-5 PMID: 33341909

Balaguer, M., Pommée, T., Farinas, J., Pinquier, J., Woisard, V., & Speyer, R. (2020). Effects of oral and oropharyngeal cancer on speech intelligibility using acoustic analysis: Systematic review. *Head & Neck*, *42*(1), 111–130. DOI: 10.1002/hed.25949 PMID: 31571334

Bandeira, A. K. C. (2004). *Qualidade de vida relacionada à voz e à deglutição após tratamento para câncer de língua* Fundação Antônio Prudente]. http://livros01.livrosgratis.com.br/cp005138.pdf

Bang, M., Haeng Lee, S., Cho, S. H., Yu, S. A., Kim, K., & Lu, Y. H., Tae Chang, G., & Yeon Min, S. (2017). Herbal Medicine Treatment for Children with Autism Spectrum Disorder: A Systematic Review. ncbi.nlm.nih.gov

Banks, J. R., & Andrews, T. (2022). Accurate and Reproducible Diagnosis of Peanut Allergy using Epitope Mapping. *Pediatrics*, *150*(Supplement 3), S23. DOI: 10.1542/peds.2022-059346FF

Bao, X., Komesidou, R., & Hogan, T. P. (2024). A review of screeners to identify risk of developmental language disorder. *American Journal of Speech-Language Pathology*, *33*(3), 1548–1571. DOI: 10.1044/2023_AJSLP-23-00286 PMID: 38324341

Barahona-Corrêa, J. B., Velosa, A., Chainho, A., Lopes, R., & Oliveira-Maia, A. J. (2018). Repetitive transcranial magnetic stimulation for treatment of autism spectrum disorder: A systematic review and meta-analysis. *Frontiers in Integrative Neuroscience*, *12*, 27. DOI: 10.3389/fnint.2018.00027 PMID: 30038561

Barker, R. (2008). *Predicting Oral Language Development in Toddlers with Significant Developmental Disabilities: The Role of Child and Parent Communication Characteristics*. Thesis, Georgia State University, https://doi.org/DOI: 10.57709/1061207

Barnett, J., Begen, F. M., Gowland, M. H., & Lucas, J. S. (2018). Comparing the eating out experiences of consumers seeking to avoid different food allergens. *BMC Public Health, 18*(1), 1263. Advance online publication. DOI: 10.1186/s12889-018-6117-y PMID: 30442121

Barnett, M. A., Gustafsson, H., Deng, M., Mills-Koonce, W. R., & Cox, M. (2012). Bidirectional Associations Among Sensitive Parenting, Language Development, and Social Competence. *Infant and Child Development, 21*(4), 374–393. DOI: 10.1002/icd.1750 PMID: 25126021

Barnhart, G., Silverwood, A., Efird, W., & Wells, K. (2023). Animal assisted interventions on therapy farms for those with autism. *The Humanistic Psychologist, 51*(2), 160–172. DOI: 10.1037/hum0000217

Barry, M. J., Nicholson, W. K., Silverstein, M., Chelmow, D., Coker, T. R., Davis, E. M., Donahue, K. E., Jaén, C. R., Li, L., Mangione, C. M., Ogedegbe, G., Rao, G., Ruiz, J. M., Stevermer, J., Tsevat, J., Underwood, S. M., & Wong, J. B.US Preventive Services Task Force. (2024). Screening for Speech and Language Delay and Disorders in Children: US Preventive Services Task Force Recommendation Statement. *Journal of the American Medical Association, 331*(4), 329–334. DOI: 10.1001/jama.2023.26952 PMID: 38261037

Básica. Política Nacional de Práticas Integrativas e Complementares no SUS - PNPIC- SUS, 1ª Ed. Brasília; 2006. 92 p. Available: < https://bvsms.saude.gov.br/bvs/saudelegis/gm/2006/prt0971_03_05_2006.html >

Basso, J. C., McHale, A., Ende, V., Oberlin, D. J., & Suzuki, W. A. (2019). Brief, daily meditation enhances attention, memory, mood, and emotional regulation in non-experienced meditators. *Behavioural Brain Research, 356*, 208–220. DOI: 10.1016/j.bbr.2018.08.023 PMID: 30153464

Bayen, S., Elliott, C., Arlorio, M., Ballins, N. Z., Birse, N., Brockmeyer, J., Chahal, S., Corradini, M. G., Hanner, R., Hann, S., Laursen, K. H., Mihailova, A., Steininger-Mairinger, T., Suman, M., Tian, L., Van Ruth, S., & Xia, J. (2024). Towards a harmonized approach for food authenticity marker validation and accreditation. *Trends in Food Science & Technology, 104550*, 104550. Advance online publication. DOI: 10.1016/j.tifs.2024.104550

Baylor, C., Burns, M., McDonough, K., Mach, H., & Yorkston, K. (2019). Teaching medical students skills for effective communication with patients who have communication disorders. *American Journal of Speech-Language Pathology, 28*(1), 155–164. DOI: 10.1044/2018_AJSLP-18-0130 PMID: 31072161

Bayuo, J., Wong, F., & Agyei, F. (2020). "on the recovery journey:" an integrative review of the needs of burn patients from immediate pre-discharge to post-discharge period using the Omaha system. *Journal of Nursing Scholarship, 52*(4), 360–368. DOI: 10.1111/jnu.12563 PMID: 32445507

Becker, B. E. (2024). Aquatic Therapy: History, Theory, and Applications. In The Use of Aquatics in Orthopedics and Sports Medicine Rehabilitation and Physical Conditioning (pp. 3-16). Routledge.

Bendowska, A., & Baum, E. (2023). The Significance of Cooperation in Interdisciplinary Health Care Teams as Perceived by Polish Medical Students. *International Journal of Environmental Research and Public Health, 20*(2), 954. DOI: 10.3390/ijerph20020954 PMID: 36673710

Beneteau, E., Paradiso, A., & Pratt, W. (2022). Telehealth experiences of providers and patients who use augmentative and alternative communication. *Journal of the American Medical Informatics Association : JAMIA, 29*(3), 462–470. DOI: 10.1093/jamia/ocab273 PMID: 34897460

Ben-Shoshan, M., DeSchryver, S., Dery, A., Mill, J., Mill, C., & O'Keefe, A. (2014). Diagnosis and management of food allergies: new and emerging options: a systematic review. *Journal of Asthma and Allergy, 141*, 141. Advance online publication. DOI: 10.2147/JAA.S49277

Benson, B. J. (2014). Domain of competence: Interpersonal and communication skills. *Academic Pediatrics, 14*(2), 55–65. DOI: 10.1016/j.acap.2013.11.016 PMID: 24602649

Berenguer, C., Martínez, E.R., De Stasio, S., & Baixauli, I. (2022). Parents' perceptions and experiences with their children's use of augmentative/alternative communication: a systematic review and qualitative meta-synthesis. *International Journal of Environmental Research and Public Health,19*, 809.n DOI: 10.3390/ijerph19138091

Berger, A., Liu, Y., Mosel, L., Champagne, K., Ruoff, M., Cornett, E., Kaye, A. D., Imani, F., Shakeri, A., Varrassi, G., Viswanath, O., & Urits, I. (2021). Efficacy of dry needling and acupuncture in the treatment of neck pain. *Anesthesiology and Pain Medicine, 11*(2). Advance online publication. DOI: 10.5812/aapm.113627 PMID: 34336626

Berghmans, B. (2018). Physiotherapy for pelvic pain and female sexual dysfunction: An untapped resource. *International Urogynecology Journal, 29*(5), 631–638. DOI: 10.1007/s00192-017-3536-8 PMID: 29318334

Berta, M., Lindgren, H., Christensson, K., Mekonnen, S., & Adefris, M. (2019). Effect of maternal birth positions on duration of second stage of labor: Systematic review and meta-analysis. *BMC Pregnancy and Childbirth, 19*(1), 466. DOI: 10.1186/s12884-019-2620-0 PMID: 31801479

Bertolozzi, M.R, Nichiata, L.Y., Takahashi, R.F., Ciosak, S.I., Hino, P., Ferreira do Val, F. & Guanillo, M.C.v(2009). The vulnerability and the compliance in Collective Health. *Revista da Escola de Enfermagem da USP, 43*(spe2),1320-1324.

Beswick, E., Park, E., Wong, C., Mehta, A., Dakin, R., Chandran, S., Newton, J., Carson, A., Abrahams, S., & Pal, S. (2020). A systematic review of neuropsychiatric and cognitive assessments used in clinical trials for amyotrophic lateral sclerosis. *Journal of Neurology, 268*(12), 4510–4521. DOI: 10.1007/s00415-020-10203-z PMID: 32910255

Betancourt, T., Keegan, K., Farrar, J., & Brennan, R. (2020). The intergenerational impact of war on mental health and psychosocial wellbeing: Lessons from the longitudinal study of war-affected youth in Sierra Leone. *Conflict and Health, 14*(1), 62. Advance online publication. DOI: 10.1186/s13031-020-00308-7 PMID: 32884581

Beukelman, D., & Mirenda, P. (2013). *Augmentative & alternative communication - supporting children & adults with complex communication needs.* Baltimore, Maryland, Ed. Paul H Brookes.

Bharathi, G., Venugopal, A., & Vellingiri, B. (2019). Music therapy as a therapeutic tool in improving the social skills of autistic children. *The Egyptian Journal of Neurology, Psychiatry and Neurosurgery, 55*(44), 1–6. DOI: 10.1186/s41983-019-0091-x

Bianquin, N., Sacchi, F., & Besio, S. (2022). Enhancing communication and participation using AAC technologies for children with motor impairments: A systematic review. *Educational Sciences and Society, 13*(1), 49–71.

Bilgin, H. (2023). Mental Health. *Mental Health (Detroit, Mich.)*, •••, 199–211. DOI: 10.69860/nobel.9786053359135.11

Bishop, D. V., Snowling, M. J., Thompson, P. A., & Greenhalgh, T.CATALISE consortium. (2016). CATALISE: A Multinational and Multidisciplinary Delphi Consensus Study. Identifying Language Impairments in Children. *PLoS One, 11*(7), e0158753. DOI: 10.1371/journal.pone.0158753 PMID: 27392128

Bishop, D., Snow, P., Thompson, P., & Greenhalgh, T. (2017). Phasc 2 of catalise: A multinational and multidisciplinary delphi consensus study of problems with language development- terminology. *Journal of Child Psychology and Psychiatry, and Allied Disciplines, 58*(10), 1068–1080. DOI: 10.1111/jcpp.12721 PMID: 28369935

Bitta, M. A., Kariuki, S. M., Gona, J., Abubakar, A., Newton, C. R., & Alcock, K. (2019). Priority mental, neurological and substance use disorders in rural Kenya: Traditional health practitioners' and primary health care workers' perspectives. *PLoS One*, *14*(7), e0220034. DOI: 10.1371/journal.pone.0220034 PMID: 31335915

Black, L. I., Vahratian, A. M., & Hoffman, H. J. (2015). Communication Disorders and Use of Intervention Services Among Children Aged 3-17 Years: United States, 2012. *NCHS Data Brief*, *205*, 1–8. PMID: 26079397

Blackstone, S. (2015). Issues and challenges in advancing effective patient-provider communication. In Blackstone, S., Beukelman, D., & Yorkston, K. (Eds.), *Patient-Provider Communication - Roles for Speech-Language Pathologists and Other Health Care Professionals* (pp. 9–35). Plural Publishing.

Blackstone, S. W. (2018). What does the patient want? *ASHA Leader*, *21*(3), 38–44. https://leader.pubs.asha.org/doi/10.1044/leader.FTR1.21032016.38. DOI: 10.1044/leader.FTR1.21032016.38

Blackstone, S. W., & Pressman, H. (2016). Patient communication in health care settings: New opportunities for augmentative and alternative communication. *Augmentative and Alternative Communication*, *32*(1), 69–79. DOI: 10.3109/07434618.2015.1125947 PMID: 26694249

Blackstone, S., Ruschke, K., Wilson-Stronks, A., & Lee, C. (2011). Converging communication vulnerabilities in health care: An emerging role for speech-language pathologists and audiologists. *Perspectives on Communication Disorders and Sciences in Culturally and Linguistically Diverse*, *18*(1), 3–11. DOI: 10.1044/cds18.1.3

Blakey, E., & Aveyard, H. (2017). Student nurses' competence in sexual health care: A literature review. *Journal of Clinical Nursing*, *26*(23-24), 3906–3916. DOI: 10.1111/jocn.13810 PMID: 28328169

Blanchfield, J. (2005). Good manufacturing practice (GMP) in the food. Institute of Food Science & Technology. In Elsevier eBooks (pp. 324–347). DOI: 10.1533/9781845690533.3.324

Bochane, M., Reijneveld, S., Krijnen, W., Schans, C., & Luinge, M. (2020). Identifying milestones in language development for young children ages 1 to 6 years. *Academic Pediatrics*, *20*(3), 421–429. DOI: 10.1016/j.acap.2019.07.003 PMID: 31306799

Boissonnault, J., Kuhn, A., Meeker, M., Strong, S., & Stephenson, R. G. (2020). An international survey of women's and pelvic health physical therapy organizational practice. *Journal of Women's Health Physical Therapy*, *44*(4), 160–175. DOI: 10.1097/JWH.0000000000000174

Bø, K., Berghmans, B., Mørkved, S., & Van Kampen, M. (Eds.). (2023). *Evidence-Based Physical Therapy for the Pelvic Floor - Bridging Science and Clinical Practice* (3rd ed.). Elsevier.

Bø, K., & Hilde, G. (2013). Does it work in the long term? — A systematic review on pelvic floor muscle training for female stress urinary incontinence. *Neurourology and Urodynamics*, *32*(3), 215–223. DOI: 10.1002/nau.22292 PMID: 22847318

Bolina, A. F., Rpdrigues, R. A. P., Tavares, D. M., & Haas, V.J. (2021). Índices de vulnerabilidade social e programático para idosos que vivem no domicilio. Enfermería Global. Nº 65 Enero 2022 P153.

Bond, C., Symes, W., Hebron, J., Humphrey, N., Morewood, G., & Woods, K. (2016). Educational interventions for children with ASD: A systematic literature review 2008-2013. [PDF]

Booker, S., & Herr, K. (2015). The state-of-"cultural validity" of self-report pain assessment tools in diverse older adults: Table 1. *Pain Medicine*, *16*(2), 232–239. DOI: 10.1111/pme.12496 PMID: 25219949

Booker, S., & Herr, K. (2016). Assessment and measurement of pain in adults in later life. *Clinics in Geriatric Medicine*, *32*(4), 677–692. DOI: 10.1016/j.cger.2016.06.012 PMID: 27741963

Booker, S., Herr, K., & Horgas, A. (2021). A paradigm shift for movement-based pain assessment in older adults: Practice, policy and regulatory drivers. *Pain Management Nursing*, *22*(1), 21–27. DOI: 10.1016/j.pmn.2020.08.003 PMID: 32948452

Borgi, M., Loliva, D., Cerino, S., Chiarotti, F., Venerosi, A., Bramini, M., Nonnis, E., Marcelli, M., Vinti, C., De Santis, C., Bisacco, F., Fagerlie, M., Frascarelli, M., & Cirulli, F. (2015). Effectiveness of a standardized equine-assisted therapy program for children with autism spectrum disorder. *Journal of Autism and Developmental Disorders*, *46*(1), 1–9. DOI: 10.1007/s10803-015-2530-6 PMID: 26210515

Borovsky, A., Thal, D., & Leonard, L. B. (2021). Moving towards accurate and early prediction of language delay with network science and machine learning approaches. *Scientific Reports*, *11*(1), 8136. DOI: 10.1038/s41598-021-85982-0 PMID: 33854086

Boso, M., Emanuele, E., Minazzi, V., Abbamonte, M., & Politi, P. (2007). Effect of long-term interactive music therapy on behavior profile and musical skills in young adults with severe autism. *Journal of Alternative and Complementary Medicine (New York, N.Y.)*, *13*(7), 709–712. DOI: 10.1089/acm.2006.6334 PMID: 17931062

Boston University Medical Group, Office of Equity, Vitality, and Inclusion, and BUMC Faculty Development and Diversity. *Inclusive language practices*. (2022). Accessed November 20, 2024. https://www.bumc.bu.edu/bumg/files/2021/10/Inclusive-Language-Practices_101821.pdf

Botting, N., & Spicer-Cain, H. (2023). The importance and challenges of improving early identification of language abilities: A commentary on Gasparini et al. (2023). *Journal of Child Psychology and Psychiatry, and Allied Disciplines*, *64*(8), 1253–1255. DOI: 10.1111/jcpp.13810 PMID: 37185876

Bowen, E., Nayfe, R., Milburn, N., Mayo, H., Reid, M., Fraenkel, L., Weiner, D., Halm, E. A., & Makris, U. (2019). Do decision aids benefit patients with chronic musculoskeletal pain? a systematic review. *Pain Medicine*, *21*(5), 951–969. DOI: 10.1093/pm/pnz280 PMID: 31880805

Bradshaw, J., Steiner, A. M., Gengoux, G., & Koegel, L. K. (2015). Feasibility and Effectiveness of Very Early Intervention for Infants At-Risk for Autism Spectrum Disorder: A Systematic Review. *Journal of Autism and Developmental Disorders*, *45*(3), 778–794. DOI: 10.1007/s10803-014-2235-2 PMID: 25218848

Brant, J. (2018). Assessment and management of cancer pain in older adults: Strategies for success. *Asia-Pacific Journal of Oncology Nursing*, *5*(3), 248–253. DOI: 10.4103/apjon.apjon_11_18 PMID: 29963586

Braun, V., & Clarke, V. (2006). Using thematic analysis in psychology. *Qualitative Research in Psychology*, *3*(2), 77–101. DOI: 10.1191/1478088706qp063oa

Brelsford, V., Meints, K., Gee, N., & Pfeffer, K. (2017). Animal-assisted interventions in the classroom—A systematic review. *International Journal of Environmental Research and Public Health*, *14*(7), 669. DOI: 10.3390/ijerph14070669 PMID: 28640200

Bronzwaer, S., Kass, G., Robinson, T., Tarazona, J., Verhagen, H., Verloo, D., Vrbos, D., & Hugas, M. (2019). Food Safety Regulatory Research Needs 2030. *EFSA Journal*, *17*(7). Advance online publication. DOI: 10.2903/j.efsa.2019.e170622 PMID: 32626400

Brosseau, L., Taki, J., Desjardins, B., Thevenot, O., Fransen, M., Wells, G., Imoto, A. M., Toupin-April, K., Westby, M., Gallardo, I. C. Á., Gifford, W., Laferrière, L., Rahman, P., Loew, L., Angelis, G. D., Cavallo, S., Shallwani, S. M., Aburub, A., Bennell, K. L., & McLean, L. (2017). The Ottawa panel clinical practice guidelines for the management of knee osteoarthritis. part one: Introduction, and mind-body exercise programs. *Clinical Rehabilitation*, *31*(5), 582–595. DOI: 10.1177/0269215517691083 PMID: 28183188

Brown, W. J., Hayman, M., Haakstad, L. A., Lamerton, T., Mena, G. P., Green, A., Keating, S. E., Gomes, G. A. O., Coombes, J. S., & Mielke, G. I. (2022). Australian guidelines for physical activity in pregnancy and postpartum. *Journal of Science and Medicine in Sport*, *25*(6), 511–519. DOI: 10.1016/j.jsams.2022.03.008 PMID: 35418334

Bruce, J., Mazuquin, B., Canaway, A., Hossain, A., Williamson, E., Mistry, P., Lall, R., Petrou, S., Lamb, S. E., Rees, S., Padfield, E., Vidya, R., & Thompson, A. M. (2021). Exercise versus usual care after non-reconstructive breast cancer surgery (UK PROSPER): Multicentre randomised controlled trial and economic evaluation. *BMJ (Clinical Research Ed.)*, *375*, e066542. DOI: 10.1136/bmj-2021-066542 PMID: 34759002

Bruce, J., Mazuquin, B., Mistry, P., Rees, S., Canaway, A., Hossain, A., Williamson, E., Padfield, E. J., Lall, R., Richmond, H., Chowdhury, L., Lait, C., Petrou, S., Booth, K., Lamb, S. E., Vidya, R., & Thompson, A. M. (2022). Exercise to prevent shoulder problems after breast cancer surgery: The PROSPER RCT. *Health Technology Assessment*, *26*(15), 1–124. DOI: 10.3310/JKNZ2003 PMID: 35220995

Bruckenthal, P., Marino, M., & Snelling, L. (2016). Complementary and integrative therapies for persistent pain management in older adults: A review. *Journal of Gerontological Nursing*, *42*(12), 40–48. DOI: 10.3928/00989134-20161110-08 PMID: 27898135

Bruehl, S., & Chung, O. Y. (2004). Interactions between the cardiovascular and pain regulatory systems: An updated review of mechanisms and possible alterations in chronic pain. *Neuroscience and Biobehavioral Reviews*, *28*(4), 395–414. DOI: 10.1016/j.neubiorev.2004.06.004 PMID: 15341037

Brumberg, J. S., Pitt, K. M., & Burnison, J. D. (2021). Emerging trends in augmentative and alternative communication access methods. *Current Physical Medicine and Rehabilitation Reports*, *9*(1), 8–17. DOI: 10.1007/s40141-021-00281-w

Buck, C., Keweloh, C., Bouras, A., & Simões, E. (2021). Efficacy of short message service text messaging interventions for postoperative pain management: Systematic review. *JMIR mHealth and uHealth*, *9*(6), e20199. DOI: 10.2196/20199 PMID: 34132646

Bulanda, M., Leśniak, M., Szałkowska, J., Madej, W., Wojtyna, A., Czarnobilska, M., Bulanda, D., & Czarnobilska, E. (2018). Component-resolved diagnosis (CRD) of food anaphylaxis. PubMed, 58(2), 89–102. DOI: 10.24425/fmc.2018.124661

Burke, J. P., & Tsiouris, J. A. (2022). Communication supports in emergency healthcare settings: A review of tools and applications. *Journal of Communication in Healthcare, 15*(3), 223–232. DOI: 10.1080/17538068.2022.2023991

Burton, A., & Shaw, R. (2015). Pain management programmes for non-English-speaking black and minority ethnic groups with long-term or chronic pain. *Musculoskeletal Care, 13*(4), 187–203. DOI: 10.1002/msc.1099 PMID: 25784618

Burton, E., Farrier, K., Galvin, R., Johnson, S., Horgan, F., Warters, A., & Hill, K. (2019). <p>physical activity programs for older people in the community receiving home care services: Systematic review and meta-analysis</p>. *Clinical Interventions in Aging, 14*, 1045–1064. DOI: 10.2147/CIA.S205019 PMID: 31239654

Cable, Amory & Domsch, Celeste. (2011). Systematic review of the literature on the treatment of children with late language emergence. *International journal of language & communication disorders / Royal College of Speech & Language Therapists*. 46. 138-54. DOI: 10.3109/13682822.2010.487883

Cadime, I., Silva, C., Ribeiro, I., & Viana, F. (2018). Early lexical development: Do day care attendance and maternal education matter? *First Language, 38*(5), 503–519. Advance online publication. DOI: 10.1177/0142723718778916

Campbell, A., Godfryd, A., Buys, D., & Locher, J. (2015). Does participation in home-delivered meals programs improve outcomes for older adults? results of a systematic review. *Journal of Nutrition in Gerontology and Geriatrics, 34*(2), 124–167. DOI: 10.1080/21551197.2015.1038463 PMID: 26106985

Canadian Task Force on Preventive Health Care. (2016). Recommendations on screening for developmental dela. *Canadian Medical Association Journal, 188*(8), 579–587. https://www.cmaj.ca/content/188/8/579.full.pdf. DOI: 10.1503/cmaj.151437 PMID: 27026672

Cano-López, I., Aliño, M., Duque, A., Martínez, P., & Meléndez, J. C. (2021). Educational level as a protective factor against the influence of depressive symptoms on cognition in older adults: Implications for functional independence during a 10-year follow-up. *International Psychogeriatrics, 33*(8), 813–825. DOI: 10.1017/S1041610221000272 PMID: 33762060

Canonica, G. W., Bachert, C., Hellings, P., Ryan, D., Valovirta, E., Wickman, M., De Beaumont, O., & Bousquet, J. (2015). Allergen Immunotherapy (AIT): a prototype of Precision Medicine. the œWorld Allergy Organization Journal, 8, 31. DOI: 10.1186/s40413-015-0079-7

Cao, S., Fisher, D., Yu, T., & Dong, H. (2019). The link between chronic pain and Alzheimer's disease. *Journal of Neuroinflammation, 16*(1), 204. Advance online publication. DOI: 10.1186/s12974-019-1608-z PMID: 31694670

Capel-Alcaraz, A. M., García-López, H., Castro-Sánchez, A. M., Fernández-Sánchez, M., & Lara-Palomo, I. C. (2023). The Efficacy of Strength Exercises for Reducing the Symptoms of Menopause: A Systematic Review. *Journal of Clinical Medicine, 12*(2), 548. DOI: 10.3390/jcm12020548 PMID: 36675477

Cardoso, A., Lima, C., & Ferreira, C. (2018). Prevalence of urinary incontinence in high-impact sports athletes and their association with knowledge, attitude and practice about this dysfunction. *European Journal of Sport Science, 18*(10), 1405–1412. DOI: 10.1080/17461391.2018.1496146 PMID: 30025510

Cardozo-Stolberg, S., Szydziak, E., Angus, L., Blake, R., Marsden, D., Venkatesh, S., & Mon, N. (2023). Geospatial mapping to target injury prevention for older adult ground-level falls: A feasibility study. *Journal of Trauma Nursing, 30*(6), 340–345. DOI: 10.1097/JTN.0000000000000753 PMID: 37937875

Carley, J., Karp, J., Gentili, A., Marcum, Z., Reid, M., Rodríguez, E., Rossi, M. I., Shega, J., Thielke, S., & Weiner, D. (2015). Deconstructing chronic low back pain in the older adult: step by step evidence and expert-based recommendations for evaluation and treatment: part iv: depression. *Pain Medicine, 16*(11), 2098–2108. DOI: 10.1111/pme.12935 PMID: 26539754

Carniel, C., Furtado, M., Vicente, J., Abreu, R., Tarozzo, R., Cardia, S., Massei, M. C. I., & Cerveira, R. (2017). Influência de fatores de risco sobre o desenvolvimento da linguagem e contribuições da estimulação precoce: Revisão integrativa da literatura. *Revista CEFAC, 19*(1), 109–118. DOI: 10.1590/1982-0216201719115616

Carragher, J., & Gormley, K. (2016). Leadership and emotional intelligence in nursing and midwifery education and practice: A discussion paper. *Journal of Advanced Nursing, 73*(1), 85–96. DOI: 10.1111/jan.13141 PMID: 27607451

Carvalho, J. L. D. S., & Nóbrega, M. D. P. S. (2017). Complementary therapies as resources for mental health in Primary Health Care. *Revista Gaúcha de Enfermagem, 38*(4), e2017–e2014. DOI: 10.1590/1983-1447.2017.04.2017-2014 PMID: 29791533

Carvalho, L., Almeida, I. Ch., Felgueiras, I., Leitão, S., Boavida, J., Santos, P. C., Serrano, A., Brito, A. T., Lança, C., Pimentel, J. S., Pinto, A. I., Grande, C., Brandão, T., & Franco, V. (2016). *Práticas recomendadas em intervenção precoce na infância: Um guia para profissionais.* Associação Nacional de Intervenção Precoce.

Casagrande, A., Fabris, F., & Girometti, R. (2020). Beyond kappa: An informational index for diagnostic agreement in dichotomous and multivalue ordered-categorical ratings. *Medical & Biological Engineering & Computing*, *58*(12), 3089–3099. DOI: 10.1007/s11517-020-02261-2 PMID: 33145661

CDC. (2014, March 28). - Developmental Disabilities Monitoring Network Surveillance Year 2010 Principal Investigators; Centers for Disease Control and Prevention (CDC). Prevalence of autism spectrum disorder among children aged 8 years - autism and developmental disabilities monitoring network, 11 sites, United States, 2010. *MMWR. Surveillance Summaries*, *63*(2), 1–21.

Çelik, A. S., & Apay, S. E. (2021). Effect of progressive relaxation exercises on primary dysmenorrhea in Turkish students: A randomized prospective controlled trial. *Complementary Therapies in Clinical Practice*, *42*, 101280. DOI: 10.1016/j.ctcp.2020.101280 PMID: 33310052

Centers for Disease Control and Prevention. (2020). National diabetes statistics report, 2020. Atlanta, GA: Centers for Disease Control and Prevention, US Department of Health and Human Services, https://www.cdc.gov/diabetes/pdfs/data/statistics/national-diabetes-statisticsreport.pdf

Centers for Disease Control and Prevention. *Health equity guiding principles for inclusive communication*. 2024. Accessed November 20, 2024. https://www.cdc.gov/healthcommunication/Health_Equity.html

Chang, Y. K., Erickson, K. I., Aghjayan, S. L., Chen, F. T., & Lin, S. (2022). The multi-domain exercise intervention for memory and brain function in late middle-aged and older adults at risk for Alzheimer's disease: A protocol for Western-Eastern Brain Fitness Integration Training trial. *Frontiers in Aging Neuroscience*, *14*, 929789. DOI: 10.3389/fnagi.2022.929789 PMID: 36062144

Chapuy, C. I., Annino, D. J., Tishler, R. B., Haddad, R. I., Snavely, A., & Goguen, L. A. (2013). Success of endoscopic pharyngoesophageal dilation after head and neck cancer treatment. *The Laryngoscope*, *123*(12), 3066–3073. DOI: 10.1002/lary.24268 PMID: 23775806

Charry-Sánchez, J. D., Pradilla, I., & Talero-Gutiérrez, C. (2018). Animal-assisted therapy in adults: A systematic review. *Complementary Therapies in Clinical Practice*, *32*, 169–180. DOI: 10.1016/j.ctcp.2018.06.011 PMID: 30057046

Chary, S. (2021). What do we need to consider for pain management?.. https://doi.org/DOI: 10.5772/intechopen.93640

Chatchumni, M., Eriksson, H., & Mazaheri, M. (2020). A scoping review of pain management education programs (PMEPS): Do they prepare nurses to deal with patients' postoperative pain? *Pain Research & Management, 2020*, 1–7. DOI: 10.1155/2020/4062493 PMID: 33123303

Checklin, M., Bain, J., Bath, L., & Lethbridge, K. (2020). Patients' Perspectives on What Makes a Better Care Experience While Undergoing Treatment for Oropharyngeal Dysphagia Secondary to Head and Neck Cancer. *Dysphagia, 35*(4), 702–716. DOI: 10.1007/s00455-019-10077-y PMID: 31748827

Chen, S. (2022). Analysis of cashew allergen in shared use of frying oil - ProQuest. https://search.proquest.com/openview/85432dc2a9662b6918c29e0100260054/1?pq-origsite=gscholar&cbl=18750&diss=y&casa_token=afrAn0hF1jAAAAAA:U1W_MiiuNMSyjhteUszXyVkxs71MIm4kQUTGzohFn9bbSv5zTbgyobdHINuFuDg6xB0j33mBalk

Chen, A. Y., Frankowski, R., Bishop-Leone, J., Hebert, T., Leyk, S., Lewin, J., & Goepfert, H. (2001). The development and validation of a dysphagia-specific quality-of-life questionnaire for patients with head and neck cancer: The M. D. Anderson dysphagia inventory. *Archives of Otolaryngology—Head & Neck Surgery, 127*(7), 870–876. PMID: 11448365

Chen, J., Lin, Y., Yan, J., Wu, Y., & Hu, R. (2018). The effects of spiritual care on quality of life and spiritual well-being among patients with terminal illness: A systematic review. *Palliative Medicine, 32*(7), 1167–1179. DOI: 10.1177/0269216318772267 PMID: 29708010

Chen, L., & Michalsen, A. (2017). Management of chronic pain using complementary and integrative medicine. *BMJ (Clinical Research Ed.), j1284*, j1284. DOI: 10.1136/bmj.j1284 PMID: 28438745

Chester, P., Ehrlich, C., Warburton, L., Baker, D., Kendall, E., & Crompton, D. (2016). what is the work of recovery oriented practice? a systematic literature review. *International Journal of Mental Health Nursing, 25*(4), 270–285. DOI: 10.1111/inm.12241 PMID: 27381002

Chia, C., Mantoo, S., & Tan, K. (2016). 'start to finish trans-institutional transdisciplinary care': A novel approach improves colorectal surgical results in frail elderly patients. *Colorectal Disease, 18*(1). Advance online publication. DOI: 10.1111/codi.13166 PMID: 26500155

Chilosi, A. M., Brovedani, P., Cipriani, P., & Casalini, C. (2023). Sex differences in early language delay and in developmental language disorder. *Journal of Neuroscience Research, 101*(5), 654–667. DOI: 10.1002/jnr.24976 PMID: 34822733

Chiu, S. T., Lai, U. H., Huang, Y. C., Leong, C. P., & Chen, P. C. (2023). Effect of various photobiomodulation regimens on breast cancer-related lymphedema: A systematic review and meta-analysis. *Lasers in Medical Science, 39*(1), 11. DOI: 10.1007/s10103-023-03959-z PMID: 38129368

Choo, C., Chew, P., Tan, P., Choo, J., Choo, A., Ho, R., & Quah, T. (2019). Health-related quality of life in pediatric patients with leukemia in Singapore: A cross-sectional pilot study. *International Journal of Environmental Research and Public Health, 16*(12), 2069. DOI: 10.3390/ijerph16122069 PMID: 31212740

Choo, H. J., Hwang, S. K., & Hynes, C. K. (2020). Musculoskeletal issues and care for pregnant and postpartum women. *Current Physical Medicine and Rehabilitation Reports, 8*(4), 493–500. DOI: 10.1007/s40141-020-00286-0

Christopulos, T. T., & Redmond, S. M. (2023). Factors Impacting Implementation of Universal Screening of Developmental Language Disorder in Public Schools. *Language, Speech, and Hearing Services in Schools, 54*(4), 1080–1102. DOI: 10.1044/2023_LSHSS-22-00169 PMID: 37459613

Cirillo, A., Collins, J., Sawatzky, B., Hamdy, R., & Dahan-Oliel, N. (2019). Pain among children and adults living with arthrogryposis multiplex congenita: A scoping review. *American Journal of Medical Genetics. Part C, Seminars in Medical Genetics, 181*(3), 436–453. DOI: 10.1002/ajmg.c.31725 PMID: 31347265

Clark, S., Bock, S., Gaeta, T. J., Brenner, B. E., Cydulka, R. K., & Camargo, C. A. (2004). Multicenter study of emergency department visits for food allergies☆. ^the ‰Journal of Allergy and Clinical Immunology/Journal of Allergy and Clinical Immunology/ the œJournal of Allergy and Clinical Immunology, 113(2), 347–352. DOI: 10.1016/j.jaci.2003.10.053

Clegg, J., & Ginsborg, J. (Eds.). (2006). *Language and Social Disadvantage: Theory into Practice* (1st ed.). Wiley.

Cleofas, J. (2024). National resilience and mental well-being among Filipino emerging adults at risk for depression: the parallel mediating role of peace of mind and life satisfaction. https://doi.org/DOI: 10.21203/rs.3.rs-5450577/v1

Cocco, R. M., Weiss, R., & Pippi, L. G. A. (2024). Análise Multicritério e Geoprocessamento no Planejamento do Sistema de Espaços Livres Urbano. *Engenharia Urbana Em Debate, 4*(2), 58–68. DOI: 10.14244/engurbdebate.v4i2.116

Coelho, F. D., Carvalho, P. H. B., Paes, S. T., & Ferreira, M. E. C. (2023). Esthetic plastic surgery and (in) satisfaction index: A current view. *Revista Brasileira de Cirurgia Plástica, 32*(1), 135–140. DOI: 10.5935/2177-1235.2017RBCP0019

Collacchi, B., Pinchaud, N., Borgi, M., & Cirulli, F. (2023). Equine-Assisted Activities (EAAs) for Children with Autism Spectrum Disorder (ASD): Positive Effects Revealed Using an Ethological Approach. *Applied Sciences (Basel, Switzerland), 13*(13), 7417. DOI: 10.3390/app13137417

Collisson, B., Graham, S., Preston, J., Rose, M., McDonald, S., & Tough, S. (2016). Risk and protective factors for late talking: An epidemiologic investigation. *The Journal of Pediatrics, 172*, 168–174.e1. DOI: 10.1016/j.jpeds.2016.02.020 PMID: 26968834

Cologon, K., Wicks, L., & Salvador, A. (2017). Supporting caregivers in developing responsive communication partnerships with their children: Extending a caregiver-led interactive language program. *Child Language Teaching and Therapy, 33*(2), 157–169. DOI: 10.1177/0265659016650978

Constantine, G. D., Graham, S., Clerinx, C., Bernick, B. A., Krassan, M., Mirkin, S., & Currie, H. (2016). Behaviours and attitudes influencing treatment decisions for menopausal symptoms in five European countries. *Post Reproductive Health, 22*(3), 112–122. DOI: 10.1177/2053369116632439 PMID: 26895640

Constantinescu, G., Rieger, J., Winget, M., Paulsen, C., & Seikaly, H. (2017). Patient Perception of Speech Outcomes: The Relationship Between Clinical Measures and Self-Perception of Speech Function Following Surgical Treatment for Oral Cancer. *American Journal of Speech-Language Pathology, 26*(2), 241–247. DOI: 10.1044/2016_AJSLP-15-0170 PMID: 28359083

Conti-Ramsden, G., & Durkin, K. (2015). What factors influence language impairment considering resilience as well as risk. *Folia Phoniatrica et Logopaedica, 67*(6), 293–299. DOI: 10.1159/000444750 PMID: 27160319

Conti-Ramsden, G., Mok, P. L., Durkin, K., Pickles, A., Toseeb, U., & Botting, N. (2018). Do emotional difficulties and peer problems occur together from childhood to adolescence? The case of children with a history of developmental language disorder (DLD). *European Child & Adolescent Psychiatry, 28*(7), 993–1004. DOI: 10.1007/s00787-018-1261-6 PMID: 30519863

Corey, J. and McQueen, K. (2017). Pain relief in areas of deprivation and conflict.. https://doi.org/DOI: 10.1093/med/9780190217518.003.0028

Corso, M., DeSouza, A., Brunton, G., Yu, H., Cancelliere, C., Mior, S., Taylor-Vaisey, A., MacLeod-Beaver, K., & Côté, P. (2022). Integrating indigenous healing practices within collaborative care models in primary healthcare in Canada: A rapid scoping review. *BMJ Open, 12*(6), e059323. DOI: 10.1136/bmjopen-2021-059323 PMID: 35710234

Coufal, K. L., & Woods, J. J. (2018). Interprofessional collaborative practice in early intervention. *Pediatric Clinics of North America, 65*(1), 143–155. DOI: 10.1016/j.pcl.2017.08.027 PMID: 29173715

Council on Children With Disabilities, Section on Developmental Behavioral Pediatrics, Bright Futures Steering Committee, Medical Home Initiatives for Children With Special Needs Project Advisory Committee. (2006). Identifying Infants and Young Children With Developmental Disorders in the Medical Home: An Algorithm for Developmental Surveillance and Screening. *Pediatrics, 118*(1), 405–420. DOI: 10.1542/peds.2006-1231 PMID: 16818591

Cowley, S. A., Tzouvara, V., & Horta Reis da Silva, T. (2023). Public Health: healthy ageing and well-being. In *Redfern's Nursing Older People*. Fifth edition. Editors: Ross, Harris, Fitzpatrick and Abley. Elsevier.

Crary, M. A., Mann, G. D., & Groher, M. E. (2005). Initial psychometric assessment of a functional oral intake scale for dysphagia in stroke patients. *Archives of Physical Medicine and Rehabilitation, 86*(8), 1516–1520. DOI: 10.1016/j.apmr.2004.11.049 PMID: 16084801

Cravello, L., Santo, S., Varrassi, G., Benincasa, D., Marchettini, P., Tommaso, M., & Caltagirone, C. (2019). Chronic pain in the elderly with cognitive decline: A narrative review. *Pain and Therapy, 8*(1), 53–65. DOI: 10.1007/s40122-019-0111-7 PMID: 30666612

Crawford, M. F. (2013). *Individuals with disabilities education improvement act of 2004 noncompliance determination complaints in commonwealth states* [Doctoral thesis Capella University. https://www.proquest.com/docview/1348696289

Crawford, C., Boller, J., Jadalla, A., & Cuenca, E. (2016). An integrative review of pain resource nurse programs. *Critical Care Nursing Quarterly, 39*(1), 64–82. DOI: 10.1097/CNQ.0000000000000101 PMID: 26633161

Creswell, J. W., & Poth, C. N. (2018). *Qualitative inquiry and research design: Choosing among five approaches* (4th ed.). SAGE Publications.

Critchley, C. J. C. (2022). Physical Therapy Is an Important Component of Postpartum Care in the Fourth Trimester. *Physical Therapy, 102*(5), pzac021. Advance online publication. DOI: 10.1093/ptj/pzac021 PMID: 35225339

Cronin, P., & Goodall, S. (2021). Measuring the impact of genetic and environmental risk and protective factors on speech, language, and communication development-evidence from australia. *International Journal of Environmental Research and Public Health, 18*(8), 4112. DOI: 10.3390/ijerph18084112 PMID: 33924666

Crosby, E., & Husk, K. (2021). Defecatory Dysfunction. *Obstetrics and Gynecology Clinics of North America*, *48*(3), 653–663. DOI: 10.1016/j.ogc.2021.05.016 PMID: 34416943

Cui, M., Ni, Q., & Wang, Q. (2023). Review of intervention methods for language and communication disorders in children with autism spectrum disorders. *PeerJ*, *11*, e15735. DOI: 10.7717/peerj.15735 PMID: 37576502

Cui, R., Liu, H., Li, M., Wang, J., Wang, L., & Han, L. (2023). Effects of "Taking the Waist as the Axis" Therapy on trunk postural control disorder after stroke: A randomized controlled trial. *Frontiers in Aging Neuroscience*, *15*, 1040277. DOI: 10.3389/fnagi.2023.1040277 PMID: 36819714

Cunha, F. P., Manso, M. C., & Ohnuma Júnior, A. A. (2024). Analysis of The Occurrence of Extreme Events in The City of Rio de Janeiro/RJ. *Revista de Gestão Social e Ambiental*, *18*(4), e04730. DOI: 10.24857/rgsa.v18n4-066

D'Cruz, K., Meikle, L., White, M., Herrmann, A., McCallum, C., & Romero, L. (2020). Tailoring education of adults with cognitive impairment in the inpatient hospital setting: A scoping review. *Australian Occupational Therapy Journal*, *68*(1), 90–102. DOI: 10.1111/1440-1630.12698 PMID: 33029784

Da Roza, T., Brandão, S., Mascarenhas, T., Jorge, R. N., & Duarte, J. A. (2015). Volume of training and the ranking level are associated with the leakage of urine in young female trampolinists. *Clinical Journal of Sport Medicine*, *25*(3), 270–275. DOI: 10.1097/JSM.0000000000000129 PMID: 25010151

Da Roza, T., de Araujo, M., Viana, R., Viana, S., Jorge, R., Bø, K., & Mascarenhas, T. (2012). Pelvic floor muscle training to improve urinary incontinence in young, nulliparous sport students: A pilot study. *International Urogynecology Journal*, *23*(8), 1069–1073. DOI: 10.1007/s00192-012-1759-2 PMID: 22552685

Da Silva, A., & De Moraes Lopes, M. (2024). Treinamento dos músculos do assoalho pélvico associado ao uso do pessário no tratamento do prolapso de órgãos pélvicos: Protocolo de revisão de escopo. *Research. Social Development*, *13*(5), e2813545704–e2813545704.

Da Silva, N. C. S., & Livramento, R. A. (2023). Intervenção Da Fisioterapia Pélvica No Tratamento Do Prolapso Genital: Revisão Integrativa. *Brazilian Journal of Implantology and Health Sciences*, *5*(5), 3402–3414. DOI: 10.36557/2674-8169.2023v5n5p3402-3414 da Silva, T. H. R. (2022). Emotional awareness and emotional intelligence. *British Journal of Community Nursing, 27*(12), 573–574. DOI: 10.12968/bjcn.2022.27.12.573 PMID: 36519463

Dahlke, S., & Hunter, K. (2021). Harnessing nursing to diminish ageism. *International Journal of Older People Nursing, 17*(2), e12417. Advance online publication. DOI: 10.1111/opn.12417 PMID: 34420260

Dallinger, V., Krishnamoorthy, G., Burton, L., Plessis, C., Pillai-Sasidharan, A., & Ayres, A. (2022). Internet-based interventions to support recovery in youth: A systematic review. *Digital Health, 8*, 205520762211290. DOI: 10.1177/20552076221129094 PMID: 36211796

Daniele, T. M., Bruin, V. M., Oliveira, D. S., Pompeu, C. M., & Forti, A. C. (2013). Associations among physical activity, comorbidities, depressive symptoms and health-related quality of life in type 2 diabetes. *Arquivos Brasileiros de Endocrinologia & Metabologia, 57*(1), 44–50. DOI: 10.1590/S0004-27302013000100006 PMID: 23440098

Das, G., & Priya, D. (2017). Family history and its influence on infants' language development. *Universal Journal of Psychology, 5*(1), 8–16. DOI: 10.13189/ujp.2017.050102

Davidoff, B. E. (2017). AAC with energy-earlier. *ASHA Leader, 22*(1), 48–53. DOI: 10.1044/leader.FTR2.22012017.48

Davies, K. E., Marshall, J., Brown, L. J. E., & Goldbart, J. (2017). Co-working: Parents' conception of roles in supporting their children's speech and language development. *Child Language Teaching and Therapy, 33*(2), 171–185. DOI: 10.1177/0265659016671169

Dawson, G. (2016). Why It's Important to Continue Universal Autism Screening While Research Fully Examines Its Impact. *JAMA Pediatrics, 170*(6), 527–528. DOI: 10.1001/jamapediatrics.2016.0163 PMID: 26882277

De Baets, L., Vets, N., Emmerzaal, J., Devoogdt, N., & De Groef, A. (2022). Altered upper limb motor behavior in breast cancer survivors and its relation to pain: A narrative review. *The Anatomical Record, 307*(2), 298–308. DOI: 10.1002/ar.25120 PMID: 36398938

De Blok, B. M. J., Vlieg-Boerstra, B. J., Elberink, J. N. G. O., & Duiverman, E. J. (2007). A framework for measuring the social impact of food allergy across Europe: A EuroPrevall state of the art paper. *Allergy, 62*(7), 733–737. DOI: 10.1111/j.1398-9995.2006.01303.x PMID: 17484733

De Groef, A., Van Kampen, M., Dieltjens, E., Christiaens, M. R., Neven, P., Geraerts, I., & Devoogdt, N. (2015). Effectiveness of postoperative physical therapy for upper-limb impairments after breast cancer treatment: A systematic review. *Archives of Physical Medicine and Rehabilitation*, *96*(6), 1140–1153. DOI: 10.1016/j.apmr.2015.01.006 PMID: 25595999

de Koning, H. J., de Ridder-Sluiter, J. G., van Agt, H. M., Reep-van den Bergh, C. M., van der Stege, H. A., Korfage, I. J., Polder, J. J., & van der Maas, P. J. (2004). A cluster-randomised trial of screening for language disorders in toddlers. *Journal of Medical Screening*, *11*(3), 109–116. DOI: 10.1258/0969141041732229 PMID: 15333268

de Oliveira Faria, S., Hurwitz, G., Kim, J., Liberty, J., Orchard, K., Liu, G., Barbera, L., & Howell, D. (2021). Identifying Patient-Reported Outcome Measures (PROMs) for Routine Surveillance of Physical and Emotional Symptoms in Head and Neck Cancer Populations: A Systematic Review. *Journal of Clinical Medicine*, *10*(18), 4162. Advance online publication. DOI: 10.3390/jcm10184162 PMID: 34575271

De Santiago Herrero, F., García-Mateos, D., Arconada Díez, I., Torres Delgado, C., & Trigo Bensusan, A. (2017). Significance of oral language delays and writing for early detection of developmental disorders. *European Psychiatry : the Journal of the Association of European Psychiatrists*, *41*(S1), S435–S435. DOI: 10.1016/j.eurpsy.2017.01.426

de Sousa, K. A., Cardoso, L. B., Pirola, F. M., Auad, L. G., & de Oliveira, A. S. (2020). Effect of manual therapies on cardiac autonomic control: a systematic review. *Manual Therapy, Posturology & Rehabilitation Journal*, 1-12. https://doi.org/DOI: 10.17784/mtprehabjournal.2021.19.804

De, A., Rajagopalan, M., Godse, K., Shankar, D. K., Zawar, V., Sharma, N., Mukherjee, S., Sarda, A., & Dhar, S. (2019). Guidelines on management of atopic dermatitis in India: An evidence-based review and an expert consensus. Indian Journal of Dermatology. *Indian Journal of Dermatology*, *64*(3), 166. DOI: 10.4103/ijd.IJD_683_18 PMID: 31148854

DeFilippis, M. (2018). The Use of Complementary Alternative Medicine in Children and Adolescents with Autism Spectrum Disorder. *Psychopharmacology Bulletin*, *48*(1), 40–63. PMID: 29382959

Deflorin, C., Hohenauer, E., Stoop, R., Van Daele, U., Clijsen, R., & Taeymans, J. (2020). Physical management of scar tissue: A systematic review and meta-analysis. *Journal of Alternative and Complementary Medicine (New York, N.Y.)*, *26*(10), 854–865. DOI: 10.1089/acm.2020.0109 PMID: 32589450

Delancey, J., Kane Low, L., Miller, J., Patel, D., & Tumbarello, J. (2008). Graphic integration of causal factors of pelvic floor disorders: An integrated life span model. *American Journal of Obstetrics and Gynecology*, *199*(6), 610.e1–610.e5. DOI: 10.1016/j.ajog.2008.04.001 PMID: 18533115

Delgado, C. E. F., Vagi, S. J., & Scott, K. G. (2005). Early Risk Factors for Speech and Language Impairments. *Exceptionality*, *13*(3), 173–191. DOI: 10.1207/s15327035ex1303_3

Dermody, G., Whitehead, L., Wilson, G., & Glass, C. (2020). The role of virtual reality in improving health outcomes for community-dwelling older adults: Systematic review. *Journal of Medical Internet Research*, *22*(6), e17331. DOI: 10.2196/17331 PMID: 32478662

Devan, H., Farmery, D., Peebles, L., & Grainger, R. (2019). Evaluation of self-management support functions in apps for people with persistent pain: Systematic review. *JMIR mHealth and uHealth*, *7*(2), e13080. DOI: 10.2196/13080 PMID: 30747715

Devi, M., Manokaran, D., Sehgal, R. K., Shariff, S. A., & Vettriselvan, R. (2025). Precision Medicine, Personalized Treatment, and Network-Driven Innovations: Transforming Healthcare With AI. In Kanthavel, R., & Dhaya, R. (Eds.), *AI for Large Scale Communication Networks* (pp. 303–322). IGI Global Scientific Publishing., DOI: 10.4018/979-8-3693-6552-6.ch014

DeVito, R. G., Craft, L., Campbell, C. A., & Stranix, J. T. (2023). Optimizing perioperative outcomes in autologous breast reconstruction. *Gland Surgery*, *12*(4), 508–515. DOI: 10.21037/gs-22-608 PMID: 37200925

Devoogdt, N., & De Groef, A. (2024). Physiotherapy management of breast cancer treatment-related sequelae. *Journal of Physiotherapy*, *70*(2), 90–105. DOI: 10.1016/j.jphys.2024.02.020 PMID: 38519340

Dias, D. C., Rondon-Melo, S., & Molini-Avejonas, D. R. (2020). Sensitivity and specificity of a low-cost screening protocol for identifying children at risk for language disorders. *Clinics (São Paulo)*, *75*, e1426. DOI: 10.6061/clinics/2020/e1426 PMID: 32294668

Digalwar, A. K., & Sangwan, K. S. (2007). Development And Validation of Performance Measures for World Class Manufacturing Practices in India. *Journal of Advanced Manufacturing Systems*, *06*(01), 21–38. DOI: 10.1142/S0219686707000887

Dillane, I., & Doody, O. (2019). Nursing people with intellectual disability and dementia experiencing pain: An integrative review. *Journal of Clinical Nursing*, *28*(13-14), 2472–2485. DOI: 10.1111/jocn.14834 PMID: 30786087

Dipietro, L., Evenson, K. R., Bloodgood, B., Sprow, K., Troiano, R. P., Piercy, K. L., Vaux-Bjerke, A., & Powell, K. E. (2019). Benefits of Physical Activity during Pregnancy and Postpartum: An Umbrella Review. *Medicine and Science in Sports and Exercise*, *51*(6), 1292–1302. DOI: 10.1249/MSS.0000000000001941 PMID: 31095086

DiSipio, T., Rye, S., Newman, B., & Hayes, S. (2013). Incidence of unilateral arm lymphoedema after breast cancer: A systematic review and meta-analysis. *The Lancet. Oncology*, *14*(6), 500–515. DOI: 10.1016/S1470-2045(13)70076-7 PMID: 23540561

Disorder, S. (•••).. . *Children (Basel, Switzerland)*, *10*(1), 122. DOI: 10.3390/children10010122

Division for Early Childhood Intervention. (2014). *DEC Recommended Practices*. https://www.dec-sped.org/dec-recommended-practices

Diz-Teixeira, P., Alonso-Calvete, A., Justo-Cousiño, L. A., González-González, Y., & Cuña-Carrera, I. D. (2023). Update on Physiotherapy in Postpartum Urinary Incontinence. A Systematic Review. *Archivos Espanoles de Urologia*, *76*(1), 29–39. DOI: 10.56434/j.arch.esp.urol.20237601.2 PMID: 36914417

Dobinson, K., & Dockrell, J. (2021). Universal strategies for the improvement of expressive language skills in the primary classroom: A systematic review. *First Language*, *41*(5), 014272372198947. DOI: 10.1177/0142723721989471

Dockrell, J. E., Forrest, C. L., Law, J., Mathers, S., & Charlton, J. (2022). Screening for Language Difficulties in Disadvantaged Populations on Entry to Early Years Education: Challenges and Opportunities. *Frontiers in Pediatrics*, *10*, 833603. DOI: 10.3389/fped.2022.833603 PMID: 35601421

Donald, K. A., Wedderburn, C. J., Barnett, W., Nhapi, R. T., Rehman, A. M., Stadler, J. A. M., Hoffman, N., Koen, N., Zar, H. J., & Stein, D. J. (2019). Risk and protective factors for child development: An observational South African birth cohort. *PLoS Medicine*, *16*(9), e1002920. DOI: 10.1371/journal.pmed.1002920 PMID: 31560687

Dornan, M., Semple, C., Moorhead, A., & McCaughan, E. (2021). A qualitative systematic review of the social eating and drinking experiences of patients following treatment for head and neck cancer. *Supportive Care in Cancer*, *29*(9), 4899–4909. DOI: 10.1007/s00520-021-06062-7 PMID: 33646367

Doucette, M., Bove, C., & Hill, S. (2024). Healing through tradition: The role of indigenous elder support in child and youth mental health in Canada. *Alternative an International Journal of Indigenous Peoples*, *20*(4), 670–681. DOI: 10.1177/11771801241289999

Draffan, E. A., & Banes, D. (2022). Augmentative and alternative communication: Emerging trends, opportunities and innovations. In Miesenberger, K., Kouroupetroglou, G., Mavrou, K., & Manduchi, R. (Eds.), *Recent Advances in Technologies for Inclusive Well-Being* (pp. 469–485). Springer., https://www.researchgate.net/publication/361677133

Drost, J. (2019). Developing the alliances to expand traditional indigenous healing practices within Alberta health services. *Journal of Alternative and Complementary Medicine (New York, N.Y.)*, *25*(S1), S69–S77. DOI: 10.1089/acm.2018.0387 PMID: 30870024

Duan, A., Zhao, H., & Zhou, C. (2024). The effects of a healthy lifestyle on depressive symptoms in older Chinese adults: The mediating role of psychological resilience. *Cureus*. Advance online publication. DOI: 10.7759/cureus.57258 PMID: 38686246

Duarte, L., Sanchez, J.G., Fonte, J., & Teodoro, A.C. (2021). A GIS pen-source application to enhance the identification of archaeological crop marks using remote sensing data. *SPIE*, v11863.

Duarte, D. C. de O., Oliveira, J. C., & de, ., Lani, J. L., Uberti, M. S., Marques, Éder T. & Abreu, M. V. S. (2021). Multi-Criteria Evaluation Applied to the Determination of Areas of Suitability for Real Estate Appreciation. Brazilian. *Journal of Cardiography*, *73*(2), 516–529.

Duff, F., Reen, G., Plunkett, K., & Nation, K. (2015). Do infant vocabulary skills predict school-age language and literacy outcomes? *Journal of Child Psychology and Psychiatry, and Allied Disciplines*, *56*(8), 848–856. DOI: 10.1111/jcpp.12378 PMID: 25557322

Dunham, M., Bonacaro, A., Schofield, P., Bacon, L., Spyridonis, F., & Mehrpouya, H. (2021). Smartphone applications designed to improve older people's chronic pain management: An integrated systematic review. *Geriatrics (Basel, Switzerland)*, *6*(2), 40. DOI: 10.3390/geriatrics6020040 PMID: 33917697

Dunn, A., Startup, H., & Cartwright-Hatton, S. (2021). Adult mental health service engagement with patients who are parents: Evidence from 15 English mental health trusts. *British Journal of Clinical Psychology*, *61*(2), 335–348. DOI: 10.1111/bjc.12330 PMID: 34609005

Dunst, C. J., Trivette, C. M., & Hamby, D. W. (2006). Technical manual for measuring and evaluating family support program quality and benefits. Winterberry Monograph Series. Winterberry Press. https://library.bsl.org.au/jspui/bitstream/1/4994/1/DunstC_Technical-manual-for-measuring-and-evaulating_Winterberry-2006.pdf

Dunst, C. J. (2020). Everyday learning opportunities of young children with and without developmental disabilities or delays. *International Journal of Early Childhood Environmental Education*, *7*(3), 23–41.

Dunst, C. J., Boyd, K., Trivette, C. M., & Hamby, D. W. (2002). Family-oriented program models and professional helpgiving practices. *Family Relations*, *51*(3), 221–229. DOI: 10.1111/j.1741-3729.2002.00221.x

Dunst, C. J., & Espe-Sherwindt, M. (2016). Family-centered practices in early childhood intervention. In Reichow, B., Boyd, B. A., Barton, E. E., & Odom, S. L. (Eds.), *Handbook of early childhood special education* (pp. 37–55). Springer. DOI: 10.1007/978-3-319-28492-7_3

Dunst, C. J., & Trivette, C. M. (2009). Capacity-Building Family-Systems Intervention Practices. *Journal of Family Social Work*, *12*(789296667), 119–143. DOI: 10.1080/10522150802713322

Dunst, C. J., Trivette, C. M., & Hamby, D. W. (2007). Meta-Analysis of family-centered helpgiving practices research. *Mental Retardation and Developmental Disabilities Research Reviews*, *13*(4), 370–378. DOI: 10.1002/mrdd.20176 PMID: 17979208

EAACI. (2023, October 12). *EAACI - News: New Clinical Guidelines for the Diagnosis of Immediate-type Food Allergies are launched.* https://eaaci.org/news/new-clinical-guidelines-for-the-diagnosis-of-immediate-type-food-allergies-are-launched/

Ebert, K. D., Ochoa-Lubinoff, C., & Holmes, M. P. (2020). Screening school-age children for developmental language disorder in primary care. *International Journal of Speech-Language Pathology*, *22*(2), 152–162. DOI: 10.1080/17549507.2019.1632931 PMID: 31262202

Ebo, D. G., Bahri, R., Tontini, C., Van Gasse, A. L., Mertens, C., Hagendorens, M. M., Sabato, V., & Elst, J. (2024). Mast cell versus basophil activation test in allergy: Current status. *Clinical and Experimental Allergy*, *54*(6), 378–387. DOI: 10.1111/cea.14487 PMID: 38686464

Eccleston, C., Fisher, E., Howard, R., Slater, R., Forgeron, P., Palermo, T., Birnie, K. A., Anderson, B. J., Chambers, C. T., Crombez, G., Ljungman, G., Jordan, I., Jordan, Z., Roberts, C., Schechter, N., Sieberg, C. B., Tibboel, D., Walker, S. M., Wilkinson, D., & Wood, C. (2021). Delivering transformative action in paediatric pain: A lancet child & adolescent health commission. *The Lancet. Child & Adolescent Health*, *5*(1), 47–87. DOI: 10.1016/S2352-4642(20)30277-7 PMID: 33064998

Eccleston, C., Fisher, E., Thomas, K., Hearn, L., Derry, S., Stannard, C., Knaggs, R., & Moore, A. (2017). Interventions for the reduction of prescribed opioid use in chronic non-cancer pain. *Cochrane Database of Systematic Reviews*, *2021*(5). Advance online publication. DOI: 10.1002/14651858.CD010323.pub3 PMID: 29130474

Edpuganti, S., Gaikwad, J. R., Maliyil, B. T., Koshy, R. R., Potdar, R., Latheef, S., & Korrapati, N. H. (2025). The not-so-sweet side of mango: Mango allergy. *Cosmoderma*, *5*, 18. Advance online publication. DOI: 10.25259/CSDM_212_2024

Eilan, N., & Associates. (Eds.). (2005) *Joint Attention: Communication and Other Minds: Issues in Philosophy and Psychology, Consciousness & Self-Consciousness Series*. Oxford, (online edn, Oxford Academic, 2010), DOI: 10.1093/acprof:oso/9780199245635.001.0001

Ekezie, F. C., Cheng, J., & Sun, D. (2018). Effects of nonthermal food processing technologies on food allergens: A review of recent research advances. *Trends in Food Science & Technology*, *74*, 12–25. DOI: 10.1016/j.tifs.2018.01.007

Elbers, S., Wittink, H., Pool, J., & Smeets, R. (2018). The effectiveness of generic self-management interventions for patients with chronic musculoskeletal pain on physical function, self-efficacy, pain intensity and physical activity: A systematic review and meta-analysis. *European Journal of Pain (London, England)*, *22*(9), 1577–1596. DOI: 10.1002/ejp.1253 PMID: 29845678

Elder, J. H., Kreider, C. M., Brasher, S. N., & Ansell, M. (2017, August 24). Clinical impact of early diagnosis of autism on the prognosis and parent-child relationships. *Psychology Research and Behavior Management*, *10*, 283–292. DOI: 10.2147/PRBM.S117499 PMID: 28883746

Eldufani, J., & Blaise, G. (2019). The role of acetylcholinesterase inhibitors such as neostigmine and rivastigmine on chronic pain and cognitive function in aging: A review of recent clinical applications. *Alzheimer's & Dementia: Translational Research & Clinical Interventions*, *5*(1), 175–183. DOI: 10.1016/j.trci.2019.03.004 PMID: 31194017

Elmajee, M., Munasinghe, C., Aljawadi, A., Elawady, K., Shuweihde, F., & Pillai, A. (2021). Posterior stabilisation without formal debridement for the treatment of non-tuberculous pyogenic spinal infection in frail and debilitated population – a systematic review and meta-analysis. *Journal of Clinical Orthopaedics and Trauma*, *15*, 9–15. DOI: 10.1016/j.jcot.2020.11.009 PMID: 33717910

Epstein, R. M., Fiscella, K., Lesser, C. S., & Stange, K. C. (2010). Why the nation needs a policy push on patient-centered health care. *Health Affairs (Project Hope)*, *29*(8), 1489–1495. DOI: 10.1377/hlthaff.2009.0888 PMID: 20679652

Eriksson, M., Westerlund, M., & Miniscalco, C. (2010). Problems and limitations in studies on screening for language delay. *Research in Developmental Disabilities*, *31*(5), 943–950. DOI: 10.1016/j.ridd.2010.04.019 PMID: 20483561

Española de Logopedia, A. Foniatria y Audiología e Ibero-Americana de Fonoaudiología. (n.d.). https://www.aelfa.org/

Espe-Sherwindt, M., & Serrano, A. M. (2016). It takes two: The role of family-centered practices in communication intervention. *Revista de Logopedia, Foniatría y Audiología*, *36*(4), 162–169. DOI: 10.1016/j.rlfa.2016.07.006

Espírito Santo, J., Moita, J., & Nunes, A. (2024). The Efficacy of Manual Therapy on Musculoskeletal Pain in Menopause: A Systematic Review. In *Healthcare* (Vol. 12, No. 18, p. 1838). MDPI. https://doi.org/DOI: 10.3390/healthcare12181838

Esseily, R., Somogyi, E., & Guellai, B. (2016). The Relative Importance of Language in Guiding Social Preferences Through Development. *Frontiers in Psychology*, *7*, 1645. DOI: 10.3389/fpsyg.2016.01645 PMID: 27812345

European Environment Agency. (2016). *Urban adaptation to climate change in Europe 2016*. EEA.

Evangeline, B., & Anitha, D. (2024). A comprehensive review on augmentative and alternative communication tools for speech-impaired individuals. In *Lecture Notes in Networks and Systems* (pp. 321–331). Springer., DOI: 10.1007/978-981-97-3973-8_20

Fabi, A., Bhargava, R., Fatigoni, S., Guglielmo, M., Horneber, M., Roila, F., Weis, J., Jordan, K., & Ripamonti, C. I.ESMO Guidelines Committee. (2020). Cancer-related fatigue: ESMO Clinical Practice Guidelines for diagnosis and treatment. *Annals of Oncology : Official Journal of the European Society for Medical Oncology*, *31*(6), 713–723. DOI: 10.1016/j.annonc.2020.02.016 PMID: 32173483

Fancourt, D., & Steptoe, A. (2019). Cultural engagement and mental health: Does socio-economic status explain the association?. Social science & medicine (1982), 236, 112425. https://doi.org/DOI: 10.1016/j.socscimed.2019.112425

Faraji, S., Najafabadi, M. G., Zandi, H. G., & Parent-Nichols, J. (2022). Water-based exercise therapy and improvement in the motor skills and cognitive function of children with autism spectrum disorder: A commentary. *Russian Open Medical Journal, 11*(1), 112. DOI: 10.15275/rusomj.2022.0112

Farias, H. S., Vargas, K. B., Marino, T. B., Souza, G. M., & Lucena, A. J. (2020). *Vulnerabilidade socioambiental no Oeste Metropolitano do Rio de Janeiro: estratégias de prevenção a riscos* (19th ed.). Espaço e Economia.

Farzad, M., MacDermid, J., Ring, D., & Shafiee, E. (2021). A scoping review of the evidence regarding assessment and management of psychological features of shoulder pain. *Rehabilitation Research and Practice, 2021*, 1–15. DOI: 10.1155/2021/7211201 PMID: 34631168

Feng, B., Hu, X., Lu, W., Wang, Y., & Ip, W. (2021). Are mindfulness treatments effective for pain in cancer patients? a systematic review and meta-analysis. *European Journal of Pain (London, England), 26*(1), 61–76. DOI: 10.1002/ejp.1849 PMID: 34369040

Feng, L., Hao, Q., Wang, S., Zhao, Y., Wu, H., Cui, Z., Zhang, J., Wang, L., Zhang, D., Zhan, X., & Wei, L. (2024). Effects of Electrical Stimulation, Pelvic Floor Muscle Exercise, and Biofeedback Program on Improving Pelvic Floor Function and Quality of Life in Postoperative Patients with Early-Stage Cervical Cancer. *The Tohoku Journal of Experimental Medicine, 264*(1), 21–29. DOI: 10.1620/tjem.2024.J044 PMID: 38897964

Fernald, A., Marchman, V., & Weisleder, A. (2012). SES differences in language processing skill and vocabulary are evident at 18 months. *Developmental Science, 16*(2), 234–248. DOI: 10.1111/desc.12019 PMID: 23432833

Fernandes, J., Fernandes, S., Almeida, A., Vareta, D., & Miller, C. (2021). Older adults' perceived barriers to participation in a falls prevention strategy. *Journal of Personalized Medicine, 11*(6), 450. DOI: 10.3390/jpm11060450 PMID: 34070987

Ferrante, G., Licari, A., Fasola, S., Marseglia, G. L., & La Grutta, S. (2020). Artificial intelligence in the diagnosis of pediatric allergic diseases. *Pediatric Allergy and Immunology, 32*(3), 405–413. DOI: 10.1111/pai.13419 PMID: 33220121

Ferreira, L. P. (2021). Terapeutas da Fala em contexto clínico: *Práticas Centradas na Família* [Master's dissertation, Instituto Politécnico do Porto]. Repositório Científico do Instituto Politécnico do Porto. https://recipp.ipp.pt/bitstream/10400.22/17254/1/DM_Liliana%20Ferrreira.pdf

Fibla, L., Kosie, J. E., Kircher, R., Lew-Williams, C., & Byers-Heinlein, K. (2022). Bilingual Language Development in Infancy: What Can We Do to Support Bilingual Families*? Policy Insights from the Behavioral and Brain Sciences*, *9*(1), 35–43. DOI: 10.1177/23727322211069312 PMID: 35224184

Finisguerra, A., Borgatti, R., & Urgesi, C. (2019). Non-invasive brain stimulation for the rehabilitation of children and adolescents with neurodevelopmental disorders: A systematic review. *Frontiers in Psychology*, *10*, 135. DOI: 10.3389/fpsyg.2019.00135 PMID: 30787895

Finke, E. H., Light, J., & Kitko, L. (2008). A systematic review of the effectiveness of nurse communication with patients with complex communication needs with a focus on the use of augmentative and alternative communication. *Journal of Clinical Nursing*, *17*(16), 2102–2115. DOI: 10.1111/j.1365-2702.2008.02373.x PMID: 18705734

Finlay, L. (2011). *Phenomenology for therapists: Researching the lived world.* Wiley-Blackwell. DOI: 10.1002/9781119975144

Fiocchi, A., Vickery, B. P., & Wood, R. A. (2021). The use of biologics in food allergy. Clinical & Experimental Allergy. *Clinical and Experimental Allergy*, *51*(8), 1006–1018. DOI: 10.1111/cea.13897 PMID: 33966304

Fitchett, R. C., Aldus, E. J., Fitchett, L. R., & Cross, J. (2018). The lived experience of head and neck cancer patients receiving curative radiotherapy: A systematic review and meta-ethnography. *Psycho-Oncology*, *27*(9), 2077–2086. DOI: 10.1002/pon.4790 PMID: 29883989

Fleischer, D. M., & Burks, A. W. (2015). Pitfalls in food allergy diagnosis: serum IGE testing. the Journal of Pediatrics/the Journal of Pediatrics, 166(1), 8–10. DOI: 10.1016/j.jpeds.2014.09.057

Flensborg-Madsen, T., Grønkjær, M., & Mortensen, E. (2019). Predictors of early life milestones: Results from the copenhagen perinatal cohort. *BMC Pediatrics*, *19*(1), 420. Advance online publication. DOI: 10.1186/s12887-019-1778-y PMID: 31703689

Food Allergies Symptoms. Diagnosis & Treatment | AAAAI. (2018, April). American Academy of Allergy Asthma & Immunology. https://www.aaaai.org/conditions-treatments/allergies/food-allergy

Food allergies. (2024, April 12). FDA. https://www.fda.gov/food/food-labeling-nutrition/food-allergies

Food allergy. (2023, August 16). www.nhs.ukNHS-UK. https://www.nhs.uk/conditions/food-allergy/

Food and agricultural organization of united nations(2023-24). Scintific advice. https://www.fao.org/food-safety/scientific-advice/food-allergens/en/

Food chain Allergen management. (2009). Google Books. https://books.google.com/books?hl=en&lr=&id=FHIoDwAAQBAJ&oi=fnd&pg=PR3&dq=Remaining+Challenges+Allergen+Detection+-+Collaboration+and+Knowledge+Sharing:&ots=xJkYxRSdmA&sig=Ie-vVVp_bdNRqlSao5TwBXElvr0

Food labelling. (2000). Google Books. https://books.google.com/books?hl=en&lr=&id=PwXnAgAAQBAJ&oi=fnd&pg=PP1&dq=Improvements+in+Allergen+Labeling+-+Multilingual+and+Pictorial+Labeling&ots=MQOIrcCzaE&sig=7sXeebe4zLDCFzNPwljNsBe-lbs

Foong, R., Dantzer, J. A., Wood, R. A., & Santos, A. F. (2021). Improving diagnostic accuracy in food allergy. Journal of Allergy and Clinical Immunology. In Practice/ the Journal of Allergy and Clinical Immunology. *In Practice*, *9*(1), 71–80. DOI: 10.1016/j.jaip.2020.09.037 PMID: 33429723

Fradley, K., Oldfield, J., Marshall, J., & Toseeb, U. (2024). Early life risk factors for adolescent mental health difficulties for individuals at risk of developmental language disorder. *Journal of Research in Special Educational Needs*, *24*(3), 713–728. DOI: 10.1111/1471-3802.12654

François, J., Audrain-Pontevia, A., Boudhraâ, S., & Vial, S. (2024). Assessing the Influence of Patient Empowerment Gained Through Mental Health Apps on Patient Trust in the Health Care Provider and Patient Compliance With the Recommended Treatment: Cross-sectional Study. *Journal of Medical Internet Research*, *26*, e48182. DOI: 10.2196/48182 PMID: 38345851

Frawley, H., Shelly, B., Morin, M., Bernard, S., Bø, K., Digesu, G., Dickinson, T., Goonewardene, S., McClurg, D., Rahnama'i, M. S., Schizas, A., Slieker-ten Hove, M., Takahashi, S., & Voelkl Guevara, J. (2021). An International Continence Society (ICS) report on the terminology for pelvic floor muscle assessment. *Neurourology and Urodynamics*, *40*(5), 1217–1260. DOI: 10.1002/nau.24658 PMID: 33844342

Fredriksen-Goldsen, K., Jen, S., Bryan, A., & Goldsen, J. (2016). Cognitive impairment, Alzheimer's disease, and other dementias in the lives of lesbian, gay, bisexual and transgender (LGBT) older adults and their caregivers: Needs and competencies. *Journal of Applied Gerontology*, *37*(5), 545–569. DOI: 10.1177/0733464816672047 PMID: 27729400

Freitas, C. M., Lopes de Carvalho, M., Ximenes, E. F., Arraes, E. F., & Gomes, J. O. (2012). Vulnerabilidade socioambiental, redução de riscos de desastres e construção da resiliência: Lições do terremoto no Haiti e das chuvas fortes na Região Serrana, Brasil. *Ciencia & Saude Coletiva*, *17*(6), 1577–1586. DOI: 10.1590/S1413-81232012000600021 PMID: 22699648

Fricke, S., Bowyer-Crane, C., Haley, A. J., Hulme, C., & Snowling, M. J. (2013). Efficacy of language intervention in the early years. *Journal of Child Psychology and Psychiatry, and Allied Disciplines*, *54*(3), 280–290. DOI: 10.1111/jcpp.12010 PMID: 23176547

Fung, K., Lyden, T. H., Lee, J., Urba, S. G., Worden, F., Eisbruch, A., Tsien, C., Bradford, C. R., Chepeha, D. B., Hogikyan, N. D., Prince, M. E. P., Teknos, T. N., & Wolf, G. T. (2005). Voice and swallowing outcomes of an organ-preservation trial for advanced laryngeal cancer. *International Journal of Radiation Oncology, Biology, Physics*, *63*(5), 1395–1399. DOI: 10.1016/j.ijrobp.2005.05.004 PMID: 16087298

Fu, W., Baldwin, T. F., Brechter, J. H., Erickson, M. R., Kobal, K., LaFay, V., Miller, T. M., & Morales, J. (2024). Effects of Educational Interventions Designed to Develop Physical Therapist Learners' Clinical Reasoning: A Systematic Review. *Physical Therapy*, *105*(3), pzae182. Advance online publication. DOI: 10.1093/ptj/pzae182 PMID: 39718199

Fu, Y., & Ji, X. (2020). Intergenerational relationships and depressive symptoms among older adults in urban China: The roles of loneliness and insomnia symptoms. *Health & Social Care in the Community*, *28*(4), 1310–1322. DOI: 10.1111/hsc.12964 PMID: 32115795

Gaalema, D. E., Savage, P. D., O'Neill, S., Bolívar, H. A., Denkmann, D., Priest, J. S., Khadanga, S., & Ades, P. A. (2022). The Association of Patient Educational Attainment With Cardiac Rehabilitation Adherence and Health Outcomes. *Journal of Cardiopulmonary Rehabilitation and Prevention*, *42*(4), 227–234. DOI: 10.1097/HCR.0000000000000646 PMID: 34840247

Gabriels, R., Pan, Z., Dechant, B., Agnew, J., Brim, N., & Mesibov, G. (2015). Randomized controlled trial of therapeutic horseback riding in children and adolescents with autism spectrum disorder. *Journal of the American Academy of Child and Adolescent Psychiatry*, *54*(7), 541–549. DOI: 10.1016/j.jaac.2015.04.007 PMID: 26088658

Gaffrey, M. S., Luby, J. L., & Barch, D. M. (2013). Towards the study of functional brain development in depression: An Interactive Specialization approach. *Neurobiology of Disease*, *52*, 38–48. DOI: 10.1016/j.nbd.2012.06.012 PMID: 22750525

Gai, J., Gomes, L., & Jansen de Càrdenas, C. (2009). Ptofobia - O medo de cair em pessoas idosas. *Acta Medica Portuguesa*, *22*, 83–88. PMID: 19341596

Gail, J., Soderberg, J., Abbott, R., Garzon, R., & Scott, C. (2022). Improving language support for infants and toddlers. Results of FIND coaching in childcare. *Infants and Young Children*, *35*(2), 91–105. https://doi.org/https://doi.org/10.1097/IYC.0000000000000214. DOI: 10.1097/IYC.0000000000000214

Gallaway, M. S., Townsend, J. S., Shelby, D., & Puckett, M. C. (2020). Pain Among Cancer Survivors. *Preventing Chronic Disease*, *17*, E54. DOI: 10.5888/pcd17.190367 PMID: 32644924

García-Sánchez, F. A., Mora, C. T. E., & Castellano, I. F. (2020). Reflexiones y estrategias de acompañamiento familiar en Atención Temprana. *Revista de Logopedia, Foniatría y Audiología*, *40*(3), 118–127. DOI: 10.1016/j.rlfa.2020.02.004

Gardner, H., Froud, K., McClelland, A., & van der Lely, H. K. (2006). Development of the Grammar and Phonology Screening (GAPS) test to assess key markers of specific language and literacy difficulties in young children. *International Journal of Language & Communication Disorders*, *41*(5), 513–540. DOI: 10.1080/13682820500442644 PMID: 17050469

Garland, E., Brintz, C., Hanley, A., Roseen, E., Atchley, R., Gaylord, S., Faurot, K. R., Yaffe, J., Fiander, M., & Keefe, F. (2020). Mind-body therapies for opioid-treated pain. *JAMA Internal Medicine*, *180*(1), 91. DOI: 10.1001/jamainternmed.2019.4917 PMID: 31682676

Gell, N., & Patel, K. (2018). Rehabilitation services use of older adults according to fall-risk screening guidelines. *Journal of the American Geriatrics Society*, *67*(1), 100–107. DOI: 10.1111/jgs.15625 PMID: 30295320

Geretsegger, M., Elefant, C., Mössler, K. A., & Gold, C. (2014). Music therapy for people with autism spectrum disorder. *Cochrane Database of Systematic Reviews*, *2016*(3), 6. DOI: 10.1002/14651858.CD004381.pub3 PMID: 24936966

Ghazi, C., Nyland, J., Whaley, R., Rogers, T., Wera, J., & Henzman, C. (2018). Social cognitive or learning theory use to improve self-efficacy in musculoskeletal rehabilitation: A systematic review and meta-analysis. *Physiotherapy Theory and Practice, 34*(7), 495–504. DOI: 10.1080/09593985.2017.1422204 PMID: 29308969

Gibson, G., Quirke, M., & Lovatt, M. (2022). The role of environmental design in enabling intergenerational support for people with dementia – what lessons can we learn from Japan. *Working with Older People (Brighton, England), 26*(3), 226–237. DOI: 10.1108/WWOP-12-2021-0064

Gil-Ibanez, B., Davies-Oliveira, J., Lopez, G., Díaz-Feijoo, B., Tejerizo-Garcia, A., & Sehouli, J. (2023). Impact of gynecological cancers on health-related quality of life: Historical context, measurement instruments, and current knowledge. *International Journal of Gynecological Cancer : Official Journal of the International Gynecological Cancer Society, 33*(11), 1800–1806. DOI: 10.1136/ijgc-2023-004804 PMID: 37696648

Gillam, S. L., Gillam, R. B., & Reece, K. (2012). Language outcomes of contextualized and decontextualized language intervention: Results of an early efficacy study. *Language, Speech, and Hearing Services in Schools, 43*(3), 276–291. DOI: 10.1044/0161-1461(2011/11-0022) PMID: 22269582

Giovannoni, G., Ford, H. L., Schmierer, K., Middleton, R., Stennett, A. M., Pomeroy, I., Fisniku, L., Scalfari, A., Bannon, C., Stross, R., Hughes, S., Williams, A., Josephs, S., Peel, C., & Straukiene, A. (2024). MS care: Integrating advanced therapies and holistic management. *Frontiers in Neurology, 14*, 1286122. DOI: 10.3389/fneur.2023.1286122 PMID: 38351950

Gluppe, S., Engh, M. E., & Bø, K. (2021). What is the evidence for abdominal and pelvic floor muscle training to treat diastasis recti abdominis postpartum? A systematic review with meta-analysis. *Brazilian Journal of Physical Therapy, 25*(6), 664–675. DOI: 10.1016/j.bjpt.2021.06.006 PMID: 34391661

Goh, S. K. Y., Griffiths, S., & Norbury, C. F. (2021). Sources of variability in the prospective relation of language to social, emotional, and behavior problem symptoms: Implications for developmental language disorder. *Journal of Abnormal Psychology, 130*(6), 676–689. DOI: 10.1037/abn0000691 PMID: 34553962

Goh, S., Persson, M., Stocks, J., Hou, Y., Welton, N., Lin, J., Hall, M. C., Doherty, M., & Zhang, W. (2019). Relative efficacy of different exercises for pain, function, performance and quality of life in knee and hip osteoarthritis: Systematic review and network meta-analysis. *Sports Medicine (Auckland, N.Z.), 49*(5), 743–761. DOI: 10.1007/s40279-019-01082-0 PMID: 30830561

Gold, C., Wigram, T., & Elefant, C. (2006). Music therapy for autistic spectrum disorder. *Cochrane Database of Systematic Reviews*, (2), CD004381. PMID: 16625601

Golden, R., Emery-Tiburcio, E., Post, S., Ewald, B., & Newman, M. (2019). Connecting social, clinical, and home care services for persons with serious illness in the community. *Journal of the American Geriatrics Society*, *67*(S2). Advance online publication. DOI: 10.1111/jgs.15900 PMID: 31074858

Gomes, N. A. C., & Gibson, M. Q. (2023). A comunicação aumentativa e alternativa para desenvolvimento da linguagem e comunicação no autismo. *Revista ISAAC*, *15*(2), 150–162. https://publicacoes.softaliza.com.br/isaac2023/article/view/7904

Gomes, V., Cajaíba, R., Costa, J., Damasceno, P., Souza, A., Goto, L., … & Figueira, S. (2023). Palliative care for the elderly in a long-stay institution in a municipality in west Pará: an experience report based on Arco de Maguerez.. https://doi.org/DOI: 10.56238/interdiinovationscrese-059

Goodwin, P. R. (2004). Food Allergen Detection Methods: A Coordinated approach. *Journal of AOAC International*, *87*(6), 1383–1390. DOI: 10.1093/jaoac/87.6.1383 PMID: 15675450

Gormley, J., & Light, J. (2019). Providing services to individuals with complex communication needs in the inpatient rehabilitation setting: The experiences and perspectives of speech-language pathologists. *American Journal of Speech-Language Pathology*, *28*(2), 456–468. DOI: 10.1044/2018_AJSLP-18-0076 PMID: 31136227

Gormley, J., & Light, J. (2021). Child-parent-provider interactions of a child with complex communication needs in an inpatient rehabilitation facility: A pilot study. *American Journal of Speech-Language Pathology*, *30*(1), 105–118. DOI: 10.1044/2020_AJSLP-20-00031 PMID: 33316177

Gouvernet, B., & Brisson, J. (2024). Menstrual health under the scientific microscope: Text mining analysis. *Women's Health (London, England)*, *20*, 17455057241290895. Advance online publication. DOI: 10.1177/17455057241290895 PMID: 39449243

Govender, R., Wood, C. E., Taylor, S. A., Smith, C. H., Barratt, H., & Gardner, B. (2017). Patient Experiences of Swallowing Exercises After Head and Neck Cancer: A Qualitative Study Examining Barriers and Facilitators Using Behaviour Change Theory. *Dysphagia*, *32*(4), 559–569. DOI: 10.1007/s00455-017-9799-x PMID: 28424898

Govindaraju, A., Lakshminarayanan, P., Sabarathinam, S., & Meganathan, H. (2020). Alternative therapies for children's with autism spectrum disorder. *International Journal of Contemporary Pediatrics*, *7*(12), 2421. DOI: 10.18203/2349-3291.ijcp20205111

Grant, E., Johnson, L., Prodromidis, A., & Giannoudis, P. V. (2021). The Impact of Peer Support on Patient Outcomes in Adults With Physical Health Conditions: A Scoping Review. *Cureus*, *13*(8), e17442. DOI: 10.7759/cureus.17442 PMID: 34589348

Graziottin, A. (2023). Female sexual dysfunction. In K. Bo, B. Berghmans, S. Mørkved, & M. Van Kampen (Eds.) *(3rd ed.), Evidence-Based Physical Therapy for the Pelvic Floor - Science and Clinical Practice (pp. 266-277). Elsevier.*

Greenslade, K. J. (2021). Using analog tasks to assess children's social communication skills. *Perspectives of the ASHA Special Interest Groups*, *6*(1), 39–54. DOI: 10.1044/2020_PERSP-20-00155

Grocke, D., & Wigram, T. (2006). *Receptive methods in music therapy: Techniques and clinical applications for music therapy clinicians, educators and students.* Jessica Kingsley Publishers.

Grogan, S. (2021). *Body Image: Understanding Body Dissatisfaction in Men, Women, and Children* (4th ed.). Routledge., DOI: 10.4324/9781003100041

Gudipally, P. R., & Sharma, G. K. (2024 Jan). Premenstrual Syndrome. [Updated 2023 Jul 17] In *StatPearls* [Internet]. StatPearls Publishing., Available from https://www.ncbi.nlm.nih.gov/books/NBK560698/

Guédeney, A., Forhan, A., Larroque, B., Agostini, M., Pingault, J., & Heude, B. (2016). Social withdrawal behaviour at one year of age is associated with delays in reaching language milestones in the eden mother-child cohort study. *PLoS One*, *11*(7), e0158426. DOI: 10.1371/journal.pone.0158426 PMID: 27391482

Güeita-Rodríguez, J., Ogonowska-Slodownik, A., Morgulec-Adamowicz, N., Martín-Prades, M. L., Cuenca-Zaldívar, J. N., & Palacios-Ceña, D. (2021). Effects of Aquatic Therapy for Children with Autism Spectrum Disorder on Social Competence and Quality of Life: A Mixed Methods Study. *International Journal of Environmental Research and Public Health*, *18*(6), 3126. DOI: 10.3390/ijerph18063126 PMID: 33803581

Guimarães, C., Cruz-Santos, A., & Almeida, L. (2013). Adaptação do Inventário Parental "Language Use Inventory (LUI)" para crianças entre 18 e 47 meses para o Português Europeu: Estudo Piloto. *Audiology - Communication Research, 18*(4), 332–338. DOI: 10.1590/S2317-64312013000400015

Guo, W., Liu, X., Zhang, Y., Chen, R., Qi, W., Deng, J., & Cui, J. (2023). Competence and perceptions of spiritual care among clinical nurses: A multicentre cross-sectional study. *Journal of Clinical Nursing, 33*(4), 1432–1443. DOI: 10.1111/jocn.16932 PMID: 37994280

Gupta, M., Cox, A., Nowak-Węgrzyn, A., & Wang, J. (2018). Diagnosis of food allergy. *Immunology and Allergy Clinics of North America, 38*(1), 39–52. DOI: 10.1016/j.iac.2017.09.004 PMID: 29132673

Gupta, U. G., & Clarke, R. E. (1996). Theory and Applications of the Delphi Technique: A Bibliography (1975–1994). *Technological Forecasting and Social Change, 53*(2), 185–211. DOI: 10.1016/S0040-1625(96)00094-7

Habimorad, P. H. L., Catarucci, F. M., Bruno, V. H. T., Silva, I. B. D., & Bernardes, L. C. (2020). Implementation of Brazil's National Policy on Complementary and Integrative Practices: Strengths and weaknesses. *Ciencia & Saude Coletiva, 25*(2), 395–405. DOI: 10.1590/1413-81232020252.11332018 PMID: 32022181

Hadizadeh-Talasaz, Z., Sadeghi, R., & Khadivzadeh, T. (2019). Effect of pelvic floor muscle training on postpartum sexual function and quality of life: A systematic review and meta-analysis of clinical trials. *Taiwanese Journal of Obstetrics & Gynecology, 58*(6), 737–747. DOI: 10.1016/j.tjog.2019.09.003 PMID: 31759521

Halfon, N., Larson, K., Lu, M., Tullis, E., & Russ, S. (2014). Lifecourse health development: Past, present and future. *Maternal and Child Health Journal, 18*(2), 344–365. DOI: 10.1007/s10995-013-1346-2 PMID: 23975451

Hammer, C. S., Morgan, P., Farkas, G., Hillemeier, M., Bitetti, D., & Maczuga, S. (2017). Late Talkers: A Population-Based Study of Risk Factors and School Readiness Consequences. *Journal of Speech, Language, and Hearing Research: JSLHR, 60*(3), 607–626. DOI: 10.1044/2016_JSLHR-L-15-0417 PMID: 28257586

Hamzah Idris, Ikhwan & Mustapha, Safinaz & Aljibori, Hakim & Al-tamimi, Adnan & Abdulrazaq Alshekhly, Mohammed & Alfiras, Mohanad. (2023). Enhancing Children's Communication Skills Through an Interactive *AR Board Game*. 1-6. .DOI: 10.1109/ICETAS59148.2023.10346447

Handberg, C., & Voss, A. K. (2018). Implementing augmentative and alternative communication in critical care settings: Perspectives of healthcare professionals. *Journal of Clinical Nursing*, *27*(1–2), 102–114. DOI: 10.1111/jocn.13851 PMID: 28401613

Hanson, E., Hellström, A., Sandvide, Å., Jackson, G., MacRae, R., Jack-Waugh, A., & Tolson, D. (2016). The extended palliative phase of dementia – an integrative literature review. *Dementia (London)*, *18*(1), 108–134. DOI: 10.1177/1471301216659797 PMID: 27460046

Harfield, S., Davy, C., McArthur, A., Munn, Z., Brown, A., & Brown, N. (2018). Characteristics of indigenous primary health care service delivery models: A systematic scoping review. *Globalization and Health*, *14*(1), 12. Advance online publication. DOI: 10.1186/s12992-018-0332-2 PMID: 29368657

Harris, A., & Williams, J. (2017). The impact of a horse riding intervention on the social functioning of children with autism spectrum disorder. *International Journal of Environmental Research and Public Health*, *14*(7), 776. DOI: 10.3390/ijerph14070776 PMID: 28708075

Harrison, L. J., & McLeod, S. (2010). Risk and protective factors associated with speech and language impairment in a nationally representative sample of 4- to 5-year-old children. *Journal of Speech, Language, and Hearing Research: JSLHR*, *53*(2), 508–529. DOI: 10.1044/1092-4388(2009/08-0086) PMID: 19786704

Hasnan, N. Z. N., Basha, R. K., Amin, N. M., Ramli, S. H. M., Tang, J. Y. H., & Aziz, N. A. (2022). Analysis of the most frequent nonconformance aspects related to Good Manufacturing Practices (GMP) among small and medium enterprises (SMEs) in the food industry and their main factors. *Food Control*, *141*, 109205. DOI: 10.1016/j.foodcont.2022.109205

Hattersley, S., Ward, R., Baka, A., & Crevel, R. W. (2014). Advances in the risk management of unintended presence of allergenic foods in manufactured food products – An overview. *Food and Chemical Toxicology*, *67*, 255–261. DOI: 10.1016/j.fct.2014.01.036 PMID: 24508586

Haylen, B., De Ridder, D., Freeman, R., Swift, S., Berghmans, B., Lee, J., Monga, A., Petri, E., Rizk, D. E., Sand, P. K., & Schaer, G. (2010). An International Urogynecological Association (IUGA)/International Continence Society (ICS) joint report on the terminology for female pelvic floor dysfunction. *International Urogynecology Journal*, *21*(1), 5–26. DOI: 10.1007/s00192-009-0976-9 PMID: 19937315

Haylen, B., Maher, C., Barber, M., Camargo, S., Dandolu, V., Digesu, A., Goldman, H. B., Huser, M., Milani, A. L., Moran, P. A., Schaer, G. N., & Withagen, M. (2016). An International Urogynecological Association (IUGA)/International Continence Society (ICS) joint report on the terminology for female pelvic organ prolapse (POP). *International Urogynecology Journal*, *27*(2), 165–194. DOI: 10.1007/s00192-015-2932-1 PMID: 26755051

Hebbeler, K., Spiker, D., & Kahn, L. (2012). Individuals With Disabilities Education Act's Early Childhood Programs: Powerful Vision and Pesky Details. *Topics in Early Childhood Special Education*, *31*(4), 199–207. DOI: 10.1177/0271121411429077

Heidlage, J. K., Cunningham, J. E., Kaiser, A. P., Trivette, C. M., Barton, E. E., Frey, J. R., & Roberts, M. Y. (2020). The effects of parent-implemented language interventions on child linguistic outcomes: A meta-analysis. *Early Childhood Research Quarterly*, *50*, 6–23. DOI: 10.1016/j.ecresq.2018.12.006

Heimes, A. S., Stewen, K., & Hasenburg, A. (2017). Psychosocial Aspects of Immediate versus Delayed Breast Reconstruction. *Breast Care (Basel, Switzerland)*, *12*(6), 374–377. DOI: 10.1159/000485234 PMID: 29456468

Helland, T., Jones, L., & Helland, W. (2017). Detecting Preschool Language Impairment and Risk of Developmental Dyslexia. *Journal of Research in Childhood Education*, *31*(2), 295–311. Advance online publication. DOI: 10.1080/02568543.2016.1274928

Hellings, D., Joosten, A., Hatfield, M., & Netto, J. (2022). Benefits and Challenges of Assistance Dogs for Families of Children on the Autism Spectrum: Mothers' Perspectives. *Qualitative Health Research*, *32*(11), 1648–1656. DOI: 10.1177/10497323221111247 PMID: 35772944

He, M., Walle, E., & Campos, J. (2015). A cross-national investigation of the relationship between infant walking and language development. *Infancy*, *20*(3), 283–305. DOI: 10.1111/infa.12071

Hemsley, B., & Balandin, S. (2014). A metasynthesis of patient-provider communication in hospital for patients with severe communication disabilities: Informing new translational research. *Augmentative and Alternative Communication*, *30*(4), 329–343. DOI: 10.3109/07434618.2014.955614 PMID: 25229213

Henderson-King, D., & Brooks, K. D. (2009). Materialism, sociocultural appearance messages, and paternal attitudes predict college women's attitudes about cosmetic surgery. *Psychology of Women Quarterly*, *33*(1), 133–142. DOI: 10.1111/j.1471-6402.2008.01480.x

Henschke, N., Lorenz, E., Pokora, R., Michaleff, Z., Quartey, J., & Oliveira, V. (2016). Understanding cultural influences on back pain and back pain research. *Best Practice & Research. Clinical Rheumatology*, *30*(6), 1037–1049. DOI: 10.1016/j.berh.2017.08.004 PMID: 29103548

Hernandez, R., Pyatak, E., Vigen, C., Jin, H., Schneider, S., Spruijt-Metz, D., & Roll, S. (2021). Understanding worker well-being relative to high-workload and recovery activities across a whole day: Pilot testing an ecological momentary assessment technique. *International Journal of Environmental Research and Public Health*, *18*(19), 10354. DOI: 10.3390/ijerph181910354 PMID: 34639654

Herrera, M., Elgueta, R., Fernández, M., Giacoman, C., Leal, D., Marshall, P., Rubio, M., & Bustamante, F. (2021). A longitudinal study monitoring the quality of life in a national cohort of older adults in Chile before and during the Covid-19 outbreak. *BMC Geriatrics*, *21*(1), 143. Advance online publication. DOI: 10.1186/s12877-021-02110-3 PMID: 33637054

Heveran, L., & Andrewes, T. (2020). Nursing measures to support the needs of haematological cancer survivors post-treatment: A literature review. *British Journal of Nursing (Mark Allen Publishing)*, *29*(3), S18–S24. DOI: 10.12968/bjon.2020.29.3.S18 PMID: 32053451

Hickey, M., LaCroix, A. Z., Doust, J., Mishra, G. D., Sivakami, M., Garlick, D., & Hunter, M. S. (2024). An empowerment model for managing menopause. *Lancet*, *403*(10430), 947–957. DOI: 10.1016/S0140-6736(23)02799-X PMID: 38458214

Hillier, A., Greher, G., Poto, N., & Dougherty, M. (2012). Positive outcomes following participation in a music intervention for adolescents and young adults on the autism spectrum. *Psychology of Music*, *40*(2), 201–215. DOI: 10.1177/0305735610386837

Hill, J., Ziviani, J., & Driscoll, C. (2020). "the connection just happens": Therapists' perspectives of canine-assisted occupational therapy for children on the autism spectrum. *Australian Occupational Therapy Journal*, *67*(6), 550–562. DOI: 10.1111/1440-1630.12680 PMID: 32510649

Hill, J., Ziviani, J., & Driscoll, C. (2020). Canine-assisted occupational therapy for children on the autism spectrum: Parents' perspectives. *Australian Occupational Therapy Journal*, *67*(5), 427–436. DOI: 10.1111/1440-1630.12659 PMID: 32201966

Hiragami, F. (2023). Developing Skills in Intra-Workplace Rehabilitation Education: II. *Open Journal of Therapy and Rehabilitation*, *11*(3), 98–121. DOI: 10.4236/ojtr.2023.113009

Hoff, E. (2006). How social contexts support and shape language development. *Developmental Review*, *26*(1), 55–88. https://doi.org/doi:10.1016/j.dr.2005.11.002. DOI: 10.1016/j.dr.2005.11.002

Hoff, E. (2013). *Language Development* (5th ed.). Cengage Learning.

Hohenberg, M., Metri, N., Firdaus, R., Simmons, D., & Steiner, G. (2021). What we need as we get older: needs assessment for the development of a community geriatrics service in an Australian context. https://doi.org/DOI: 10.21203/rs.3.rs-156168/v1

Holm, A., Karlsson, V., Nikolajsen, L., & Dreyer, P. (2021). Strengthening and supporting nurses' communication with mechanically ventilated patients in the intensive care unit: Development of a communication intervention. *International Journal of Nursing Studies Advances*, *3*, 100025. DOI: 10.1016/j.ijnsa.2021.100025 PMID: 38746735

Hoornweg, D., Sugar, L., & Gomez, C. L. T. (2011). Cities and greenhouse gas emissions: Moving forward. *Environment and Urbanization*, *23*(1), 207–227. DOI: 10.1177/0956247810392270

Hopf, S. C., & White, D. (2021). Supporting communication access in healthcare: An interprofessional approach to training. *Perspectives of the ASHA Special Interest Groups*, *6*(4), 838–847. DOI: 10.1044/2021_PERSP-21-00120

Hoque, F., Akhter, S., & Mannan, M. (2021). Risk factors identification of speech and language delay in children in a tertiary level hospital: A pilot study. *World Journal of Advanced Research and Reviews*, *11*(1), 103–112. DOI: 10.30574/wjarr.2021.11.1.0323

Horne, A. W., & Missmer, S. A. (2022). Pathophysiology, diagnosis, and management of endometriosis. *BMJ (Clinical Research Ed.)*, *379*, e070750. DOI: 10.1136/bmj-2022-070750 PMID: 36375827

Horwitz, S. M., Irwin, J. R., Briggs-Gowan, M. J., Bosson Heenan, J. M., Mendoza, J., & Carter, A. S. (2003). Language delay in a community cohort of young children. *Journal of the American Academy of Child and Adolescent Psychiatry*, *42*(8), 932–940. DOI: 10.1097/01.CHI.0000046889.27264.5E PMID: 12874495

Hulme, C., Snowling, M. J., West, G., Lervåg, A., & Melby-Lervåg, M. (2020). Children's Language Skills Can Be Improved: Lessons From Psychological Science for Educational Policy. *Current Directions in Psychological Science*, *29*(4), 372–377. DOI: 10.1177/0963721420923684

Hume, K., Steinbrenner, J., Odom, S., Morin, K., Nowell, S., Tomaszewski, B., Szendrey, S., McIntyre, N., Yücesoy-Özkan, S., & Savage, M. (2021). Evidence-Based Practices for Children, Youth, and Young Adults with Autism: Third Generation Review. *Journal of Autism and Developmental Disorders, 51*(11), 4013–4032. DOI: 10.1007/s10803-020-04844-2 PMID: 33449225

Hunter, K. U., Schipper, M., Feng, F. Y., Lyden, T., Haxer, M., Murdoch-Kinch, C.-A., Cornwall, B., Lee, C. S. Y., Chepeha, D. B., & Eisbruch, A. (2013). Toxicities Affecting Quality Of Life After Chemo-Imrt Of Oropharyngeal Cancer: Prospective Study Of Patient-Reported, Observer-Rated, And Objective Outcomes. International Journal Of Radiation Oncology*Biology*Physics 85, 935–940. Https://Doi.Org/10.1016/J.Ijrobp.2012.08.030

Hurley-Wallace, A., Nowotny, E., Schoth, D., & Liossi, C. (2021). Online multidisciplinary interventions for paediatric chronic pain: A content analysis. *European Journal of Pain (London, England), 25*(10), 2140–2154. DOI: 10.1002/ejp.1827 PMID: 34155745

Hurtig, R., Alper, R. M., Bryant, K. N. T., Davidson, K. R., & Bilskemper, C. (2019). Improving patient safety and patient-provider communication. *Perspectives of the ASHA Special Interest Groups, 4*(5), 1017–1027. DOI: 10.1044/2019_PERS-SIG12-2019-0021 PMID: 34113718

Hutchins, S. D. (2020). SLP Brings AAC to COVID-19 Patients. *Leader Live*, https://leader.pubs.asha.org/do/10.1044/leader.LML.25062020.26/full/

Ihara, E., & Vakalahi, H. (2011). Spirituality: The essence of wellness among Tongan and Samoan elders. *Journal of Religion & Spirituality in Social Work, 30*(4), 405–421. DOI: 10.1080/15426432.2011.619916

Iliescu, M. G., Stanciu, L. E., Uzun, A. B., Cristea, A. E., Motoască, I., Irsay, L., Iliescu, D. M., Vari, T., Ciubean, A. D., Caraban, B. M., Ciufu, N., Azis, O., & Ciortea, V. M. (2024). Assessment of Integrative Therapeutic Methods for Improving the Quality of Life and Functioning in Cancer Patients—A Systematic Review. *Journal of Clinical Medicine, 13*(5), 1190. DOI: 10.3390/jcm13051190 PMID: 38592012

Insalaco, W. and Hobelmann, J. (2023). Behavioral and self-directed treatments for opioid use disorder., 730-758. https://doi.org/DOI: 10.1093/oxfordhb/9780197618431.013.26

Institute for Quality and Efficiency in Health Care (IQWiG). (2023, August 21). Overview: Food allergies. InformedHealth.org - NCBI Bookshelf. https://www.ncbi.nlm.nih.gov/books/NBK447107/

International Organization of Physiotherapists in Pelvic & Women's Health [IOP-PWH] (2013). Scope of practice. https://themamasphysio.com/wp-content/uploads/2022/01/womens_health_pt_-_scope_of_practice.pdf

International Organization of Physiotherapists in Pelvic & Women's Health [IOP-PWH], (2023). Recommendations for Education in Pelvic and Women's Health fields. https://ioppwh-website.s3.eu-west-2.amazonaws.com/IOPPWH+Education+Recommendations+June+2023.pdf

IPCC. (2022). *Climate Change 2022: Impacts, Adaptation, and Vulnerability. Contribution of Working Group II to the Sixth Assessment Report of the Intergovernmental Panel on Climate Change*. Cambridge University Press.

Jacobson, M. C. (2018). The experience of head and neck cancer survivorship (including laryngectomy): An integrated biopsychosocial model. *Current Opinion in Supportive and Palliative Care*, *12*(1), 65–73. DOI: 10.1097/SPC.0000000000000322 PMID: 29232259

James, R., Sigafoos, J., Green, V. A., Lancioni, G. E., O'Reilly, M. F., Lang, R., Davis, T., Carnett, A., Achmadi, D., Gevarter, C., & Marschik, P. B. (2015). Music therapy for individuals with autism spectrum disorder: A systematic review. *Review Journal of Autism and Developmental Disorders*, *2*(1), 39–54. DOI: 10.1007/s40489-014-0035-4

Jasemi, M., Valizadeh, L., Zamanzadeh, V., & Keogh, B. (2017). A concept analysis of holistic care by hybrid model. *Indian Journal of Palliative Care*, *23*(1), 71. DOI: 10.4103/0973-1075.197960 PMID: 28216867

Jethava, V., Kadish, J., Kakonge, L., & Wiseman-Hakes, C. (2022). Early Attachment and the Development of Social Communication: A Neuropsychological Approach. *Frontiers in Psychiatry*, *13*, 838950. DOI: 10.3389/fpsyt.2022.838950 PMID: 35463524

Jimenez-Arberas, E., Casais-Suarez, Y., Fernandez-Mendez, A., Menendez-Espina, S., Rodriguez-Menendez, S., Llosa, J. A., & Prieto-Saborit, J. A. (2024). Evidence-based implementation of the family-centered model and the use of tele-intervention in early childhood services: A systematic review. *Health Care*, *12*(1), 112. DOI: 10.3390/healthcare12010112 PMID: 38201017

Jiménez-Picón, N., Romero-Martín, M., Ponce-Blandón, J., Ramírez-Baena, L., Palomo-Lara, J., & Gómez-Salgado, J. (2021). The relationship between mindfulness and emotional intelligence as a protective factor for healthcare professionals: Systematic review. *International Journal of Environmental Research and Public Health*, *18*(10), 5491. DOI: 10.3390/ijerph18105491 PMID: 34065519

Johnson, M. (2019). The landscape of chronic pain: Broader perspectives. *Medicina, 55*(5), 182. DOI: 10.3390/medicina55050182 PMID: 31117297

Jones, H. E., Faulkner, H. R., & Losken, A. (2022). The Psychological Impact of Aesthetic Surgery: A Mini-Review. *Aesthetic Surgery Journal Open Forum*. Vol. 4 https://doi.org/DOI: 10.1093/asjof/ojac077

Jones, E., Speyer, R., Kertscher, B., Denman, D., Swan, K., & Cordier, R. (2018). Health-Related Quality of Life and Oropharyngeal Dysphagia: A Systematic Review. *Dysphagia, 33*(2), 141–172. DOI: 10.1007/s00455-017-9844-9 PMID: 28866854

Jones, K., Kearney, M., & Best, M. (2024). Effect of a spiritual care training program to build knowledge, competence, confidence and self-awareness among Australian health and aged care staff: An exploratory study. *Journal of Religion and Health, 63*(1), 274–288. DOI: 10.1007/s10943-023-01990-6 PMID: 38206559

Joo, J., & Liu, M. (2021). Nurses' barriers to caring for patients with covid-19: A qualitative systematic review. *International Nursing Review, 68*(2), 202–213. DOI: 10.1111/inr.12648 PMID: 33420749

Jullien, S. (2021). Screening for language and speech delay in children under five years. *BMC Pediatrics, 21*(S1, Suppl 1), 362. DOI: 10.1186/s12887-021-02817-7 PMID: 34496812

Jung, M., & Matthews, A. (2021). Understanding nurses' experiences and perceptions of end-of-life care for cancer patients in Korea: A scoping review. *Journal of Palliative Care, 36*(4), 255–264. DOI: 10.1177/08258597211027021 PMID: 34182840

Jurček, A. and Urek, M. (2021). Integrating the needs of LGBT+ older adults into health and social care education., 81-88. https://doi.org/DOI: 10.26493/978-961-293-129-2.81-88

Kaiser, A., Chow, J., & Cunningham, J. (2022). A Case for Early Language and Behavior Screening: Implications for Policy and Child Development. *Policy Insights from the Behavioral and Brain Sciences, 9*(1), 120–128. DOI: 10.1177/23727322211068886

Kalita, J. J., Buragohain, P., Mosahari, P. V., & Bora, U. (2019). Food allergens: Detection and management. In Apple Academic Press eBooks (pp. 243–279). DOI: 10.1201/9780429242793-11

Kang, K., & Joung, J. (2020). Outcomes of consumer involvement in mental health nursing education: An integrative review. *International Journal of Environmental Research and Public Health, 17*(18), 6756. DOI: 10.3390/ijerph17186756 PMID: 32948052

Kang, Y., & Demiris, G. (2017). Self-report pain assessment tools for cognitively intact older adults: Integrative review. *International Journal of Older People Nursing, 13*(2), e12170. Advance online publication. DOI: 10.1111/opn.12170 PMID: 28980440

Karim, M., Smith, A., Halgamuge, S., & Islam, M. (2008). A comparative study of manufacturing practices and performance variables. *International Journal of Production Economics, 112*(2), 841–859. DOI: 10.1016/j.ijpe.2007.07.005

Karthika, S., b, a., & Bakker, C. (2025). A qualitative study on psychiatric social workers in mental health profession., 150-156. https://doi.org/DOI: 10.26524/royal.228.31

Kemp, H., Laycock, H., Costello, A., & Brett, S. (2019). Chronic pain in critical care survivors: A narrative review. *British Journal of Anaesthesia, 123*(2), e372–e384. DOI: 10.1016/j.bja.2019.03.025 PMID: 31126622

Kendall, K. A., Kosek, S. R., & Tanner, K. (2014). Quality-of-life scores compared to objective measures of swallowing after oropharyngeal chemoradiation. *The Laryngoscope, 124*(3), 682–687. DOI: 10.1002/lary.24344 PMID: 23929736

Kern, P., Wolery, M., & Aldridge, D. (2007). Use of songs to promote independence in morning greeting routines for young children with autism. *Journal of Autism and Developmental Disorders, 37*(7), 1264–1271. DOI: 10.1007/s10803-006-0272-1 PMID: 17120150

Khammissa, R., Ballyram, R., Fourie, J., Bouckaert, M., Lemmer, J., & Feller, L. (2020). Selected pathobiological features and principles of pharmacological pain management. *The Journal of International Medical Research, 48*(5), 0300060520903653. Advance online publication. DOI: 10.1177/0300060520903653 PMID: 32408839

Khan, A., Spector, N. D., Baird, J. D., Ashland, M., Starmer, A. J., Rosenbluth, G., Garcia, B. M., Litterer, K. R., Rogers, J. E., Dalal, A. K., Lipsitz, S., Yoon, C. S., Zigmont, K. R., Guiot, A., O'Toole, J. K., Patel, A., Bismilla, Z., Coffey, M., Langrish, K., & Landrigan, C. P. (2018). Patient safety after implementation of a coproduced family centered communication programme: Multicenter before and after intervention study. *BMJ (Clinical Research Ed.), 363*, k4764. Advance online publication. DOI: 10.1136/bmj.k4764 PMID: 30518517

Khan, M., Banerjee, S., Muskawad, S., Maity, R., Chowdhury, S. R., Ejaz, R., Kuuzie, E., & Satnarine, T. (2024). The impact of artificial intelligence on allergy diagnosis and treatment. *Current Allergy and Asthma Reports, 24*(7), 361–372. DOI: 10.1007/s11882-024-01152-y PMID: 38954325

Khokale, R. S., Mathew, G., Ahmed, S., Maheen, S., Fawad, M., Bandaru, P., Zerin, A., Nazir, Z., Khawaja, I., Sharif, I., Abdin, Z. U., & Akbar, A. (2023). Virtual and Augmented Reality in Post-stroke Rehabilitation: A Narrative Review. *Cureus, 15*(4), e37559. DOI: 10.7759/cureus.37559 PMID: 37193429

Khor, P., Vearing, R., & Charlton, K. (2021). The effectiveness of nutrition interventions in improving frailty and its associated constructs related to malnutrition and functional decline among community-dwelling older adults: A systematic review. *Journal of Human Nutrition and Dietetics, 35*(3), 566–582. DOI: 10.1111/jhn.12943 PMID: 34494314

Kilmer, M., Hong, M., Randolph, D., Reichel, A., Huetter, S., Bowden, M., & Kilmer, C. (2024). Animal-assisted therapy in pediatric autism spectrum disorder: A case report. *The Nurse Practitioner, 49*(3), 31–39. DOI: 10.1097/01.NPR.0000000000000151 PMID: 38386471

Kim, H., Jung, S., Kim, H., & Abraham, I. (2020). Systematic review of longitudinal studies on chemotherapy-associated subjective cognitive impairment in cancer patients. *Psycho-Oncology, 29*(4), 617–631. DOI: 10.1002/pon.5339 PMID: 32017297

Kirn, D., Koochek, A., Reid, K., Berens, Å., Travison, T., Folta, S., & Fielding, R. (2015). The vitality, independence, and vigor in the elderly 2 study (vive2): Design and methods. *Contemporary Clinical Trials, 43*, 164–171. DOI: 10.1016/j.cct.2015.06.001 PMID: 26044464

Kittitongsophon, W., Wangwonsin, A., & Jariya, W. (2023). Factors influencing parents' behaviours to promote early childhood development of 1–3-year-old children with delayed language development in thailand. *Journal of Public Health Dentistry, 21*(1), 150–160. DOI: 10.55131/jphd/2023/210111

Kiyoshi-Teo, H., Northrup-Snyder, K., Davis, M., Garcia, E., Leatherwood, A., & Izumi, S. (2020). Qualitative descriptions of patient perceptions about fall risks, prevention strategies and self-identity: Analysis of fall prevention motivational interviewing conversations. *Journal of Clinical Nursing, 29*(21-22), 4281–4288. DOI: 10.1111/jocn.15465 PMID: 32810908

Klatte, S. I., Bloemen, M., Groot, A., Mantel, T. M., Ketelaar, M., & Gerrits, E. (2024). Collaborative working in speech and language therapy for children with DLD—What are parents' needs? *International Journal of Language & Communication Disorders, 59*(1), 340–353. DOI: 10.1111/1460-6984.12951 PMID: 37715545

Klatte, S. I., Ketelaar, M., Groot, A., Bloemen, M., & Gerrits, E. (2023). Collaboration: How does it work according to therapists and parents of young children? A systematic review. *Child: Care, Health and Development*, *50*(1), 1–20. DOI: 10.1111/cch.13167 PMID: 37724049

Klatte, S. I., Lyons, R., Davies, K., Harding, S., Marshall, J., McKean, C., & Roulstone, S. (2020). Collaboration between parents and SLTs produces optimal outcomes for children attending speech and language therapy: Gathering the evidence. *International Journal of Language & Communication Disorders*, *00*(0), 1–11. DOI: 10.1111/1460-6984.12538 PMID: 32383829

Klein, I., Kalichman, L., Chen, N., & Susmallian, S. (2021). A pilot study evaluating the effect of early physical therapy on pain and disabilities after breast cancer surgery: Prospective randomized control trail. *The Breast : Official Journal of the European Society of Mastology*, *59*, 286–293. DOI: 10.1016/j.breast.2021.07.013 PMID: 34340163

Koch, S. C., Riege, R. F., Tisborn, K., Biondo, J., Martin, L., & Beelmann, A. (2019). Effects of dance movement therapy and dance on health-related psychological outcomes. A meta-analysis update. *Frontiers in Psychology*, *10*, 1806. DOI: 10.3389/fpsyg.2019.01806 PMID: 31481910

Kodak, T., & Bergmann, S. (2020). Autism Spectrum Disorder: Characteristics, Associated Behaviors, and Early Intervention. *Pediatric Clinics of North America*, *67*(3), 525–535. DOI: 10.1016/j.pcl.2020.02.007 PMID: 32443991

Kokorelias, K., Gignac, M. A. M., Naglie, G., & Cameron, J. I. (2019). Towards a universal model of family centered care: A scoping review. *BMC Health Services Research*, *19*(1), 564. DOI: 10.1186/s12913-019-4394-5 PMID: 31409347

Komesidou, R., Feller, M. J., Wolter, J. A., Ricketts, J., Rasner, M. G., Putman, C. A., & Hogan, T. P. (2022). Educators' Perceptions of Barriers and Facilitators to the Implementation of Screeners for Developmental Language Disorder and Dyslexia. *Journal of Research in Reading*, *45*(3), 277–298. DOI: 10.1111/1467-9817.12381 PMID: 36250042

Konstantinou, G. N., Pampoukidou, O., Sergelidis, D., & Fotoulaki, M. (2025). Managing Food Allergies in Dining Establishments: Challenges and Innovative Solutions. *Nutrients*, *17*(10), 1737. DOI: 10.3390/nu17101737 PMID: 40431476

Kozlowski, D., Hutchinson, M., Hurley, J., Rowley, J., & Sutherland, J. (2017). The role of emotion in clinical decision making: An integrative literature review. *BMC Medical Education*, *17*(1), 255. Advance online publication. DOI: 10.1186/s12909-017-1089-7 PMID: 29246213

Kraaijenga, S. A., Lapid, O., van der Molen, L., Hilgers, F. J., Smeele, L. E., & van den Brekel, M. W. (2016). Feasibility and potential value of lipofilling in post-treatment oropharyngeal dysfunction. *The Laryngoscope*, *126*(12), 2672–2678. DOI: 10.1002/lary.26003 PMID: 27076387

Krier, J. C., Green, T. D., & Kruger, A. (2018). Youths in foster care with language delays: Prevalence, causes, and interventions. *Psychology in the Schools*, *55*(5), 523–538. DOI: 10.1002/pits.22129

Kumar, M., Sharan, S., Kishore, S., Gupta, A., & Kumar, A. (2022). Prevalence of speech and language delay in children (0-3 years) and its associated risk factors in a tertiary care teaching hospital of eastern india. *International Journal of Health Sciences*, •••, 1778–1784. DOI: 10.53730/ijhs.v6nS6.9917

Kwok, E., Bootsma, J., Cahill, P., & Rosenbaum, P. (2021). A scoping review of qualitative studies on parents' perspectives on speech, language, and communication interventions. *Disability and Rehabilitation*, *44*(25), 8084–8093. DOI: 10.1080/09638288.2021.1989061 PMID: 34669539

Kwon, C., Lee, B., Suh, H., Chung, S., & Kim, J. (2018). Efficacy and safety of auricular acupuncture for cognitive impairment and dementia: a systematic review. *Evidence-Based Complementary and Alternative Medicine*, 2018(1). https://doi.org/ DOI: 10.1155/2018/3426078

Lafer, M., Achlatis, S., Lazarus, C., Fang, Y., Branski, R. C., & Amin, M. R. (2013). Temporal measurements of deglutition in dynamic magnetic resonance imaging versus videofluoroscopy. *The Annals of Otology, Rhinology, and Laryngology*, *122*(12), 748–753. DOI: 10.1177/000348941312201204 PMID: 24592577

LaGasse, A. B. (2017). Social outcomes in children with autism spectrum disorder: A review of music therapy outcomes. *Patient Related Outcome Measures*, *8*, 23 32. DOI: 10.2147/PROM.S106267 PMID: 28260959

Landa, R. J. (2018). Efficacy of early interventions for infants and young children with, and at risk for, autism spectrum disorders. *International Review of Psychiatry (Abingdon, England)*, *30*(1), 25–39. DOI: 10.1080/09540261.2018.1432574 PMID: 29537331

Landauer, M., Juhola, S., & Söderholm, M. (2015). Inter-Relationships Between Adaptation and Mitigation: A Systematic Literature Review. *Climatic Change*, *131*(4), 505–517. DOI: 10.1007/s10584-015-1395-1

Landi, G., Pakenham, K., Boccolini, G., Grandi, S., & Tossani, E. (2020). Health anxiety and mental health outcome during Covid-19 lockdown in Italy: The mediating and moderating roles of psychological flexibility. *Frontiers in Psychology, 11*, 2195. Advance online publication. DOI: 10.3389/fpsyg.2020.02195 PMID: 32982888

Lang, H., France, E., Williams, B., Humphris, G., & Wells, M. (2013). The psychological experience of living with head and neck cancer: A systematic review and meta-synthesis. *Psycho-Oncology, 22*(12), 2648–2663. DOI: 10.1002/pon.3343 PMID: 23840037

Langner, J., & Fukkink, R. G. (2022). A realist synthesis of interprofessional collaborative practices in early intervention for children with speech, language and communication needs. *International Journal of Language & Communication Disorders, 58*(2), 516–541. DOI: 10.1111/1460-6984.12789 PMID: 36217271

Lang, R., McLay, L., & Rispoli, M. (2023). Advanced language models: Potential to improve augmentative and alternative communication for individuals with intellectual and developmental disabilities. *Advances in Neurodevelopmental Disorders, 7*(3), 481–484. DOI: 10.1007/s41252-023-00350-5

Lara-Ramos, A., Álvarez-Salvago, F., Fernández-Lao, C., Galiano-Castillo, N., Ocón-Hernández, O., Mazheika, M., Salinas-Asensio, M. M., Mundo-López, A., Arroyo-Morales, M., Cantarero-Villanueva, I., & Artacho-Cordón, F. (2021). Widespread pain hypersensitivity and lumbopelvic impairments in women diagnosed with endometriosis. *Pain Medicine, 22*(9), 1970–1981. DOI: 10.1093/pm/pnaa463 PMID: 33675228

Lauder, G. (2017). A review of intravenous lidocaine infusion therapy for paediatric acute and chronic pain management.. DOI: 10.5772/66771

LaVela, S., Heinemann, A., Etingen, B., Mišković, A., Locatelli, S., & Chen, D. (2015). Relational empathy and holistic care in persons with spinal cord injuries. *The Journal of Spinal Cord Medicine, 40*(1), 30–42. DOI: 10.1080/10790268.2015.1114227 PMID: 26833180

Law, J., McCartney, E., & Roulstone, S. (2019). *The United Kingdom Vignette in McKean C, Murphy C & Thordardottir E (eds.) Managing children with developmental language disorder: theory and practice across Europe and beyond.* Abingdon: Routledge, pp. 497-509

Law, James & Boyle, James & Harris, F & Harkness, A & Nye, C. (1998). Screening for Speech and Language Delay: A Systematic Review of the Literature. (Winchester, England). 2. 1-184. .DOI: 10.3310/hta2090

Law, J., Boyle, J., Harris, F., Harkness, A., & Nye, C. (2000). The feasibility of universal screening for primary speech and language delay: Findings from a systematic review of the literature. *Developmental Medicine and Child Neurology*, *42*(3), 190–200. DOI: 10.1111/j.1469-8749.2000.tb00069.x PMID: 10755459

Law, J., Garrett, Z., & Nye, C. (2004). The Efficacy of Treatment for Children With Developmental Speech and Language Delay/Disorder: A Meta-Analysis. *Journal of Speech, Language, and Hearing Research: JSLHR*, *47*(4), 924–943. DOI: 10.1044/1092-4388(2004/069) PMID: 15324296

Law, J., McKean, C., Murphy, C., & Thordardottir, E. (Eds.). (2019). *Managing children with developmental language disorder: Theory and practice across europe and beyond*. Routledge. DOI: 10.4324/9780429455308

Lazarus, C. L. (2009). Effects of chemoradiotherapy on voice and swallowing. *Current Opinion in Otolaryngology & Head & Neck Surgery*, *17*(3), 172–178. DOI: 10.1097/MOO.0b013e32832af12f PMID: 19337126

Lazarus, C. L., Husaini, H., Jacobson, A. S., Mojica, J. K., Buchbinder, D., Okay, D., & Urken, M. L. (2014). Development of a new lingual range-of-motion assessment scale: Normative data in surgically treated oral cancer patients. *Dysphagia*, *29*(4), 489–499. DOI: 10.1007/s00455-014-9534-9 PMID: 24810704

Lazarus, C. L., Ward, E. C., & Yiu, E. M. (2007). Speech and swallowing following oral, oropharyngeal, and nasopharyngeal cancers. In *Head and Necl Cancer - treatment, rehabilitation, and outcomes* (pp. 103–122). Plural Publishing.

Leal Filho, W., Mifsud, M., Molthan-Hill, P., & Nagy, J, G., Ávila, L.V. & Salvia, A.L. (. (2019). O ceticismo das mudanças climáticas nas universidades: Um estudo global. *Sustainability*, *11*, 2981. DOI: 10.3390/su11102981

LeBlanc, L., Belanger, S., & Andrews, D., & Charach. (2016). Take home message of Task Force report: NOT the strong recommendation against developmental screening, BUT the need for rigorous research and practice [letter]. *Canadian Medical Association Journal*, *20*(188).

Ledezma, J. M., & Correa, J. C. P. (2023). Definition and evaluation of good manufacturing practices for plastic injection molding. *Energy Efficiency*, *16*(4), 24. Advance online publication. DOI: 10.1007/s12053-023-10103-x

Lee, B., Park, S., Kwon, H. J., Hwang, G. S., & Kim, M. (2023, January 4). Integrative treatment program for the treatment of children with autism spectrum disorder: A prospective observational case series. *Frontiers in Neurology*, *13*, 1017005. DOI: 10.3389/fneur.2022.1017005 PMID: 36686506

Lee, J., Kaat, A. J., & Roberts, M. Y. (2022). Involving caregivers of autistic toddlers in early intervention: Common practice or exception to the norm? *American Journal of Speech-Language Pathology, 31*(4), 1755–1770. DOI: 10.1044/2022_AJSLP-21-00246 PMID: 35749738

Lee, J., & Porretta, D. L. (2013). Enhancing the motor skills of children with autism spectrum disorders: A pool-based approach. *Journal of Physical Education, Recreation & Dance, 84*(1), 41–45. DOI: 10.1080/07303084.2013.746154

Lee, S. (2023). Exploring the role of resilience and optimism during the covid-19 pandemic in older European adults. *Research on Aging, 45*(9-10), 643–653. DOI: 10.1177/01640275231152570 PMID: 36696282

Lee, S., Oh, E., & Hong, G. (2018). Comparison of factors associated with fear of falling between older adults with and without a fall history. *International Journal of Environmental Research and Public Health, 15*(5), 982. DOI: 10.3390/ijerph15050982 PMID: 29757960

Leeuwen, K., Loon, M., Nes, F., Bosmans, J., Vet, H., Ket, J., & Ostelo, R. (2019). What does quality of life mean to older adults? a thematic synthesis. *PLoS One, 14*(3), e0213263. DOI: 10.1371/journal.pone.0213263 PMID: 30849098

Lehrer, S. B., Ayuso, R., & Reese, G. (2002). Current understanding of food allergens. *Annals of the New York Academy of Sciences, 964*(1), 69–85. DOI: 10.1111/j.1749-6632.2002.tb04133.x PMID: 12023195

Leighton, S., Rodriguez, K., Nieforth, L., & O'Haire, M. (2023). Service dogs for autistic children and family system functioning: A constant comparative analysis. *Frontiers in Psychiatry, 14*, 1210095. Advance online publication. DOI: 10.3389/fpsyt.2023.1210095 PMID: 37520226

Leis, J., & Morrison, C. (2021). An integrative review of arts-based strategies for addressing pain and substance use disorder during the opioid crisis. *Health Promotion Practice, 22*(1, suppl), 44S–52S. DOI: 10.1177/1524839921996065 PMID: 33942641

Leite, C. S. C. (2018). *Benefícios da intervenção precoce: Perspetiva de famílias portuguesas* [Doctoral thesis, Universidade do Minho]. Repositório da Universidade do Minho. https://hdl.handle.net/1822/56328

Levey, S. (2024). *Introdution to Language Development* (3rd ed.). Plural Publishing Inc.

Levickis, P., Conway, L., Smith, J., & Bennetts, S. (2022). *Parent–Child Interaction and Its Impact on Language Development.* In J. Law, S. Reilly, & C. McKean (Eds.), Language Development: Individual Differences in a Social Context (pp. 166–192). chapter, Cambridge: Cambridge University Press. DOI: 10.1017/9781108643719.010

Levinson, W., Roter, D. L., Mullooly, J. P., Dull, V. T., & Frankel, R. M. (1997). Physician-patient communication. The relationship with malpractice claims among primary care physicians and surgeons. *Journal of the American Medical Association, 277*(7), 553–559. DOI: 10.1001/jama.1997.03540310051034 PMID: 9032162

Levy, S., & Hyman, S. (2015). Complementary and Alternative Medicine Treatments for Children with Autism Spectrum Disorders. *Child and Adolescent Psychiatric Clinics of North America, 24*(1), 117–143. DOI: 10.1016/j.chc.2014.09.004 PMID: 25455579

Lewis, P., Gaffney, R., & Wilson, N. (2017). A narrative review of acute care nurses' experiences nursing patients with intellectual disability: Underprepared, communication barriers and ambiguity about the role of caregivers. *Journal of Clinical Nursing, 26*(11-12), 1473–1484. DOI: 10.1111/jocn.13512 PMID: 27533751

Libertus, K., & Violi, D. (2016). Sit to talk: Relation between motor skills and language development in infancy. *Frontiers in Psychology, 7*. Advance online publication. DOI: 10.3389/fpsyg.2016.00475 PMID: 27065934

Li, C., Tang, N., Yang, L., Zeng, Q., Yu, T., Pu, X., Wang, J., & Zhang, H. (2023). Effect of caregiver burden on anticipatory grief among caregivers of elderly cancer patients: Chain mediation role of family functioning and resilience. *Frontiers in Psychology, 13*, 1020517. Advance online publication. DOI: 10.3389/fpsyg.2022.1020517 PMID: 36704702

Li, D., & BouZeid, E. (2013). Synergistic interactions between urban heat islands and heat waves: The impact in cities is larger than the sum of its parts. *Journal of Applied Meteorology and Climatology, 52*(9), 2051–2064. DOI: 10.1175/JAMC D-13-02.1

Lieberman, J. A., & Sicherer, S. H. (2010). The diagnosis of food allergy. *American Journal of Rhinology & Allergy, 24*(6), 439–443. DOI: 10.2500/ajra.2010.24.3515 PMID: 21144222

Lima, A., Nóbrega, H., Filho, J., Cordeiro, A., Sobral, R., & Oliveira, K. (2024). Evolution and challenges of telemedicine in children's health: an integrative review.. https://doi.org/DOI: 10.56238/sevened2023.007-086

Lim, H. A. (2010). Effect of "developmental speech and language training through music" on speech production in children with autism spectrum disorders. *Journal of Music Therapy*, *47*(1), 2–26. DOI: 10.1093/jmt/47.1.2 PMID: 20635521

Lim, H., & Draper, E. (2011). The effects of music therapy incorporated with applied behavior analysis verbal behavior approach for children with autism spectrum disorders. *Journal of Music Therapy*, *48*(4), 532–550. DOI: 10.1093/jmt/48.4.532 PMID: 22506303

Lim, S., Levickis, P., & Eadie, P. (2022). Associations between early childhood education and care (ecec) attendance, adversity and language outcomes of 2-year-olds. *Journal of Early Childhood Research*, *20*(4), 565–579. DOI: 10.1177/1476718X221087078

Lim, X., Yap, A., Mahendran, R., & Yu, J. (2021). The interplay between anxiety, fear, protective behaviors, compassion, and resilience among older adults during a covid-19 lockdown: A structural equation modeling study. *Translational Behavioral Medicine*, *11*(5), 1172–1178. DOI: 10.1093/tbm/ibaa143 PMID: 33793946

Linares-Orama, N. (2005). Language-learning disorders and youth incarceration. *Journal of Communication Disorders*, *38*(4), 311–319. DOI: 10.1016/j.jcomdis.2005.02.006 PMID: 15862813

Linders, Y. F., Lentz, L. R., Blom, W. M., Michelsen-Huisman, A., Strikwerda, J., Van Dijk, L. M., Knulst, A. C., Houben, G. F., Van Os-Medendorp, H., & Holleman, B. C. (2023). Precautionary allergen labeling: Current communication problems and potential for future improvements. *Food Control*, *147*, 109561. DOI: 10.1016/j.foodcont.2022.109561

Lindström, B., & Eriksson, M. (2020). Complexity, Reductionism and the Biomedical Model. In *Health Promotion in Health Care – Vital Theories and Research* (pp. 57–70). Springer., DOI: 10.1007/978-3-030-63135-2

Lin, I., Wang, C., Lin, Y., Chen, H., & Lin, L. (2022). Simulation-based holistic education in physiotherapy interns to increase empathy toward older adults and individuals with disabilities. *BMC Geriatrics*, *22*(1), 795. Advance online publication. DOI: 10.1186/s12877-022-03500-x PMID: 36224529

Lin, L., Li, H., Yang, J., Hao, X., Yan, S., Wang, Y., Yu, F.-T., Shi, G.-X., & Liu, C. (2021). Acupuncture for psychological disorders caused by chronic pain: A review and future directions. *Frontiers in Neuroscience*, *14*, 626497. Advance online publication. DOI: 10.3389/fnins.2020.626497 PMID: 33584181

Linstone, H. A., & Turoff, M. (2002). *The Delphi Method: techniques and applications*. Listone and Turof.

Li, P., Sheng, L., Ye, Y., Wang, J. S., Geng, S., Ning, D., & Sun, X. (2025). Allergenicity of alternative proteins: research hotspots, new findings, evaluation strategies, regulatory status, and future trends: a bibliometric analysis. *Critical Reviews in Food Science and Nutrition*, *65*(9), 1749–1760. DOI: 10.1080/10408398.2023.2299748 PMID: 38189352

Liszkowski, U. (2011). Three lines in the emergence of prelinguistic communication and social cognition. *Journal of Cognitive Education and Psychology*, *10*(1), 32–43. DOI: 10.1891/1945-8959.10.1.32

Liu, W., Yang, Q., Wang, Z., Wang, J., Min, F., Yuan, J., Tong, P., Li, X., Wu, Y., Gao, J., & Chen, H. (2025). Quantitative food allergen risk assessment: Evolving concepts, modern approaches, and industry implications. *Comprehensive Reviews in Food Science and Food Safety*, *24*(2), e70132. DOI: 10.1111/1541-4337.70132 PMID: 39929606

Liu, X. L., Zahrt, D. M., & Simms, M. D. (2018). An Interprofessional Team Approach to the Differential Diagnosis of Children with Language Disorders. *Pediatric Clinics of North America*, *65*(1), 73–90. DOI: 10.1016/j.pcl.2017.08.022 PMID: 29173721

Liu, Y. C., Hung, T. T., Konara Mudiyanselage, S. P., Wang, C. J., & Lin, M. F. (2022). Beneficial Exercises for Cancer-Related Fatigue among Women with Breast Cancer: A Systematic Review and Network Meta-Analysis. *Cancers (Basel)*, *15*(1), 151. DOI: 10.3390/cancers15010151 PMID: 36612147

Llambias, C., Magill-Evans, J., Smith, V., & Warren, S. (2016). Equine-assisted occupational therapy: Increasing engagement for children with autism spectrum disorder. The American journal of occupational therapy, 70(6), 7006220040p1-7006220040p9. DOI: 10.5014/ajot.2016.020701

Locke, J., Lawson, G., Beidas, R., Aarons, G., Xie, M., Lyon, A., Stahmer, A., Seidman, M., Frederick, L., Oh, C., Spaulding, C., Dorsey, S., & Mandell, D. (2019). Individual and organizational factors that affect implementation of evidence-based practices for children with autism in public schools: A cross-sectional observational study. *Implementation Science : IS*, *14*(1), 29. DOI: 10.1186/s13012-019-0877-3 PMID: 30866976

Lokapavani, Y., Krishna, S. R., & Madhavi, K. (2014). Influence of pre operative physical therapy education and exercise on post operative shoulder range of motion and functional activites in subjects with modified radical mastectomy. *International Journal of Physiotherapy*, *1*(4), 170–177. DOI: 10.15621/ijphy/2014/v1i4/54556

López-Calvo, R., Montero-Barrantes, M., González-Vargas, M., Henderson-García, M., & Víquez-Barrantes, D. (2025). Allergen Management in Costa Rican Food Industries: Challenges and Future Actions. *Food and Humanity*, *100502*, 100502. Advance online publication. DOI: 10.1016/j.foohum.2025.100502

Lopez, K. M. J., Lyons, R., Novogrodsky, R., Baena, S., Feilberg, J., Harding, S., Kelić, M., Klatte, I. S., Mantel, T. C., Tomazin, M. O., Ulfsdottir, T. S., Zajdó, K., & Rodriguez-Ortiz, I. R. (2021). Exploring parental perspectives of childhood speech and language disorders across 10 countries: A pilot qualitative study. *Journal of Speech, Language, and Hearing Research: JSLHR*, *64*(5), 1739–1747. DOI: 10.1044/2020_JSLHR-20-00415 PMID: 33823117

López-Liria, R., Torres-Álamo, L., Vega-Ramírez, F. A., García-Luengo, A. V., Aguilar-Parra, J. M., Trigueros-Ramos, R., & Rocamora-Pérez, P. (2021). Efficacy of Physiotherapy Treatment in Primary Dysmenorrhea: A Systematic Review and Meta-Analysis. *International Journal of Environmental Research and Public Health*, *18*(15), 7832. DOI: 10.3390/ijerph18157832 PMID: 34360122

Lousada, M., Valente, A., & Mendes, A. (2017). Validation of a Paediatric Speech and Language Screening (RALF). *Folia Phoniatrica et Logopaedica*, *68*(6), 247–251. DOI: 10.1159/000479928 PMID: 29176312

Luby, J. L., Gaffrey, M. S., Tillman, R., April, L. M., & Belden, A. C. (2014). Trajectories of preschool disorders to full DSM depression at school age and early adolescence: Continuity of preschool depression. *The American Journal of Psychiatry*, *171*(7), 768–776. DOI: 10.1176/appi.ajp.2014.13091198 PMID: 24700355

Lumley, M., & Schubiner, H. (2019). Psychological therapy for centralized pain: An integrative assessment and treatment model. *Psychosomatic Medicine*, *81*(2), 114–124. DOI: 10.1097/PSY.0000000000000654 PMID: 30461545

Luo, H., Li, J., Zhang, Q., Cao, P., Ren, X., Fang, A., Liao, H., & Liu, L. (2018). Obesity and the onset of depressive symptoms among middle-aged and older adults in China: Evidence from the CHARLS. *BMC Public Health*, *18*(1), 909. DOI: 10.1186/s12889-018-5834-6 PMID: 30041632

Luze, G. J., Linebarger, D. L., Greenwood, C. R., Carta, J. J., Walker, D., Leitschuh, C., & Atwater, J. B. (2001). Developing a general outcome measure of growth in expressive communication of infants and toddlers. *School Psychology Review*, *30*(3), 383–406. DOI: 10.1080/02796015.2001.12086122

Lyons, N., Cooper, C., & Lloyd-Evans, B. (2021). A systematic review and meta-analysis of group peer support interventions for people experiencing mental health conditions. *BMC Psychiatry, 21*(1), 315. Advance online publication. DOI: 10.1186/s12888-021-03321-z PMID: 34162340

Lyons, S. A., Burney, P. G., Ballmer-Weber, B. K., Fernandez-Rivas, M., Barreales, L., Clausen, M., Dubakiene, R., Fernandez-Perez, C., Fritsche, P., Jedrzejczak-Czechowicz, M., Kowalski, M. L., Kralimarkova, T., Kummeling, I., Mustakov, T. B., Lebens, A. F., Van Os-Medendorp, H., Papadopoulos, N. G., Popov, T. A., Sakellariou, A., & Le, T. (2019). Food allergy in adults: Substantial variation in prevalence and causative foods across Europe. Journal of Allergy and Clinical Immunology. In Practice/ the œJournal of Allergy and Clinical Immunology. *In Practice, 7*(6), 1920–1928.e11. DOI: 10.1016/j.jaip.2019.02.044 PMID: 30898689

MacGuillion, M., Pine, J., Herbert, J., & Matthews, D. (2017). A randomised controlled trial to test the effect of promoting caregiver contingent talk on language development in infants from diverse socioeconomic status backgrounds. *Journal of Child Psychology and Psychiatry, and Allied Disciplines, 58*(10), 1122–1131. DOI: 10.1111/jcpp.12725 PMID: 28429816

Madigan, S., Prime, H., Graham, S. A., Rodrigues, M., Anderson, N., Khoury, J., & Jenkins, J. M. (2019). Parenting behavior and child language: A meta-analysis. *Pediatrics, 144*(4), e20183556. DOI: 10.1542/peds.2018-3556 PMID: 31551396

Madya, R., Malik, M., & Suparno, S. (2019). The impact of socioeconomic status (SES) on early childhood language development. *Advances in Social Science, Education and Humanities Research, 296*, 140–145. DOI: 10.2991/icsie-18.2019.26

Maenner MJ, Warren Z, Williams AR, Amoakohene E, Bakian AV, Bilder DA, Durkin MS, Fitzgerald RT, Furnier SM, Hughes MM, Ladd-Acosta CM, McArthur D, Pas ET, Salinas A, Vehorn A, Williams S, Esler A, Grzybowski A, Hall-Lande J, Nguyen RHN, Pierce K, Zahorodny W, Hudson A, Hallas L, Mancilla KC, Patrick M, Shenouda J, Sidwell K, DiRienzo M, Gutierrez J, Spivey MH, Lopez M, Pettygrove S, Schwenk YD, Washington A, Shaw KA. (2023) Prevalence and Characteristics of Autism Spectrum Disorder Among Children Aged 8 Years - Autism and Developmental Disabilities Monitoring Network, 11 Sites, United States, 2020. MMWR Surveill Summ. 24;72(2):1-14. . PMID: 36952288; PMCID: PMC10042614.DOI: 10.15585/mmwr.ss7202a1

Maenner, M. J., Shaw, K. A., Bakian, A. V., Bilder, D. A., Durkin, M. S., Esler, A., Furnier, S. M., Hallas, L., Hall-Lande, J., Hudson, A., Hughes, M. M., Patrick, M., Pierce, K., Poynter, J. N., Salinas, A., Shenouda, J., Vehorn, A., Warren, Z., Constantino, J. N., & Cogswell, M. E. (2021, December 3). Prevalence and Characteristics of Autism Spectrum Disorder Among Children Aged 8 Years - Autism and Developmental Disabilities Monitoring Network, 11 Sites, United States, 2018. *MMWR. Surveillance Summaries, 70*(11), 1–16. DOI: 10.15585/mmwr.ss7011a1 PMID: 34855725

Maestas, N., Mullen, K., & Powell, D. (2016). The effect of population aging on economic growth, the labor force and productivity.. https://doi.org/DOI: 10.3386/w22452

Maguire, D., McCormack, D., Downes, C., Teggart, T., & Fosker, T. (2021). The impact of care-related factors on the language and communication needs of looked after and adopted children/young people. *Developmental Child Welfare, 3*(3), 235–255. DOI: 10.1177/25161032211021436

Mahoney, G., & MacDonald, J. D. (2007a). *Autism and developmental delays in young children: The responsive teaching curriculum for parents and professionals, Curriculum guide*. Pro-ed.

Mahoney, G., & MacDonald, J. D. (2007b). Autism and developmental delays in young children. [file:///C:/Users/Utilizador/Downloads/Autism_and_Developmental_Delays_in_Young_Children.pdf]. *International Journal of Early Childhood Special Education, 1*, 1.

Mahoney, N., Wilson, N., Buchanan, A., Milbourn, B., Hoey, C., & Cordier, R. (2019). Older male mentors: Outcomes and perspectives of an intergenerational mentoring program for young adult males with intellectual disability. *Health Promotion Journal of Australia, 31*(1), 16–25. DOI: 10.1002/hpja.250 PMID: 30959560

Ma, J., Yu, J., Jia, Y., Luo, Z., Yang, X., Li, H., & Long, F. (2025). Fermented Apple Juice Reduces the Susceptibility of Offspring Mice to Food Allergy Exacerbated by Maternal High-Fat Diet. *Nutrients, 17*(11), 1927. DOI: 10.3390/nu17111927 PMID: 40507196

Major allergens: The Big Nine – School Nutrition Association. (2022). School Nutrition Association. https://schoolnutrition.org/resource/major-allergens-the-big-nine/

Maksimović, S., Marisavljević, M., Stanojević, N., Ćirović, M., Punišić, S., Adamović, T., Đorđević, J., Krgović, I., & Subotić, M. (2023). Importance of Early Intervention in Reducing Autistic Symptoms and Speech-Language Deficits in Children with Autism

Malcolm, R., Ecks, S., & Pickersgill, M. (2017). 'it just opens up their world': Autism, empathy, and the therapeutic effects of equine interactions. *Anthropology & Medicine, 25*(2), 220–234. DOI: 10.1080/13648470.2017.1291115 PMID: 28513182

Mallari, B., Spaeth, E., Goh, H., & Boyd, B. (2019). Virtual reality as an analgesic for acute and chronic pain in adults: A systematic review and meta-analysis. *Journal of Pain Research, 12*, 2053–2085. DOI: 10.2147/JPR.S200498 PMID: 31308733

Malta, F. S., & Marques, C. (2021). E. Socio-Environmental Vulnerability Index: An Application to Rio de Janeiro-Brazil. *International Journal of Public Health, 66*, 1–11. DOI: 10.3389/ijph.2021.584308 PMID: 34744556

Manduchi, B., Che, Z., Ringash, J. G., Fitch, M. I., Howell, D., & Martino, R. (2024). Patient-reported outcome measures for dysphagia in head and neck cancer: A systematic review and appraisal of content validity and internal structure. *Head & Neck, 46*(4), 951–972. DOI: 10.1002/hed.27693 PMID: 38356437

Manikantan, K., Khode, S., Sayed, S. I., Roe, J., Nutting, C. M., Rhys-Evans, P., Harrington, K. J., & Kazi, R. (2009). Dysphagia in head and neck cancer. *Cancer Treatment Reviews, 35*(8), 724–732. DOI: 10.1016/j.ctrv.2009.08.008 PMID: 19751966

Manso, M. (2010). Pragmatic language development and educational style in neglected children. *Children and Youth Services Review, 32*(7), 1028–1034. DOI: 10.1016/j.childyouth.2010.04.008

Manso, M. (2012). Morphosyntactic development and educational style of parents in neglected children. *Children and Youth Services Review, 34*(1), 311–315. DOI: 10.1016/j.childyouth.2011.10.028

Manso, M., García-Baamonde, M. E., & Alonso, M. B. (2011). Design of a language stimulation program for children suffering abuse. *Children and Youth Services Review, 33*(7), 1325–1331. DOI: 10.1016/j.childyouth.2011.03.003

Marks, K. P., & Glascoe, F. P. (2016, February 1). USPSTF did not "connect the dots" between early detection and intervention. Pediatrics. *American Academy of Pediatrics*. DOI: 10.1542/peds.2015-4039A

Marquez-Garcia, A. V., Magnuson, J., Morris, J., Iarocci, G., Doesburg, S., & Moreno, S. (2021). Music therapy in autism spectrum disorder: A systematic review. *Review Journal of Autism and Developmental Disorders, 9*(2), 1–17.

Martin, C., Bakker, C., Breth, M., Gao, G., Lee, K., Lee, M., Tiase, V. L., Tunby, L. J., Wyatt, T. H., & Janeway, L. (2020). The efficacy of mobile health interventions used to manage acute or chronic pain: A systematic review. *Research in Nursing & Health*, *44*(1), 111–128. DOI: 10.1002/nur.22097 PMID: 33341989

Masek, L. R., McMillan, B. T. M., Paterson, S. J., Tamis-LeMonda, C. S., Golinkoff, R. M., Hirsh-Pasek, K. (2021) Where language meets attention: How contingent interactions promote learning. *Developmental Review*, 60, 0273-2297. DOI: 10.1016/j.dr.2021.100961

Masini E, Loi E, Vega-Benedetti AF, Carta M, Doneddu G, Fadda R, Zavattari P. (2020) An Overview of the Main Genetic, Epigenetic and Environmental Factors Involved in Autism Spectrum Disorder Focusing on Synaptic Activity. Int J Mol Sci. 5;21(21):8290. . PMID: 33167418; PMCID: PMC7663950.DOI: 10.3390/ijms21218290

Mas, J. M., Canadas, M., Balcells-Balcells, A., Gine, C., Serrano, A. M., & Dunst, C. J. (2018). Psychometric properties of the Spanish version of the family-centred practices scale for use with families of young children receiving early childhood intervention. *Journal of Applied Research in Intellectual Disabilities*, *31*(5), 851–861. DOI: 10.1111/jar.12442 PMID: 29532976

Mataqi, M., & Aslanpour, Z. (2019). Factors influencing palliative care in advanced dementia: A systematic review. *BMJ Supportive & Palliative Care*, *10*(2), 145–156. DOI: 10.1136/bmjspcare-2018-001692 PMID: 30944119

Mateos-Moreno, D., & Atencia-Doña, L. (2013). Effect of a combined dance/movement and music therapy on young adults diagnosed with severe autism. *The Arts in Psychotherapy*, *40*(5), 465–472. DOI: 10.1016/j.aip.2013.09.004

Math, S., Nirmala, M., Moirangthem, S., & Kumar, N. (2015). Disaster management: Mental health perspective. *Indian Journal of Psychological Medicine*, *37*(3), 261–271. DOI: 10.4103/0253-7176.162915 PMID: 26664073

McFadd, E. D., & Hustad, K. C. (2020). Communication modes and functions in children with cerebral palsy. *Journal of Speech, Language, and Hearing Research: JSLHR*, *63*(6), 1776–1792. DOI: 10.1044/2020_JSLHR-19-00228 PMID: 32459163

McGuire, D., Kaiser, K., Haisfield-Wolfe, M., & Iyamu, F. (2016). Pain assessment in noncommunicative adult palliative care patients. *The Nursing Clinics of North America*, *51*(3), 397–431. DOI: 10.1016/j.cnur.2016.05.009 PMID: 27497016

McHorney, C. A., Bricker, D. E., Kramer, A. E., Rosenbek, J. C., Robbins, J., Chignell, K. A., Logemann, J. A., & Clarke, C.Conceptual Foundation and Item Development. (2000). The SWAL-QOL outcomes tool for oropharyngeal dysphagia in adults: I. Conceptual foundation and item development. *Dysphagia*, *15*(3), 115–121. DOI: 10.1007/s004550010012 PMID: 10839823

McHorney, C. A., Bricker, D. E., Robbins, J., Kramer, A. E., Rosenbek, J. C., & Chignell, K. A. (2000). The SWAL-QOL outcomes tool for oropharyngeal dysphagia in adults: II. Item reduction and preliminary scaling. *Dysphagia*, *15*(3), 122–133. DOI: 10.1007/s004550010013 PMID: 10839824

McHorney, C. A., Robbins, J., Lomax, K., Rosenbek, J. C., Chignell, K., Kramer, A. E., & Bricker, D. E. (2002). The SWAL-QOL and SWAL-CARE outcomes tool for oropharyngeal dysphagia in adults: III. Documentation of reliability and validity. *Dysphagia*, *17*(2), 97–114. DOI: 10.1007/s00455-001-0109-1 PMID: 11956835

McKean, C., Reilly, S., Bavin, E., Bretherton, L., Cini, E., Conway, L., Cook, F., Eadie, P., Prior, M., Wake, M., & Mensah, F. (2017). Language outcomes at 7 years: Early predictors and co-occurring difficulties. *Pediatrics*, *139*(3), e20161684. Advance online publication. DOI: 10.1542/peds.2016-1684 PMID: 28179482

McKenna, D. H.Jr, Sumstad, D., Bostrom, N., Kadidlo, D. M., Fautsch, S., McNearney, S., DeWaard, R., McGlave, P. B., Weisdorf, D. J., Wagner, J. E., McCullough, J., & Miller, J. S. (2007). Good manufacturing practices production of natural killer cells for immunotherapy: A six-year single-institution experience. *Transfusion*, *47*(3), 520–528. DOI: 10.1111/j.1537-2995.2006.01145.x PMID: 17319835

McLeod, S., & Harrison, L. J. (2009). Epidemiology of speech and language impairment in a nationally representative sample of 4- to 5-year-old children. *Journal of Speech, Language, and Hearing Research: JSLHR*, *52*(5), 1213–1229. DOI: 10.1044/1092-4388(2009/08-0085) PMID: 19403947

McMaughan, D., Oloruntoba, O., & Smith, M. (2020). Socioeconomic status and access to healthcare: Interrelated drivers for healthy aging. *Frontiers in Public Health*, *8*, 231. Advance online publication. DOI: 10.3389/fpubh.2020.00231 PMID: 32626678

Mcnally, S., & Quigley, J. (2014). An irish cohort study of risk and protective factors for infant language development at 9 months. *Infant and Child Development*, *23*(6), 634–649. DOI: 10.1002/icd.1861

Meehan, E., & Carter, B. (2021). Moving with pain: What principles from somatic practices can offer to people living with chronic pain. *Frontiers in Psychology*, *11*, 620381. Advance online publication. DOI: 10.3389/fpsyg.2020.620381 PMID: 33569028

Mehanna, H., West, C. M., Nutting, C., & Paleri, V. (2010). Head and neck cancer—Part 2: Treatment and prognostic factors. *BMJ (Clinical Research Ed.)*, *341*(sep28 2), c4690. DOI: 10.1136/bmj.c4690 PMID: 20876637

Melgarejo, M., Lind, T., Stadnick, N., Helm, J., & Locke, J. (2020). Strengthening Capacity for Implementation of Evidence-Based Practices for Autism in Schools: The Roles of Implementation Climate, School Leadership and Fidelity. *The American Psychologist*, *75*(8), 1105–1115. DOI: 10.1037/amp0000649 PMID: 33252948

Melo, L., Silva, B., Nitschke, R., & Viegas, S. (2023). Virtual social networks and health technologies in the daily life of clients and households: Care and health promotion. *Ciencia & Saude Coletiva*, *28*(8), 2193–2202. DOI: 10.1590/1413-81232023288.05252023 PMID: 37531528

Memaryan, N., Rassouli, M., & Mehrabi, M. (2016). Spirituality concept by health professionals in Iran: a qualitative study. *Evidence-Based Complementary and Alternative Medicine*, 2016(1). https://doi.org/DOI: 10.1155/2016/8913870

Menezes, C., Silva, A., Santos, A., Gonçalves, D., Teles, E., Silva, E., … & Maciel, K. (2024). Colágeno como agente de mudança na osteoartrite: perspectivas de uma revisão integrativa.. https://doi.org/DOI: 10.58871/CONSAMU24.C43

Mercer, J. (2013). Holding therapy: A harmful mental health intervention. *Focus on Alternative and Complementary Therapies*, *18*(2), 70–76. DOI: 10.1111/fct.12024

Mercier, J., Dumoulin, C., & Carrier-Noreau, G. (2023). Pelvic floor muscle rehabilitation for genitourinary syndrome of menopause: Why, how and when? *Climacteric*, *26*(4), 302–308. DOI: 10.1080/13697137.2023.2194527 PMID: 37019140

Merle, J. L., Cook, C. R., Locke, J. J., Ehrhart, M. G., Brown, E. C., Davis, C. J., & Lyon, A. R. (2023). Teacher attitudes toward evidence-based practices: Exploratory and confirmatory analyses of the school-adapted evidence-based practice attitude scale. *Implementation Research and Practice*, *4*, 26334895221151026. Advance online publication. DOI: 10.1177/26334895221151026 PMID: 37091537

Mesko, P. J., Eliades, A. B., Christ-Libertin, C., & Shelestak, D. (2011). Use of picture communication aids to assess pain location in pediatric postoperative patients. *Journal of Perianesthesia Nursing*, *26*(6), 395–404. DOI: 10.1016/j.jopan.2011.09.006 PMID: 22099132

Messing, B. P., Ward, E. C., Lazarus, C., Ryniak, K., Kim, M., Silinonte, J., Gold, D., Thompson, C. B., Pitman, K. T., Blanco, R., Sobel, R., Harrer, K., Ulmer, K., Neuner, G., Patel, K., Tang, M., & Lee, G. (2019). Establishing a Multidisciplinary Head and Neck Clinical Pathway: An Implementation Evaluation and Audit of Dysphagia-Related Services and Outcomes. *Dysphagia*, *34*(1), 89–104. DOI: 10.1007/s00455-018-9917-4 PMID: 29922848

Milazzo, T., Yuan, M., Graham, A., Kim, P., Gallo, L., Uhlman, K., Thoma, A., Coroneos, C., & Voineskos, S. (2024). Reporting of patient-reported outcomes amongst randomized clinical trials in plastic surgery: A systematic review using CONSORT-PRO. *Journal of Plastic, Reconstructive & Aesthetic Surgery; JPRAS*, *99*, 110–121. DOI: 10.1016/j.bjps.2024.09.022 PMID: 39368267

Mileu, N., & Queirós, M. (2018). Integrating risk assessment into spatial planning: Risk The decision support system. *ISPRS International Journal of Geo-Information*, *7*(5), 184–202. DOI: 10.3390/ijgi7050184

Milsom, I., Altman, D., Cartwright, R., Lapitan, M., Nelson, R., Sjöström, S., & Tikkinen, K. (2023). Epidemiology of urinary incontinence (UI) and other lower urinary tract symptoms (LUTS), pelvic organ prolapse (POP) and anal (AI) incontinence. In: L. Cardozo, E. Rovner, A. Wagg, A. Wein, P. Abrams (Eds.) 7th International Consultation on Incontinence. International Continence Society. https://www.ics.org/ici7/session/7310

Moller, A. S., Odell-Miller, H., & Wigram, T. (2002). Indications in music therapy: Evidence from assessment that can identify the expectations of music therapy as a treatment for autistic spectrum disorder (ASD); meeting the challenge of evidence based practice. *British Journal of Music Therapy*, *16*(1), 11–28. DOI: 10.1177/135945750201600104

Monaci, L., De Angelis, E., Montemurro, N., & Pilolli, R. (2018). Comprehensive overview and recent advances in proteomics MS based methods for food allergens analysis. *Trends in Analytical Chemistry*, *106*, 21–36. DOI: 10.1016/j.trac.2018.06.016

Mondal, A., Sharma, R., Abiha, U., Ahmad, F., Karan, A. L., Jayaraj, R., & Sundar, V. (2023). A Spectrum of Solutions: Unveiling Non-Pharmacological Approaches to Manage Autism Spectrum Disorder. ncbi.nlm.nih.gov

Mondal, N., Bhat, B., Plakkal, N., Thulasingam, M., Ajayan, P., & Poorna, D. (2016). Prevalence and risk factors of speech and language delay in children less than three years of age. *Journal of Comprehensive Pediatrics*, *7*(2). Advance online publication. DOI: 10.17795/compreped-33173

Mora, C. T. E., García, L. R., & Sánchez, F. A. G. (2023). *Guía de intervención logopédica en atención temprana centrada en la familia*. Editorial Síntesis.

Moreira, M. O. (2020). A Comunicação como um direito humano. *Revista Científica Multidisciplinar Núcleo do Conhecimento, 4*(6), 17-35. https://www.nucleodoconhecimento.com.br/comunicacao/direito-humano

Moreland, B., Durbin, L., Kasper, J., & Mielenz, T. (2018). Rehabilitation utilization for falls among community-dwelling older adults in the United States in the national health and aging trends study. *Archives of Physical Medicine and Rehabilitation, 99*(8), 1568–1575. DOI: 10.1016/j.apmr.2018.02.009 PMID: 29545001

Morgan, S., & O'Byrne, D. A. (2023). How Autism Assistance Canines Enhance the Lives of Autistic Children. INQUIRY. *Inquiry : a Journal of Medical Care Organization, Provision and Financing, 60*, 00469580231195029. Advance online publication. DOI: 10.1177/00469580231195029 PMID: 37615078

Morone, N. (2019). Not just mind over matter: Reviewing with patients how mindfulness relieves chronic low back pain. *Journal of Evidence-based Integrative Medicine, 24*, 2515690X19838490. Advance online publication. DOI: 10.1177/2515690X19838490 PMID: 30942087

Mortada (2024) Evidence-Based Complementary and Alternative Medicine in Current Medical Practice. Cureus 16(1): e52041. DOI DOI: 10.7759/cureus.52041

Moser, C. O. N. (1998). The asset vulnerability framework: Reassessing urban poverty reduction strategies. *World Development, 26*(1), 1–19. DOI: 10.1016/S0305-750X(97)10015-8

Moustakas, C. (1994). *Phenomenological research methods*. SAGE Publications. DOI: 10.4135/9781412995658

Mtewa, A. G., Chikowe, I., Kumar, S., Ngwira, K. J., & Lampiao, F. (2020). Good manufacturing practices and safety issues in functional food industries. In Springer eBooks (pp. 613–628). DOI: 10.1007/978-3-030-42319-3_27

Muhinyi, A., & Rowe, M. L. (2019). Shared reading with preverbal infants and later language development. *Journal of Applied Developmental Psychology, 64*, 101053. Advance online publication. DOI: 10.1016/j.appdev.2019.101053

Mulcair, G., Pietranton, A. A., & Williams, C. (2018). The international communication project: Raising global awareness of communication as a human right. *International Journal of Speech-Language Pathology, 20*(1), 34–38. DOI: 10.1080/17549507.2018.1422023 PMID: 29355390

Murniati, N., Al Aufa, B., Kusuma, D., & Kamso, S. (2022). A scoping review on biopsychosocial predictors of mental health among older adults. *International Journal of Environmental Research and Public Health, 19*(17), 10789. DOI: 10.3390/ijerph191710909 PMID: 36078627

Murray, S., & Hopf, S. C. (2022). Attitudes toward the use of low-tech AAC in acute settings: A systematized review. *Augmentative and Alternative Communication, 38*(3), 184–195. DOI: 10.1080/07434618.2022.2122870 PMID: 36128661

Music Therapy Handbook. https://books.google.pt/books?hl=pt-PT&lr=&id=mfnhBQAAQBAJ&oi=fnd&pg=PP1&dq=music+therapy&ots=0l7lwb413X&sig=y6-8hXKsOXS9OVzKMYrPO4YasKM&redir_esc=y#v=onepage&q=music%20therapy&f=false

Muthukumar, J., Selvasekaran, P., Lokanadham, M., & Chidambaram, R. (2020). Food and food products associated with food allergy and food intolerance – An overview. *Food Research International, 138*, 109780. DOI: 10.1016/j.foodres.2020.109780 PMID: 33288166

Mytko, A. (2024). *Vulnerabilidade do sistema urbano costeiro frente a ameaças relacionadas à mudança climática*. PUC-Rio. DOI: 10.17771/PUCRio.acad.68292

Nader, T., Rothenberg, S., Averbach, R., Charles, B., Fields, J. Z., & Schneider, R. H. (2000). Improvements in chronic diseases with a comprehensive natural medicine approach: A review and case series. *Behavioral Medicine (Washington, D.C.), 26*(1), 34–46. DOI: 10.1080/08964280009595751 PMID: 10971882

Nahin, R., Boineau, R., Khalsa, P., Stussman, B., & Weber, W. (2016). Evidence-based evaluation of complementary health approaches for pain management in the United States. *Mayo Clinic Proceedings, 91*(9), 1292–1306. DOI: 10.1016/j.mayocp.2016.06.007 PMID: 27594189

Nascimento, S. L., Surita, F. G., & Cecatti, J. G. (2012). Physical exercise during pregnancy: A systematic review. *Current Opinion in Obstetrics & Gynecology, 24*(6), 387–394. DOI: 10.1097/GCO.0b013e328359f131 PMID: 23014142

Nath, S. (2024, July 19). (2024). Advancements in food quality monitoring: Integrating biosensors for precision detection. [RSC Publishing]. *Sustainable Food Technology, 2*(4), 976–992. Advance online publication. DOI: 10.1039/D4FB00094C

Naughton, C. A. (2018). Patient-centered communication. *Pharmacy (Basel, Switzerland), 6*(1), 18–25. DOI: 10.3390/pharmacy6010018 PMID: 29438295

Navarro-Brazález, B., Vergara-Pérez, F., Prieto-Gómez, V., Sánchez-Sánchez, B., Yuste-Sánchez, M. J., & Torres-Lacomba, M. (2021). What influences women to adhere to pelvic floor exercises after physiotherapy treatment? A qualitative study for individualized pelvic health care. *Journal of Personalized Medicine*, *11*(12), 1368. DOI: 10.3390/jpm11121368 PMID: 34945840

Nawabi, F., Krebs, F., Vennedey, V., Shukri, A., Lorenz, L., & Stock, S. (2021). Health Literacy in Pregnant Women: A Systematic Review. *International Journal of Environmental Research and Public Health*, *18*(7), 3847. DOI: 10.3390/ijerph18073847 PMID: 33917631

Ndubisi, N. O., Jantan, M., Hing, L. C., & Ayub, M. S. (2005). Supplier selection and management strategies and manufacturing flexibility. *Journal of Enterprise Information Management*, *18*(3), 330–349. DOI: 10.1108/17410390510592003

Neil-Sztramko, S., Teggart, K., Moore, C., Sherifali, D., Fitzpatrick-Lewis, D., Coletta, G., Phillips, S. M., Newbold, K. B., Alvarez, E., Kuspinar, A., Kennedy, C. C., Santaguida, P. L., & Ganann, R. (2022). Community-based group physical activity and/or nutrition interventions to promote mobility in older adults: An umbrella review. *BMC Geriatrics*, *22*(1), 539. Advance online publication. DOI: 10.1186/s12877-022-03170-9 PMID: 35768770

Nekhlyudov, L., Lacchetti, C., Davis, N. B., Garvey, T. Q., Goldstein, D. P., Nunnink, J. C., Ninfea, J. I. R., Salner, A. L., Salz, T., & Siu, L. L. (2017). Head and Neck Cancer Survivorship Care Guideline: American Society of Clinical Oncology Clinical Practice Guideline Endorsement of the American Cancer Society Guideline. *Journal of Clinical Oncology*, *35*(14), 1606–1621. DOI: 10.1200/JCO.2016.71.8478 PMID: 28240970

Nettleton, S., Woods, B., Burrows, R., & Kerr, A. (2009). Food allergy and food intolerance: Towards a sociological agenda. *Health*, *13*(6), 647–664. DOI: 10.1177/1363459308341433 PMID: 19841024

New test improves diagnosis of allergies. (2024, October 24). ScienceDaily. https://www.sciencedaily.com/releases/2024/10/241015141449.htm

News-Medical. (2024, February 23). The future of food allergy Management: New technologies and treatments. https://www.news-medical.net/health/The-Future-of-Food-Allergy-Management-New-Technologies-and-Treatments.aspx

Newton, E. R., & May, L. (2017). Adaptation of Maternal-Fetal Physiology to Exercise in Pregnancy: The Basis of Guidelines for Physical Activity in Pregnancy. *Clinical medicine insights. Women's health*, *10*, 1179562X17693224. https://doi.org/DOI: 10.1177/1179562X17693224

Nicolau, C., Mendes, L., Ciríaco, M., Ferreira, B., Baixinho, C. L., Fonseca, C., Ferreira, R., & Sousa, L. (2022). Educational Intervention in Rehabilitation to Improve Functional Capacity after Hip Arthroplasty: A Scoping Review. *Journal of Personalized Medicine*, *12*(5), 656. DOI: 10.3390/jpm12050656 PMID: 35629079

Niknejad, B., Bolier, R., Henderson, C.Jr, Delgado, D., Kozlov, E., Löckenhoff, C., & Reid, M. (2018). Association between psychological interventions and chronic pain outcomes in older adults. *JAMA Internal Medicine*, *178*(6), 830. DOI: 10.1001/jamainternmed.2018.0756 PMID: 29801109

Nimer, J., & Lundahl, B. (2007). Animal-assisted therapy: A meta-analysis. *Anthrozoos*, *20*(3), 225–238. DOI: 10.2752/089279307X224773

Nio, R. A., Esteban, P. R., De Faria Catarina, T., & Conrado, C. (2017). Allergen management as a key issue in food safety. In CRC Press eBooks (pp. 195–241). DOI: 10.1201/9781315153414-6

Norbury, C. F., Gooch, D., Wray, C., Baird, G., Charman, T., Simonoff, E., Vamvakas, G., & Pickles, A. (2016). The impact of nonverbal ability on prevalence and clinical presentation of language disorder: Evidence from a population study. *Journal of Child Psychology and Psychiatry, and Allied Disciplines*, *57*(11), 1247–1257. DOI: 10.1111/jcpp.12573 PMID: 27184709

Norton, C., Whitehead, W., Bliss, D., Harari, D., & Lang, J. (2010). Conservative Management of Fecal Incontinence in Adults Committee of the International Consultation on Incontinence. Management of fecal incontinence in adults. *Neurourology and Urodynamics*, *29*(1), 199–206. DOI: 10.1002/nau.20803 PMID: 20025031

Nowak-Węgrzyn, A., & Albin, S. (2015). Oral immunotherapy for food allergy: Mechanisms and role in management. Clinical & Experimental Allergy. *Clinical and Experimental Allergy*, *45*(2), 368–383. DOI: 10.1111/cea.12382 PMID: 25077670

Nund, R. L., Rumbach, A. F., Debattista, B. C., Goodrow, M. N., Johnson, K. A., Tupling, L. N., Scarinci, N. A., Cartmill, B., Ward, E. C., & Porceddu, S. V. (2015). Communication changes following non-glottic head and neck cancer management: The perspectives of survivors and carers. *International Journal of Speech-Language Pathology*, *17*(3), 263–272. DOI: 10.3109/17549507.2015.1010581 PMID: 25764915

Nund, R. L., Ward, E. C., Scarinci, N. A., Cartmill, B., Kuipers, P., & Porceddu, S. V. (2014). The lived experience of dysphagia following non-surgical treatment for head and neck cancer. *International Journal of Speech-Language Pathology*, *16*(3), 282–289. DOI: 10.3109/17549507.2013.861869 PMID: 24345002

Nyatuka, D., & Harpe, R. (2021). Service design as a catalyst for patient-centered ehealth innovation. *International Journal of Information System Modeling and Design*, *12*(3), 62–85. DOI: 10.4018/IJISMD.20210701.oa1

O'Brien, B. C., Harris, I. B., Beckman, T. J., Reed, D. A., & Cook, D. A. (2014). Standards for reporting qualitative research: A synthesis of recommendations. *Academic Medicine*, *89*(9), 1245–1251. DOI: 10.1097/ACM.0000000000000388 PMID: 24979285

O'Haire, M., McKenzie, S., Beck, A., & Slaughter, V. (2013). Social behaviors increase in children with autism in the presence of animals compared to toys. *PLoS One*, *8*(2), e57010. DOI: 10.1371/journal.pone.0057010 PMID: 23468902

Ogonowska-Slodownik, A., Jakobowicz, O., Alexander, L., Marinho-Buzelli, A. R., Devion, C., & Morgulec-Adamowicz, N. (2024). Aquatic Therapy in Children and Adolescents with Disabilities: A Scoping Review. *Children (Basel, Switzerland)*, *11*(11), 1404. DOI: 10.3390/children11111404 PMID: 39594979

Okamura, I., Matsuyama, N., Yasui, K., Hirayama, F., & Ikeda, T. (2017). Clinical utility of the basophil activation test for analysis of allergic transfusion reactions: A pilot study. *Vox Sanguinis*, *112*(2), 114–121. DOI: 10.1111/vox.12471 PMID: 28070919

Okoye, C., M Obialo-Ibeawuchi, C., A Obajeun, O., Sarwar, S., Tawfik, C., Subhan Waleed, M., Ullah Wasim, A., Mohamoud, I., Y Afolayan, A., & N Mbaezue, R. (2023). Early Diagnosis of Autism Spectrum Disorder: A Review and Analysis of the Risks and Benefits.

Olij, B., Barmentloo, L., Smilde, D., Velde, N., Polinder, S., Schoon, Y., & Erasmus, V. (2019). Factors associated with participation of community-dwelling older adults in a home-based falls prevention program. *International Journal of Environmental Research and Public Health*, *16*(6), 1087. DOI: 10.3390/ijerph16061087 PMID: 30917618

Olszewska, K., Ptak, A., Rusak, A., Dębiec-Bąk, A., & Stefańska, M. (2024). Changes in the scar tissue structure after cesarean section as a result of manual therapy. *Advances in clinical and experimental medicine: Official organ Wroclaw. Medicina Universitaria*, *33*(4), 387–395. DOI: 10.17219/acem/169236 PMID: 37665082

Ortolani, C., & Pastorello, E. A. (2006). Food allergies and food intolerances. Baillière's Best Practice & Research. Clinical Gastroenterology/Baillière's. *Best Practice & Research. Clinical Gastroenterology*, *20*(3), 467–483. DOI: 10.1016/j.bpg.2005.11.010 PMID: 16782524

Ottosson, S., Laurell, G., & Olsson, C. (2013). The experience of food, eating and meals following radiotherapy for head and neck cancer: A qualitative study. *Journal of Clinical Nursing, 22*(7-8), 1034–1043. DOI: 10.1111/jocn.12151 PMID: 23480499

Owens, R. (2014). *Language disorders: a functional approach to assessment and intervention* (6th ed.). Pearson.

Owens, R. (2016). *Language development: An introduction* (8th ed.). Pearson.

Owens, R. E. (2016). *Language Development: An Introduction* (9th ed.). Pearson.

Padilha, C. O. S., & De Oliveira, W. F. (2013). Representação social do terapeuta comunitário no Sistema Único de Saúde. *Ciencia & Saude Coletiva, 18*(8), 2211–2220. DOI: 10.1590/S1413-81232013000800005 PMID: 23896903

Pak, N. S., Chow, J. C., Dillehay, K. M., & Kaiser, A. P. (2023). Long-Term Effects of Early Communication Interventions: A Systematic Review and Meta-Analysis. *Journal of Speech, Language, and Hearing Research: JSLHR, 66*(8), 2884–2899. DOI: 10.1044/2023_JSLHR-22-00711 PMID: 37418755

Papadopoulos, N. G., Agache, I., Bavbek, S., Bilo, B. M., Braido, F., Cardona, V., Custovic, A., Demonchy, J., Demoly, P., Eigenmann, P., Gayraud, J., Grattan, C., Heffler, E., Hellings, P. W., Jutel, M., Knol, E., Lötvall, J., Muraro, A., Poulsen, L. K., & Akdis, C. A. (2012). Research needs in allergy: An EAACI position paper, in collaboration with EFA. *Clinical and Translational Allergy, 2*(1), 21. Advance online publication. DOI: 10.1186/2045-7022-2-21 PMID: 23121771

Pappa, E., Chatzikonstantinidou, S., Chalkiopoulos, G., Papadopoulos, A., & Niakas, D. (2015). Health-related quality of life of the Roma in Greece: The role of socio-economic characteristics and housing conditions. *International Journal of Environmental Research and Public Health, 12*(6), 6669–6681. DOI: 10.3390/ijerph120606669 PMID: 26075724

Parker, A., Beresford, B., Dawson, V., Elphick, H., Fairhurst, C., Hewitt, C., Scantlebury, A., Spiers, G., Thomas, M., Wright, K., & McDaid, C. (2019). Oral melatonin for non-respiratory sleep disturbance in children with neurodisabilities: Systematic review and meta-analyses. *Developmental Medicine and Child Neurology, 61*(8), 880–890. DOI: 10.1111/dmcn.14157 PMID: 30710339

Parrinello, G., Fontana, D. E., & Villalta, D. (2025). An overview of hidden food allergens: Need for change to the priority food allergen lists? *European Annals of Allergy and Clinical Immunology, 57*(2), 51–67. DOI: 10.23822/EurAnnACI.1764-1489.370 PMID: 39450657

Pask, S., Dell'Olio, M., Murtagh, F., & Boland, J. (2020). The effects of opioids on cognition in older adults with cancer and chronic noncancer pain: A systematic review. *Journal of Pain and Symptom Management*, *59*(4), 871–893.e1. DOI: 10.1016/j.jpainsymman.2019.10.022 PMID: 31678462

Pasupuleti, M. (2024). Resilient innovations: leading the way in disaster management and recovery., 1-25. https://doi.org/DOI: 10.62311/nesx/77639

Patel, A. V., Friedenreich, C. M., Moore, S. C., Hayes, S. C., Silver, J. K., Campbell, K. L., Winters-Stone, K., Gerber, L. H., George, S. M., Fulton, J. E., Denlinger, C., Morris, G. S., Hue, T., Schmitz, K. H., & Matthews, C. E. (2019). American College of Sports Medicine Roundtable Report on Physical Activity, Sedentary Behavior, and Cancer Prevention and Control. *Medicine and Science in Sports and Exercise*, *51*(11), 2391–2402. DOI: 10.1249/MSS.0000000000002117 PMID: 31626056

Patel, B. Y., & Volcheck, G. W. (2015). Food allergy: Common causes, diagnosis, and treatment. *Mayo Clinic Proceedings*, *90*(10), 1411–1419. DOI: 10.1016/j.mayocp.2015.07.012 PMID: 26434966

Patel, K., & Chotai, N. (2011). Documentation and records: Harmonized GMP requirements. *Journal of Young Pharmacists : JYP*, *3*(2), 138–150. DOI: 10.4103/0975-1483.80303 PMID: 21731360

Patterson JM, Lawton M. (2023). Dysphagia Advances in Head and Neck Cancer. Curr Otorhinolaryngol Rep. Feb 15:1-8. . Epub ahead of print. PMID: 36816911; PMCID: PMC9930077.DOI: 10.1007/s40136-023-00445-6

Patton, M. Q. (2002). *Qualitative research and evaluation methods* (3rd ed. ed.). Thousand Oaks, CA: Sage Publications.

Paul, B., Kirubakaran, R., Isaac, R., Dozier, M., Grant, L., & Weller, D.RESPIRE Collaboration. (2023). A systematic review of the theory of planned behaviour interventions for chronic diseases in low health-literacy settings. *Journal of Global Health*, *13*, 04079. DOI: 10.7189/jogh.13.04079 PMID: 37681679

Pauloski, B. R., Rademaker, A. W., Lazarus, C., Boeckxstaens, G., Kahrilas, P. J., & Logemann, J. A. (2009). Relationship between manometric and videofluoroscopic measures of swallow function in healthy adults and patients treated for head and neck cancer with various modalities. *Dysphagia*, *24*(2), 196–203. DOI: 10.1007/s00455-008-9192-x PMID: 18956228

Pauloski, B. R., Rademaker, A. W., Logemann, J. A., Lazarus, C. L., Newman, L., Hamner, A., MacCracken, E., Gaziano, J., & Stachowiak, L. (2002). Swallow function and perception of dysphagia in patients with head and neck cancer. *Head & Neck*, *24*(6), 555–565. DOI: 10.1002/hed.10092 PMID: 12112553

Pendergast, D. R., Moon, R. E., Krasney, J. J., Held, H. E., & Zamparo, P. (2015). Human Physiology in an Aquatic Environment. *Comprehensive Physiology*, *5*(4), 1705–1750. DOI: 10.1002/j.2040-4603.2015.tb00655.x PMID: 26426465

Perloff, R. M. (2014). Social Media Effects on Young Women's Body Image Concerns: Theoretical Perspectives and an Agenda for Research. *Sex Roles*, *71*(11-12), 363–377. DOI: 10.1007/s11199-014-0384-6

Perry, A., Lee, S. H., Cotton, S., & Kennedy, C. (2016). Therapeutic exercises for affecting post-treatment swallowing in people treated for advanced-stage head and neck cancers. *Cochrane Database of Systematic Reviews*, *2016*(8), CD011112. Advance online publication. DOI: 10.1002/14651858.CD011112.pub2 PMID: 27562477

Peters, B., O'Brien, K., & Fried-Oken, M. (2022). AAC use and service delivery experiences of people with ALS in the United States. *Disability and Rehabilitation. Assistive Technology*, *17*(7), 762–771. DOI: 10.1080/17483107.2022.2149866 PMID: 36448513

Picariello, G., Mamone, G., Addeo, F., & Ferranti, P. (2011). The frontiers of mass spectrometry-based techniques in food allergenomics. Journal of Chromatography a. *Journal of Chromatography. A*, *1218*(42), 7386–7398. DOI: 10.1016/j.chroma.2011.06.033 PMID: 21737089

Pimentel, F. (2006). *Qualidade de vida e Oncologia*. Almedina.

Pinto M. & Serrano, A.M. (2022). Perceção dos profissionais acerca da participação das famílias no apoio pelas equipas de intervenção precoce. *Zero-a-Seis*, 24 (n. Especial), 740-768. DOI: 10.5007/1518-2924.2022.e83100

Pinto, M. J. S. (2018). *Participação das famílias no apoio prestado pelo Sistema Nacional de Intervenção Precoce na Infância* [Doctoral thesis, Universidade do Minho]. Repositório da Universidade do Minho. https://hdl.handle.net/1822/65351

Pires, T. P., Costa, R., & Viana, R. (2020a). Effects of pelvic floor muscle training in pregnant women. *Porto Biomedical Journal*, *5*(5), e077. DOI: 10.1097/j.pbj.0000000000000077 PMID: 33195869

Pires, T., Pires, P., Moreira, H., Gabriel, R., Viana, S., & Viana, R. (2020c). Assessment of pelvic floor muscles in sportswomen: Quality of life and related factors. *Physical Therapy in Sport*, *43*, 151–156. DOI: 10.1016/j.ptsp.2020.02.015 PMID: 32200260

Pires, T., Pires, P., Moreira, H., & Viana, R. (2020b). Prevalence of urinary incontinence in high-impact sport athletes: A systematic review and meta-analysis. *Journal of Human Kinetics, 73*(1), 279–288. DOI: 10.2478/hukin-2020-0008 PMID: 32774559

Pires, T., Pires, P., Moreira, M., Gabriel, R., João, P., Viana, S., & Viana, R. (2020d). Pelvic Floor Muscle Training in Female Athletes: A Randomized Controlled Pilot Study. *International Journal of Sports Medicine, 41*(4), 264–270. DOI: 10.1055/a-1073-7977 PMID: 31935774

Pispati, V., Africawala, A. N., & Varghese, S. (2019). Developmental Screening of Children of Migrant Construction Workers in Mumbai. *Indian Journal of Human Development, 13*(1), 109–114. DOI: 10.1177/0973703019839820

Poms, R. E., Klein, C. L., & Anklam, E. (2004). Methods for allergen analysis in food: A review. Food Additives & Contaminants. *Food Additives and Contaminants, 21*(1), 1–31. DOI: 10.1080/02652030310001620423 PMID: 14744677

Popich, E., Louw, B., & Eloff, I. (2006). The need for collaboration in early communication intervention: Whom do parents consult regarding the prevention of communication disorders? *Early Child Development and Care, 176*(7), 675–692. DOI: 10.1080/03004430500206395

Poulos, R., Boon, M., George, A., Liu, K., Mak, M., Maurice, C., Palesy, D., Pont, L. G., Poulos, C. J., Ramsey, S., Simpson, P., Steiner, G. Z., Villarosa, A. R., Watson, K., & Parker, D. (2020). Preparing for an aging Australia: The development of multidisciplinary core competencies for the Australian health and aged care workforce. *Gerontology & Geriatrics Education, 42*(3), 399–422. DOI: 10.1080/02701960.2020.1843454 PMID: 33252017

Prat, J., & Mutch, D. G. (2018). Pathology of cancers of the female genital tract including molecular pathology. *International Journal of Gynaecology and Obstetrics: the Official Organ of the International Federation of Gynaecology and Obstetrics, 143*(S2), 93–108. DOI: 10.1002/ijgo.12617 PMID: 30306579

Prelock, P. J., & Nelson, N. W. (2012). Language and Communication in Autism: An Integrated View. *Pediatric Clinics of North America, 59*(1), 129–145. DOI: 10.1016/j.pcl.2011.10.008 PMID: 22284798

Prezerakos, P. (2018). Nurse managers' emotional intelligence and effective leadership: A review of the current evidence. *The Open Nursing Journal, 12*(1), 86–92. DOI: 10.2174/1874434601812010086 PMID: 29997711

Pritchard, A. (1969). Statistical bibliography or bibliometrics? *The Journal of Documentation, 25*(4), 348–349.

Probyn, K., Bowers, H., Mistry, D., Caldwell, F., Underwood, M., Patel, S., Sandhu, H. K., Matharu, M., & Pincus, T. (2017). Non-pharmacological self-management for people living with migraine or tension-type headache: A systematic review including analysis of intervention components. *BMJ Open*, *7*(8), e016670. DOI: 10.1136/bmjopen-2017-016670 PMID: 28801425

Professional, C. C. M. (2024, March). Food allergies. Cleveland Clinic. https://my.clevelandclinic.org/health/diseases/9196-food-allergies

Püsküllüoğlu, M., Tomaszewski, K. A., Grela-Wojewoda, A., Pacholczak-Madej, R., & Ebner, F. (2022). Effects of Transcutaneous Electrical Nerve Stimulation on Pain and Chemotherapy-Induced Peripheral Neuropathy in Cancer Patients: A Systematic Review. *Medicina (Kaunas, Lithuania)*, *58*(2), 284. DOI: 10.3390/medicina58020284 PMID: 35208610

Putri, A. P., & Lu, Y. Y. (2024). Maternal Health Literacy in Pregnant Women: A Concept Analysis. *Maternal and Child Health Journal*, *28*(8), 1272–1282. DOI: 10.1007/s10995-024-03945-z PMID: 38864987

Queirós, A., Moreira, S., Silva, A., Costa, R., & Lains, J. (2013). Contributo para a Adaptação e Validação da Eat Assessment Tool (EAT-10) e da Functional Oral Intake Scale (FOIS). *Revista da Sociedade Portuguesa de Medicina de Reabilitação*, *2*(24), 25–30.

Raby, K. L., Freedman, E., Yarger, H. A., Lind, T., & Dozier, M. (2019). Enhancing the language development of toddlers in foster care by promoting foster parents' sensitivity: Results from a randomized controlled trial. *Developmental Science*, *22*(2), e12753. DOI: 10.1111/desc.12753 PMID: 30230658

Rahmani, A., Lai, J., Jafarlou, S., Yunusova, A., Rivera, A., Labbaf, S., . . . Borelli, J. (2020). Personal mental health navigator: harnessing the power of data, personal models, and health cybernetics to promote psychological well-being. https://doi.org//arxiv.2012.09131DOI: 10.48550

Rampazo, É. P., Rehder-Santos, P., Catai, A. M., & Liebano, R. E. (2024). Heart rate variability in adults with chronic musculoskeletal pain: A systematic review. *Pain Practice*, *24*(1), 211–230. DOI: 10.1111/papr.13294 PMID: 37661339

Ravid, D., Bar-On, A., & Dattner, E. (2013). Linguistics in the service of communication disorders: *New frontiers. AILA Review*, *26*, 79–99. Advance online publication. DOI: 10.1075/aila.26.06rav

Rd, H. W. (2024, March 7). The 9 most common food allergies. Healthline. https://www.healthline.com/nutrition/common-food-allergies

Rd, J. C. M. (2024, April 3). The 9 most common food allergies. Verywell Health. https://www.verywellhealth.com/the-most-common-food-allergies-1324134

Reed, B. R. (2021). What are key considerations when selecting high-tech AAC? *Leader Live*, https://leader.pubs.asha.org/do/10.1044/2021-high-tech-aac/full/

Reed, J., Hirsh-Pasek, K., & Golinkoff, R. M. (2016). Meeting Children Where They Are: Adaptive Contingency Builds Early Communication Skills. In Witt, P. (Ed.), *Communication and Learning - Handbooks of Communication Science* (pp. 601–627). Gruyter Mouton. DOI: 10.1515/9781501502446-025

Reed, P., Osborne, L. A., Whittall, C. M., & Emery, S. (2021). Impact of patient motivation on compliance and outcomes for incontinence. *Physiotherapy*, *113*, 100–106. DOI: 10.1016/j.physio.2020.10.003 PMID: 34563914

Regenhardt, R., Takase, H., Lo, E., & Lin, D. (2020). Translating concepts of neural repair after stroke: Structural and functional targets for recovery. *Restorative Neurology and Neuroscience*, *38*(1), 67–92. DOI: 10.3233/RNN-190978 PMID: 31929129

Rehn, A. K., Caruso, V. R., & Kumar, S. (2023). The effectiveness of animal assisted therapy for children and adolescents with autism spectrum disorder: A systematic review. *Complementary Therapies in Clinical Practice*, *50*, 101719. DOI: 10.1016/j.ctcp.2022.101719 PMID: 36599281

Reilly, S., Wake, M., Ukoumunne, O., Bavin, E., Prior, M., Cini, E., Conway, L., Eadie, P., & Bretherton, L. (2010). Predicting language outcomes at 4 years of age: Findings from early language in victoria study. *Pediatrics*, *126*(6), e1530–e1537. DOI: 10.1542/peds.2010-0254 PMID: 21059719

Reis da Silva, T. (2024b). The Evolution of Nursing for Older Adult: A Historical Perspective. *Associative J Health Sci.* 3(3). AJHS. 000561. 2024. DOI: . Link: https://crimsonpublishers.com/ajhs/pdf/AJHS.000561.pdfDOI: 10.31031/AJHS.2024.03.000561

Reis da Silva, T. H (2024c). Oncology and Cancer Medicine: Understanding the complexities in Older Patients. *Biomed J Sci & Tech Res* 55(3)-2024. DOI: https://doi.org/DOI: 10.26717/BJSTR.2024.55.008720

Reis da Silva, T. H. (2024a). Chapter 8 – Emotional Intelligence in Teaching Geriatric Nursing: Humanising Technology for Compassionate Care in Higher Education. In Tikadar, S.; Liu, H.; Bhattacharya, P.; Bhattacharya, S. *Humanizing Technology With Emotional Intelligence*. Pp. 141-160. IGI Global Scientific Publishing. https://doi.org/DOI: 10.4018/979-8-3693-7011-7.ch008

Reis da Silva, T. H. (2024e). Chapter 12 – Emotional Intelligence in Integrative Medicine: Enhancing Patient-Centred Care Through Humanised Technology. In Tikadar, S.; Liu, H.; Bhattacharya, P.; Bhattacharya, S. *Humanizing Technology With Emotional Intelligence*. Pp. 263-280. IGI Global Scientific Publishing. https://doi.org/DOI: 10.4018/979-8-3693-7011-7.ch012

Reis da Silva, T. H. (2024h). Chapter 11 - Integrating business essentials into Gerontological Nursing: Enhancing Care for Older Adults in Diverse Settings. In Sedky, A. *Resiliency Strategies for Long-Term Business Success*. Pp. 283-316. IGI Global. DOI: https://doi.org/DOI: 10.4018/979-8-3693-9168-6.ch011

Reis da Silva, T. H. (2024i). Chapter 6 – Navigating Healthcare Complexity: Integrating Business Fundamentals into Nursing Leadership. In Sedky, A. *Resiliency Strategies for Long-Term Business Success*. Pp. 145-168. IGI Global. https://doi.org/DOI: 10.4018/979-8-3693-9168-6.ch006

Reis da Silva, T. H. (2024j). Death and Its Significance in Nursing Practice. *Palliat Med Care Int J*. 2024; 4(3): 555640. DOI: https://juniperpublishers.com/pmcij/pdf/PMCIJ.MS.ID.555640.pdf

Reis da Silva, T. H. (2023a). Ageing in place: Ageing at home and in the community. *British Journal of Community Nursing*, *28*(5), 213–214. DOI: 10.12968/bjcn.2023.28.5.213 PMID: 37130715

Reis da Silva, T. H. (2023b). Falls assessment and prevention in the nursing home and community. *British Journal of Community Nursing*, *28*(2), 68–72. DOI: 10.12968/bjcn.2023.28.2.68 PMID: 36735363

Reis da Silva, T. H. (2023c). Moving and Handling in the Community. *British Journal of Community Nursing*, *28*(8), 369. DOI: 10.12968/bjcn.2023.28.8.369 PMID: 37527217

Reis da Silva, T. H. (2024d). Enhancing the mental health of refugees and asylum seekers through music interventions. *Mental Health Practice*. Advance online publication. DOI: 10.7748/mhp.2024.e1717

Reis da Silva, T. H. (2024f). Loneliness in older adults. *British Journal of Community Nursing*, *29*(2), 60–66. DOI: 10.12968/bjcn.2024.29.2.60 PMID: 38300245

Reis da Silva, T. H. (2024g). Falls prevention in older people and the role of nursing. *British Journal of Community Nursing*, *29*(7), 335–339. DOI: 10.12968/bjcn.2024.0005 PMID: 38963269

Reis da Silva, T. H. (2024k). Prevalence of elder abuse: A narrative review. *British Journal of Community Nursing*, *29*(9), 442–446. DOI: 10.12968/bjcn.2024.0004 PMID: 39240800

Reis da Silva, T. H. (2025b). Emotional Intelligence and AI in Geriatric Nursing: Bridging Technology and Compassionate Care. In Jermsittiparsert, K., & Marzo, R. R. (Eds.), *Physical Health, Mental Health, and Human Well-Being in the Age of AI*. IGI Global Scientific Publishing., DOI: 10.4018/979-8-3693-6190-0.ch10

Reis da Silva, T. H. (2025e). Exploring loneliness: Conceptualisation and impact in older adults. *British Journal of Community Nursing*, *30*(4), 188–195. DOI: 10.12968/bjcn.2024.0025

Reis da Silva, T. M. (2025a). Designing for Longevity: Economic Perspectives on Age-Friendly Housing and Urban Development. In Gölçek, A. (Ed.), *Perspectives on the Economics of Aging* (pp. 151–176). IGI Global Scientific Publishing., DOI: 10.4018/979-8-3693-7753-6.ch006

Reis da Silva, T. M. (2025c). Fostering Emotional Resilience and Mindful Leadership in Gerontology Nursing: A Model for Change and Innovation. In Baez, M. (Ed.), *Strategic Approaches to Mindful Leadership and Change Management* (pp. 259–280). IGI Global Scientific Publishing., https://doi.org/10.4018/979-8-3693-7066-7.ch009

Reis da Silva, T. M. (2025f). Fostering Emotional Intelligence for Competency Development in Nursing Education. In Aldosemani, T., Lytras, M., & Ordóñez de Pablos, P. (Eds.), *Innovative Educational Frameworks for Future Skills and Competencies* (pp. 39–62). IGI Global Scientific Publishing., https://doi.org/10.4018/979-8-3693-7555-6.ch002

Reis da Silva, T. M. (2025i). Teaching With Adaptability: Cognitive and Pedagogical Strategies for Geriatric Nursing. In Yalçın, M., Uslukaya, A., & Demirdiş, B. (Eds.), *Holistic Approaches to Teacher Development: Leadership, Pedagogical Practices, and Cognitive Insights* (pp. 205–234). IGI Global Scientific Publishing., DOI: 10.4018/979-8-3373-0472-4.ch009

Reis da Silva, T. M. H. (2025g). The Role of Emotional Intelligence in Promoting Mental Peace, Healthy Work Environments, and Emotional Well-Being Among Entrepreneurs. In Tunio, M. N. (Ed.), *Supporting Psychological and Emotional Well-being Among Entrepreneurs*. IGI Global Scientific Publishing., DOI: 10.4018/979-8-3693-3673-1.ch21

Reis da Silva, T. M., Hammett, R., & Low, G. (2025). Emotional Intelligence in Business: Enhancing Leadership, Collaboration, and Performance. In Sedky, A. (Ed.), *Building Business Knowledge for Complex Modern Business Environments* (pp. 149–178). IGI Global Scientific Publishing., DOI: 10.4018/979-8-3693-6447-5.ch006

Rejeb, A., Keogh, J. G., Zailani, S., Treiblmaier, H., & Rejeb, K. (2020). Blockchain Technology in the Food Industry: A review of potentials, challenges and future research directions. *Logistics (Basel)*, *4*(4), 27. DOI: 10.3390/logistics4040027

Ren, Y., Kebede, M. A., Ogunleye, A. A., Emerson, M. A., Evenson, K. R., Carey, L. A., Hayes, S. C., & Troester, M. A. (2022). Burden of lymphedema in long-term breast cancer survivors by race and age. *Cancer*, *128*(23), 4119–4128. DOI: 10.1002/cncr.34489 PMID: 36223240

Renz, H., Allen, K. J., Sicherer, S. H., Sampson, H. A., Lack, G., Beyer, K., & Oettgen, H. C. (2018). Food allergy. *Nature Reviews. Disease Primers*, *4*(1), 17098. Advance online publication. DOI: 10.1038/nrdp.2017.98 PMID: 29300005

Rett, M. T., Moura, D. P., Oliveira, F. B. D., Domingos, H. Y. B., Oliveira, M. M. F. D., Gallo, R. B. S., & Silva, W. M. D.Junior. (2022). Physical therapy after breast cancer surgery improves range of motion and pain over time. *Fisioterapia e Pesquisa*, *29*(1), 46–52. DOI: 10.1590/1809-2950/21001929012022en

Ribeiro, M. M., Andrade, A., & Nunes, I. (2021). Physical exercise in pregnancy: Benefits, risks and prescription. *Journal of Perinatal Medicine*, *50*(1), 4–17. DOI: 10.1515/jpm-2021-0315 PMID: 34478617

Ricci, L., Villegente, J., Loyal, D., Ayav, C., Kivits, J., & Rat, A. C. (2022). Tailored patient therapeutic educational interventions: A patient-centred communication model. *Health Expectations*, *25*(1), 276–289. DOI: 10.1111/hex.13377 PMID: 34816546

Rinaldi, S., Caselli, M. C., Cofelice, V., D'Amico, S., De Cagno, A. G., Della Corte, G., Di Martino, M. V., Di Costanzo, B., Levorato, M. C., Penge, R., Rossetto, T., Sansavini, A., Vecchi, S., & Zoccolotti, P. (2021). Efficacy of the Treatment of Developmental Language Disorder: A Systematic Review. *Brain Sciences*, *11*(3), 407. DOI: 10.3390/brainsci11030407 PMID: 33806938

Rizzo, A. (2016). The Role of Exercise and Rehabilitation in the Cancer Care Plan. *Journal of the Advanced Practitioner in Oncology*, *7*(3), 339–342. DOI: 10.6004/jadpro.2016.7.3.20 PMID: 29152403

Roberts, M. Y., Curtis, P. R., Sone, B. J., & Hampton, L. H. (2019). Association of parent training with child language development: A systematic review and meta-analysis. *JAMA Pediatrics, 173*(7), 671–680. DOI: 10.1001/jamapediatrics.2019.1197 PMID: 31107508

Roberts, M. Y., & Kaiser, A. P. (2011). The Effectiveness of Parent-Implemented Language Interventions: A Meta-Analysis. *American Journal of Speech-Language Pathology, 20*(3), 180–199. DOI: 10.1044/1058-0360(2011/10-0055) PMID: 21478280

Rodgers, M. M., Alon, G., Pai, V. M., & Conroy, R. S. (2019). Wearable technologies for active living and rehabilitation: Current research challenges and future opportunities. *Journal of Rehabilitation and Assistive Technologies Engineering, 6*, 2055668319839607. DOI: 10.1177/2055668319839607 PMID: 31245033

Rogers, R., Pauls, R., Thakar, R., Morin, M., Kuhn, A., Petri, E., Fatton, B., Whitmore, K., Kingsberg, S. A., & Lee, J. (2018). An International Urogynecological Association (IUGA)/International Continence Society (ICS) joint report on the terminology for the assessment of sexual health of women with pelvic floor dysfunction. *International Urogynecology Journal, 29*(5), 647–666. DOI: 10.1007/s00192-018-3603-9 PMID: 29577166

Rogers, S. N. (2016). Improving quality-of-life questionnaires in head and neck cancer. *Expert Review of Quality of Life in Cancer Care, 1*(1), 61–71. DOI: 10.1080/23809000.2016.1142357

Rogers, S., & Dawson, G. (2010). *Early start denver model for young children with autism: Promoting language, learning, and engagement*. The Guilford Press.

Rogus-Pulia, N. M., Pierce, M., Mittal, B. B., Zecker, S. G., & Logemann, J. (2015). Bolus effects on patient awareness of swallowing difficulty and swallow physiology after chemoradiation for head and neck cancer. *Head & Neck, 37*(8), 1122–1129. DOI: 10.1002/hed.23720 PMID: 24841209

Rose, G. L., Stewart, E. M., Clifford, B. K., Bailey, T. G., Rush, A. J., Abbott, C. R., Hayes, S. C., Obermair, A., & McCarthy, A. L. (2023). Efficacy of exercise interventions for women during and after gynaecological cancer treatment–a systematic scoping review. *Supportive Care in Cancer, 31*(6), 342. DOI: 10.1007/s00520-023-07790-8 PMID: 37195433

Ross, G. M. S., Bremer, M. G. E. G., & Nielen, M. W. F. (2018). Consumer-friendly food allergen detection: moving towards smartphone-based immunoassays. Analytical and Bioanalytical Chemistry/Analytical & Bioanalytical Chemistry, 410(22), 5353–5371. DOI: 10.1007/s00216-018-0989-7

Rossignol, D. A., & Frye, R. E. (2011). Melatonin in autism spectrum disorders: A systematic review and meta-analysis. *Developmental Medicine and Child Neurology*, *53*(9), 783–792. DOI: 10.1111/j.1469-8749.2011.03980.x PMID: 21518346

Rostad, H., Utne, I., Grov, E., Puts, M., & Halvorsrud, L. (2017). Measurement properties, feasibility and clinical utility of the doloplus-2 pain scale in older adults with cognitive impairment: A systematic review. *BMC Geriatrics*, *17*(1), 257. Advance online publication. DOI: 10.1186/s12877-017-0643-9 PMID: 29096611

Ruchat, S. M., Mottola, M. F., Skow, R. J., Nagpal, T. S., Meah, V. L., James, M., Riske, L., Sobierajski, F., Kathol, A. J., Marchand, A.-A., Nuspl, M., Weeks, A., Gray, C. E., Poitras, V. J., Jaramillo Garcia, A., Barrowman, N., Slater, L. G., Adamo, K. B., Davies, G. A., & Davenport, M. H. (2018). Effectiveness of exercise interventions in the prevention of excessive gestational weight gain and postpartum weight retention: A systematic review and meta-analysis. *British Journal of Sports Medicine*, *52*(21), 1347–1356. DOI: 10.1136/bjsports-2018-099399 PMID: 30337461

Ruggeri, A., Dancel, A., Johnson, R., & Sargent, B. (2020). The effect of motor and physical activity intervention on motor outcomes of children with autism spectrum disorder: A systematic review. *Autism*, *24*(3), 544–568. DOI: 10.1177/1362361319885215 PMID: 31782658

Rush, D. D. & Shelden, M'L. L. (2011). *The Early Childhood Coaching Handbook*. Paul H Brookes Publishing Co.

Rustichelli, D., Castiglia, S., Gunetti, M., Mareschi, K., Signorino, E., Muraro, M., Castello, L., Sanavio, F., Leone, M., Ferrero, I., & Fagioli, F. (2013). Validation of analytical methods in compliance with good manufacturing practice: A practical approach. *Journal of Translational Medicine*, *11*(1), 197. DOI: 10.1186/1479-5876-11-197 PMID: 23981284

Sabaghi, M., & Jamali, S. N. (2024). Advancements, challenges, and future prospects of nanobiosensors in food packaging for allergen detection. *Journal of Food Measurement and Characterization*, *18*(5), 3444–3457. Advance online publication. DOI: 10.1007/s11694-024-02416-x

Sagen, J. S., Kjeken, I., Habberstad, A., Linge, A. D., Simonsen, A. E., Lyken, A. D., Irgens, E. L., Framstad, H., Lyby, P. S., Klokkerud, M., Dagfinrud, H., & Moe, R. H. (2024). Patient Involvement in the Rehabilitation Process Is Associated with Improvement in Function and Goal Attainment: Results from an Explorative Longitudinal Study. *Journal of Clinical Medicine*, *13*(2), 320. DOI: 10.3390/jcm13020320 PMID: 38256454

Sakamoto, J., Ward, H., Vissoci, J., & Eucker, S. (2018). Are nonpharmacologic pain interventions effective at reducing pain in adult patients visiting the emergency department? a systematic review and meta-analysis. *Academic Emergency Medicine*, *25*(8), 940–957. DOI: 10.1111/acem.13411 PMID: 29543359

Salati, S. A., Alsulaim, L., Alharbi, M. H., Alharbi, N. H., Alsenaid, T. M., Alaodah, S. A., Alsuhaibani, A. S., & Albaqami, K. A. (2023). Postmastectomy Pain Syndrome: A Narrative Review. *Cureus*, *15*(10), e47384. DOI: 10.7759/cureus.47384 PMID: 38021812

Sampath, V., Abrams, E. M., Adlou, B., Akdis, C., Akdis, M., Brough, H. A., Chan, S., Chatchatee, P., Chinthrajah, R. S., Cocco, R. R., Deschildre, A., Eigenmann, P., Galvan, C., Gupta, R., Hossny, E., Koplin, J. J., Lack, G., Levin, M., Shek, L. P., . . . Renz, H. (2021). Food allergy across the globe. ^the ‰Journal of Allergy and Clinical Immunology/Journal of Allergy and Clinical Immunology/ the œJournal of Allergy and Clinical Immunology, 148(6), 1347–1364. DOI: 10.1016/j.jaci.2021.10.018

Sampson, H. A. (2016). Food allergy: Past, present and future. *Allergology International*, *65*(4), 363–369. DOI: 10.1016/j.alit.2016.08.006 PMID: 27613366

Sánchez, F. A. G. (2019). Neurociencias y atención temprana. In Mora, C. T. E., & García, L. R. (Eds.), *Prácticas de atención temprana centradas en la familia y en entornos naturales* (pp. 33–50). UNED.

Sánchez, K., Spittle, A., Cheong, J., Thompson, D., Doyle, L., Anderson, P., & Morgan, A. (2018). Language in 2-year-old children born preterm and term: A cohort study. *Archives of Disease in Childhood*, *104*(7), 647–652. DOI: 10.1136/archdischild-2018-315843 PMID: 30470685

Sansavini, A., Favilla, M. E., Guasti, M. T., Marini, A., Millepiedi, S., Di Martino, M. V., Vecchi, S., Battajon, N., Bertolo, L., Capirci, O., Carretti, B., Colatei, M. P., Frioni, C., Marotta, L., Massa, S., Michelazzo, L., Pecini, C., Piazzalunga, S., Pieretti, M., & Lorusso, M. L. (2021). Developmental Language Disorder: Early Predictors, Age for the Diagnosis, and Diagnostic Tools. A Scoping Review. *Brain Sciences*, *11*(5), 654. DOI: 10.3390/brainsci11050654 PMID: 34067874

Santos, A. F., Riggioni, C., Du Toit, G., & Skypala, I. (2025). An algorithm for the diagnosis and management of IgE-mediated food allergy, 2024 update. https://doi.org/DOI: 10.1111/all.16321

Sapage, S., & Cruz-Santos, A. (2021). Portuguese Early Literacy Screening Tool-RaLEPE: Pilot Study. *Revista de Investigación en Logopedia*, *11*(2), e71711. DOI: 10.5209/rlog.71711

Saral, D., Olcay, S., & Ozturk, H. (2023). Spectrum Disorder: When There is no Cure, There are Countless of Treatments. *Journal of Autism and Developmental Disorders, 53*(12), 4901–4916. DOI: 10.1007/s10803-022-05745-2 PMID: 36222992

Sathe, S. K., & Sharma, G. M. (2009). Effects of food processing on food allergens. *Molecular Nutrition & Food Research, 53*(8), 970–978. DOI: 10.1002/mnfr.200800194 PMID: 19603400

Satnarine, T., Makkoukdji, N., Pundit, V., Vignau, A., Sharma, P., Warren, D., Kleiner, G., & Gans, M. (2025). Peanut Allergy Diagnosis: Current Practices, Emerging Technologies, and Future Directions. *Allergies, 5*(1), 4. DOI: 10.3390/allergies5010004

Sawyer, S., & Tapia, A. (2005). The sociotechnical nature of mobile computing work: Evidence from a study of policing in the United States. *International Journal of Technology and Human Interaction, 1*(3), 1–14. DOI: 10.4018/jthi.2005070101

Schauberger, E. M., & Singh, A. M. (2020). Food allergy management. *Journal of Food Allergy, 2*(1), 59–63. DOI: 10.2500/jfa.2020.2.200021 PMID: 39022156

Scher, C., Petti, E., Meador, L., Cleave, J., Liang, E., & Reid, M. (2020). Multidimensional pain assessment tools for ambulatory and inpatient nursing practice. *Pain Management Nursing, 21*(5), 416–422. DOI: 10.1016/j.pmn.2020.03.007 PMID: 32448737

Schlosser, R., & Koul, K. (2023). Advances in augmentative and alternative communication research for individuals with autism spectrum disorder: Moving research and practice forward. *Augmentative and Alternative Communication, 39*(1), 2–6. DOI: 10.1080/07434618.2023.2181214 PMID: 36994996

Schmidt, M. A. R., & Barbosa, G. R. (2016). Use of artificial neural networks in initial ponderation of AHP techniques applied to analysis of watershed vulnerability. *Boletim de Ciências Geodésicas, 22*(3), 511–525. DOI: 10.1590/S1982-21702016000300029

Schoen, S. A., Lane, S. J., Mailloux, Z., May-Benson, T., Parham, L. D., Smith Roley, S., & Schaaf, R. C. (2019). A systematic review of ayres sensory integration intervention for children with autism. *Autism Research, 12*(1), 6–19. DOI: 10.1002/aur.2046 PMID: 30548827

Schwartzberg, E., & Silverman, M. (2013). Effects of music-based social stories on comprehension and gencralization of social skills in children with autism spectrum disorders: A randomized effectiveness study. *The Arts in Psychotherapy, 40*(3), 331–337. DOI: 10.1016/j.aip.2013.06.001

Scribner, E. (2013) Exploring Different Factors of Language Development. Awards for Excellence in Student Research & Creative Activity - Documents. 1. https://thekeep.eiu.edu/lib_awards_2013_docs/1

Scurrah, A., Shiner, C., Stevens, J., & Faux, S. (2017). Regional nerve blockade for early analgesic management of elderly patients with hip fracture – a narrative review. *Anaesthesia*, *73*(6), 769–783. DOI: 10.1111/anae.14178 PMID: 29278266

Secord, E. A. MD. (2021, May). Food Allergies: practice Essentials, background, pathophysiology. https://emedicine.medscape.com/article/135959-overview?form=fpf

Sela, Y., Grinberg, K., & Nissanholtz-Gannot, R. (2020). Attracting Israeli nursing students to community nursing. *Israel Journal of Health Policy Research*, *9*(1), 44. Advance online publication. DOI: 10.1186/s13584-020-00400-6 PMID: 33059759

Senger, J. B., Kadle, R. L., & Skoracki, R. J. (2023). Current Concepts in the Management of Primary Lymphedema. *Medicina (Kaunas, Lithuania)*, *59*(5), 894. DOI: 10.3390/medicina59050894 PMID: 37241126

Shariat, A., Najafabadi, M. G., Dos Santos, I. K., Anastasio, A. T., Milajerdi, H. R., Hassanzadeh, G., & Nouri, E. (2024). The Effectiveness of Aquatic Therapy on Motor and Social Skill as Well as Executive Function in Children With Neurodevelopmental Disorder: A Systematic Review and Meta-analysis. *Archives of Physical Medicine and Rehabilitation*, *105*(5), 1000–1007. DOI: 10.1016/j.apmr.2023.08.025 PMID: 37690741

Sharma, B., & Deshmukh, R. (2023). An overview of nanotechnological approaches for the diagnosis and treatment of allergic illness. *Current Pharmaceutical Design*, *29*(26), 2050–2061. DOI: 10.2174/1381612829666230828104015 PMID: 37641985

Sheldrick, R. C., & Perrin, E. C. (2013). Evidence-Based Milestones for Surveillance of Cognitive, Language, and Motor Development. *Academic Pediatrics*, *13*(6), 577–586. DOI: 10.1016/j.acap.2013.07.001 PMID: 24238685

Shelton, A., Allen, J., Mercer, V., Crenshaw, J., & Franz, J. (2024). Questionnaires of self-perception poorly correlate with instability elicited by walking balance perturbations. *PLoS One*, *19*(12), e0315368. DOI: 10.1371/journal.pone.0315368 PMID: 39666738

Sherrington, C., Whitney, J. C., Lord, S. R., Herbert, R. D., Cumming, R. G., & Close, J. C. (2008). Effective exercise for the prevention of falls: A systematic review and meta-analysis. *Journal of the American Geriatrics Society*, *56*(12), 2234–2243. DOI: 10.1111/j.1532-5415.2008.02014.x PMID: 19093923

Shipton, E., Bate, F., Garrick, R., Steketee, C., Shipton, E., & Visser, E. (2018). Systematic review of pain medicine content, teaching, and assessment in medical school curricula internationally. *Pain and Therapy*, *7*(2), 139–161. DOI: 10.1007/s40122-018-0103-z PMID: 30058045

Shropshire, M., Stapleton, S., Dyck, M., Kim, M., & Mallory, C. (2018). Non-pharmacological interventions for persistent, noncancer pain in elders residing in long-term care facilities: An integrative review of the literature. *Nursing Forum*, *53*(4), 538–548. DOI: 10.1111/nuf.12284 PMID: 30242833

Shuang-Shuang, X., & Ma, X. (2023). Mechanisms of physical exercise effects on anxiety in older adults during the covid-19 lockdown: An analysis of the mediating role of psychological resilience and the moderating role of media exposure. *International Journal of Environmental Research and Public Health*, *20*(4), 3588. DOI: 10.3390/ijerph20043588 PMID: 36834282

Shu, Z., Xiao, J., Dai, X., Yu, H., & Liu, Y. (2021). Effect of family "upward" intergenerational support on the health of rural elderly in China: Evidence from Chinese longitudinal healthy longevity survey. *PLoS One*, *16*(6), e0253131. DOI: 10.1371/journal.pone.0253131 PMID: 34143838

Sicherer, S. H. (2011). Epidemiology of food allergy. The Journal of Allergy and Clinical Immunology/Journal of Allergy and Clinical Immunology. *The Journal of Allergy and Clinical Immunology*, *127*(3), 594–602. DOI: 10.1016/j.jaci.2010.11.044 PMID: 21236480

Silva & Peixoto. (2008) Rastreio e prevalência das perturbações da comunicação num agrupamento de escolas. *Revista da Faculdade de Ciências da Saúde*. Porto. ISSN 1646-0480. 5 (2008) 272-282.

Silva, K., Correia, R., Lima, M., Magalhães, A., & Sousa, L. (2011). Can dogs prime autistic children for therapy? evidence from a single case study. *Journal of Alternative and Complementary Medicine (New York, N.Y.)*, *17*(7), 655–659. DOI: 10.1089/acm.2010.0436 PMID: 21689015

Silver, J. K., Dodurgali, M. R., & Gavini, N. (2024). Artificial Intelligence in Medical Education and Mentoring in Rehabilitation Medicine. *American Journal of Physical Medicine & Rehabilitation*, *103*(11), 1039–1044. DOI: 10.1097/PHM.0000000000002604 PMID: 39016292

Simental, A. A.Jr, & Carrau, R. L. (2004). Assessment of swallowing function in patients with head and neck cancer. *Current Oncology Reports*, *6*(2), 162–165. DOI: 10.1007/s11912-004-0028-z PMID: 14751094

Sim, F., O'Dowd, J., Thompson, L., Law, J., Macmillan, S., Affleck, M., Gillberg, C., & Wilson, P. (2013). Language and social/emotional problems identified at a universal developmental assessment at 30 months. *BMC Pediatrics*, *13*(1), 206. DOI: 10.1186/1471-2431-13-206 PMID: 24330767

Simms, M. D., & Jin, X. (2015). (in review). Autism, Language Disorder, and Social (Pragmatic) Communication Disorder: DSM-V and Differential Diagnoses. *Pediatrics*, *36*(8), 355–362. PMID: 26232465

Simões, M. C. B. (2011). *Rotinas familiares privilegiadas na comunicação de crianças com perturbação do espectro do autismo. Uma perspectiva parental* [Monografia, Universidade Atlântida]. Repositório Científico Universidade Atlântida.

Sindher, S., Long, A. J., Purington, N., Chollet, M., Slatkin, S., Andorf, S., Tupa, D., Kumar, D., Woch, M. A., O'Laughlin, K. L., Assaad, A., Pongracic, J., Spergel, J. M., Tam, J., Tilles, S., Wang, J., Galli, S. J., Nadeau, K. C., & Chinthrajah, R. S. (2018). Analysis of a large standardized food challenge data set to determine predictors of positive outcome across multiple allergens. *Frontiers in Immunology*, *9*, 2689. Advance online publication. DOI: 10.3389/fimmu.2018.02689 PMID: 30538699

Singer, A., & Ravi, R. (2015). Complementary and alternative treatments for autism part 2: Identifying and avoiding non-evidence-based treatments. *AMA Journal of Ethics*, *17*(4), 375–380. DOI: 10.1001/journalofethics.2015.17.4.sect2-1504 PMID: 25901708

Singer, I., Klatte, I. S., Vries, R., Lugt, R., & Gerrits, E. (2022). Using co-design to develop a tool for shared goal-setting with parents in speech and language therapy. *International Journal of Language & Communication Disorders*, *57*(6), 1281–1303. DOI: 10.1111/1460-6984.12753 PMID: 35859264

Sinn, F. S., Charters, E., Stone, D., Janabi, M., & Bogaardt, H. (2020). Responsiveness of the EAT-10 to Clinical Change in Head and Neck Cancer Patients with Dysphagia. *International Journal of Speech-Language Pathology*, *22*(1), 78–85. DOI: 10.1080/17549507.2019.1596312 PMID: 31032643

Sissons, J., Blakemore, E., Shafi, H., Skotny, N., & Lloyd, D. (2022). calm with horses? a systematic review of animal-assisted interventions for improving social functioning in children with autism. *Autism*, *26*(6), 1320–1340. DOI: 10.1177/13623613221085338 PMID: 35403450

Siu, A. L. (2015). Screening for Speech and Language Delay and Disorders in Children Aged 5 Years or Younger: US Preventive Services Task Force Recommendation Statement. *Pediatrics*, *136*(2), e474–e481. DOI: 10.1542/peds.2015-1711 PMID: 26152670

Skuban, E. (2010) *Language impairment and child adjustment in high-risk, low-income toddlers: moderating influences of parenting and emotion regulation.* Doctoral Dissertation, University of Pittsburgh. https://d-scholarship.pitt.edu/8134/

Smith, C. A., Parton, C., King, M., & Gallego, G. (2020). Parents' experiences of information-seeking and decision-making regarding complementary medicine for children with autism spectrum disorder: A qualitative study. *BMC Complementary Medicine and Therapies*, *20*(1), 1–13. DOI: 10.1186/s12906-019-2805-0 PMID: 32020887

Snow, P. (2021) Psychosocial Adversity in Early Childhood and Language and Literacy Skills in Adolescence: The Role of Speech Language Pathology in Prevention, Policy, and Practice. *Perspectives of the ASHA Special Interest Groups,* 6, 253–261. https://pubs.asha.org 37.189.29.156

Snowling, M. J., Nash, H. M., Gooch, D. C., Hayiou-Thomas, M. E., & Hulme, C. (2019). Developmental Outcomes for Children at High Risk of Dyslexia and Children With Developmental Language Disorder. *Child Development*, *90*(5), e548–e564. DOI: 10.1111/cdev.13216 PMID: 30676649

Soares, A., Silva, K., & Zuanetti, P. (2017). Variáveis de risco para o desenvolvimento da linguagem associadas à prematuridade. *Audiology - Communication Research*, *22*(0). Advance online publication. DOI: 10.1590/2317-6431-2016-1745

Sobhgol, S. S., Priddis, H., Smith, C. A., & Dahlen, H. G. (2019). The Effect of Pelvic Floor Muscle Exercise on Female Sexual Function During Pregnancy and Postpartum: A Systematic Review. *Sexual Medicine Reviews*, *7*(1), 13–28. DOI: 10.1016/j.sxmr.2018.08.002 PMID: 30301705

Sociedade Portuguesa de Terapia da Fala. (n.d.). *Linguagem na criança.* https://sptf.org.pt/departamento-linguagem-na-crianca/

Soimah, S. and Utami, S. (2023). The emotional intelligent and social support as predictor of stress at work among nurses during post pandemic., 145-152. https://doi.org/DOI: 10.2991/978-94-6463-186-9_18

So, K. K. H., & To, C. (2022). Systematic Review and Meta-Analysis of Screening Tools for Language Disorder. *Frontiers in Pediatrics*, *10*, 801220. Advance online publication. DOI: 10.3389/fped.2022.801220 PMID: 35281230

So, L., Miller, E., & Eastwood, J. (2021). Exploring mothers' experience of a linguistic feedback technology for children at risk of poor language development: Qualitative pilot study. *JMIR Pediatrics and Parenting*, *4*(3), e27049. DOI: 10.2196/27049 PMID: 34463633

Soldatova, L., & Mirza, N. (2019). Long-Term Voice and Swallowing Outcomes for Oral and Oropharyngeal Cancer Following Primary or Adjuvant Chemoradiation. *The Annals of Otology, Rhinology, and Laryngology, 3489419842256*(9), 802–810. Advance online publication. DOI: 10.1177/0003489419842256 PMID: 31007044

Soltani, S., Moghadam, M. M., Amani, S., Akbari, S., Shiani, A., & Soofi, M. (2022). Socioeconomic disparities in using rehabilitation services among Iranian adults with disabilities: A decomposition analysis. *BMC Health Services Research, 22*(1), 1449. DOI: 10.1186/s12913-022-08811-8 PMID: 36447232

Sosa, A. V. (2016). Association of the Type of Toy Used During Play With the Quantity and Quality of Parent-Infant Communication. *JAMA Pediatrics, 170*(2), 132–137. DOI: 10.1001/jamapediatrics.2015.3753 PMID: 26720437

Sourvinos, S., Mavropoulos, A., Kasselimis, D. S., Korasidi, A., Voukouni, A. L., Papadopoulos, P., Vlaseros, S., Damianos, G., Potagas, C., & Damianos, D. (2021). Brief Report: Speech and Language Therapy in Children with ASD in an Aquatic Environment: the ASLT (Aquatic Speech and Language Therapy) Program. *Journal of Autism and Developmental Disorders, 51*(4), 1406–1416. DOI: 10.1007/s10803-020-04629-7 PMID: 32748193

Souza, A., Santos, P., Cachoeira, F., & Beal, S. (2023). Interprofessionality in health care.. https://doi.org/DOI: 10.56238/globalhealthprespesc-037

Spanoudaki, M., Giaginis, C., Karafyllaki, D., Papadopoulos, K., Solovos, E., Antasouras, G., Sfikas, G., Papadopoulos, A. N., & Papadopoulou, S. K. (2023). Exercise as a promising agent against cancer: Evaluating its anti-cancer molecular mechanisms. *Cancers (Basel), 15*(21), 5135. DOI: 10.3390/cancers15215135 PMID: 37958310

Speech Pathology Australia. (2024). *Let's talk about speech pathology*. https://www.speechpathologyaustralia.org.au/

Spicer-Cain, H., Camilleri, B., Hasson, N., & Botting, N. (2023). Early Identification of Children at Risk of Communication Disorders: Introducing a Novel Battery of Dynamic Assessments for Infants. *American Journal of Speech-Language Pathology, 32*(2), 523–544. DOI: 10.1044/2022_AJSLP-22-00040 PMID: 36787149

Sreeram, A., Cross, W., & Townsin, L. (2021). Effect of recovery-based interventions on recovery knowledge and attitudes of mental health professionals, regarding recovery-oriented practice: A quantitative narrative review. *International Journal of Mental Health Nursing, 30*(5), 1057–1069. DOI: 10.1111/inm.12897 PMID: 34109703

Stahmer, A., Dababnah, S. & Rieth, S. (2019) Considerations in implementing evidence-based early autism spectrum disorder interventions in community settings. Pediatr Med;2:18 | DOI: 10.21037/pm.2019.05.01

Stansfeld, S. A., Clark, C., Rodgers, B., Caldwell, T., & Power, C. (2011). Repeated exposure to socioeconomic disadvantage and health selection as life course pathways to mid-life depressive and anxiety disorders. *Social Psychiatry and Psychiatric Epidemiology*, *46*(7), 549–558. DOI: 10.1007/s00127-010-0221-3 PMID: 20383489

Stans, S. E. A., Dalemans, R. J. P., Roentgen, U. R., Smeets, H. W. H., & Beurskens, A. J. H. M. (2018). Who said dialogue conversations are easy? The communication between communication vulnerable people and health-care professionals: A qualitative study. *Health Expectations*, *21*(5), 848–857. DOI: 10.1111/hex.12679 PMID: 29671920

Starmer, H., & Edwards, J. (2019). Clinical Decision Making with Head and Neck Cancer Patients with Dysphagia. *Seminars in Speech and Language*, *40*(3), 213–226. DOI: 10.1055/s-0039-1688979 PMID: 31158905

Steinbrenner, J. R., Hume, K., Odom, S. L., Morin, K. L., Nowell, S. W., Tomaszewski, B., Szendrey, S., & McIntyre, N. S. YücesoyÖzkan, S., & Savage, M. N. (2020). Evidence-Based Practices for Children, Youth, and Young Adults with Autism. FPG Child Development Institute.

Stepanian, N., Larsen, M. H., Mendelsohn, J. B., Mariussen, K. L., & Heggdal, K. (2023). Empowerment interventions designed for persons living with chronic disease - a systematic review and meta-analysis of the components and efficacy of format on patient-reported outcomes. *BMC Health Services Research*, *23*(1), 911. DOI: 10.1186/s12913-023-09895-6 PMID: 37626346

Strand, L., Gundrosen, K., Lein, T., Laekeman, M., Lobbezoo, F., Defrin, R., & Husebø, B. (2018). Body movements as pain indicators in older people with cognitive impairment: A systematic review. *European Journal of Pain (London, England)*, *23*(4), 669–685. DOI: 10.1002/ejp.1344 PMID: 30450680

Strand, N. H., D'Souza, R., Gomez, D. A., Whitney, M. A., Attanti, S., Anderson, M. A., & Maloney, J. A. (2024). Pain during menopause. *Maturitas*, *108135*. Advance online publication. DOI: 10.1016/j.maturitas.2024.108135 PMID: 39500125

Su, C. Y. (1997). Aspiration and speech shunt stenosis in near-total laryngectomy patients. *European Archives of Oto-Rhino-Laryngology*, *254*(8), 401–404. DOI: 10.1007/BF01642559 PMID: 9332898

Suchodoletz, Waldemar. (2011). Early identification of children with developmental language disorders - When and how?. *Zeitschrift für Kinder- und Jugendpsychiatrie und Psychotherapie*. 39. 377-84; 384. .DOI: 10.1024/1422-4917/a000136

Sultan, A., Monga, A., Lee, J., Emmanuel, A., Norton, C., Santoro, G., Hull, T., Berghmans, B., Brody, S., & Haylen, B. (2017). An International Urogynecological Association (IUGA)/International Continence Society (ICS) joint report on the terminology for female anorectal dysfunction. *International Urogynecology Journal, 28*(1), 5–31. DOI: 10.1007/s00192-016-3140-3 PMID: 27774569

Suntai, Z., Won, C., & Noh, H. (2020). Access barrier in rural older adults' use of pain management and palliative care services: A systematic review. *The American Journal of Hospice & Palliative Care, 38*(5), 494–502. DOI: 10.1177/1049909120959634 PMID: 32959683

Swain, C. T., Drummond, A. E., Boing, L., Milne, R. L., English, D. R., Brown, K. A., van Roekel, E. H., Dixon-Suen, S. C., Lynch, M. J., Moore, M. M., Gaunt, T. R., Martin, R. M., Lewis, S. J., & Lynch, B. M. (2022). Linking physical activity to breast cancer via sex hormones, part 1: The effect of physical activity on sex steroid hormones. *Cancer Epidemiology, Biomarkers & Prevention, 31*(1), 16–27. DOI: 10.1158/1055-9965.EPI-21-0437 PMID: 34670800

Swami, V., & Furnham, A. (2008). *The Psychology of Physical Attraction* (1st ed.). Routledge.

T C. J. (2024, February 28). Food allergy vs. food intolerance: What's the difference? Mayo Clinic. https://www.mayoclinic.org/diseases-conditions/food-allergy/expert-answers/food-allergy/faq-20058538

Tamis-LeMonda, C. S., Kuchirko, Y., & Song, L. (2014). Why Is Infant Language Learning Facilitated by Parental Responsiveness? *Current Directions in Psychological Science, 23*(2), 121–126. DOI: 10.1177/0963721414522813

Tang, S., Tse, M., Leung, S., & Fotis, T. (2019). The effectiveness, suitability, and sustainability of non-pharmacological methods of managing pain in community-dwelling older adults: A systematic review. *BMC Public Health, 19*(1), 1488. Advance online publication. DOI: 10.1186/s12889-019-7831-9 PMID: 31703654

Taveira, L., Gaspar, A. C., Pinto, M., Dias, J. C., Mendes, J., Martins, A. L., & Prata, J. (2023). Intervenção em Comunicação Aumentativa. In Alves, D. C., Correia, P., Cruz, S., Fonseca, J., Ibrahim, S., Lopes, I., Lousada, M., Oliveira, P., & Pinto, C. (Eds.), *Compendium de Terapia da Fala – Avaliar e intervir com evidência* (pp. 933–1024). Sociedade Portuguesa de Terapia da Fala.

Taylor, S. L., & Lehrer, S. B. (1996). Principles and characteristics of food allergens. Critical Reviews in Food Science and Nutrition, 36(sup001), 91–118. DOI: 10.1080/10408399609527761

Taylor, H. S., Adamson, G. D., Diamond, M. P., Goldstein, S. R., Horne, A. W., Missmer, S. A., Snabes, M. C., Surrey, E., & Taylor, R. N. (2018). An evidence-based approach to assessing surgical versus clinical diagnosis of symptomatic endometriosis. *International Journal of Gynaecology and Obstetrics: the Official Organ of the International Federation of Gynaecology and Obstetrics*, *142*(2), 131–142. DOI: 10.1002/ijgo.12521 PMID: 29729099

Taylor, H. S., Kotlyar, A. M., & Flores, V. A. (2021). Endometriosis is a chronic systemic disease: Clinical challenges and novel innovations. *Lancet*, *397*(10276), 839–852. DOI: 10.1016/S0140-6736(21)00389-5 PMID: 33640070

Tazreean, R., Nelson, G., & Twomey, R. (2022). Early mobilization in enhanced recovery after surgery pathways: Current evidence and recent advancements. *Journal of Comparative Effectiveness Research*, *11*(2), 121–129. DOI: 10.2217/cer-2021-0258 PMID: 35045757

Te Kaat-van den Os, D., Jongmans, M., Volman, M. C. J. M., & Lauteslager, P. E. M. (2017). Parent-implemented language interventions for children with developmental delay: A systematic review. *Journal of Policy and Practice in Intellectual Disabilities*, *14*(2), 129–137. DOI: 10.1111/jppi.12181

Tennfjord, M. K., Gabrielsen, R., & Tellum, T. (2021). Effect of physical activity and exercise on endometriosis-associated symptoms: A systematic review. *BMC Women's Health*, *21*(1), 355. DOI: 10.1186/s12905-021-01500-4 PMID: 34627209

The Joint Comission. (2022). *National Patient Safety Goals| The Joint Commission*. https://www.jointcommission.org/standards/national-patient-safety-goals/

Thomas, E., Battaglia, G., Patti, A., Brusa, J., Leonardi, V., Palma, A., & Bellafiore, M. (2019). Physical activity programs for balance and fall prevention in elderly: A systematic review. *Medicine*, *98*(27), e16218. DOI: 10.1097/MD.0000000000016218 PMID: 31277132

Threats, T. T. (2007). Use of the ICF in dysphagia management. *Seminars in Speech and Language*, *28*(4), 323–333. DOI: 10.1055/s-2007-986529 PMID: 17935017

Thunberg, G., Buchholz, M., & Nilsson, S. (2016). Strategies that assist children with communicative disability during hospital stay: Parents' perceptions and ideas. *Journal of Child Health Care*, *20*(2), 224–233. DOI: 10.1177/1367493514568298 PMID: 25676537

Thurman, A. (2017). *Parent-child interaction: how it impacts language and literacy skills*, Graduate Research Papers. 617. https://scholarworks.uni.edu/grp/617

Tobin, G., & Montz, B. (1997). *Natural hazards*. Guilford.

Tomasello, M. (2003). *Constructing a language: A usage-based theory of language acquisition*. Harvard University Press.

Tomblin, J. B., Smith, E., & Zhang, X. (1997). Epidemiology of specific language impairment: Prenatal and perinatal risk factors. *Journal of Communication Disorders*, *30*(4), 325–344. DOI: 10.1016/S0021-9924(97)00015-4 PMID: 9208366

Topia, M., & Hocking, C. (2012). Enabling development and participation through early provision of augmentative and alternative communication. *New Zealand Journal of Occupational Therapy*, *59*(1), 24–30.

Torres-Cueco, R., & Nohales-Alfonso, F. (2021). Vulvodynia—It is time to accept a new understanding from a neurobiological perspective. *International Journal of Environmental Research and Public Health*, *18*(12), 6639. DOI: 10.3390/ijerph18126639 PMID: 34205495

Triska, V. L. (2016) *The Comorbidity of Communication and Psychological Disorders: An analysis of the origin and prevalence of children presenting with comorbid language, speech, and psychological disorders*. Student Research Submissions. 139. https://scholar.umw.edu/student_research/139

Tsai, Y., Browne, G., & Inder, K. (2020). The effectiveness of interventions to improve pain assessment and management in people living with dementia: A systematic review and meta-analyses. *Journal of Advanced Nursing*, *77*(3), 1127–1140. DOI: 10.1111/jan.14660 PMID: 33222273

Tsai, Y., Yang, P., Yang, Y., Lin, M., & Wang, Y. (2020). Prevalence and risk factors of falls among community-dwelling older people: Results from three consecutive waves of the national health interview survey in Taiwan. *BMC Geriatrics*, *20*(1), 529. Advance online publication. DOI: 10.1186/s12877-020-01922-z PMID: 33297968

Tulviste, T., & Schults, A. (2020). Parental reports of communicative development at the age of 36 months: The Estonian CDI-III. *First Language*, *40*(1), 64–83. DOI: 10.1177/0142723719887313

Turnbull, J. L., Adams, H. N., & Gorard, D. A. (2014). Review article: The diagnosis and management of food allergy and food intolerances. *Alimentary Pharmacology & Therapeutics*, *41*(1), 3–25. DOI: 10.1111/apt.12984 PMID: 25316115

Turnbull, K., & Justice, M. (2016). *Language Development From Theory to Practice* (3rd ed.). Pearson.

Turner, J. S., Pettit, K. E., Buente, B. B., Humbert, A. J., Perkins, A. J., & Kline, J. A. (2016). Medical student use of communication elements and association with patient satisfaction: A prospective observational pilot study. *BMC Medical Education, 16*(1), 150–158. DOI: 10.1186/s12909-016-0671-8 PMID: 27209065

Turner, P. (2018). Facilitators and barriers to holistic practice, an osteopathic perspective. *IJCAM, 11*(2). Advance online publication. DOI: 10.15406/ijcam.2018.11.00355

Turton, B., Williams, S., Burton, C., & Williams, L. (2017). Arts-based palliative care training, education and staff development: A scoping review. *Palliative Medicine, 32*(2), 559–570. DOI: 10.1177/0269216317712189 PMID: 28604224

Tyler, S., & Moench, M. (2012). A framework for urban climate resilience. *Climate and Development, 4*(4), 311–326. DOI: 10.1080/17565529.2012.745389

UNDRR. (2019). *United Nations Office for Disaster Risk Reduction*. United Nations.

United Nations. (2008). *Final report of the Ad Hoc Committee on a Comprehensive and Integral International Convention on the Protection and Promotion of the Rights and Dignity of Persons with Disabilities | United Nations Enable*. Accessed November 20, 2024.https://www.un.org/development/desa/disabilities/final-report-of-the-ad-hoc-committee-on-a-comprehensive-and-integral-international-convention-on-the-protection-and-promotion-of-the-rights-and-dignity-of-persons-with-disabilities.html

Upasen, R., Saengpanya, W., Awae, W., & Prasitvej, P. (2024). The influence of resilience and social support on mental health of older adults living in community: A cross-sectional study. *BMC Psychology, 12*(1), 397. Advance online publication. DOI: 10.1186/s40359-024-01892-6 PMID: 39020436

Urisu, A., Ebisawa, M., Mukoyama, T., Morikawa, A., & Kondo, N. (2011). Japanese guideline for food allergy. *Allergology International, 60*(2), 221–236. DOI: 10.2332/allergolint.11-RAI-0329 PMID: 21636968

Vachon-Presseau, É., Centeno, M., Ren, W., Berger, S., Tétreault, P., Ghantous, M., Baria, A., Farmer, M., Baliki, M. N., Schnitzer, T. J., & Apkarian, A. (2016). The emotional brain as a predictor and amplifier of chronic pain. *Journal of Dental Research, 95*(6), 605–612. DOI: 10.1177/0022034516638027 PMID: 26965423

Vaismoradi, M., Skär, L., Söderberg, S., & Bondas, T. (2016). Normalizing suffering: A meta-synthesis of experiences of and perspectives on pain and pain management in nursing homes. *International Journal of Qualitative Studies on Health and Well-being*, *11*(1), 31203. DOI: 10.3402/qhw.v11.31203 PMID: 27173102

Valade, F., Béliveau, M.-J., Breault, C., Chabot, B., & Labelle, F. (2023). Individual and cumulative risk factors in developmental language disorder: A case-control study. *Clinical Child Psychology and Psychiatry*, *28*(1), 398–414. DOI: 10.1177/13591045221113389 PMID: 35797616

van Agt, H. M., van der Stege, H. A., de Ridder-Sluiter, H., Verhoeven, L. T., & de Koning, H. J. (2007). A cluster-randomized trial of screening for language delay in toddlers: Effects on school performance and language development at age 8. *Pediatrics*, *120*(6), 1317–1325. DOI: 10.1542/peds.2006-3145 PMID: 18055682

van Agt, H. M., van der Stege, H. A., de Ridder-Sluiter, J. G., & de Koning, H. J. (2007). Detecting language problems: Accuracy of five language screening instruments in preschool children. *Developmental Medicine and Child Neurology*, *49*(2), 117–184. DOI: 10.1111/j.1469-8749.2007.00117.x PMID: 17253998

Van Bilsen, J., Szłapka, E. S., Ojalvo, D. L., Willemsen, L. E. M., Antunes, C. M., Molina, E., Smit, J. J., & Wróblewska, B. (2017). Application of the adverse outcome pathway (AOP) concept to structure the available in vivo and in vitro mechanistic data for allergic sensitization to food proteins. *Clinical and Translational Allergy*, *7*(1), 13. Advance online publication. DOI: 10.1186/s13601-017-0152-0 PMID: 28507730

van der Schuit, M., Segers, E., van Balkom, H., & Verhoeven, L. (2011). Early language intervention for children with intellectual disabilities: A neurocognitive perspective. *Research in Developmental Disabilities*, *32*(2), 705–712. DOI: 10.1016/j.ridd.2010.11.010 PMID: 21159487

van Manen, M. (2016). *Researching lived experience: Human science for an action sensitive pedagogy* (2nd ed.). Routledge.

Van Wijk, F., & Knippels, L. (2007). Initiating mechanisms of food allergy: Oral tolerance versus allergic sensitization. *Biomedicine and Pharmacotherapy*, *61*(1), 8–20. DOI: 10.1016/j.biopha.2006.11.003 PMID: 17218079

Vandana, P., Simkin, D. R., Hendren, R. L., & Arnold, L. E. (2023). Autism Spectrum Disorder and Complementary-Integrative Medicine. *Child and Adolescent Psychiatric Clinics of North America*, *32*(2), 469–494. DOI: 10.1016/j.chc.2022.08.004 PMID: 37147047

Varghese, S. M., Parisi, S., Singla, R. K., & Begum, A. S. A. (2022). Food safety and quality control in food industry. In Springer briefs in molecular science (pp. 31–44). DOI: 10.1007/978-3-031-06304-6_5

Vasilescu, A., Nunes, G., Hayat, A., Latif, U., & Marty, J. (2016). Electrochemical affinity biosensors based on disposable Screen-Printed electrodes for detection of food allergens. *Sensors (Basel), 16*(11), 1863. DOI: 10.3390/s16111863 PMID: 27827963

Vendramini, A., Azevedo, R., Reiners, A., Mendes, P., & Segri, N. (2017). Factors associated with fall prevention practices in older adults. *Escola Anna Nery, 21*(2). Advance online publication. DOI: 10.5935/1414-8145.20170044

Vergeldt, T. F., Weemhoff, M., IntHout, J., & Kluivers, K. B. (2015). Risk factors for pelvic organ prolapse and its recurrence: A systematic review. *International Urogynecology Journal, 26*(11), 1559–1573. DOI: 10.1007/s00192-015-2695-8 PMID: 25966804

Verhoeckx, K. C., Vissers, Y. M., Baumert, J. L., Faludi, R., Feys, M., Flanagan, S., Herouet-Guicheney, C., Holzhauser, T., Shimojo, R., Van Der Bolt, N., Wichers, H., & Kimber, I. (2015). Food processing and allergenicity. *Food and Chemical Toxicology, 80*, 223–240. DOI: 10.1016/j.fct.2015.03.005 PMID: 25778347

Vettriselvan, R., Deepan, A., Jaiswani, G., Balakrishnan, A., & Sakthivel, R. (2025). Health Consequences of Early Marriage: Examining Morbidity and Long-Term Wellbeing. In Uddin, E. (Ed.), *Social, Political, and Health Implications of Early Marriage* (pp. 189–212). IGI Global Scientific Publishing., DOI: 10.4018/979-8-3693-3394-5.ch008

Viana, F.; Cadime, I.; Silva, C. (…) Monteiro, J. (2017*) MacArthut-Bates inventários de desenvolvimento comunicativo.* Luso info Edutora.

Viana, R., Viana, S., Neto, F., & Mascarenhas, T. (2015). Adaptation and validation of the King's Health Questionnaire in Portuguese women with urinary incontinence. *International Urogynecology Journal, 26*(7), 1027–1033. DOI: 10.1007/s00192-015-2628-6 PMID: 25653033

Victoria Sandham, Anne E. Hill & Fiona Hinchliffe (2021): The current practices of Australian speech-language pathologists in providing communication services to children with autism spectrum disorder, International Journal of Speech-Language Pathology, DOI: To link to this article: https://doi.org/DOI: 10.1080/17549507.2021.1923800

Vieira, D., & Monteiro, E. (2010). Head and neck cancer: contribution for the analysis of the rehabilitation needs. *Revista da Faculdade de Ciências da Saúde, 7*, 108-121. http://hdl.handle.net/10284/2984

Vieira, D. O., Antunes, E. B., Dinis-Ribeiro, M., & Monteiro, E. (2020). Psychometric validity of the Portuguese version of SWAL-QOL for head and neck cancer. *Revista de Logopedia, Foniatría y Audiología*.

Vieira, D., & Antunes, B. E. (2017). Clinical characteristics of dysphagia-related quality of life questionnaires. *Revista de Investigación en Logopedia, 2*, 157–188.

Vincent, L. A., Peterson, T. C., Barros, V. R., Marino, M. B., Rusticucci, M., Carrasco, G., Ramirez, E., Alves, L. M., Ambrizzi, T., Berlato, M. A., Grimm, A. M., Marengo, J. A., Molion, L., Moncunill, D. F., Rebello, E., Anunciação, Y. M. T., Quintana, J., Santos, J. L., Baez, J., & Karoly, D. (2005). Observed trends in indices of daily temperature extremes in South America 1960-2000. *Journal of Climate, 18*(23), 5011–5023. DOI: 10.1175/JCLI3589.1

Vincenzo, J., Patton, S., Lefler, L., Falvey, J., McElfish, P., Curran, G., & Wei, J. (2021). Older adults' perceptions regarding the role of physical therapists in fall prevention: A qualitative investigation. *Journal of Geriatric Physical Therapy, 45*(3), E127–E136. DOI: 10.1519/JPT.0000000000000304 PMID: 33782360

Vissirini, F.S.B., Reis, P.T.B., Cunha, F.P., Gondim, F.R., Ohuma JR.A.A. Formiga, R.M. (2023). Urban Vulnerability and the Tools Required for Hydro-Meteorological Risk Disaster Management. *Journal of Environmental Management and Sustainability, 12*(2), 1-37, e22616.

Vitoula, K., Venneri, A., Varrassi, G., Paladini, A., Sykioti, P., Adewusi, J., & Zis, P. (2018). Behavioral therapy approaches for the management of low back pain: An up-to-date systematic review. *Pain and Therapy, 7*(1), 1–12. DOI: 10.1007/s40122-018-0099-4 PMID: 29767395

Vocci, M., Gallo, I., Spiri, W., Borgato, M., & Fontes, C. (2021). Vulnerabilities of nurses in an intensive care unit: An integrative review. *Revista Brasileira de Enfermagem, 74*(3), e20200724. Advance online publication. DOI: 10.1590/0034-7167-2020-0724 PMID: 34161500

Vogel, S.W., Mullins, K.L., & Kumar, S. (2024). Art therapy for children and adolescents with autism: a systematic review. *International Journal of Art Therapy*.

Voineskos, S. H., Nelson, J. A., Klassen, A. F., & Pusic, A. L. (2018). Measuring Patient-Reported Outcomes: Key Metrics in Reconstructive Surgery. *Annual Review of Medicine*, *69*(1), 467–479. DOI: 10.1146/annurev-med-060116-022831 PMID: 29414263

Wade, M., Zeanah, C. H., Fox, N. A., & Nelson, C. A. (2020). Social communication deficits following early-life deprivation and relation to psychopathology: A randomized clinical trial of foster care. *Journal of Child Psychology and Psychiatry, and Allied Disciplines*, *61*(12), 1360–1369. DOI: 10.1111/jcpp.13222 PMID: 32222079

Wake, M., Levickis, P., Tobin, S., Zens, N., Law, J., Gold, L., Ukoumunne, O. C., Goldfeld, S., Le, H. N., Skeat, J., & Reilly, S. (2012). Improving outcomes of preschool language delay in the community: Protocol for the Language for Learning randomised controlled trial. *BMC Pediatrics*, *12*(1), 96. DOI: 10.1186/1471-2431-12-96 PMID: 22776103

Wallace, I. F., Berkman, N. D., Watson, L. R., Coyne-Beasley, T., Wood, C. T., Cullen, K., & Lohr, K. N. (2015). Screening for Speech and Language Delay in Children 5 Years Old and Younger: A Systematic Review. *Pediatrics*, *136*(2), e448–e462. DOI: 10.1542/peds.2014-3889 PMID: 26152671

Walle, E., & Campos, J. (2014). Infant language development is related to the acquisition of walking. *Developmental Psychology*, *50*(2), 336–348. DOI: 10.1037/a0033238 PMID: 23750505

Wang, M., Sung, H., & Liu, J. (2022). Population aging and its impact on human wellbeing in China. *Frontiers in Public Health*, *10*, 883566. Advance online publication. DOI: 10.3389/fpubh.2022.883566 PMID: 35419339

Wang, R., Wang, M., Zhou, J., Wu, D., Ye, J., Sun, G., & Sun, X. (2021). Saponins in Chinese herbal medicine exerts protection in myocardial ischemia–reperfusion injury: Possible mechanism and target analysis. *Frontiers in Pharmacology*, *11*, 570867. Advance online publication. DOI: 10.3389/fphar.2020.570867 PMID: 33597866

Wang, Y., Zhang, S., Peng, P., He, W., Zhang, H., Xu, H., & Liu, H. (2023). The effect of myofascial therapy on postpartum rectus abdominis separation, low back and leg pain, pelvic floor dysfunction: A systematic review and meta-analysis. *Medicine*, *102*(44), e35761. DOI: 10.1097/MD.0000000000035761 PMID: 37932976

Ward, E., & Van As-Brooks, C. (2007). *Head and Neck Cancer: Treatment, Rehabiliation, and Outcomes*. Plural Publishing Inc.

Ward, R., Clark, A., Campbell, S., Graham, B., Kullberg, A., Manji, K., & Keady, J. (2018). The lived neighborhood: Understanding how people with dementia engage with their local environment. *International Psychogeriatrics, 30*(6), 867–880. DOI: 10.1017/S1041610217000631 PMID: 28462764

Warner, R. (2017). *Intersubjectivity as a precursor to literacy: revisiting the home-school study of language and literacy development.* Thesis in Doctor of Philosophy The University of Texas at Austin. https://repositories.lib.utexas.edu/server/api/core/bitstreams/457c869a-d1db-4e84-a211-7f8d99ee05e4/content

Warner, K., Keville, S., Hockley, J., & Ludlow, A. (2023). Experiences of equine assisted therapy for females with autism spectrum disorders. *Advances in Autism, 9*(2), 150–164. DOI: 10.1108/AIA-10-2021-0040

Warren, C. M., Dyer, A. A., Otto, A. K., Smith, B. M., Kauke, K., Dinakar, C., & Gupta, R. S. (2017). Food Allergy–Related Risk-Taking and Management Behaviors among Adolescents and Young Adults. Journal of Allergy and Clinical Immunology. In Practice/the Journal of Allergy and Clinical Immunology. *In Practice, 5*(2), 381–390.e13. DOI: 10.1016/j.jaip.2016.12.012 PMID: 28132799

Weare, K. (2015). Rehabilitation after gynecological cancer treatment. *International Journal of Gynaecology and Obstetrics: the Official Organ of the International Federation of Gynaecology and Obstetrics, 131*(S2), S164–S166. DOI: 10.1016/j.ijgo.2015.06.015 PMID: 26433675

Wei, G., Farooq, J., & Kumar, A. (2020). Impact of mind-body treatment interventions on quality of life in neurofibromatosis patients: A systematic review and meta-analysis. *Dermatologic Therapy, 34*(1). Advance online publication. DOI: 10.1111/dth.14613 PMID: 33258517

Weisberg, D. S., Hirsh-Pasek, K., Golinkoff, R. M., Kittredge, A. K., & Klahr, D. (2016). Guided play: Principles and practices. *Current Directions in Psychological Science, 25*(3), 177–182. DOI: 10.1177/0963721416645512

Weiss, R., & Pippi, L. G. (2019). Análise multicritério na definição de vulnerabilidade ambiental. *TerraPlural, 13*(3), 272–295. DOI: 10.5212/TerraPlural.v.13i3.0018

Wells, G. (2007). Semiotic mediation, dialogue and the construction of knowledge. *Human Development, 50*(5), 244–247. DOI: 10.1159/000106414

Wen, G., Singh, D., Mesbah, N., Hanafi, A., & Azwan, A. (2021). Fall awareness behaviour and its associated factors among Malaysian community dwelling older adults. https://doi.org/DOI: 10.21203/rs.3.rs-54230/v2

Wetherby, A., Warren, S., & Reichle, J. (1998) *Transitions in Prelinguistic Communication*. Volume 7 de Communication and language intervention series. Brookes Publishing

Wetherby, A. M., Guthrie, W., Hooker, J. L., Delehanty, A., Day, T. N., Woods, J., Pierce, K., Manwaring, S. S., Thurm, A., Ozonoff, S., Petkova, E., & Lord, C. (2021). The Early Screening for Autism and Communication Disorders: Field-testing an autism-specific screening tool for children 12 to 36 months of age. *Autism*, *25*(7), 2112–2123. DOI: 10.1177/13623613211012526 PMID: 33962531

Wheeler, B. L., Shultis, C. L., & Polen, D. W. (2005). Clinical training guide for the student music therapist. Barcelona: Gilsum.

Wheeler, B. (2015). Music therapy as a profession. In Wheeler, B. (Ed.), *Music therapy handbook* (pp. 5–16). The Guilford Press.

Wideman, T., Edwards, R., Walton, D., Martel, M., Hudon, A., & Seminowicz, D. (2019). The multimodal assessment model of pain. *The Clinical Journal of Pain*, *35*(3), 212–221. DOI: 10.1097/AJP.0000000000000670 PMID: 30444733

Wigram, T., & Gold, C. (2006). Music therapy in the assessment and treatment of autistic spectrum disorder: Clinical application and research evidence. *Child: Care, Health and Development*, *32*(5), 535–542. DOI: 10.1111/j.1365-2214.2006.00615.x PMID: 16919132

Wiklander, P., Fröberg, A., & Lundvall, S. (2023). Searching for the alternative: A scoping review of empirical studies with holistic perspectives on health and implications for teaching physical education. *European Physical Education Review*, *29*(3), 351–368. DOI: 10.1177/1356336X221147813

Wilkinson, L., & Gathani, T. (2022). Understanding breast cancer as a global health concern. *The British Journal of Radiology*, *95*(1130), 20211033. DOI: 10.1259/bjr.20211033 PMID: 34905391

Wingood, M., Kiyoshi-Teo, H., Scott, A., Caulley, J., Wilson, B., Council, S., & Vincenzo, J. (2024). Demographic comparisons of self-reported fall risk factors among older adults attending outpatient rehabilitation. *Clinical Interventions in Aging*, *19*, 1287–1300. DOI: 10.2147/CIA.S456894 PMID: 39050519

Wójcik, M., Szczepaniak, R., & Placek, K. (2022). Physiotherapy Management in Endometriosis. *International Journal of Environmental Research and Public Health*, *19*(23), 16148. DOI: 10.3390/ijerph192316148 PMID: 36498220

Wong, D. S. H., & Santos, A. F. (2024). The future of food allergy diagnosis. *Frontiers in Allergy*, *5*, 1456585. Advance online publication. DOI: 10.3389/falgy.2024.1456585 PMID: 39575109

World Bank. (2011). *Guide to climate change adaptation in cities*. World Bank.

World Federation of Music Therapy. (2024, July 30th). About WFMT. Retrieved from https://www.wfmt.info/about

World Health Organization. (2018). *WHO recommendations on intrapartum care for a positive childbirth experience*. World Health Organization.

World Health Organization. (2024). *Disability*. Accessed November 20, 2024. https://www.who.int/news-room/fact-sheets/detail/disability-and-health

Wright, H., Hall, S., Hames, A., Hardiman, J., Mills, R., & Mills, D.PAWS Project Team. (2015). Pet dogs improve family functioning and reduce anxiety in children with autism spectrum disorder. *Anthrozoos*, *28*(4), 611–624. DOI: 10.1080/08927936.2015.1070003

Wu, X., Liu, Y., Zhu, D., Wang, F., Ji, J., & Yan, H. (2021). Early prevention of complex decongestive therapy and rehabilitation exercise for prevention of lower extremity lymphedema after operation of gynecologic cancer. *Asian Journal of Surgery*, *44*(1), 111–115. DOI: 10.1016/j.asjsur.2020.03.022 PMID: 32402630

Xiao, N., Shinwari, K., Kiselev, S., Huang, X., Li, B., & Qi, J. (2023). Effects of Equine-Assisted Activities and Therapies for Individuals with Autism Spectrum Disorder: Systematic Review and Meta-Analysis. *International Journal of Environmental Research and Public Health*, *20*(3), 2630. DOI: 10.3390/ijerph20032630 PMID: 36767996

Xin, W., Xu, D., Dou, Z., Jacques, A., Umbella, J., & Hill, A. M. (2024). Effectiveness of Community-Based Rehabilitation (CBR) Centers for Improving Physical Fitness for Community-Dwelling Older Adults: A Systematic Review and Meta-Analysis. *Annals of Rehabilitation Medicine*, *48*(1), 5–21. DOI: 10.5535/arm.23148 PMID: 38433005

Xiong, T., Chen, H., Luo, R., & Mu, D. (2016). Hyperbaric oxygen therapy for people with autism spectrum disorder (ASD). *Cochrane Database of Systematic Reviews*, *2016*(11), 10. DOI: 10.1002/14651858.CD010922.pub2 PMID: 27737490

Xu, Y., Chakraborti, M., Zhang, T., Eng, K., Mohan, A., & Prpa, M. (2025). Your voice is your voice: supporting self-expression through speech generation and LLMs in AAC. arXiv preprint arXiv:2503.17479. https://arxiv.org/abs/2503.17479

Xu, H., Stjernswärd, S., & Glasdam, S. (2021). Psychosocial experiences of frontline nurses working in hospital-based settings during the covid-19 pandemic - a qualitative systematic review. *International Journal of Nursing Studies Advances*, *3*, 100037. DOI: 10.1016/j.ijnsa.2021.100037 PMID: 34308373

Xu, J., Wang, Y., Cheung, J., & Yin, Y. (2024). Analysis of the chain mediation effect between intergenerational support and mental health of older adults in urban China: A structural equation model. *BMC Geriatrics*, *24*(1), 323. Advance online publication. DOI: 10.1186/s12877-024-04883-9 PMID: 38589808

Xu, X., Luckett, T., Wang, A., Lovell, M., & Phillips, J. (2018). Cancer pain management needs and perspectives of patients from Chinese backgrounds: A systematic review of the Chinese and English literature. *Palliative & Supportive Care*, *16*(6), 785–799. DOI: 10.1017/S1478951517001171 PMID: 29338806

Yamamoto, R., & Yamamoto, T. (2007). Effectiveness of the treatment-phase of two-phase complex decongestive physiotherapy for the treatment of extremity lymphedema. *International Journal of Clinical Oncology*, *12*(6), 463–468. DOI: 10.1007/s10147-007-0715-5 PMID: 18071866

Yamanaka, M. (2018). A concept analysis of self-management of cancer pain. *Asia-Pacific Journal of Oncology Nursing*, *5*(3), 254–261. DOI: 10.4103/apjon.apjon_17_18 PMID: 29963587

Yang, C.-H., Hossain, S. Z., & Sitharthan, G. (2013). Collaborative practice in early childhood intervention from the perspectives of service providers. *Infants and Young Children*, *26*(1), 57–73. DOI: 10.1097/IYC.0b013e3182736cbf

Yang, E. J., Lim, J. Y., Rah, U. W., & Kim, Y. B. (2012). Effect of a pelvic floor muscle training program on gynecologic cancer survivors with pelvic floor dysfunction: A randomized controlled trial. *Gynecologic Oncology*, *125*(3), 705–711. DOI: 10.1016/j.ygyno.2012.03.045 PMID: 22472463

Yang, F. A., Wu, P. J., Su, Y. T., Strong, P. C., Chu, Y. C., & Huang, C. C. (2024). Effect of kinesiology taping on breast cancer-related lymphedema: A systematic review and meta-analysis of randomized controlled trials. *Clinical Breast Cancer*, *24*(6), 541–551.e1. Advance online publication. DOI: 10.1016/j.clbc.2024.04.013 PMID: 38834497

Yang, S., & Chang, M. (2019). Chronic pain: Structural and functional changes in brain structures and associated negative affective states. *International Journal of Molecular Sciences*, *20*(13), 3130. DOI: 10.3390/ijms20133130 PMID: 31248061

Yang, X., Li, H., Zhao, Q., Han, R., Xiang, Z., & Gao, L. (2022). Clinical Practice Guidelines That Address Physical Activity and Exercise During Pregnancy: A Systematic Review. *Journal of Midwifery & Women's Health*, *67*(1), 53–68. DOI: 10.1111/jmwh.13286 PMID: 34841649

Yang, Y. J., Siao, M. R., Tsai, F. T., & Luo, H. J. (2015). Effect of physical activity interventions on children and adolescents with autism spectrum disorder: A systematic review and meta-analysis. *Physiotherapy*, *101*, e1685–e1686. DOI: 10.1016/j.physio.2015.03.091

Yang, Y., Yao, M., Yang, Y., & Lin, T. (2024). Self-management experiences in fall prevention among community-dwelling older adults in China: A descriptive qualitative study. *Annals of Medicine*, *56*(1), 2392878. Advance online publication. DOI: 10.1080/07853890.2024.2392878 PMID: 39320983

Yan, X., Wu, W., Chen, X., Xu, G., Yu, S., & Li, S. (2023). Intergenerational caregiving on mental health of middle-aged and older adults in China: Empirical insights. *Frontiers in Public Health*, *11*, 1224062. Advance online publication. DOI: 10.3389/fpubh.2023.1224062 PMID: 37483932

Yeh, G., & Horwitz, R. (2017). Integrative medicine for respiratory conditions. *The Medical Clinics of North America*, *101*(5), 925–941. DOI: 10.1016/j.mcna.2017.04.008 PMID: 28802471

Yesildere Saglam, H., & Orsal, O. (2020). Effect of exercise on premenstrual symptoms: A systematic review. *Complementary Therapies in Medicine*, *48*, 102272. DOI: 10.1016/j.ctim.2019.102272 PMID: 31987230

Yin, H., Tse, M., & Wong, F. (2015). Systematic review of the predisposing, enabling, and reinforcing factors which influence nursing administration of opioids in the postoperative period. *Japan Journal of Nursing Science*, *12*(4), 259–275. DOI: 10.1111/jjns.12075 PMID: 25781037

Young Carson, B. (2014). An Evaluation of the Attitudes Teachers Have Towards Adopting Evidence-Based Practices for Students with Autism in Preschool Classrooms.

Yue, X. (2023). Exploring the economic implications and challenges of an ageing population in the UK and China. *Lecture Notes in Education Psychology and Public Media*, *9*(1), 358–367. DOI: 10.54254/2753-7048/9/20230260

Yu, W., Freeland, D. M. H., & Nadeau, K. C. (2016). Food allergy: Immune mechanisms, diagnosis and immunotherapy. *Nature Reviews. Immunology*, *16*(12), 751–765. DOI: 10.1038/nri.2016.111 PMID: 27795547

Zahari, Z., Ishak, A., & Justine, M. (2020). The effectiveness of patient education in improving pain, disability and quality of life among older people with low back pain: A systematic review. *Journal of Back and Musculoskeletal Rehabilitation*, *33*(2), 245–254. DOI: 10.3233/BMR-181305 PMID: 31356191

Zainordin, N. H., Karim, N. A., Shahril, M. R., & Abd Talib, R. (2021). Physical Activity, Sitting Time, and Quality of Life among Breast and Gynaecology Cancer Survivors. *Asian Pacific Journal of Cancer Prevention : APJCP*, *22*(8), 2399–2408. DOI: 10.31557/APJCP.2021.22.8.2399 PMID: 34452552

Zambrana, I. M., Pons, F., Eadie, P., & Ystrom, E. (2014). Trajectories of language delay from age 3 to 5: Persistence, recovery and late onset. *International Journal of Language & Communication Disorders*, *49*(3), 304–316. DOI: 10.1111/1460-6984.12073 PMID: 24382196

Zanobini, M., & Solari, S. (2019). Effectiveness of the Program "Acqua Mediatrice di Comunicazione" (Water as a Mediator of Communication) on Social Skills, Autistic Behaviors and Aquatic Skills in ASD Children. *Journal of Autism and Developmental Disorders*, *49*(10), 4134–4146. DOI: 10.1007/s10803-019-04128-4 PMID: 31267291

Zebralla, V., Wichmann, G., Pirlich, M., Hammermüller, C., Berger, T., Zimmermann, K., Neumuth, T., Mehnert-Theuerkauf, A., Dietz, A., Hinz, A., & Wiegand, S. (2021). Dysphagia, voice problems, and pain in head and neck cancer patients. *European Archives of Oto-Rhino-Laryngology*, *278*(10), 3985–3994. DOI: 10.1007/s00405-020-06584-6 PMID: 33452920

Zebron, S., Mhute, I., & Constantine Chando Musingafi, M. (2015). Classroom Challenges: Working with Pupils with Communication Disorders. *Journal of Education and Practice*, v6 n9 p181\11

Zeidan, F., & Vago, D. (2016). Mindfulness meditation–based pain relief: A mechanistic account. *Annals of the New York Academy of Sciences*, *1373*(1), 114–127. DOI: 10.1111/nyas.13153 PMID: 27398643

Zhang, A.. (2010). Clinical Studies with Traditional Chinese Medicine in the Past Decade: A Review. *Chinese Journal of Integrative Medicine*, *16*(1), 1–7.

Zhang, M., Chen, C., Zhou, X., Wang, X., Wang, B., Huan, F., & Liu, J. (2024). The impact of accelerating population aging on service industry development: Evidence from China. *PLoS One*, *19*(6), e0296623. DOI: 10.1371/journal.pone.0296623 PMID: 38843199

Zhang, S. (2021). Chemotherapy-induced peripheral neuropathy and rehabilitation: A review. *Seminars in Oncology*, *48*(3), 193–207. DOI: 10.1053/j.seminoncol.2021.09.004 PMID: 34607709

Zhao, M., Yi, L., & Wang, Z. (2022). Mercury and mercury-containing preparations: History of use, clinical applications, pharmacology, toxicology, and pharmacokinetics in traditional Chinese medicine. *Frontiers in Pharmacology*, *13*, 807807. Advance online publication. DOI: 10.3389/fphar.2022.807807 PMID: 35308204

Zhou, F., He, S., Sun, H., Wang, Y., & Zhang, Y. (2021). Advances in epitope mapping technologies for food protein allergens: A review. *Trends in Food Science & Technology*, *107*, 226–239. DOI: 10.1016/j.tifs.2020.10.035

Zhu, B., Gu, H., Mao, Z., Beeraka, N. M., Zhao, X., Anand, M. P., Zheng, Y., Zhao, R., Li, S., Manogaran, P., Fan, R., Nikolenko, V. N., Wen, H., Basappa, B., & Liu, J. (2024). Global burden of gynaecological cancers in 2022 and projections to 2050. *Journal of Global Health*, *14*, 04155. DOI: 10.7189/jogh.14.04155 PMID: 39148469

Zhu, X., Du, Q., Li, Y., Zhu, Y., Ge, C., & Chen, J. (2025). Activating the souls of the older adults: Insights into the psychological well-being of older adults through social interactions in the Guangdong - Hong Kong - Macao greater bay area. *Frontiers in Public Health*, *13*, 1461481. Advance online publication. DOI: 10.3389/fpubh.2025.1461481 PMID: 40109420

Ziegler, S. A., & Hadders-Algra, M. (2020). Coaching approaches in early intervention and pediatric rehabilitation. *Developmental Medicine and Child Neurology*, *62*(5), 569–574. DOI: 10.1111/dmcn.14493 PMID: 32065385

Zoccante, L., Marconi, M., Ciceri, M. L., Gagliardoni, S., Gozzi, L. A., Sabaini, S., Di Gennaro, G., & Colizzi, M. (2021). Effectiveness of equine-assisted activities and therapies for improving adaptive behavior and motor function in autism spectrum disorder. *Journal of Clinical Medicine*, *10*(8), 1726. DOI: 10.3390/jcm10081726 PMID: 33923582

Zubow, L., & Hurtig, R. (2013). A demographic study of AAC/AT needs in hospitalized patients. *Perspectives on Augmentative and Alternative Communication*, *22*(2), 79–90. DOI: 10.1044/aac22.2.79

Zubow, L., & Hurtig, R. (2021). The role of speech-language pathologists in improving communication access in healthcare settings. *Communication Disorders Quarterly*, *42*(4), 215–225. DOI: 10.1177/1525740120975805

Zwakhalen, S., Docking, R., Gnass, I., Sirsch, E., Stewart, C., Allcock, N., & Schofield, P. (2018). Pain in older adults with dementia. *Schmerz (Berlin, Germany)*, *32*(5), 364–373. DOI: 10.1007/s00482-018-0290-x PMID: 29931391

About the Contributors

Adérito Seixas is a physiotherapist, higher education teacher and clinical educator. Currently, alongside his work as a full time Professor on a Physiotherapy Graduate course and Master Program at Escola Superior de Saúde Fernando Pessoa (Porto, Portugal), he is carrying out research for his PhD, focusing in the biomechanical and thermophysiological assessment of the foot in diabetic patients at risk to develop foot ulcers, and has supervised over 100 graduate and master students in research activities. His research interests lie in evidence-based practice, assessment of the neuro-musculoskeletal system in a clinical, sporting and occupational context, and in the role of cognitive assessment in human adaptation to performance situations. He maintains editorial and reviewer activities in several international scientific journals indexed in reference databases. He has been member of the scientific or technical committee of 29 international and 9 national events, has edited 2 books, and has published 68 articles in scientific journals, 26 book chapters in international publishers, 38 full articles/abstracts in international conferences, and has authored or co-authored over 60 oral communications in international congresses.

Rita Alegria has been a Speech and Language Therapist since 2000. She holds a PhD in "Language Disorders and Development, Specialty Language Disorders". Since 2008, Rita has been a lecturer at Escola Superior de Saúde Fernando Pessoa. In addition to her teaching role, Rita serves as a clinical supervisor, a scientific reviewer in her field, and a guest lecturer at national and international congresses. She is a published author and co-author in national and international journals. Her PhD research focused on speech therapy in a water-based setting for patients with UVFP or bilateral VFN. As a former high-level competitive swimmer, she has a deep understanding of biomechanics in water and has applied these insights to speech therapy interventions in aquatic settings. Over the last 20 years, she has incorporated these skills into her private practice, offering voice and communication skills coaching in water for singers, actors, and individuals with speech and language disorders.

Daniela Oliveira Vieira completed her PhD degree in language development and perturbation in 2022 at Fernando Pessoa University, her SLP specialist at 2021 at Fernando Pessoa Health School, her Master's Degree in Oncology in 2010 at the University of Porto's Abel Salazar Biomedical Sciences Institute and her Degree in Speech Therapy in 2008 at the Fernando Pessoa University. She is an Adjunt Professor at Fernando Pessoa Health School. Published 6 articles in specialized journals. She has 2 book chapters and 1 book. Organized 5 events. Participated in 11 events. Supervised 5 master's thesis(es) and co-supervised 2. Supervised 8 bachelor's/ master's thesis(es) and co-supervised 1. Participated as technical development in 2 project(s). She works in the area(s) of Medical and Health Sciences, with an emphasis on Health Sciences and Medical and Health Sciences. In her professional activities, she has interacted with 15 collaborators in co-authoring scientific papers. In her Ciência Vitae CV, the most frequent terms used to contextualise her scientific, technological and artistic-cultural production are: rehabilitation; speech therapy; head and neck; dysphagia; quality of life; questionnaire; oncology.

***

Sachi Dubey, pursuing B. Technology in Food Technology at University Institute of Chemical Technology (UICT), Kavayitri Bahinabai Chaudhari North Maharashtra University (KBCNMU), Jalgaon, Maharashtra, she is poised to explore the cutting-edge research and innovative topics within the field of Food Technological Trends and Innovation. As a first-time student, she brings a fresh perspective and a keen interest in expanding her knowledge and skills. With a strong academic performance and involvement in National Conference on Recent Trends in Chemical Engineering and Technology and certification in Advanced Food Packaging, she is eager to engage with the vast network of researchers and scholars associated with IGI Global. Aspiring to leverage the resources and opportunities provided by IGI Global, she also aims to further develope her expertise and contribute to the advancement of knowledge in areas of Food Science and Technology.

Mário Esteves is currently a full professor at School of Health Fernando Pessoa. He holds a degree in Physiotherapy (2010), an MSc in Adapted Physical Activity (2013), and a Ph.D. in Physiotherapy (2022).

Clarinda Fernanda da Silva Festas holds a PhD in Physical Activity and Health (2010) a Master's in Sport Sciences – Physical Activity for the Elderly (2002) from the Faculty of Sport, University of Porto, a Licentiate degree in Specialised Higher Studies in Teaching and Administration (1998) and a Bachelor's degree in

Physiotherapy (1988) from the Polytechnic Institute of Porto, School of Health. Member of RISE-Health, Fernando Pessoa Health School_University Fernando Pessoa. Coordinating Professor and director at the Fernando Pessoa Health School. Published 14 articles in specialised journals and 8 book chapters. Organised 16 events and participated in 73 events. She has supervised 1 PhD thesis, 4 Master's dissertations, and 20 undergraduate/Bachelor's final projects. She has been involved as a Researcher in 2 projects. Throughout her professional activities, she has collaborated with 77 co-authors in scientific works. In her Ciência Vitae profile, the most frequently used terms in the context of her scientific, technological, and artistic-cultural production include: Women Health; Uro-gynaecological re-education; Urinary incontinence; Breast cancer; Breast reconstruction. Elderly

Ajaygiri Goswami has 22 years of teaching and research experience. His area of interest is biodiesel, environmental biotechnology and wastewater engineering. He has worked on different statutory committees at KBC North Maharashtra University.

Tiago Horta Reis da Silva, SFHEA, FRSM, FFNMRCSI Lecturer in Nursing Education (AEP), King's College London. Tiago Horta Reis da Silva is an accomplished Lecturer in Nursing Education at the Florence Nightingale Faculty of Nursing, Midwifery & Palliative Care, King's College London. He brings a multidisciplinary academic background, holding a BSc in Nursing, a BSc and MSc in Traditional Chinese Medicine, an MSc in Emotional Intelligence, Counselling and NLP, a Master of Business Administration (MBA), and a Master of Arts in Clinical Education. His academic and clinical expertise is further grounded in practical experience within both the UK's National Health Service (NHS) and a range of higher education institutions. At King's College London, Reis da Silva plays a central role in the design, development, and delivery of undergraduate and postgraduate programmes in Adult Nursing. His responsibilities span curriculum enhancement, pedagogical leadership, interprofessional education, and student admissions and assessments. He also contributes to cross-modular teaching and supports strategic academic initiatives in nursing education. A prolific academic, Reis da Silva has authored over 100 peer-reviewed publications, including original research articles, book chapters, and professional commentaries in high-impact journals such as the British Journal of Community Nursing, Journal of Prescribing Practice, Emergency Nurse, and Journal of Kidney Care. His recent scholarship addresses critical topics in gerontological nursing, such as falls prevention, frailty, loneliness, emotional intelligence, ageing in place, pharmacokinetics, and safeguarding older adults. His contributions are shaping contemporary debates on nursing leadership, curriculum innovation, and integrative approaches to gerontological care. Reis da Silva is recognised as a Senior Fellow of the Higher Education Academy (SFHEA) for his sustained contribution to academic practice and mentoring in nursing education. He is also a Fellow of the Royal Society of Medicine (FRSM) and a Fellow for

Faculty of Nursing and Midwifery at the Royal College of Surgeons in Ireland (FFNMRCSI). His current research interests include: Interdisciplinary strategies for falls prevention among older adults. Emotional intelligence and leadership development in nursing education. Holistic and integrative models of care for older populations. AI-enhanced tools for geriatric nursing assessment. Reis da Silva is dedicated to advancing scholarship, promoting inclusive and person-centred care, and fostering the next generation of nursing professionals through evidence-informed teaching and impactful research.

Sunil J. Kulkarni has done his PhD in Chemical Engineering with focus on adsorption for wastewater treatment. He has done his Masters in chemical engineering from Tatyasaheb Kore Institute of Engineering and Technology, Warananagar. He has worked as an Assistant Professor in Chemical Engineering Department of Datta Meghe College of Engineering, Airoli, Navi Mumbai, India for 13 years. He has total 25 years of teaching and research experience. Dr. Sunil is involved with different academic activities across the universities in Maharashtra. His area of investigation in doctoral studies is phenol and heavy metal removal from waste water. He has also worked on kinetics and isotherms of various sorption operations. His area of research includes adsorption, clean technology and environmental biotechnology. He is on the reviewer board of many international journals and reviewed many international papers. He is also governing body member, promotional editor and executive member of many reputed international journals. Currently he is working as Professor and head in chemical engineering at GIT, Lavel, India.

Maria Conceição Manso currently works at the Faculty of Health Sciences; she is a researcher at RISE-Health, Associate Professor at Faculty of Health Sciences, Fernando Pessoa University, Fernando Pessoa Teaching and Culture Foundation) and UFP I3ID (both subdivisions: Energy, Environment and Health Research (FP-ENAS) and FP-BHS) at the University of Fernando Pessoa and at LAQV-REQUIMTE, University of Porto. Maria Conceição has done research in food science and engineering, and currently in health, mainly but not only in Dentistry and Environment and Health.

R. Vettriselvan an Associate Professor, AMET University, specialised in HRM and Marketing. He is acting as Mentor, Saraswathi Institute of Medical Sciences, Hapur. He served as Review Board member, National Council for Higher Education, Malawi, Head of the Department, School of Commerce and Management Studies, St. Eugene University, Zambia, and Director, Research and Publication, St. John the Baptist University, Malawi. He has published 25 books and 100+ articles in peer reviewed journals and edited book chapters. Under his guidance two have completed and five are pursuing their PhD.

Ramachandren Ramya, is a seasoned healthcare administrator dedicated to enhancing public health systems and empowering communities through outreach programs. With extensive experience and academic qualifications in Public Administration and Hospital Management, she serves as Vice Chairperson at Saraswathi Institute of Medical Sciences, Hapur driving excellence in healthcare delivery and education. Through her leadership and initiatives via charitable trusts, she addresses healthcare disparities and promotes community welfare, embodying a commitment to social impact and public health advancement.

Palanivel Rathinasabapathi Velmurugan is associated with BSBI, Berlin, as a professor in the Human Resource Management and Finance Stream. Prior to joining BSBI, he held the designation "Head" Faculty of Management at Sharda University, Uzbekistan, Central Asia, and "Dean of Arts" assignments at DMI St. John the Baptist University, Malawi, Central Africa. Also, he has been associated earlier with DMI St. Eugene University in Zambia, MAM Business School and various Engineering Colleges in India. He has a Ph.D. in Management from Mannonmanium Sundaranar University in India. Besides this, he holds an MBA Degree from SRM University in India and a BE Chemical Engineering degree from Annamalai University in India. Also, he completed six NPTEL Certificate Programs conducted by various IITs in India. He brings with him 15 years of rich working experience in teaching and research. Furthermore, he has a keen interest in the Case Method of teaching and research. He is an academic out of passion. Not only that, but he also takes a keen interest in guiding Ph.D. students. He has supervised three Ph.D. research scholars under his supervision at DMI St. Eugene University in Zambia.

Fátima Santos is currently a full professor at School of Health Fernando Pessoa. She holds a degree in Physiotherapy (1999), MSc in Adapted Physical Activity (2005), and a PhD in Sports Science (2012).

Selvalakshmi V is an academician, educator, researcher,POSH Trainer and mentor currently serving Professor,Saveetha School of Management, SIMATS,Chennai.With more than two decades of rich experience, her experience and interest likes in the fields of research,incubation, entrepreneurship and have published more than 35 research papers and 5 books. She has served as one of the Expert Committee member for course development at NAHEP – IPD,Dapoli and have reviewed a full book under Taylor and Francis Publication.

Index

A

B

C

D

E

F

G

H

I

K

L

M

N

O

P

Q

R

S

W

www.ingramcontent.com/pod-product-compliance
Lightning Source LLC
LaVergne TN
LVHW062339300926
849161LV00007B/1749
* 9 7 9 8 3 6 9 3 6 4 3 2 1 *